American Medical Association

Physicians dedicated to the health of America

Healthcare

.... Resource and

.... Reference Guide

Editor
Lorri A. Zipperer, MA

Deputy Editor
Brian P. Pace, MA

Division of Library and Information Management

Cataloging Data

Healthcare resource and reference guide / editor,
        Lorri A.Zipperer; deputy editor, Brian P. Pace.
                p. cm.

            Includes bibliographical references and index.
            ISBN 0-89970-554-5

            1. Health Services--United States--encyclopedias.
2. Medicine--United States--encyclopedias. 3.
Societies, Medical--United States--encyclopedias.
4. American Medical Association. I. Zipperer,
Lorri, A., 1959-   . II. Pace, Brian P., 1961-   . III.
American Medical Association. Division of Library
and Information Management.
W 13 H4345 1993

Copies may be ordered from:
Order Department: OP 311793
American Medical Association
P.O.Box 109050

Chicago, IL 60610

For credit card orders, call toll-free
800 621-8335

ISBN 0-89970-554-5

BB21: 93-70:3: 593

Introduction and Acknowledgements

The *Healthcare Resource and Reference Guide* (The Guide) grew out of experience.

The American Medical Association (AMA) library has had a reference and referral center for many years. In 1992 it handled over 100,000 phone inquiries from physicians, hospitals, medical and allied health students, and various other health care professionals as well as the public. Many of these questions were straightforward in nature and were answerable by the 'right' book of lists. In an attempt to address this type of information need for the small professional office or the physician without convenient access to a hospital library, The Guide was developed.

The questions most frequently posed to the center by health professionals served as a framework in compiling The Guide. However, The Guide does not intend to be representative of every organization related to medicine. The organizations listed here are those that are inquired about consistently at the AMA library.

This publication was envisioned as a prototype, therefore it is recognized that some relevant information may have been omitted, and user input would appreciated in defining those gaps. Please direct corrections, suggestions and comments for The Guide to the AMA's Division of Library and Information Management.

The AMA does not except responsibility, nor should this publication serve as endorsement for any of the organizations, schools or therapies listed herein.

Please keep in mind that legal opinions and policy statements can change often. Consult with an attorney, or, in regard to policy, the AMA directly for the most current information.

How To Use:

The Guide is organized alphabetically, broken into general subject headings used for a specific area. (i.e cancer instead of neoplasms.) American Medical Association and government publications were used to expand upon the subject listings included. The references to specific essays are generalized, for simplicity of use and space. Overall, the sources from which materials were pulled are noted in three-digit abbreviations at the end of each essay. (see the reference list at the end of the book.)

Acknowledgements: The following individuals deserve honorable mention:

Brian Pace, MA.: Brian is primary editor for the in-house referral directory from which the Guide was developed, and was, therefore, a logical, and willing deputy editor.

Marie Bates: Her knowledge of AMA greatly contributed to the AMA section.

Maribeth Diamond: She came in at the last minute to help with proofing and desk-top publishing operation.

Norman Frankel, PhD, MLS: Provided overall support, editorial work, helpful suggestions, and patience in seeing the project home.

Barbara Hopper: Her knowledge of both the AMA and the arena of medicine contributed to making editorial decisions much easier.

Fred Hunter: His knowledge of AMA publishing methods and familiarity with the desk-top publishing software used proved to be invaluable.

George Kruto: Formulated the index to the publication.

Anne White Michalski, MLS: Provided both amounts of departmental support beyond the call-of-duty, and technical knowledge that aided in making informed editorial decisions.

Michael Tarpey: Input huge amounts of text material.

as well as the various departments, divisions and individuals of the American Medical Association that produced the many Association publications used herein.

Support: Members of the staff of the Division of Library and Information Management: Sandra Schefris MLS, Yolanda Davis-Ellis, Mary Sugrue, Sharon Ali, Marguerite Fallucco, Mary Kay Tinerella; as well as those outside the AMA: Debbie Wright MLS, Rebecca Corliss MLS, Joan Odgen MLS, Laura Sklanski MLS, and Helen Treblenski MLS, were also of great help.

I thank them all.

Lorri Zipperer, MA. editor

Seeing Ignorance is the curse of God,
Knowledge the wing wherewith we fly to
heaven.

Shakespeare, W.
The Second Part of King Henry the IV.
Act IV; scene 7; line 79

Abbreviated Injury Scale

Abbreviated Injury Scale
(Released every 5 years--Current revision 1990)
American Association of Automotive Medicine
2350 E. Devon Ave., Suite 205
Des Plaines, IL 60018
708/390-8927

Abbreviation of Specialties

Alphabetic Codes for American Medical Directory:
AMA Codes for Self Designation of Practice
Specialties

A   Allergy

ADL   Adolescent Medicine

ADM   Addiction Medicine

AI   Allergy & Immunology

ALI   Allergy & Immunology/Diagnostic Laboratory Immunology

AM   Aerospace Medicine

AN   Anesthesiology

APM   Anesthesiology, Pain Management

AS   Surgery, Abdominal

ATP   Pathology, Anatomic

BBK   Pathology, Blood Banking

CCA   Anesthesiology, Critical Care

CCM   Critical Care Medicine

CCP   Pediatric Critical Care

CCS   Surgery, Critical Care

CD   Cardiovascular Disease

CDS   Surgery, Cardiovascular

CHN   Neurology, Child

CHP   Psychiatry, Child

CLP   Pathology, Clinical

CN   Neurology, Clinical Neurophysiology

CRS   Surgery, Colon & Rectal

D   Dermatology

DDL   Dermatology Immunology/Diagnostic Laboratory Immunology

DIA   Diabetes

DMP   Dermatopathology

DR   Radiology, Diagnostic

EM   Emergency Medicine

END   Endocrinology

FOP   Pathology, Forensic

FP   Family Practice

FPG   Family Practice, Geriatric Medicine

FPS   Facial Plastic Surgery, Otolaryngology

FSM   Family Medicine, Sports Medicine

GE   Gastroenterology

GO   Gynecological Oncology

GP   General Practice

GPM   Preventive Medicine, General

GS   Surgery, General

GYN   Gynecology

HEM   Hematology

HMP   Pathology, Hematology

HNS   Surgery, Head & Neck

HSO   Orthopedic Surgery, Hand Surgery

HSP   Plastic Surgery, Hand Surgery

ICE   Internal Medicine Cardiac Electrophysiology

ID   Infectious Diseases

IG   Immunology

ILI   Internal Medicine/Diagnostic Laboratory Immunology

IM   Internal Medicine

IMG   Internal Medicine, Geriatrics

LM   Legal Medicine

MFM   Maternal & Fetal Medicine

MM   Medical Microbiology

N   Neurology

NCC   Neurological Surgery, Critical Care

NEP   Nephrology

NM   Nuclear Medicine

NP   Pathology, Neuropathology

NPM   Neonatal-Perinatal Medicine

NR   Nuclear Radiology

NS   Surgery, Neurological

NSP   Neurology, Pediatric Surgery

NTR   Nutrition

OAR   Orthopedic Surgery, Adult Reconstructive Orthopedics

OBG	Obstetrics & Gynecology
OBS	Obstetrics
OCC	Obstetrics & Gynecology/Critical Care Medicine
OM	Occupational Medicine
OMO	Orthopedic Surgery, Musculoskeletal Oncology
ON	Oncology, Medical
OP	Orthopedic Surgery, Pediatric Orthopedics
OPH	Ophthalmology
ORS	Surgery, Orthopedic
OSM	Orthopedic Surgery, Sports Medicine
OSS	Orthopedic Surgery, Spine Surgery
OT	Otology
OTO	Otolaryngology
OTR	Orthopedic Surgery, Trauma
P	Psychiatry
PA	Pharmacology, Clinical
PCH	Pathology, Chemical
PCP	Pathology, Cytopathology
PD	Pediatrics
PDA	Pediatric Allergy
PDC	Pediatric Cardiology
PDE	Pediatric Endocrinology
PDP	Pediatric Pulmonology
PDR	Radiology, Pediatric
PDS	Surgery, Pediatric
PEM	Pediatric Emergency Medicine
PG	Pediatric Gastroenterology
PH	Public Health
PHO	Pediatric Hematology
PH	Public Health
PHO	Pediatric Hematology-Oncology
PIP	Pathology, Immunopathology
PLI	Pediatrics/Diagnostic Laboratory Immunology
PM	Physical Medicine & Rehabilitation
PN	Pediatric Nephrology
PP	Pathology, Pediatric Pathology

PS	Surgery, Plastic
PTH	Pathology, Anatomic/Clinical
PUD	Pulmonary Disease
PYA	Psychoanalysis
PYG	Psychiatry, Geriatric
R	Radiology
REN	Reproductive Endocrinology
RHU	Rheumatology
RIP	Pathology, Radioisotopic
RO	Radiation Oncology
TRS	Surgery, Traumatic
TS	Surgery, Thoracic
U	Surgery, Urological
UM	Undersea Medicine
VIR	Radiology, Vascular and Interventional
VS	Surgery, Vascular (DUS)

2 digit codes for Medicare forms:
Contact local Medicare carriers

Abdominal Surgery

American Society of Abdominal Surgeons
675 Main Street, Melrose, MA 02176
617/665-6102

Abortion

AMA Policy. Abortion: The AMA reaffirms that (1) abortion is a medical procedure and should be performed only by a duly licensed physician and surgeon in conformance with standards of good medical practice and the Medical Practice Act of his state; and (2) no physician or other professional personnel shall be required to perform an act violative good medical judgment. Neither physician, hospital, nor hospital personnel shall be required to perform any act violative of personally held moral principles. In these circumstances, good medical practice requires only that the physician or other professional withdraw from the case, so long as the withdrawal in consistent with good medical practice.

JAMA Article of Note: Induced Termination of Pregnancy Before and After Roe v Wade. Trends in the Mortality and Morbidity of Women. Council on Scientific Affairs, American Medical Association. JAMA. 1992 Dec 12; 268(22): 3231-39
The mortality and morbidity of women who terminated their pregnancy before the 1973 Supreme Court decision in Roe v Wade are compared with post-Roe v Wade mortality and

morbidity. Mortality date before 1973 are from the National Center for Health Statistics; data from 1973 through 1985 are from the Centers for Disease Control and The Alan Guttmacher Institute. Trends in serious abortion-related complications between 1970 and 1990 are based on data from the Joint Program for the Study of Abortion and from the National Abortion Federation. Deaths from illegally induced abortion declined between 1940 and 1972 in part because of the introduction of antibiotics to manage sepsis and the widespread use of effective contraceptives. Deaths from legal abortion declined fivefold between 1973 and 1985 (from 3.3 deaths to 0.4 death per 100,000 procedures), reflecting increased physicians education and skills, improvements in medical technology, and, notably, the earlier termination of pregnancy. The risk of death from legal abortion is higher among minority women and women over the age of 35 years, and increases with gestational age. Legal-abortion mortality between 1979 and 1985 was 0.6 death per 100,000 procedures, more than 10 times lower than the 9.1 maternal deaths per 100,000 live births, between 1979 and 1986. Serious complications from legal abortion are rare. Most women who have a single abortion with vacuum aspiration experience few if any subsequent problems getting pregnant or having healthy children. Less is known about the effects of multiple abortions on future fecundity. Adverse emotional reactions to abortion are rare; most women experience relief and reduced depression and distress.

"Public Health Policy Implications of Abortion"
American College of Obstetricians and Gynecologists
409 12th Street, SW, Washington, DC 20024-2188
202/638-5577

Abortion Clinics, Referral to

Planned Parenthood Federation of America
810 Seventh Ave., New York, NY 10019
212/541-7800
Contact local Planned Parenthood
Contact local department of health

Academic Health

Association of Academic Health Centers
1400 16th St., NW, Suite 410
Washington, DC 20036
202/265-9600

Accent Reduction

American Speech-Language-Hearing Association
10801 Rockville Pike, Rockville, MD 20852
301/897-5700
800/638-TALK - Referral to a speech pathologist

Accreditation

American Federation for Medical Accreditation
515 N. State St, Chicago, IL 60610
312/464-4670

Continuing Medical Education
Accreditation Council for Continuing Medical Education
PO Box 245, Lake Bluff, IL 60044
708/295-1490

Graduate Medical Education
Accreditation Council for Graduate Medical Education
515 N. State St, Chicago, IL 60610
312/464-4920

Hospitals, Ambulatory surgical facilities, Long-term nursing homes
Joint Commission on Accreditation of Healthcare Organizations
One Renaissance Blvd.
Oakbrook Terrace, IL 60181
708/916-5600

Medical schools
AMA Department of Undergraduate Medical Education
515 N. State St, Chicago, IL 60610
312/464-4691

Acne

Skincare Help Line
800/222-SKIN (800/222-7546)

Acoustic Neuroma

Acoustic Neuroma Association
PO Box 398, Carlisle, PA 17013
717/249-4783

Acupuncture

Acupuncture has been part of Chinese medicine for thousands of years. Its proponents state that the body's vital energy (Ch'i or Qi) circulates through "meridians" along the surface of the body. They also state that illness and disease result from imbalances or interruptions of Ch'i, which can be corrected by acupuncture. The treatment is applied to "acupuncture points," which are said to be located along the meridians. The existence of meridians or acupuncture points has never been scientifically validated.

Traditional acupuncture, as now practiced, involves the insertion of stainless steel needles into various body areas. Low-frequency current may be applied to the needles to produce grater stimulation. Other procedures used separately or together include
- moxibustion (burning or floss or herbs applied to the skin);
- injection of sterile water, procaine, morphine, vitamins or homeopathic solutions through the inserted needles;
- placement of needles in the external ear (auriculotherapy); and
- acupressure (use of manual pressure).
Some practitioners espouse the traditional Chinese view of health and disease and consider acupuncture and its variations a valid approach to the full gamut of disease. Others reject these trappings and claim that acupuncture offers a simple way to achieve pain relief.

Acupuncture was introduced to the United States in about 1825 but generated little interest until President Richard M. Nixon's 1972 visit to China. Since then it has been promoted for the treatment of pain and a wide variety of other problems.

All states permit acupuncture to be performed – some by physicians alone, some by lay

acupuncturists under medical supervision, and some by unsupervised laypersons. In 1990 the National Accreditation Commission for Schools and colleges of Acupuncture and Oriental Medicine was recognized by the U.S. Secretary of education as an accrediting agency. This recognition is not based upon the scientific validity of what is taught but upon other criteria. Many insurance companies cover acupuncture treatment if performed by a licensed physician, but Medicare and Medicaid generally do not. Acupuncture needles are considered "investigational" devices by the FDA and are not approved for the treatment of any disease. (ALT)

Acupuncturist

Administers specific therapeutic treatment of symptoms and disorders amenable to acupuncture procedures, as specifically indicated by supervising physician: Reviews patient's medical history, physical findings, and diagnosis made by physician to ascertain symptoms or disorder to be treated. Selects needles of various lengths, according to location of insertion. Inserts needles at locations of body known to be efficacious to certain disorders, utilizing knowledge of acupuncture points and their functions. Leaves needles in patient for specific length of time, according to symptom or disorder treated, and removes needles. Burns bark of mugwort tree in small strainer to administer moxibustion treatment. Covers insertion are with cloth and rubs strainer over cloth to impart heat and assist in relieving patient's symptoms. (DOT)

American Academy of Medical Acupuncturists
5820 Wilshire Blvd, Suite 500
Los Angeles, CA 90036
800/521-2262

National Commission for the
Certification for Acupuncture
1424 16th St. NW,/Suite 105
Washington, DC 20036
202/232-1404

Addiction Medicine/Addictionology

American Society on Addiction Medicine
5225 Wisconsin Ave, NW, Suite 409
Washington, DC 20015
202/244-8948

Adolescence

Missing Child Hotline 800/843-5678
9 AM-Midnight
National Center for Missing and Exploited Children
101 Wilson Blvd. Suite 550, Arlington, VA 22201
703/235-3900

Runaway Hotline
800/231-6946

National Committee on Youth Suicide Prevention
666 Fifth Ave., 13th Floor, New York, NY 10103
212/677-6666

Suicide Hotline/Chicago Runaway Switchboard
800/621-3230

Adolescent Health

Adolescence: Medical Education for Adolescent Health

Medical Education
Although specialty medical education in adolescent medicine is strong, many primary care physicians feel that they lack the necessary skills and information to manage the complex biopsycho-social problems of adolescents. Medical organizations should develop creative, new educational approaches for teaching the principles and techniques of adolescent health care to nonspecialists who see the majority of adolescents in office practices.

Greater involvement of medical students and residents in community field experiences would increase physician sensitivity to the broad nature of adolescent health problems. Valuable field experience could include working with schools, drug rehabilitation programs, correctional facilities, or volunteer groups that sponsor adolescent health programs, such as health hot lines and mentoring programs.

Education modules could be developed for entire office-based medical practices that include the medical, clerical, and nursing staff. The modules would sensitize all office staff to the need and concerns of adolescents and develop their skills when dealing with adolescents. The goals of this approach would be increased utilization of medical services by adolescents, greater satisfaction with medical services, and increased compliance by adolescents.

The American Academy of Child and Adolescent Psychiatry recently completed Project Prevention: An Intervention Initiative. This interdisciplinary effort educates psychiatrists and other health professionals about risk factors and intervention strategies for the prevention of mental health disorders and alcohol and drug abuse. The project report can be found in the monograph, Prevention of Mental Disorders, Alcohol and Other Drug Use in Children and Adolescents.

The American Academy of Pediatrics provides an educational newsletter, Adolescent Health Update: A Clinical Guide for Pediatricians. Each issue includes information on topics related to the practice of adolescent medicine as well as a list of selected resources for professionals and families. The AAP is also involved in The Adolescent Wellness Program, a joint effort with Health Learning Systems, Inc., and Lederle Laboratories to educate pediatricians about adolescent wellness (including, for example, issues of depression, alcohol and substance use, and sexuality). Information about these programs can be obtained by writing American Academy of Pediatrics, 141 Northwest Point Boulevard, PO Box 927, Elk Grove Village, IL 60009-0927.

The American College of Obstetrics and Gynecology recently published a two-volume guide entitled Adolescent Sexuality: Guides for Professional Involvement. The guide offers a wide range of materials that can be used in lectures and presentations on adolescent sexuality and family life education. Included are articles, fact sheets, references, slides, sample handouts, and supplementary material. The guide can be

purchased from the ACOG Distribution Center, PO Box 91180, Washington, DC 20090.

Partnership and Advocacy
Because most adolescent health problems cut across medicine, education, juvenile justice, and social service, the development and dissemination of successful programs require interdisciplinary cooperation and coordination. Although much has been done on behalf of adolescents, many recent initiatives have had a limited impact because they were developed and implemented without the support and input of others working in the same area. Organized medicine must continue to develop partnerships with the many groups involved in adolescent health. More effective advocacy and use of resources results from a strong unified voice.

The AMA and the National Association of State Boards of Education (NASBE), with support from the Centers for Disease Control, are cosponsoring the National Commission on the Role of the School and the Community in Improving Adolescent Health. The purpose of the Commission is to raise national consciousness about the need for educational and health reforms, as well as to motivate communities to reform, invest in, and reinforce school efforts. Additional information can be obtained by writing either the AMA Department of Adolescent Health, 515 N. State Street, Chicago, IL 60610, or NASBE, 1012 Cameron Street, Alexandria, VA 22314.

In 1988, the AMA established the AMA Adolescent Health Coalition, consisting of 31 organizations involved in adolescent health. The members of the coalition represent medical specialty societies, government agencies, private foundations, and membership organizations in the health and social service professions. The Coalition provides a vehicle for disseminating information about adolescent health and discussing major issues and initiatives in the area.

Many specialty and state medical societies have successfully advocated for comprehensive health education curricula and prevention programs in unintentional injury, adolescent drug use, unintended pregnancy, and other areas of adolescent health.

The American Association of Neurological Surgeons and the Congress Of Neurological Surgeons sponsor a National Health and Spinal Cord Injury Prevention Program in 35 states. The program includes a presentation and discussion in high schools about spinal cord injuries. It also includes follow-up activities on the local level, public education programs, and a legislative educational program. Further information can be obtained by writing National Head and Spinal Cord Injury Prevention Program of the AANS/CNS, 22 S. Washington Street, Park Ridge, IL 60068.

The American College Of Obstetrics And Gynecology (ACOG) and the American Academy Of Family Physicians (AAFP) with support from the AMA Auxiliary are sponsoring a public service program to combat adolescent pregnancy. The campaign uses radio and TV public service announcements in English and Spanish, featuring adolescents who have had unintended

pregnancies. Information can be obtained by writing the American College of Obstetrics and Gynecology, Office of Public Information, 409 12th Street S.W., Washington, DC 20024-2188.

The American Academy Of Pediatrics is involved with the national "Health Children" program, funded by the Robert Wood Johnson Foundation. The program offers nonfinancial assistance to help communities provide health services to all "children who need them, and to do so at reduced cost through imaginative and efficient use of resources already available in the community". Further information can be obtained by writing the American Academy of Pediatrics, 141 Northwest Point Boulevard, PO Box 927 Elk Grove Village, IL 60009-0927.

Better organization and coordination of resources is critically needed at the national, state, and local levels. The development of a coordinating council in the federal government to monitor funding and public policy related to adolescent health should be considered. In addition, organized medicine should also promote and participate in state- and community-level coordinating committees consisting of public and private groups involved in health, education youth service, advocacy, and policy making.

Organized medicine will continue its role and expand its vigilance to ensure that adolescents receive the health education and health services they need to become healthy and productive adults. In the future, organized medicine is likely to become increasingly involved in issues related to (a) adolescents' access to health care services (e.g., Medicaid coverage, services to underserved youth, availability of school-based health centers, drug testing of students, and confidentiality issues), (b) the coordination and integration of health, education, and social services for adolescents, and (c) preventive services for adolescents.(ADK)

Gans, JE, McManus, MA, Newacheck, P. *Adolescent Health Care: Use, Cost, and Problems of Access*; American Medical Association; Chicago. 1991. 87 pp. OP018091. ISBN 0-89970-413-1

Gans, JE. *America's Adolescents: How Healthy are They?*; American Medical Association; Chicago. 1990. 89 pp. OP012690 ISBN 0-89970-385-2

"Code Blue: Uniting for Healthier Youth" paperback, 52pp A report by school boards across the US of recommendations to improve the health of adolescents.

Society for Adolescent Medicine 19401 E. US Highway 40/Suite 120, Independence, MO 64055 816/795-8336

National Association of State Boards of Education 1012 Cameron St., Alexandria, VA 22314 703/684-4000

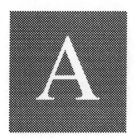

Guidelines for Adolescent Preventive Services (GAPS):
GAPS is a comprehensive set of recommendations that provides a framework for the organization and the content of preventive health services. The guidelines are unique because they emphasize health guidance and the prevention of behavioral and emotional disorders in addition to traditional biomedical conditions.

AMA Department of Adolescent Health
515 N. State St, Chicago, IL 60610
312/464-5570

Adoption
National Adoption Center
1218 Chestnut Street, Philadelphia, PA 19107
215/925-0200

Advertisements - Television & Radio
Complaints & Inquiries:
Federal Trade Commission
Pennsylvania Avenue at Sixth St., NW
Washington, DC 20580
202/326-2222

Aerospace Medicine
Aerospace Medical Association
320 S. Henry Street, Alexandria, VA 22314
703/739-2240

Board Certification in Aerospace Medicine
American Board of Preventive Medicine
Department of Community Medicine,
Wright State University
PO Box 927, Dayton OH 45401
513/278-6915

Aesculapius, Staff of
Graphic of staff and single serpent incorporated in the AMA logo is the Staff of Aesculapius NOT the caduceus (which is the winged staff of Hermes [Roman--Mercury] entwined with two serpents)

One Snake Or Two?

Robert E. Rakel, MD "A Piece of My Mind" JAMA. 1985 April 26; 253(16): 2369

The staff of Aesculapius has represented medicine since about 800 BC, and most authorities support its use as the symbol of medicine. The Encyclopaedia Britannica agrees: "This staff is the only true symbol of medicine."

Why, then, is the caduceus, which had never been chosen to represent medicine until after 1800, so frequently being adopted as the symbol of medicine? And is the twin-serpent magic wand of Hermes (later the Roman Mercury), messenger of the gods and protector of merchants and thieves, an appropriate symbol for the medical profession?

The word caduceus is derived from a Greek root meaning "herald's wand." The Romans were said to have used caduceus as badge of neutrality among heralds seeking peaceful negotiations with the enemy.

Hart[1] notes that the beginning of the use of the caduceus as a medical as a medical symbol in the United States dates back to 1856, when it was selected by the US Marine Hospital Service to designate the noncombatant nature of the medical corps. The Surgeon General's crest of 1818, which was designed for this purpose and contained the single-snake staff of Aesculapius, was somehow ignored. This omission was compounded in 1871, when the caduceus became the symbol of the Public Health Service, and in 1902, when it was adopted by the US Army Medical Corps.

The popularity of the caduceus today is probably attributable to its being more aesthetically appealing than the staff of Aesculapius. The symmetry of the wings atop a staff and the double snakes is more balanced than the staff and single snake of Aesculapius.

Purists, however, fervently profess and staunchly defend the staff of Aesculapius, emphasizing that from its inception it has represented the ideals of medicine. It is not clear whether Aesculapius was famous physicians who practiced in Thessaly, Greece, around 1200 BC and who subsequently was deified, or whether he was just a Greek god without human origin. In any event, more than 300 temples incorporating many therapeutic measures that remain popular today - such as diet, rest, drugs, and massage - were established in his honor throughout Greece and Rome[2].

There is general agreement among scholars that the snake, whether it be one or two around a staff, is an appropriate symbol for the healing art. In addition to representing wisdom, learning, and fertility, it stands for longevity and restoration of health. The snake, after all, appears to regenerate by shedding its skin, thereby assuming a new life. The serpent also was considered a potent force against disease and was thought to protect children from epidemics if they touched its skin.

The debate begins over whether Aesculapius or Hermes is the most appropriate representative of medicine. The Greek lyric poet Pindar described Aesculapius in this way:

A gentle craftsman who drove pain away,
Soother of cruel pangs, a joy to men,
Bringing them golden health.[3]

Aesculapius provides medicine with a purely ethical and noncommercial image, in contrast to Hermes, the god of commerce, who is usually depicted with a full purse. The cunning and craftiness of Hermes also made him the protector of thieves and outlaws, an association medicine may well wish to avoid. In Homer's "Hymn to Hermes," Apollo says:

This among the Gods shall be your gift...
To be considered as the Lord of those
    who swindle,
housebreak, sheepsteal and shop-lift.
A schemer subtle beyond all belief....[4]

Hermes is not only associated with the marketplace and a fat purse, he is also a god of dreams, magic, and sleep. His image adorns graves, and he is said to conduct departed souls to Hades - a role physicians should rightfully shun. The number 4 was sacred to Mercury, so the

Romans named the fourth day of the week "dies murcurii," or Wednesday, in his honor.[5] It is probably only a coincidence that this has become known as the physician's favorite "day off" - or perhaps this is Mercury's most legitimate tie to the medical profession.

Aesculapius, the god of medicine, was never represented as using the caduceus. Indeed, his staff first appears in history around 800 BC as a staff or rod around which a single snake is entwined[5] Greek mythology explains this staff by describing how Aesculapius discovered a magical herb when he observed a snake rejuvenate a previously dead companion by placing the herb in its mouth.[6]

The caduceus, representing neutrality, noncombatant, and peace, will remain the symbol for military medicine. It will, no doubt, also continue to be embraced by others who prefer for aesthetic reasons its balance and symmetry.

There is insufficient reason, however, for it to be the symbol for all of medicine. Those who respect the past and value the circumstances under which symbols are born will prefer the staff of Aesculapius, insisting that it more accurately reflects the ideals of the profession.

References
1. Hart GD: The earliest medical use of the caduceus. Can Med Assoc J 1972;107:1107-1110.
2. Schouten J: The Rod and Serpent of Asklepios. New Yorker, Elsevier North Holland Inc, 1967.
3. Hamilton E: Mythology. Boston, Little Brown & Co, 1942.
4. Ingpen R, Peck WE (eds): The Complete Works of Percy Bysshe Shelley. New York, Charles Scribner's Sons, 1928.
5. Stenn F: The symbol of medicine. Q Bull Northwestern Univ Med Sch 1958;32:74-87.
6. Bunn JT: Origin of the caduceus motif. JAMA 1967;202:163-167.

Aging
American Medical Association white paper on elderly health. Report of the Council on Scientific Affairs [published erratum appears in Arch Intern Med 1991 Feb; 151(2): 265] Arch-Intern-Med 1990 Dec; 150:(12): 2459-72

Administration on Aging
330 Independence Ave. SW, Rm. 4640,
Washington, DC 20201
202/619-0641

"American Aging: Trends and Projections"
Federal Council on the Aging
Room 4342, 330 Independence Ave. SW
Washington, DC 20201
202/619-2451

American Association for International Aging
1511 K St. NW, Suite 443, Washington, DC 20005
202/638-6815

American Health Assistance Foundation
15825 Shady Grove Road, Rockville, MD 20850
800/227-7998

Children of Aging Parents (CAPS)
2761 Trenton Road, Levittown, PA 19056
Living at Home
565 W. Howard, Evanston, IL 60202
708/570-7066

National Institute on Aging
National Institutes of Health
Department of Health and Human Services
9000 Rockville Pike, MD 20892
301/496-1752

Aging, State Departments of
Alabama Commission on Aging
136 Catoma St., 2nd Floor
Montgomery, AL 36130
205/242-5743

Alaska Department of Administration
Older Alaskan Commission
State Office Building, 7th Floor, PO Box C,
Juneau, AK 99811-0209
907/465-3250

Arizona Department of Economic Security
Division of Social Services,
Aging and Adult Administration
1717 W Jefferson St, Phoenix, AZ 85007
602/542-4446

Arkansas Department of Human Services
Division of Aging and Adult Services
Donaghey Plaza S, PO Box 1437
Little Rock, AR 72203
501/682-2441

California Health and Welfare Agency
Department of Aging, 1600 K St.
Sacramento, CA 95814
916/322-5290

Colorado Department of Social Services
Division of Aging and Adult Services
1575 Sherman St., 8th Floor, Denver, CO 80203
303/866-2580

Connecticut Department on Aging
175 Main St, Hartford, CT 06106
203/566-3238

Delaware Department of
Health and Social Services
Division of Aging, Delaware State Hospital
1901 N. DuPont Highway, New Castle, DE 19720
302/421-6791

District of Columbia Office on Aging
1424 K St, NW, 2nd Floor, Washington, DC 20005
202/724-5622

Florida Department of Health
and Rehabilitative Services
Office of Aging and Adult Services
1317 Winewood Blvd.
Tallahassee, FL 32399-0700
904/488-8922

Georgia Department of Human Resources
Division of Aging Services
47 Trinity Ave, SW, Atlanta, GA 30334-2102
404/894-2023

Hawaii Executive Office on Aging
Old Federal Building
335 Merchant St, Room 241, Honolulu, HI 96813
808/548-2593

Idaho Executive Office on Aging
Statehouse, Room 108, Boise, ID 83720
208/334-3833

Illinois Department of Aging
421 E Capitol Ave, Springfield, IL 62702
217/785-2870

Indiana Department of Human Services
Division of Aging Services
PO Box 7083, Indianapolis, IN 46207-7083
317/232-7020

Iowa Department of Elder Affairs
236 Jewett Bldg, Des Moines, IA 50319
515/281-5187

Kansas Department on Aging
915 SW Harrison, Room 122-S
Topeka, KS 66612-1500
913/296-4986

Kentucky Human Resources Cabinet
Department for Social Services
Aging Services Division
275 E. Main St, Frankfort, KY 40621
502/564-6930

Louisiana Governor's Office of Elderly Affairs
4328 Bennington Drive
PO Box 80374, Baton Rouge, LA 70898-0374
504/925-1700

Maine Department of Human Services
Elderly and Adult Services Bureau
State House, Station 11, Augusta, ME 04333
207/289-2561

Maryland Office on Aging
301 W Preston St, Room 1004
Baltimore, MD 21201
301/225-1100

Massachusetts Executive Office
of Economic Affairs
Department of Elder Affairs
38 Chauncey St, Boston, MA 02111
617/727-7750

Michigan Office of Services to the Aging
611 W Ottawa St, 3rd Floor, PO Box 30026,
Lansing, MI 48909
517/373-7876

Minnesota Department of Human Services Aging
Program Division
444 Lafayette Road, St. Paul, MN 55155
612/296-2770

Mississippi Office of the Governor Aging Council
421 W Pascagoula St, Jackson, MS 39203
601/949-2070

Missouri Department of Social Services
Division of Aging
615 Howerton Court, Jefferson City, MO 65109
314/751-3082

Montana Office of the Governor
Aging Services Bureau
Capitol Station, Helena, MT 59620
406/444-3111

Nebraska Department on Aging
301 Centennial Mall S, 5th Floor
PO Box 95044, Lincoln, NE 68509-5044
402/471-2306

Nevada Department of Human Resources
Aging Service Division
340 N 11th St, Suite 114, Las Vegas, NV 89101
702/486-3572

New Hampshire Department of Health and Human
Service
Division of Elderly and Adult Services
6 Hazen Drive, Concord, NH 03301
603/271-4394

New Jersey Department of Community Affairs
Division on Aging
101 S Broad St, CN 800, Trenton, NJ 08625
609/292-4833

New Mexico State Agency on Aging
La Villa Rivera Bldg
224 E Palace Ave, Santa Fe, NM 87501
505/827-7640

New York State Office for the Aging
Agency Bldg 2, Empire State Plaza
Albany, NY 12223
518/474-4425

North Carolina Department of Human Services
Division of Aging
693 Palmer Drive, Raleigh, NC 27603-2001
919/733-3983

North Dakota Department of Human Services
Division on Aging Services
State Capitol, Judicial Wing, Bismarck, ND 58505
701/224-4130

Ohio Department of Aging
50 W Broad St, 9th Floor
Columbus, OH 43266-0501
614/466-5500

Oklahoma Department of Human Services
Aging Services Division
Sequoyah Memorial Office Bldg,
2400 N Lincoln Blvd
PO Box 25352, Oklahoma City, OK 73125
405/521-2327

Oregon Department of Human Resources
Division of Senior and Disabled Services
313 Public Services Bldg, Salem, OR 97310
503/378-4728

Pennsylvania Department of Aging
231 State St, Harrisburg, PA 17120
717/783-1924

Puerto Rico Department of Social Services
Division of Geriatrics
PO Box 11398, Santurce, PR 00910
809/722-7400

Rhode Island Department of Elderly Affairs
160 Pine St, Providence, RI 02903
401/277-2894

South Carolina Commission on Aging
400 Arbor Lake Drive, Suite B-500
Columbia, SC 29223
803/735-0210

South Dakota Department of Social Services
Office of Program Management
Adult Services and Aging Department
Kneip Bldg, 700 Governors Drive
Pierre, SD 57501-2291
605/773-3656

Tennessee Commission on Aging
706 Church St, Suite 201
Nashville, TN 37243-0860
615/741-2056

Texas Department on Aging
1949 IH 35 S, PO Box 12786, Capitol Station,
Austin, TX 78741
512/444-2727

Utah Department of Human Services
Division of Aging and Adult Services
120 North 200 West, PO Box 45500
Salt Lake City, UT 84145-5500
801/538-3910

Vermont Agency of Human Services
Office on Aging and Disability
State Complex, 103 S Main St.
Waterbury, VT 05676
802/241-2400

Virginia Department of Mental Health, Mental
Retardation, and Substance
Abuse Services, Division of Geriatric Services
109 Governor St.
Richmond, VA 23219
804/786-4837

Washington Department of Social and Health
Services
Bureau of Aging and Adult Services
Mail Stop OB-44, Olympia, WA 98504
206/753-3768

West Virginia Department of Health and Human
Resources
Aging Commission
State Capitol--Holy Grove, Charleston, WV 25305
304/348-3317

Wisconsin Department of Health
and Social Services
Division of Community Services, Bureau on Aging
1 W Wilson St, PO Box 7850
Madison, WI 53707
608/266-2536

Wyoming Department of Health
Aging Division
Hathaway Bldg, Room 139, Cheyenne, WY 82002
307/777-7986

AIDS

AIDS Archive
Gerber Hart Library and Archive
3352 N. Paulina, Chicago, IL 60657
312/883-3003

"Business Response to Aids"
An initiative by the Centers for Disease Control
and Prevention to provide work-place awareness
and educational materials to companies that wish
to increase their effectiveness in this area.
800-458-5231

Clinical Trials Information
800/TRIALS-A
(800/874-2572 M-F 9:00am-7:00pm EST)

JAMA Article of Note: Ethical Issues Involved in
Growing AIDS Crisis" Council on Ethical and
Judicial Affairs. JAMA. 1988 Mar 4; 259(9): 1360-1.

"HIV Early Care: Guidelines for Physicians"
AMA Department of HIV/AIDS
515 North State Street, Chicago, IL 60610
312/464-5563

Rapoza, N. *HIV/AIDS Infection and Disease:
Monographs for Physicians and Other Health Care
Workers* American Medical Association; Chicago
1989. 202 pp. (16 monographs in one volume)
ISBN 0-89970-376-3 OP014690

JAMA Theme Issue: AIDS
JAMA. 1992 July 22/29; 268(4):
AIDS has been a selected topic of JAMA (see also
June 21, 1985 & March 4, 1988 issues) on several
occasions. This recent issue focuses on clinical
articles regarding, for example, tuberculosis and
HIV-infected drug users, contraceptive sponge
use and HIV prevention, and a discussion of
residents' attitudes toward caring for persons with
AIDS.

AIDS-Education

American Alliance for Health, Physical Education,
Recreation and Dance
1900 Association Dr., Reston, VA 22091
703/476-3400

Child Welfare League of America
Foster Care: Infected Children
Publications and Videos
440 First Street, MW, Suite 310
Washington D.C. 20001
202/638-2952

Free facts on AIDS write:
American Red Cross/ Public Health Service
AIDS
Suite 700, 155 Wilson Blvd.
Rosslyn, VA 22209

Public Health Service
Office of Public Affairs, Room 721-H
200 Independence Ave. SW
Washington, DC 20201

"Living with AIDS," (Videotape regarding home health care for AIDS patients):
National Center for Homecare
Education and Research
350 Fifth Ave., New York, NY 10011
212/560-3300

National PTA
700 N. Rush, Chicago, IL 60610
312/787-0977

Surgeon General's pamphlet:
"AIDS"
PO Box 14252, Washington, DC 20044
for bulk orders 800/458-5231

"Teens and AIDS: Playing It Safe":
American Council on Life Insurance, Dept. 190,
1001 Pennsylvania Ave. NW
Washington, DC 20004

AIDS-Education for Health Care Professionals

AIDS Foundation of Chicago (AIDS information and referral service for health professionals)
1332 N. Halsted/Suite 303, Chicago, IL 60622
312/642-3763; Hours: M-Th 9-1pm/Fri 1-5pm

National HIV Telephone Consulting Service:
a consultation service for doctors and other health professionals who have questions about providing care to people with HIV infections or AIDS:
800/933-3413

AIDS-Hotlines-National

AZT Hotline
800/843-9388

CAIN (Computerized AIDS Information Network)
San Francisco AIDS Foundation
54 Tenth St., San Francisco, CA 94103
415/864-4376

Centers for Disease Control and Prevention/American Social Health Association
800/342-AIDS

Clinical Trials Information
800/TRIALS-A (M-F 9:00am-7:00pm EST)

Johns Hopkins AIDS Service
(Information on AIDS drug trials)
301/955-4345
(Describes trial eligibility requirements)

National AIDS Information Clearinghouse
(operated by the Centers for Disease Control)
Box 6003, Rockville, MD 20850
800/458-5231

National AIDS Hotline
800/342-2437
Spanish
800/344-7432
Hearing Impaired (TTY-TDD line)
800/243-7889

National AIDS Testing
800/356-2437

National Association of People with AIDS
202/483-7979

National Gay Task Force/Gay Lesbian Crisisline
800/221-7044

Physician Link, list of MDs with expertise in AIDS treatment and research
800/344-5500

Statistics on AIDS
(tape recorded message set up by the Centers for Disease Control and Prevention

National Statistics
404/330-3020
State and City Statistics
404/330-3022
Statistics by Transmission Categories
404/330-3021

Teen staffed AIDS hotline
800/234-TEEN 5-9 PM EDT/ 2-6 PM PDT
Monday through Saturday

U.S. Public Health Service Hotline
800/342-2437 (recorded message)
800/342-7514
(questions answered, information on NIH experimental AIDS treatment)

AIDS-Hotlines-Statewide

Alabama
800/228-0469 (M-F 8 AM-8 PM)

Alaska
800/478-2437 (M-F 9 AM-6 PM)

Arizona
602/402-9396 (M-F 8 AM-5 PM)

Arkansas
800/448-8305

California
California, Northern
415/864-4376; 800/367-2437

California, Southern
213/871-AIDS: 800/922-2437

Colorado
303/831-6268; 800/252-2437

Connecticut
Department of Health, AIDS Coordinator
203/566-5058
Statewide Hotline 800/342-AIDS

Delaware
800/422-0429

DC, Washington
DC AIDS Task Force 202/332-5295
Hotline 202/332-2437

Florida
AIDS Center One 800/325-5371 (Ft. Lauderdale)
Health Crisis Network 305/634-4780 (Miami)
Statewide Hotline 800/352-2437

Georgia
AID Atlanta 404/872-0600
Statewide Hotline 800/551-2728

Hawaii
800/922-1313

Idaho
208-345-2277

Illinois
800/243-2437
(will provide list of free and
confidential testing sites)
Chicago: Howard Brown Clinic
945 W. George, Chicago, IL 60657
312/871-5777 (fee for test)

Indiana
800/848-2437 (Mon-Sat, 10 AM-8 PM)

Iowa
800/445-2437 (7 days/24 hours)

Kansas
800/232-0040 (M-F. 9 AM-9 PM)

Kentucky
800/654-2437 (M-F, 8 AM.-8 PM)

Louisiana
800/992-4379 (M-F, 2 PM-10 PM;S-S, 2 PM-8 PM)

Maine
800/851-2437 (M-F, 9 AM-5 PM)

Maryland
Baltimore Health Education Resource
Organization
301/945-AIDS
Statewide Hotline: 800/638-6252

Massachusetts
Boston: Fenway Community Health Center
617/267-7573
Statewide Hotline: 800/235-2331

Michigan
800/872-2437
(M-F 9 AM-9 PM;S-S 9 AM-5 PM)

Minnesota
612/870-0700 (Minneapolis-St. Paul)
800/248-2437

Mississippi
800/537-0851 (24 hours)

Missouri
800/533-2437 (24 hours)

Montana
800/233-6668 (24 hours)

Nebraska
800/782-2437 (9 AM-11 PM)

Nevada
800-842-2437

New Hampshire
800/872-8909
(M-F, 8:30 AM-4:30 PM)

New Jersey
Highland Park:: Hyacinth Foundation
201/246-8439
Statewide Hotline: 800/624-2377

New Mexico
800/545-2437

New York
212/807-6016
800/541-2437
New York City: 800/462-1884

North Carolina
800/342-2437
(M-F, 9 AM-5 PM)

North Dakota
800/472-2180
(M-F, 8 AM-5 PM)

Ohio
800/332-2437
(M-F, 9 AM-11 PM; S-S, 9 AM- 6 PM)

Oklahoma
800/535-2437 (24 hours)

Oregon
800/777-2437
(M-F, 10 AM-9 PM; S-S, noon-6 PM)

Pennsylvania
800/662-6080, (M-F, 8 AM-4:30 PM)
Philadelphia: 215/232-8055

Puerto Rico
809/765-1010

Rhode Island
800-726-3010
(M-F, 9:30 AM-8 PM)
Spanish
800/442-7432
(M-F, 4:30 PM-8 PM)

South Carolina
800/322-2437 (24 hours)

South Dakota
800/592-1861
(M-F, 8 AM-5 PM)

Tennessee
800/525-2437
(M-F, 8 AM- 4:30 PM)

Texas
800/299-2437
(M-F, 8 AM-12 PM, 1 PM-5 PM)
Houston 713/792-3245

Utah
800/366-2437 (24 hours)
Salt Lake City 801/538-6094
(24 hours)

Vermont
800/882-2437
(M-F, 8 AM-4:30 PM)

Virginia
800/533-4138
(M-F, 8:30 AM- 5 PM)

Virgin Islands
809-773-2437

Washington
800/272-2437
(M-F, 8 AM-5 PM)

West Virginia
800/642-8244
(M-F, 8:30 AM- 8 PM)

Wisconsin
Milwaukee: 414/273-2437
800/334-2437
(M-F, 9 AM- 9 PM; S-S 11 AM-5 PM)

Wyoming
800/327-3577
(M-F, 8 AM-5 PM)

AIDS, Policy
AMA Board of Trustees report YY
"Prevention and Control of AIDS - an Interim
Report"

Centers for Disease Control and Prevention
There are several compilations of MMWR reports
that reflect AIDS policies of the CDC.

New AIDS Definition

AMNews 1/18/1993

The number of people diagnosed with AIDS will
jump under the new disease definition that took
effect Jan. 1. It lists a CDC count of 200 as the
AIDS-defining standard and adds pulmonary
tuberculosis, recurrent pneumonia and invasive
cervical cancer to the list of defining conditions.
Under this definition, an estimated 90,000

Americans will be diagnosed with full-blown AIDS
in 1993, almost double the current number.

Citation for new definition: Centers for Disease
Control and Prevention. 1993 Revised
classification system for HIV infection and
expanded surveillance case definition for AIDS
among adolescents and adults. MMWR
1992;41(No. RR-17)

1987 Revision of the Adult Case Definition of AIDS for Surveillance Purposes
An illness in an adult characterized by one or
more of the following indicator diseases,
depending on the laboratory evidence of HIV
infection, as follows:
- Without laboratory evidence regarding HIV
infection. If laboratory test for HIV were not
performed or gave inconclusive results, and if
there were no other identifiable causes of
immunodeficiency that disqualify diseases as
indicators, then any disease listed indicated
AIDS if it were diagnosed by a definitive
method: candida esophagitis, tracheitis, or
bronchopulmonary infection; extrapulmonary
cryptococcus; persistent cryptosporidiosis with
diarrhea; persistent systemic cytomegalovirus
infection; persistent herpes simplex; Kaposi's
sarcoma; primary lymphoma of the brain;
disseminated Mycobacterium avium;
Pneumocystis carinii pneumonia; progressive
multifocal leukoencephalopathy; toxoplasmosis
of the brain.
- With laboratory evidence for HIV infection.
Regardless of the presence of other causes of
immunodeficiency, in the presence of laboratory
evidence for HIV infection, any disease listed
above in Section I or immediately following, if
diagnosed definitively, indicates a diagnosis of
AIDS: disseminated histoplasmosis; persistent
isosporiasis diarrhea; non-Hodgkins lymphoma
of B-cell or unknown immunologic phenotype;
disseminated mycobacterial disease; recurrent
salmonella septicemia; wasting syndrome. If
there is laboratory evidence for HIV infection,
the following indicator diseases diagnoses
presumptively can also be used to define AIDS:
candidiasis of the esophagus; cytomegalovirus
retinitis; Kaposi's sarcoma; disseminated
mycobacterial disease; pneumocystis
pneumonia; toxoplasmosis of the brain.
- With laboratory evidence against HIV infection.
With laboratory test results negative for HIV, the
following condition can be used to diagnose
"AIDS":no other cause of immunodeficiency and
PCP and a depressed number of blood CD4
helper lymphocytes.(HIV)

"Guidelines for HIV-Infected Children"
American Academy of Pediatrics
141 Northwest Point Blvd.
Elk Grove Village, IL 60007
708/228-5005
800/433-9016

Air Pollution

Air Pollution Control Association
PO Box 2861, Pittsburgh, PA 15230
412/232-3444

Environmental Protection Agency
401 M St, SW, Washington, DC 20460
Public Information 202/382-4454

Alcoholism

*AMA Policy: Alcoholism as a Disability:
(1) The AMA believes it is important for
professional and layman alike to
recognize that alcoholism is in and of
itself a disabling and handicapped
condition. (2) The AMA encourages the
availability of appropriate services to
persons suffering from multiple
disabilities or multiple handicaps,
including alcoholism. (3) The AMA
endorses the position that printed and
audiovisual materials pertaining to the
subject of people suffering from both
alcoholism and other disabilities include
the terminology "alcoholic person with
multiple disabilities or alcoholic person
with multiple disabilities or alcoholic
person with multiple handicaps."
Hopefully, this language clarification will
reinforce the concept that alcoholism is
in and of itself a disabling and
handicapping conditions.*

AL-ANON Family Group Headquarters
1372 Broadway, 7th Floor, New York, NY 10018
212/302-7240

Alcohol Education for Youth
1500 Western Ave., Albany, NY 12203
514/456-3800

Alcoholics Anonymous World Services
468 Park Avenue South, New York, NY 10016
212/686-1100

American Society on Addiction Medicine
12 W 21st St., New York, NY 10010
212/206-6770

Children of Alcoholics Foundation
200 Park Avenue, 31st Floor, New York, NY 10166
212/949-1404

*AMA Policy Dual Disease Classification
of Alcoholism: The AMA reaffirms it
policy endorsing the dual classification
of alcoholism under both the psychiatric
and medical sections of the International
Classification of Diseases.*

Drunk Driving

Mothers Against Drunk Driving
PO Box 541688, Dallas, TX 75354-1688
214/744-6233

National Commission Against Drunk Driving
114 Connecticut Ave. NW, Suite 804, Washington,
DC 20036
202/452-0130

National Safety Council
1121 Spring Lake Drive, Itasca, IL 60143-3201
708/285-1121 (brochure available)

JAMA Theme Issue: Alcohol
JAMA. 1986 Sept 19; 256(11)
JAMA's second issue devoted to alcohol use,
abuse and alcoholism (see also October 12,
1984), spotlights advertising and alcohol use,
various treatments for alcohol abuse and
alcoholism, women and alcohol, plus book reviews
of publications on the subject.

National Clearinghouse for Alcohol Information
Good Executive Blvd., Wilco Bldg., Suite 402,
Box 2345, Rockville, MD 20852
301/468-2600

National Council on Alcoholism
800/NCA-CALL (800/622-2255)

National Institute of Alcohol Abuse and Alcoholism
National Clearinghouse for Alcohol Information
9000 Rockville Pike
Bethesda, MD 20892
301/443-3860

National Referral
800/ALCOHOL (800/252-6465)

Allergy

American Academy of Allergy and Immunology
611 E. Wells St., Milwaukee, WI 53202
414/272-6071
Hotline: 800/822-2762

American Academy of Otolaryngic Allergy
8455 Colesville Rd., Suite 745
Silver Spring, MD 20910
301/588-1800

American College of Allergy and Immunology
800 E. Northwest Hwy, Ste. 1080
Palatine, IL 60067
708/359-2800

American Board of Allergy and Immunology
University City Science Center
3624 Market St., Philadelphia, PA 19104
215/349-9466

National Institute of Allergy and Infectious
Diseases
Public Response, 9000 Rockville Pike
Bethesda, MD 20892
301/496-5717

JAMA Theme Issue: Allergic and Immunologic Diseases. JAMA. 1992 Nov 25; 268(20) Preface - deShazo, RD ed, Smith, RL associate ed. *Primer*
This JAMA *Primer on Allergic and Immunologic Diseases* represents a continuing effort to provide up-to-date information on applied immunology Although the JAMA *Primer* traditionally has been directed toward medical students and copies are sent to all US medical students, previous editions have been equally popular with graduate physicians. This interest in the *Primer* reflects the central role of immunologic processes in health and disease, the rapidly changing data-base in the field, and the user-friendly format that we have tried to preserve in the Third edition. (see also JAMA. 1987 Nov 27; 258(20) and JAMA. 1982 Nov 26; 248(20)).

Wheat and Gluten Intolerance
Celiac Sprue Society
PO Box 31700, Omaha, NE 68131-0700
402/558-0600

Allied Health
Accreditation:
Committee on Allied Health
Education and Accreditation
515 N. State St, Chicago, IL 60610
312/464-4660

Includes the following fields:

Anesthesiologist's Assistant
Athletic Trainer
Cardiovascular Technologist
Cytotechnologist
Diagnostic Medical Sonographer - Ultrasound
Electroneurodiagnostic Technologist
Emergency Medical Technician - Paramedic
Histologic Technologist/Technician
Medical Assistant
Medical Illustrator
Medical Laboratory Technician (Associate Degree)
Medical Laboratory Technician (Certificate)
Medical Record Administrator
Medical Record Technician
Medical Technologist
Nuclear Medicine Technologist
Occupational Therapist
Occupational Therapy Assistant
Ophthalmic Medical Assistant
Perfusionist
Physician's Assistant
Radiation Therapy Technologist
Radiographer
Respiratory Therapist
Respiratory Therapy Technician
Specialist in Blood Bank Technology
Surgeon's Assistant
Surgical Technologist
Ultrasound - Diagnostic Medical Sonographer

CAHEA Accreditation
Definition, Purpose, Benefits: Accreditation is a process of external peer review in which a private, nongovernmental agency or association grants public recognition to an institution or specialized program of study that meets certain established qualifications and educational standards, as determined through initial and subsequent periodic evaluations.

The purpose of the accreditation process is to provide a professional judgment of the quality of the educational institution or program and to encourage its continued improvement.

General public and governmental acceptance of the CAHEA system is indicated by the fact that federal agencies and nongovernmental foundations use the lists of CAHEA-accredited programs to determine eligibility for some special institutional and student grants and financial aid. In addition, many health care facilities require job applications to be graduates of a program accredited by CAHEA. Accreditation in an assurance of acceptable quality in education, in that accredited programs are required to meet certain national standards established by the professional in the field and their communities of interest.

By stating that an institution has met established standards, accreditation provides benefits in the following areas:
• Students. Helps prospective students to identify institutions and programs that meet standards established by and for the field in which they are interested. Assists students who wish to transfer from one institution to another.
• Institutions. Protects against internal and external pressures to modify programs for reasons that are not educationally sound. Involves faculty and staff in comprehensive program and institutional evaluation and planning. Stimulates self-improvement by providing nationally acceptable standards against which the institution can evaluate the program it sponsors.
• Society. Assists the process of professional certification, registration or licensure by providing reasonable assurance of quality educational preparation for such credentialing; provides one of several consideration used as a basis of determining eligibility for some types of Federal assistance; and helps to identify institutions and programs for the investment of public and private funds.
Recognizing Health Occupations: National organizations desiring AMA recognition of a health occupation, for the purposes of eventual collaboration with the AMA in sponsorship of accreditation of educational programs by CAHEA, should use the Guideline for Development of New Health Occupations (AMA House of Delegates, December 1969). The Guidelines may be obtained from the Secretary, Council on Medical Education, AMA, 515 N. State, Chicago, IL 60610.

Before considering the establishment of a new allied health occupation and the development of minimum standards for an educational program for this occupation, the following questions are to be addressed:
• What services are needed by the patients?
• How can these services be provided most effectively?
• Can the people in existing health occupations provide these services most efficiently?
• If not, what new allied health occupation is needed?
• What, exactly, are the tasks which this new allied health occupation will be expected to perform?
• What educational program is needed to develop the proficiency to perform these tasks?

Establishing Collaborative Relationships:
When a new allied health occupation has been formally recognized by the AMA Council on Medical Education as an emerging health occupation, the Division of Allied Health Education and Accreditation (DAHEA) assists interested allied health organizations and medical specialty societies in achieving collaborative status, in writing Essentials for adoption, in establishing policies and procedures necessary for accreditation of programs by CAHEA. The CAHEA document entitled Collaborative Relationships discusses establishing a collaborative relationship with organizations for a new health occupation, for an established health profession with educational programs presently accredited by CAHEA, and for an established health profession with educational programs not presently accredited by CAHEA. The method for dissolving collaborative relationships is also described. Once the collaborative relationship is established, the collaborating organization or organizations draft and adopt Essentials.

Application for Accreditation: Accreditation is a voluntary process. Evaluation of an allied health educational program is undertaken only with specific authorization from the chief executive office of the sponsoring institution. An application form is submitted to AMA/DAHEA and a Self-Study Report is prepared by the program and forwarded to the review committee. A decision is made at this point on whether the program may be accreditable and whether it should be visited. DAHEA staff and/or review committee staff provide consultation to programs throughout the process.

Self-Study: Ideally, ongoing internal review, analysis, and assessment of the entire range of educational operations, including ancillary services that contribute to accomplishing valid objectives, should be conducted by faculty and other appropriate members of the academic community. This type of self-study (also called self-analysis or self-assessment) is required of programs requesting to be considered or accreditation by CAHEA. Review committees and DAHEA provide self-study materials to guide the evaluation of the program within its institutional setting. These materials usually include an outline of the Self-Study Report, which is "keyed" to the Essentials. Some review committee conduct workshops on the self-study and analysis process.

Self-Study Report: The self-study requirements of the review committee frequently contain specific instructions for preparing the report. Programs are advised that the report need contain only enough representative documentation to substantiate compliance with the Essentials, as clarified in the Guidelines. The report should also contain a qualitative self-assessment (analysis) based on applications of the Essentials, which concludes with changes anticipated to strengthen the program.

The institution/program may conduct a self-study which exceeds in depth and breadth the needs of the accreditation process. In this case, the needs of the latter are singled out and presented in the Self-Study Report.

Site Visit: The program is visited by a team assembled by the review committee staff. The site visit process provides the opportunity to validate and/or clarify the contents of the Self-Study Report and to determine the extent to which the allied health program seeking accreditation complies with the Essentials.

Site Visit Report: Review committees specify the format and content of the Site Visit Report. In the usual procedure, the Site Visit Report is submitted to the review committee staff, which sends copies of the report to the chief executive officer of the sponsoring institution and to the program director to provide an opportunity for comment and the correction of factual errors and conclusions. The written materials provided to the institution identify program strengths and areas of concern. Specific Essentials are cited if noncompliance is identified.

Review Committee Evaluation: After the program has had adequate time to respond to the factual content of the Site Visit Report, the program is placed on the agenda for the next review committee meeting. Review committees meet two or three times annually and occasionally by teleconference. During these meetings, the review committees consider each current application for initial or continuing accreditation.

A DAHEA staff member attends each review committee meeting as a representative of CAHEA. This individual is responsible for providing assistance to the review committee and help in assuring that CAHEA's policies and procedures are observed.

CAHEA Subcommittee: Accreditation recommendations are reviewed by a CAHEA subcommittee. This group gives special attention to recommendations for placing programs on probation or for withdrawing or withholding accreditation. It is not the function or purpose of a subcommittee to duplicate the work of review committees in making an independent assessment of each program's relative compliance with the Essentials. Subcommittee reviews are designed to provide assurance that established CAHEA and review committee policies and practices have been followed and that due process has been observed in arriving at accreditation recommendations. The subcommittee also examine suggestions and recommendations for program improvement that may be perceived as inappropriate intrusion into the administrative prerogatives of a program and its sponsoring institution.

Accreditation by CAHEA: Once the subcommittee work is completed, CAHEA convenes in plenary session to receive the recommendations resulting from the subcommittee reviews and to award or deny accreditation to applicant programs. If CAHEA finds itself unable to support a review committee recommendation, CAHEA action is deferred and the recommendation is returned to the review committee for further consideration.

Fees and Cost-Benefits: The cost-benefits derived from accreditation fees are substantial. Accreditation processes within the collaborative system provided by CAHEA and the review committees are a low-cost high-value service.

In addition to the broad benefits cited earlier are the following:

- professional evaluation by competent faculty and practitioners
- assurance that the institution's programs compare favorably with others nationwide assurance that the students should qualify for entry into their profession upon graduation
- assurance that students should qualify for entry into their profession upon graduation.
- assurance that faculty should be motivated to maintain continuous self-analysis of the strengths inherent in the program and of the dimensions that merit improvement or further development.
- gaining the fresh perspectives of other competent educators and practitioners which enhances creativity among faculty and administration.

Programs pay to review committee an annual accreditation fee to help offset review committee operating expenses. Programs also cover expenses associated with the American Medical Association's support of the operation of CAHEA and the maintenance of the national allied health education accreditation archives which are vital to program graduates and state regulating agencies concerned with the allied health professions.

Confidentiality in the Accreditation Process: Meticulous efforts are made by all components of the peer review process to maintain the confidentiality of information collected during the entire accreditation review and to avoid conflicts of interest. Materials, such as the Self-Study Report and the Site Visit Report, are to be read and discussed only by members of the visiting team, the review committee, CAHEA, and other authorized persons. It is further recognized that these materials are the property of the sponsoring institution which is free to share or distribute them as it chooses.

Ensuring Due Process: In order to ensure due process for all parties involved in the accreditation and operation of allied health educational programs, CAHEA and the review committees have disseminated clear descriptions of the rights of the parties involved and of their recourse should they feel that those rights have been denied.

CAHEA makes available to the public its criteria or standard for accreditation, reports of its operations, lists of accredited educational programs, and notification of programs no longer accredited.(ACC)

Allied Health Education Directory 20th ed. Committee on Allied Health Education and Accreditation, Chicago. 1992 ISBN 0-89970-420-4 OP417592

American Society of Allied Health Professions 1101 Connecticut Avenue, NW Suite 700, Washington, DC 20036 202/857-1150

Alzheimer's Disease

Alzheimer's Disease and Related Disorders Association
70 E. Lake St., Chicago, IL 60601
800/272-3900

Brain Donors:
McLean Hospital Brain Bank, 115 Mill St., Belmont, MA 02178
617/855-2400

THA (Tetrahydroaminocridine) Study
800/621-0379, 800/572-6037 (IL only)

Ambulances

American Ambulance Association (AAA)
3814 Auburn Blvd, Suite 70
Sacramento, CA 95821
916/483-3827

Ambulatory Care Organizations

Accreditation Association for Ambulatory Health Care
9933 Lawler Avenue, Skokie, IL 60077
708/676-9610

American Society of Outpatient Surgery
3960 Park Blvd, Suite E, San Diego, CA 92103
619/692-9918

Ambulatory Health Care Accreditation
Unlike the requirements of state licensure laws, which must be met before a facility can operate, accreditation is voluntary. Facilities that seek accreditation are committed to providing the highest achievable quality of care for patients, a goal that is widely advocated and supported by organized medicine and encouraged by third-party payers.

Two organizations accredit freestanding ambulatory surgical centers: the Accreditation Association for Ambulatory Health Care, Inc., and the Joint Commission on Accreditation of Health Care Organizations, Division of Ambulatory Health Care. (The American Association for Accreditation of Ambulatory Plastic Surgery Facilities, Inc., inspects and accredits both office-based and freestanding plastic surgery facilities.) Both the AAAHC and the JCAHO have developed similar programs and standards with the technical assistance of recognized health care professionals active in ambulatory care. The underlying purpose and philosophy of both programs provides that:

- Surveys are conducted by a team that evaluates the operation of the facility and shares its experience and knowledge about techniques used by similar facilities that enhance patient care and efficiency of administrative systems;
- Standards are developed that reflect that state of the art and are surveyable; and
- Ongoing research in aspects of standards development and quality assurance is maintained.

Facilities must be operational for one year before being eligible for accreditation. The standards offer a systematic approach to designing organizational systems and establishing policies and procedures for the new facility. To date, the Accreditation Association for Ambulatory Health Care, Inc., has been more active than the JCAHO in working with freestanding ambulatory surgical centers.(EST)

National Association for Ambulatory Care
21 Michigan St, Grand Rapids, MI 49503
616/949-2138

Amputation

American Amputee Foundation, Inc.
PO Box 55218, Hillcrest Station
Little Rock, AR 72225
501/666-2523

Amputee Services Association
6613 North Clark St., Chicago, IL 60626
312/274-2044

National Odd Shoe Exchange
2242 W. Keim Drive, Phoenix, AZ 85015
602/246-8725

Amyotrophic Lateral Sclerosis

Amyotrophic Lateral Sclerosis Association
21021 Ventura Blvd., Suite 321
Woodland Hills, CA 91364
818/990-2151

Anatomical Dolls

Eymann Anatomically Correct Dolls
3645 Scarsdale Ct., Sacramento, CA 95827
916/362-8503

Hal's Pals
Susan Anderson
PO Box 3490, Winter Park, CO 80482
303/726-8388

Patient Puppets
Tacey Lawrence
40 Home St., Winnipeg, Manitoba
Canada R3G1W6
204/942-7291

West River Sexual Abuse Treatment Center
AumaneNA Family Guidance Service
PO Box 1572, 924 N. Maple
Rapid City, SD 57709
605/342-4303

Anesthesiologists' Assistant

History: The concept of an anesthesiologist's assistant (AA) was initiated in 1969 at Case Western Reserve University in Cleveland, Ohio and at Emory University in Atlanta, Georgia. Having been advised of the programs' purposes and operations, by 1975 the American Society of Anesthesiologists (ASA) was supportive of the emerging profession. The Emory University curriculum was designed to result in a Master of Medical Science degree. Case Western Reserve offered a Bachelor of Science degree, designed largely as a pre-medicine curriculum that would provide students with a marketable body of clinical knowledge and skills.

In 1976, the ASA petitioned the AMA Council on Medical Education (CME) for recognition of the anesthesiologist's assistant as an emerging health profession. CME's recognition followed in 1978.

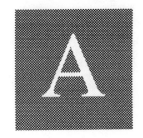

This authorized the initiation of an ad hoc committee within the ASA to work collaboratively with AMA's then Department of Allied Health Education and Accreditation on the development of a body of educational standards (Essentials). Due to differences in opinion about the level of the credential and about the need for graduates in this field, in 1981 the ASA withdrew from its collaboration with the AMA in the development of accreditation standards.

By 1982, the Association for Anesthesiologists' Assistants Education (AAAE, originally called the "Association of Anesthesiologist's Assistant Training Programs") was created and incorporated. The following year the AAAE and the American Academy of Anesthesiologists' Assistants (AAAA) petitioned the AMA Council on Medical Education to recognize them as collaborative sponsors for the programs designed to educate anesthesiologists' assistants. In 1984 the AMA Council on Medical Education reinstated its recognition of the anesthesiologist's assistants profession. Essentials for the education and training of anesthesiologists' assistants were adopted in 1987 by the CME, the AAAE, and the AAAA.

Occupational Description: The anesthesiologist's assistant (AA) functions under the direction of a licensed and qualified anesthesiologist, principally in medical centers. The AA assists the anesthesiologist in collecting preoperative data, such as taking an appropriate health history and performing an appropriate physical examination; in performing various preoperative tasks, such as the insertion of intravenous and arterial lines, central venous pressure monitors, special catheters; in airway management and drug administration for induction and maintenance of anesthesia; in administering supportive therapy, such as intravenous fluids and vasodilators; in providing recovery room care and in performing other functions or tasks relating to care in an intensive care unit or pain clinic; in providing anesthesia monitoring services; and in performing administrative functions and tasks, such as staff education.

Job Description: In addition to the duties described in the occupational description above, AAs provide technical support according to established protocols. This support includes first-level maintenance of anesthesia equipment; skilled operation of special monitors, including echocardiographs, electroencephalographs, special analyzers, evoked-potential apparatuses, autotransfusion devices, mass spectrometers, and intraaortic balloon pumps; the operation and maintenance of bedside electronic computer-based monitors; supervised laboratory functions associated with anesthesia and operating room care; and cardiopulmonary resuscitation.

Employment Characteristics: Studies have indicated that anesthesiologist's assistants are likely to be employed by hospitals with 200 beds and larger and with staffs of 15 or more anesthesiologists, nurse anesthetists and anesthesiologist's assistants; which use a team approach to anesthesia service; which have facilities for open heart surgery; and which have a graduate medical residency training program for anesthesiologists.

The normal work week for the majority of AAs is comparable to that of the supervising anesthesiologist. Salaries vary depending on the experience and education of the graduate, the economy of the given region, the time demands on the AAs work schedule and scope of responsibilities. Starting salaries are in the upper-forty to mid-fifty thousand dollar range.(ALL)

AMA Allied Health Department
312/464-4622

American Academy of
Anesthesiologists' Assistants
PO Box 33876, Decatur, GA 30033-0876
404/727-5910

Anesthesiology

Anesthesiologist: administers anesthetics to render patients insensible to pain during surgical, obstetrical, and other medical procedures: Examines patient to determine degree of surgical risk, and type of anesthetic and sedation to administer, and discusses findings with medical practitioner concerned with case. Positions patient on operating table and administers local, intravenous, spinal, caudal, or other anesthetic according to prescribed medical standards. Institutes remedial measures to counteract adverse reactions or complications. Records type and amount of anesthetic and sedation administered and condition of patient before, during, and after anesthesia. May instruct medical students and other personnel in characteristics and methods of administering various types of anesthetics, signs, and symptoms of reactions and complications, and emergency measures to employ.(DOT)

American Board of Anesthesiology
100 Constitution Plaza, Hartford, CT 06103
203/522-9857

American Society of Anesthesiologists
520 N. Northwest Highway, Park Ridge, IL 60068
708/825-5586

Anesthesiology, Ambulatory

Society of Ambulatory Anesthesiology
520 N. Northwest Highway, Park Ridge, IL 60068
708/825-5586

Animal Rights

American Association for Laboratory
Animal Science
70 Timber Creek Drive, Suite 5
Cordova, TN 38018
901/754-8620

Animal Resource Program Branch
(Division of Research Resources)
Westwood Building
Room 853, 5335 Westbard Avenue
Bethesda, MD 20892
301/496-5175

The Center for Alternatives to Animal Testing
Johns Hopkins School of Hygiene and
Public Health

615 N. Wolfe St., Baltimore, MD 21205
301/955-3343

Foundation for Biomedical Research
818 Connecticut Ave., N.W., Suite 303,
Washington, DC 20006
202/457-0654

JAMA Article of Note: Use of Animals in Biomedical Research: The Challenge and the Response JAMA. 1989 Nov 17; 262(19): 2716-20 Human vs. Animal Rights. In Defense of Animal Research. For centuries, opposition has been directed against the use of animals for the benefit of humans. For more than four centuries in Europe, and for more than a century in the United States, this opposition has targeted scientific research that involves animals. More recent movements in support of animal rights have arisen in an attempt to impede, if not prohibit, the use of animals in scientific experimentation. These movements employ various means that range from information and media campaigns to destruction of property and threats against investigators. The latter efforts have resulted in the identification of more militant animal rights bands as terrorist groups. The American Medical Association has long been a defender of humane research that employs animals, and it is very concerned about the efforts of animal rights and welfare groups to interfere with research. Recently, the Association prepared a detailed analysis of the controversy over the use of animals in research, and the consequences for research and clinical medicine if the philosophy of animal rights activists were to prevail in society. This article is a condensation of the Association's analysis. (also known as "White Paper" on Animal Research:)

Use of animals in medical education. Council on Scientific Affairs, American Medical Association. JAMA. 1991 Aug 14; 266(6): 836-7
The use of animals in general medical education is essential. Although several adjuncts to the use of animals are available, none can completely replace the limited use of animals in the medical curriculum. Students should be made aware of an institution's policy on animal use in the curriculum before matriculation, and faculty should make clear to all students the learning objectives of any educational exercise that uses animals. The Council on Scientific Affairs recognizes the necessity for the responsible and humane treatment of animals and urges all medical school faculty members to discuss this moral and ethical imperative with their students.

Animal Therapy (Pets used for therapy)

Humane Society of the United States
2100 L St., NW, Washington, DC 20037
202/452-1100

Latham Foundation
Latham Plaza Building
Clement and Schiller Streets, Alameda, CA 94501

National Association for the Advancement of
Humane Education
PO Box 98, East Haddam, CT 06423
203/434-8666

Anorexia Nervosa
Anorexia Nervosa and Associated Disorders
Box 271, Highland Park, IL 60035
708/831-3438

Anorexia Nervosa and Related Eating Disorders
PO Box 5102, Eugene, OR 97405
503/344-1144

BASH (Bulimia Anorexia Self Help)
c/o Deaconess Hospital
6150 Oakland Avenue, St. Louis, MO 63139
800/762-3334
St. Louis area 314/768-3838 or 768-3292

Anxiety
Pass Group (Panic Attack Sufferers'
Support Group)
1042 East 105th Street, Brooklyn, NY 11236
718/763-0190

Art
American Physicians Art Association
76 Forest Road, Asheville, NC 28803
704/274-0748

Art Therapy
Art Therapist: Plans and conducts art therapy
programs in public and private institutions to
rehabilitate mentally and physically disabled
clients: Confers with members of medically
oriented team to determine physical and
psychology needs of client. Devises art therapy
program to fulfill physical and psychological
needs. Instructs individuals and groups in use of
various art materials, such as paint, clay, and
yarn. Appraises client's art projection and
recovery progress. Reports finding to other
members of treatment team and counsels on
client's response until art therapy is discontinued.
Maintains and repairs art materials and
equipment.(DOT)

American Art Therapy Association
1202 Allanson Road, Mundelein, IL 60060
708/949-6064

Arthritis
Arthritis, sometimes referred to as "rheumatism,"
is a general term applied to more than a hundred
different conditions characterized by aches and
pains of joints, muscles, and/or fibrous tissues.
Close to forty million Americans suffer from one
form of arthritis or another. Although scientific
medical care cannot cure the common forms of
arthritis, pain and disability can be controlled or
minimized with appropriate and timely care.

Arthritis is a fertile field for quackery. As with many
chronic diseases, the major forms of arthritis are
subject to considerable variation in severity. If a
spontaneous remission takes place following use
of an unconventional measure, the individual may
incorrectly conclude that the measure was
effective. Many people try unconventional
remedies because friends have recommended
them. (ALT)

Arthritis Foundation
1314 Spring St. NW
Atlanta, GA 30309
404/872-7100

National Institute of Arthritis and Musculoskeletal
and Skin Diseases
9000 Rockville Pike, Bethesda, MD 20892
301/468-3235

Arthroscopy
Arthroscopy Association of North America
2250 East Devon Ave, Suite 101
Des Plaines, IL 60018
708/299-9444

Artificial Organs
American Society for Artificial Internal Organs
PO Box C, Boca Raton, FL 33429
305/391-8589

Asbestos
Asbestos Information Association of North America
1745 Jefferson Davies Hwy., CS 4, Suite 509,
Arlington, VA 22202
703/979-1150

Asbestos Victims of America
2715 Porter Street, Soquel, CA 95073
408/476-3646

Asbestos removal, health hazards, and the EPA.
Council on Scientific Affairs, American Medical
Association. JAMA. 1991 Aug 7; 266(5): 696-7
Resolution 193 (A-90), which was adopted by the House of
Delegates of the American Medical Association, called on the
Council on Scientific Affairs to study the situation regarding
asbestos abatement, the risks to health, and the
appropriateness of Environmental Protection Agency
regulations, policies, and control measures. This report
reviews the current status of asbestos abatement as applied
to schools and public buildings, which currently accounts for
the major expenditure of public funds.

Asthma and Allergy
Asthma and Allergy Foundation of America
1717 Massachusetts Ave., NW, Suite 305,
Washington, D.C. 20036
202/265-0265

American Academy of Allergy and Immunology
414/272-6071 8:00-5:00,
hotline: 800/822-ASMA

National Jewish Hospital/
National Asthma Center Denver
800/222-LUNG, 8:30-5:00, MST

Ataxia
National Ataxia Foundation
15500 Wayzata Blvd., Suite 600
Wayzata, MN 55391
612/473-7666

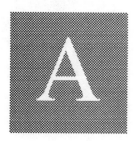

Athletic Associations, Medical

American Medical Golf Association
PO Box 841, Alton, IL 62002
618/462-6841

American Medical Joggers Association
PO Box 4704, North, Hollywood, CA 91607
818/706-2049

Surfer's Medical Association
2396 48th Ave., Great Highway
San Francisco, CA 94116
415/566-4687

American Medical Tennis Association .
PO Box 841, Alton, IL 62002-0841
618/462-6841

Athletic Trainer

History: Work on establishing standards for
athletic training educational programs was
initiated in 1959 by the National Athletic Trainers
Association (NATA). In 1969, the NATA
Committee on Curriculum Development approved
the first two programs. By 1979 there were 23
undergraduate programs and two graduate
programs approved by the NATA. In 1982, the
NATA Certification Committee completed a role
delineation study that led to the NATA Profession
Education Committee's development of an
"entry-level" list of 175 competencies. Another role
delineation study was conducted in 1989,
resulting in a 1990 revision of the athletic
training-entry-level competencies. By 1991, the
NATA approved 78 undergraduate and 13
graduate athletic training educational programs.

During 1989, the NATA, through its Professional
Education Committee, applied to the American
Medical Association Council on Medical Education
for recognition of athletic training as allied health
occupation. Recognition was granted on June 22,
1990.

In October of 1990, an initial meeting was
conducted in Chicago for the development of the
Essentials for the accreditation of educational
programs for athletic trainers. Individuals
attending that meeting represented the American
Medical Association's Division of Allied Health
Education and Accreditation, the American
Academy of Pediatrics, the American Academy of
Family Physicians, the American Orthopaedic
Society for Sports Medicine, and the National
Athletic Trainers, Inc.

In late 1991, the Essentials were submitted for
adoption to the Council on Medical Education of
the American Medical Association and to the
sponsors of the Review Committee established for
the profession: the American Academy of Family
Physician; the American Academy of Pediatrics;
and the National Athletic Trainers Association.

Occupational Description: The athletic trainer, with
the consultation and supervision of attending
and/or consulting physicians, is an integral part of
the health care system associated with sports.
Through preparation in both academic and
practical experience, the athletic trainer provides a
variety of services, including injury prevention,
recognition, immediate care, treatment, and
rehabilitation after athletic trauma.

Job Description: Role delineation studies
conducted by the profession in 1982 and in 1989
concluded that the role of an athletic trainer
includes, but may not be limited to, six major
domains: prevention; recognition and evaluation;
management and treatment; rehabilitation;
organization and administration; and education
and counseling.

Employment Characteristics: Athletic trainers
typically provide their services in one or more of
the following settings: secondary schools; colleges
and universities; professional athletic organization;
private or hospital-based clinics.(ALL)

AMA Allied Health Department
312/464-4696

National Athletic Trainers Association, Inc
2952 Stemmons, Dallas, TX 75247
214/637-6282

Audio-Visuals, Medical

Anatomical Wall Chart Co.
8221 N. Kimball, Skokie, IL 60076
708/679-4700 800/621-7500

Audio Digest
1577 E. Chevy Chase Dr., Glendale, CA 91206
213/245-8505

Medical Group Management Association
104 Inverness Terrace East
Englewood, CO 80112-5306
303/799-1111 or 303/397-7888

National Audio Visual Center
8700 Edgeworth Dr.
Capitol Heights, MD 20743-3701
301/763-1896

National Library of Medicine, Audio-Visual Section
8600 Rockville Pike, Bethesda, MD 20894
301/496-6095

Audiology

Audiologist: Determines type and degree of
hearing impairment and implements habilitation
and rehabilitation services for patient: Administers
and interprets variety to tests, such as air and
bone conduction, and speech reception and
discrimination tests, to determine type and degree
of hearing impairment, site of damage, and effects
on comprehension and speech. Evaluates tests
results in relation to behavioral, social,
educational, and medical information obtained
from patients, families, teachers, speech
pathologists and other professionals to determine
communication problems related to hearing
disability. Plans and implements prevention,
habilitation, or rehabilitation services, including
hearing aid selection and orientation, counseling,
auditory training, lip reading, language habilitation,
speech conservation, and other treatment
programs developed in consultation with speech
pathologist and other professionals. May refer
patient to physician or surgeon if medical
treatment is determined necessary. May conduct
research in physiology, pathology, biophysics, or
psychophysics of auditory systems, or design and
develop clinical and research procedures and
apparatus. May act as consultant to educational,

medical, legal, and other professional groups.
May teach art and science of audiology and direct
scientific projects.(DOT)

Academy of Rehabilatative Audiology (ARA)
c/o Dr. Carol L. De Filippo
Central Michigan University
Ronan Hall 307, Mount Pleasant, MI 48859

Autism

Autism Society of America
8601 Georgia Ave, Suite 503
Silver Spring, MD 20910
301/565-0433

Automobile Safety - Medical Aspects

Association for the Advancement
of Automotive Medicine
2350 E. Devon Ave., Suite 205
Des Plaines, IL 60018
708/390-8927

National Highway Traffic Safety Administration
HTS-10, US Department of Transportation
400 7th St., SW,
Room 5130, Washington, DC 20590
202/426-9294

Auto Safety Hotline
800/424-9393; 202/426-0123 (in DC)

Aviation

For referral to FAA authorized physician:
Federal Aviation Administration
Department of Transportation
800 Independence Avenue SW
Washington, DC 20591
202/267-3484

Aviation Medicine

Aerospace Medical Association
320 S. Henry Street, Alexandria, VA 22314
703/739-2240

Board Certification in Aerospace Medicine
American Board of Preventive Medicine
Department of Community Medicine
Wright State University
PO Box 927, Dayton OH 45401
513/278-6915

Civil Aviation Medical Association
1305 Vine St, Paso Robles, CA 93446
805/238-0366

Flying Physicians Association
PO Box 17841, Kansas City, MO 64134
816/763-9336 816/966-4003

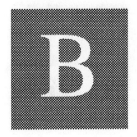

Baby Sitting
Baby Sitting Safety Kit
National Safety Council
1121 Spring Lake Drive, Itasca, IL 60143-3201
708/285-1121

Back
American Back Society, (interdisciplinary organization)
2647 E. 14th St., Suite 401, Oakland, CA 94601
415/536-9929

Bell's Palsy
"Facial Nerve Problems" (booklet)
Send stamped, self-addressed envelope to:
American Academy of Otolaryngology-Head & Neck Surgery
1 Prince Street, Alexandria, VA 22314
703/836-4444

Better Business Bureau
Local Better Business Bureaus keep track of complaints against businesses and may issue reports when many people complain about a company (i.e. clinics, imaging centers). Can issue occasional pamphlets related to health frauds and quackery. This Council has also teamed with the FDA to issue educational materials urging advertising managers to screen out misleading ads for health products. (ALT)

Council of Better Business Bureaus
4200 Wilson Blvd., Arlington, VA 22203
703/276-0100

Betty Ford Center
Betty Ford Center
39000 Bob Hope Dr., Rancho Mirage, CA 92270
800/854-9211

Bibliographies, Medical
Current Bibliographies in Medicine from the The National Library of Medicine
The National Library of Medicine
Public Services Division: Bethesda, Maryland 20894
Superintendent of Document Series Number HE 20.3615/2
i.e., (full SU-Doc number HE 20.3615/2-88-1)

1992
92-1 "Methods for Voluntary Weight Loss and Control"
January 1985 - December 1991
-- prepared by K.M. Scannell and S.M. Pilch;
1119 citations

92-2 "Laboratory Animal Welfare"
January 1991 - December 1991
-- prepared by F.P. Gluckstein; 86 citations

92-3 "Adolescent Alcoholism"
January 1986 - April 1992
-- prepared by P. Tillman; 928 citations

92-4 "Gallstones and Laparoscopic Cholescystetomy"
January 1989 - August 1992
-- prepared by P.S. Tillman and S.C. Kalser;
683 citations

92-5 "Saliva as a Diagnostic Fluid"
January 1982 - April 1992
-- prepared by M.H. Glock, P.A. Heller, and D. Malamud; 2298 citations

92-6 "Silicone Implants"
January 1989 - July 1992
-- prepared by J. Hunt and J. van de Kamp;
985 citations

92-7 "Seafood Safety"
January 1990 - July 1992
-- prepared by F.P. Gluckenstein; 961 citations

92-8 "Impotence"
January 1986 - September 1992
-- prepared by M.E. Beratan; 956 citations

1991
91-1 "Laboratory Animal Welfare"
January 1990 - December 1990
-- prepared by F.P. Gluckstein; 89 citations

91-2 "Therapy-Related Second Cancers"
January 1986 - March 1991
-- prepared by N. Miller; 880 citations

91-3 "Nutrition and AIDS"
January 1986 - April 1991
-- prepared by R.L. Fordner and S. Evans;
668 citations

91-4 "Medical Waste Disposal"
January 1986 - January 1991
-- prepared by J. van de Kamp; 629 citations

91-5 "Transmissible Subacute Spongiform Encephalopathies: Transmission Between Animals and Man"
January 1986 - May 1991
-- prepared by F.P. Gluckstein; 148 citations

91-6 "Dental Restorative Materials"
January 1986 - June 1991
-- prepared by L.D. Ulincy; 779 citations

91-7 "Adverse effects of fluoxetine (Prozac)"
January 1987 - June 1991
-- prepared by J.S. Martyniuk; 270 citations

91-8 "Treatment of Panic Disorder With and Without Agoraphobia"
January 1985 - July 1991
-- prepared by K. Patrias and B.E. Wolfe;
1448 citations

91-9 "Pain, Anesthesia, and Analgesia in Common Laboratory Animals"
June 1988 - October 1991
-- Prepared by F.P. Gluckstein; 474 citations

91-10 "Diagnosis and Treatment of Depression in Later-Life"
January 1980 - September 1991
-- prepared by M.H. Glock and L.S. Schneider: 886 citations

91-11 "Acoustic Neuroma"
January 1986 - October 1991
-- prepared by R.L. Gordner, R. Eldridge and D.M. Parry; 1112 citations

91-12 "Regional Medical Programs"
January 1964 - December 1977
-- prepared by M.H. Glock; 602 citations

91-13 "Diagnosis and Treatment of Early Melanoma"
January 1983 - November 1991
-- prepared by K. Patrias and A.N. Moshell; 447 citations

91-14 "Postpartum Depression"
January 1984 - December 1991
-- prepared by J.P. Hunt; 729 citations

91-15 "Electromagnetic Fields"
January 1989 - October 1991
-- prepared by M.E. Beratan; 733 citations

91-16 "Triglyceride, High Density Lipoprotein and Coronary Heart Disease"
January 1989 - February 1992
-- prepared by N. Miller and P.T. Einhorn; 1636 citations

91-17 "Health Effects of Global Warming"
January 1986 - December 1991
-- prepared by J. van de Kamp; 175 citations

91-18 "Seasonal Affective Disorder"
January 1986 - December 1991
-- prepared by L.J. Klein; 402 citations

91-19 "Biomedical Effects of Volcanoes"
January 1980 - September 1991
-- prepared by C.B. Love; 697 citations

1990
90-1 "Surgery for Epilepsy"
January 1985 - February 1990"
-- prepared by K. Patrias & W. H. Theodore; 681 citations

90-2 "Sleep Disorders of Older People"
January 1985 through March 1990
-- prepared by L.J. Klein, L.D. Ulincy, and A.A. Monjan; 725 citations

90-3 "Adjuvant Therapy for Colon and Rectum Cancer"
January 1985 - April 1990
-- prepared by K. Patrias and J. M. Hamilton; 491 citations

90-4 "Intravenous Immunoglobulin: Prevention and Treatment of Disease"
January 1986 - April 1990"
-- prepared by M. E. Beratan and H. B. Dickler; 888 citations

90-5 "Laboratory Animal Welfare"
December 1988 - December 1989
-- prepared by F. P. Gluckstein; 86 citations

90-6 "Treatment of Early-Stage Breast Cancer"
January 1985 - May 1990"
-- prepared by N. Miller and F. Andrew Dorr; 668 citations

90-7 "Cocaine, Pregnancy, and the Newborn"
January 1988 - March 1990
-- prepared by C. B. Love; 468 citations

90-8 "Fish Oils"
January 1989 - July 1990"
-- prepared by J. van de Kamp; 653 citations

90-9 "Alzheimer's Disease and the Family"
January 1986-July 1990"
-- prepared by J.S. Martyniuk; 343 citations

90-10 "Clinical Use of Botulinum Toxin"
January 1987 - September 1990
-- prepared by F.P. Gluckstein and M. Hallett; 318 citations

90-11 "Diagnosis and Management of Asymptomatic Primary Hyperparathyroidism"
January 1986 - September 1990
-- prepared by K.Patrias and J.E. Fradkin; 1057 citations

90-12 "Prison Health Care"
January 1986 - September 1990
-- prepared by Ronald L. Gordner; 1132 Citations

90-13 "Bovine Somatotropin"
January 1985 - October 1990
-- prepared by F.P. Gluckstein, M. Glock, and J.G. Hill; 1097 citations

90-14 "Adverse Effects of Aspartame"
January 1986 - December 1990
-- prepared by J. van de Kamp; 167 citations

90-15 "Patient Education for Self-Care: The Role of Nurses"
January 1983 - November 1990"
-- prepared by P.S. Tillman; 468 citations

90-16 "Blood Substitutes"
January 1986 - December 1990
-- prepared by J. van de Kamp; 744 citations

90-17 "Hospital Technology Assessment"
January 1984 - December 1990"
-- prepared by A. Carbery-Fox, L.J. Klein, and T. Meikle; 784 citations

90-18 "Gastrointestinal Surgery for Severe Obesity"
January 1986 - December 1990"
-- prepared by M.H. Glock and W.R. Foster; 548 citations

90-19 "Human-Pet Relations"
January 1983 - December 1990
-- prepared by J. Hunt; 385 citations

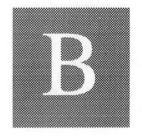

1989

89-1 "Therapeutic Endoscopy and Bleeding Ulcers
January 1980 - December 1988
-- prepared by K. Patrias and F. Hamilton

89-2 "History of Neurosurgery"
January 1970 - December 1988
-- prepared by Y.K. Rhee; 402 citations

89-3 "Laboratory Animal Welfare"
October 1987 - November 1988
-- prepared by F.P. Gluckstein; 86 citations

89-4 "Oral Complications of Cancer Therapies"
January 1980 - February 1989
-- prepared by E.J. Abrams and P.C. Fox;
288 citations

89-5 "Modeling in Biomedical Research:
Applications to Studies in
Cardiovascular/Pulmonary Function and Diabetes"
January 1986 - March 1989
-- prepared by F. P. Gluckstein; 830 citations

89-6 "Sunlight, Ultraviolet Radiation and the Skin"
January 1984 - April 1989
-- prepared by K. Patrias and A. N. Moshell; 521
citations

89-7 "Health Benefits of Fish Oils"
January 1985 - May 1989
-- prepared by J. van de Kamp and S.J. Jackson;
576 citations

89-8 "Behavioral and Mental Disorders of the
Homeless"
January 1983 - May 1989
-- prepared by J.S. Martyniuk; 294 citations

89-9 "Toxoplasmosis in Man and Animals"
January 1987 - May 1989
-- prepared by F.P.Gluckstein; 986 citations

89-10 "Anthropometric Measures of Malnutrition in
Children"
January 1955 - March 1989
-- prepared by K.J. Parker; 529 citations

89-11 "Treatment of Destructive Behaviors in
Persons with
Developmental Disabilities"
January 1966 - August 1989
-- prepared by K. Patrias and D. B. Gray; 751
citations

89-12 "Post-Polio Syndrome"
January 1967 - September 1989
-- prepared by L.J. Klein; 223 citations

89-13 "Exercise and the Elderly"
January 1986 - July 1989
-- prepared by M.E. Beratan; 1050 citations

89-14 "Noise and Hearing Loss"
January 1985 - December 1989
-- prepared by M. Glock and R.F. Naunton;
757 citations

89-15 "Care and Use of Laboratory Animals"
January 1985 - December 1989
-- prepared by F.P. Gluckstein; 230 citations

89-16 "Alcoholism and the Family"
January 1988 - December 1989"
-- prepared by C.B. Love; 292 citations

89-17 "Chronic Fatigue:
January 1980 - December 1989"
-- prepared by J.P. Hunt; 285 citations

89-18 "Growth Hormones and Short Stature"
January 1983 - September 1989
-- prepared by P.S. Tillman; 470 citations

89-19 "Medication and the Elderly. Part 1:
Treatment Issues"
January 1985 through December 1989
-- prepared by J. van de Kamp; 1017 citations

89-20 "Medication and the Elderly. Part 2: Specific
Diseases"
January 1985 through December 1989
-- prepared by J. van de Kamp; 867 citations

1988

88-1 "Pregnancy in Older Women"
January 1983 - December 1987
-- prepared by J.Kamp; 327 citations

88-2 "Prevention and Treatment of Kidney Stones"
January 1983 - February 1988
-- prepared by E.J. Abrams and M. Lange;
524 citations

88-3 "Cochlear Implants"
January 1983 - March 1988
-- prepared by K. Patrias and R.F. Naunton;
420 citations

88-4 "Dental Implants"
January 1980 - April 1988
-- prepared by E.J. Abrams, A.A. Rizzo, T.E.
Valega, and A.D. Guckes: 622 citations

88-5 "Perioperative Red Cell Transfusion"
January 1985 - May 1988
-- prepared by L. Klein and P.R. McCurdy;
803 citations

88-6 "Pain, Anesthesia, and Analgesia in
Common Laboratory Animals"
January 1987 - May 1988
-- prepared by F.P. Gluckstein; 178 citations

88-7 "Adolescent Suicide"
January 1986 - June 1988
-- prepared by J.S. Martyniuk; 475 citations

88-8 "Invertebrates in Biomedical Research"
January 1985 - July 1988
-- prepared by F.P. Gluckstein; 503 citations

88-9 "Urinary Incontinence in Adults:
January 1983 - September 1988
-- prepared by K. Patrias and E.C. Hadley;
707 citations

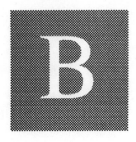

88-10 "Indoor Air Pollution. Part 1: Radon"
January 1984 - July 1988
-- prepared by J. van de Kamp; 353 citations

88-11 "Indoor Air Pollution. Part II: Household and Occupational Pollutants, Excluding Radon."
January 1984 - July 1988
-- prepared by J. van de Kamp; 1847 citations

88-12 "Vaccine-Preventable Diseases of Childhood"
January 1986 - August 1988
-- prepared by L. Klein; 748 citations

88-13 "Bacterial, Viral, and Parasitic Foodborne Infections and Intoxications"
January 1986 - October 1988
-- prepared by F.P. Gluckstein; 662 citations

88-14 "Sjogren's Syndrome"
January 1985 - December 1988
-- prepared by K. Patrias, P.C. Fox and S.P. Heyse; 185 citations

88-15 "Sport Psychology"
January 1986 - December 1988
-- prepared by J.S. Martyniuk; 576 citations

88-16 "Institutional Ethics Committees"
January 1975 - December 1988
-- prepared by A.F. Kiger; 434 citations

88-17 "Lyme Disease"
January 1985 - December 1988
-- prepared by K. Scannell and F.P. Gluckenstein: 850 citations

88-18 "Wrongful Life: Birth as the Result of Negligence"
January 1970 - September 1988
-- prepared by M.E. Beratan; 627 citations

88-19 "Social and Economic Aspects of Dialysis"
January 1977 - October 1988
-- prepared S.J. Jackson: 727 citations

88-20 "Health Education and Promotion for Minorities"
January 1983 - December 1988
-- prepared by P.S. Tillman; 381 citations

Billing, Electronic

American Medical Informatics Association
4915 St. Elmo Ave, Suite 302
Bethesda, MD 20814
301/657-1291

Billings and Collections

Collection fundamentals: A good collection system does not evolve by accident, but requires careful advance planning to establish an effective routine and adhere to that routine. The success of a collection system is measured by its collection ratio - the percentage of fees charged which is actually collected. Many physicians maintain a collection ratio in excess of 90 percent.

Three principles are vital to achieving a high collection percentage:
• Make certain that patients understand what they are paying for, and appreciate that the fee is commensurate with the services rendered.
• Make it convenient for patients to pay at the time of treatment, and encourage them to do so.
• Send bills punctually and regularly; follow up on unpaid bills.

A frank and open discussion of the fee in advance of treatment is the best way of making certain that patients understand and accept treatment costs. The patient is buying medical services and is entitled to know their price, just as he would expect to know the price of an automobile or a new suit before buying. The patient who has been warned in advance about an expensive procedure is less likely to react with shock when he sees the bill, and is more likely to pay promptly.

The best way to explain medical charges is to itemize each bill. Statements which lump all charges under the heading "For professional services" are virtually disappearing as insurance companies and other third party carriers insist on itemized accounts of services rendered.

The charge slip provides a simple means of itemizing services, and is widely used. This form, usually used in triplicate, lists the various services the doctor commonly performs, and differs from specialty to specialty.

At the start of the office visit, the patient is either given a charge slip to take with him into the examining room or it is attached to the chart and is in the exam room for the physician. When the doctor completes his examination or treatment, he indicates the services performed, together with the charge. The patient returns the slip to the front desk on the way out.

The charge slip not only informs the receptionist of what was done so she can make appropriate entries on the patient's financial record, but gives her the opportunity to request payment. Many patients are prepared to pay on the spot for routine office visits but leave without doing so because no one gave them a chance.

A simple statement by the receptionist, such as "The charge for today will be $15," is all that's necessary. If the patient responds with payment, the need for future bill, and its expense, will be reduced.

The patient who pays before leaving is given a receipted charge slip as a record of payment, the other copies being retained for the office record. If the patient is not prepared to pay at the time of service, it is a good idea to hand him an envelope addressed to the office, with the request that he mail in his payment as soon as possible. In this case, a copy of the charge slip can be placed in the envelope as a reminder of the amount owed.

If the patient asked to be billed, the information from the charge slip is transferred to the patient's ledger card. At billing time, the ledger card is photocopied, inserted into a window envelope so the patient's name and address are visible, and mailed to the patient as an itemized statement of his account.

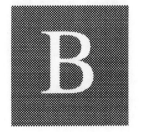

When bills are sent out is less important than regularity and punctuality. Regularity of billing helps to prevent patients from falling behind in their payments, and also insures a steady cash flow to the medical office (thereby enabling the doctor to pay his bills). Punctuality in billing encourages prompt payment. The doctor who bills erratically, perhaps allowing several months to elapse between statements, must expect patients to treat their responsibilities similarly. It is natural for the patient to think: "If the doctor doesn't attach much importance to the bill, then I won't either." The longer payment is delayed, the harder it is to collect.

Prompt payment will also be encouraged if the statement specifies the date on which payment is due. A business reply envelope should always be enclosed with the statement. The envelope emphasizes that the doctor expects payment, and makes it easier for the patient to pay.

Some physicians prefer to get the billing out of the way in one monthly batch. Others send out statements semi-monthly - on the first and fifteenth. Some follow a cyclical billing pattern in which statements go to patients in certain sections of the alphabet on certain dates each month. The choice of billing time is a matter of the individual physician's preference.

Following up on collections:
When regular itemized statements have been sent and payment has not been received, a collection follow-up program should routinely come into play. In devising such a program, it is important to understand some of the reasons that patients don't pay. While there are a number of causes, these three are probably the most common:
• Negligence
• Inability to pay
• Unwillingness to pay
When a patient is negligent and puts off payment for no good reason, the physician himself may be partly to blame. He may have been negligent in his own billing responsibilities. Failure to bill promptly and regularly will only encourage negligent patients in their bad habits.

Many people tend to pigeon-hole their doctor bills, postponing payment until their other debts have been paid. One of the benefits of collection follow-up is that it educates patients to treat medical bills as they do any other kind of indebtedness - paying what they owe when it is due.

Some patients who would like to pay are sometimes temporarily unable to do so, and will ask to take care of the bill in installments. The physician who agrees to accept payment in more than three installments will come under the provisions of the Federal Truth in Lending law. Complying with the filing and disclosure provisions of this law will require extensive paperwork that could significantly increase the cost of billing. Failure to comply is punishable by both civil and criminal penalties.

The doctor can avoid involvement with Truth in Lending because of installment payments by not making any agreement for deferred payment, and by simply charging on a 30-day basis. Even if the patient pays only a portion of the bill, each succeeding statement should show only the balance due. Neither the physician nor the employees should agree in writing or verbally to installments. If a patient offers installments, the response should be, "Please pay whatever you can each month."

Alternatively, a physician may agree to accept installment payments and not come within the scope of the law, providing the payments are not made in more than three installments, and remembering that the first payment counts as an installment.

Some doctors would like to levy an "interest," "service," or "carrying" charge on the patient's unpaid balance in order to encourage prompt payment and improve their collection ratio. Still others try to achieve the same goals by offering discounts for cash payment. These physicinas should be aware that charging interest or offering cash discounts that exceed five percent will also require compliance with the Truth in Lending law.

Doctors who wish to make a service charge, a finance charge, accept installment payments, or offer discounts for payments in cash should contact their lawyer for assistance in meeting the requirements of federal credit statutes.

In addition to the patients who are negligent about paying, and those who are unable to do so, there are some patients who are unwilling to pay. Among the common causes for unwillingness to pay are disgruntlement with the size of the bill, or unhappiness with some aspect of the service the patient has received. In these cases, the unwillingness is a symptom and should be treated as such. Talking over the situation with the patient will elicit the real problem and is the first step to obtaining payment.

Finally, there is the rare patient who is a "deadbeat." The vast majority of patients want to pay their bills, and only fail to do so for some specific reason. The deadbeat doesn't intend to pay, and probably never did. The usual collection measures are of little avail, and the best policy is to turn the account over to a collection agency, or even consider instituting suit.

Keeping in mind the basic causes of nonpayment, the doctor's follow-up collection system should accomplish the following:
• Remind the negligent patient of his financial obligation for treatment.
• Determine the specific reason that payment hasn't been made.
• Get patient with a reason for nonpayment into the office to discuss the problem and work out a solution.
Adequate credit information, obtained in advance of treatment, is a basic aid in collection follow-up. At the time of the patient's first visit, the medical office should routinely fill out a form designated for patient information. The information should be updated at least annually to make sure it is current, and will form the basis for later collection efforts, As one collection adage puts it: "An account properly opened is half collected."

Such information can be secured quickly, and with no affront to the patient. In some offices, inquiries are made about patients' charge accounts, since these are good credit indices. It is poor policy to ask about banks and bank accounts. Superficial

signs of prosperity should not color an evaluation of the patient's financial status. When a substantial sum is involved and there is some question of whether the patient can afford the financial obligation, the credit rating can be checked with the local credit bureau. Obviously, it's easier for the doctor in a small town to gauge his patient's ability to pay than it is for a city physician.

Every physician will want to work out his own "collection timetable" which determines what collection steps are taken and when.

The following collection letters should be signed by the staff member who is handling the follow-up process, with a title such as Financial Secretary, Bookkeeper, or Business Manager.

The first collection letter reminding the patient that he is receiving a second statement could read as follows:

There must be a reason why you haven't paid your bill of $____. Won't you call us about your account today? Maybe we can help.

Or

Does your statement contain an error? If so, give us a call so we can correct it.
Otherwise, why not send your check for $____ today so we can keep your account current. Thank you.

The second letter, to be sent in the third month after service, should be along these lines:

I'm sure there is a good reason why we have not heard from you about your past due bill of $____.
Telephone me this week, because arrangements must be made to avoid collection action.

Or

Your past due account:$____.
Apparently you have overlooked payment of your account, which is several weeks past due.
It will only take a minute to slip a check into the enclosed envelope and bring your account up to date. Thank you.

To make sure this second letter is opened and read, send it in a plain envelope without the office return address, write the patient's address by hand, and use a stamp instead of a postage meter.

Here is a suggestion for the final letter before turning the account over to a collection agency:

Unless we can agree on a plan to settle your overdue account of $____, it will be turned over to a professional collection service.
You have 10 ten days to contact this office.

Remember, when a physician's office states that it will turn an account over to a collection agency and fails to do so, that office's credibility will be destroyed and will also be in violation of federal collection statutes.

Handwritten thank-you notes to patients who make a honest effort to settle large bills in small amounts are seen as nice touch from a busy physician's office. The note can be a very simple: "Your partial payments on your account show a splendid spirit of cooperation! Thank you." This can promote patient goodwill and encourage continued payment.

A record should be kept of collection efforts with a particular account, but remember never to include financial information in the medical record. Also, bear in mind that it is unethical to refuse to transfer a patient's records for non-payment of a bill.

When an office has established a collection policy, instituted the records needed, and worked out a collection timetable, a method of spotting those accounts which are delinquent or about to become so, is needed. An Accounts Receivable Aging Record is an invaluable guide to accounts which need some action.

The aging record shows exactly how many dollars are in an office's accounts that are 30, 60, 90 and more days past due. If a practice is on a manual bookkeeping system, a pegboard, for example, accounts should be aged at least once a quarter. Every month is much better if time permits. If a computer billing system is in use, a report is normally generated on a monthly basis.

To prepare an aging record, take all the ledger cards that have a balance and enter the amounts due on each account in the appropriate columns, i.e.; 60 days past due, etc. Add each column to determine the total amount in each age category. Figure the percent of accounts receivable in each category by dividing the total accounts receivable into the total at the bottom of each column.

A complete aging record will have three important items of information:
• A patient-by-patient listing of those accounts which require collection follow-up.
• An overall picture of your collection system's effectiveness. Any MD will have two month's accounts receivable, but if many accounts are running two and a half to three months past due, he should start reviewing his entire system of billing and collecting to spot the trouble and correct it.
• An estimate of the real worth of an office's accounts receivable. For example, at the time of this writing, an account that is six months overdue is worth about fifty to sixty cents on the dollar, according to collection specialists, and after twelve months, it is worth only about thirty cents. (BUS)

Bioethics
Hastings Center
255 Elm Road, Briarcliff Manor, NY 10510
914/762-8500

Joseph and Rose Kennedy Institute of Ethics
National Reference Center for Bioethics Literature,
Georgetown University, Washington, DC 20057
800/MED-ETHX (800-633-3849)

President's Commission for the Study of Ethical
Problems in Medicine and Biomedicine Behavioral
Research Report:
Government Printing Office
Washington, DC 20402
202/783-3238

Biofeedback

A technique in which a person uses information
about a normally unconscious body function, such
as blood pressure, to gain conscious control over
that function. Biofeedback training may help in the
treatment of stress-related conditions, including
certain types of hypertension, anxiety and
migraine. (ENC)

Biofeedback Training

Biofeedback training is a technique in which a
person uses information about a body function to
attempt to gain control over that function. The
practitioner connects the patient to an electronic
device that measures blood pressure, pulse rate,
muscle tension, skin temperature, perspiration,
brain waves, or other various bodily functions. The
patient receives information (feedback) on the
changing levels of these activities from alterations
in the instrument's signals, such as a flashing
light, fluctuating needle, sound that rises or falls in
pitch, or variable display on a television monitor.
Relaxation techniques are used to effect changes
in the signal and to identify which methods are
most effective. The patient may ultimately learn to
control the body function subconsciously without
the machine.(ALT)
Association of Applied Physiology
and Biofeedback
10200 W. 44th Ave., #304
Wheat Ridge, CO 80303
303/422-8436

Biomedical Engineering - Careers

Alliance for Engineering in Medicine and Biology
1101 Connecticut Ave., NW, Suite 700,
Washington DC 20036
202/857-1199

Biomedical Engineering Society
PO Box 2399, Culver City, CA 90231
213/206-6443

Birth Control

free pamphlet on contraception:
American College of Obstetricians and
Gynecologists
409 12th Street, SW
Washington, DC 20024-2188
202/638-5577

Birth Defects

Association of Birth Defect Children
3526 Emerywood Lane, Orlando, FL 32812
407/859-2821

March of Dimes Birth Defects Foundation
1275 Mamaroneck Ave., White Plains, NY 10605
914/428-7100

National Easter Seal Society
70 E. Lake St., Chicago, IL 60601
312/726-6200

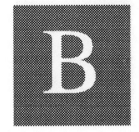

Blind

American Council of the Blind
1010 Vermont Ave. NW, Suite 1100
Washington, DC 20005
202/467-5081 or 800/424-8666

American Council of Blind Parents
Knoll Webb, 14400 Cedar
University Heights, OH 44121
216/381-1822

Eye Bank Association of America
1725 Eye St., NW, St. 308
Washington, D.C. 20006
202/775-4999

Guide Dog Foundation for the
Blind Training Center
371 E. Jericho Turnpike, Smithtown, NY 11787
516/265-2121

Helen Keller National Center for Deaf/Blind Youths
and Adults
111 Middle Neck Rd., Sands Point, NY 11050
516/944-8900

Leader Dog for the Blind
1039 S. Rochester Road
Rochester Hills, MI 48603
313/651-9011

Lion's Club International
300 22nd St., Oak Brook, IL 60657
708/986-1700

National Alliance of Blind Students
1010 Vermont Avenue, NW, Suite 1100,
Washington, DC 20005
800/424-8666

National Library Service for the Blind and
Physically Handicapped
Library of Congress, 1291 Taylor St., NW,
Washington, DC 20542
202/287-5100 (in DC)
800/424-8567

National Society to Prevent Blindness
500 E. Remington Rd., Schaumberg, IL 60173
708/843-2020
800/221-3004

Blindness, Societies to Prevent, Statewide

Arkansas Society to Prevent Blindness
400 W Capitol, Little Rock, AR 72201
501/376-6217

National Society to Prevent Blindness Southern
California Division
300 Carlsbad Village Drive, Suite 222
Carlsbad, CA 92008
619/399-8090

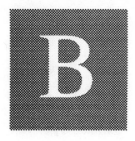

Northern California Society to Prevent Blindness
4200 California St, San Francisco, CA 94118
415/387-0934

Colorado Society to Prevent Blindness
3500 E 12th Ave, Denver, CO 80206
303/399-8090

Connecticut Society to Prevent Blindness
1275 Washington St, Middletown, CT 06457
203/347-6800

National Society to Prevent Blindness
Florida Affiliate
5501 W Gray St, Tampa, FL 33609
813/874-2020

Georgia Society to Prevent Blindness
2025 Peachtree Road, NE, Atlanta, GA 30309
404/355-0182

Indiana Society to Prevent Blindness
1425 E 86th St, Indianapolis, IN 46204
317/259-8163

Iowa Society to Prevent Blindness
1111 9th St, Suite 250, Des Moines, IA 50314
515/244-4341

Kentucky Society to Prevent Blindness
101 W Chestnut St, Louisville, KY 40202
502/584-6127

National Society to Prevent Blindness
Massachusetts Affiliate
375 Concord Ave, Belmont, MA 02178
617/489-0007

National Society to Prevent Blindness
Mississippi Affiliate
115 Broadmoor Dr, Jackson, MS 39206
601/362-6985

National Society to Prevent Blindness
Nebraska Affiliate
120 N 69th St, Suite 203, Omaha, NE 68132
402/551-2198

National Society to Prevent Blindness New Jersey
Affiliate
200 Centennial Ave, Piscataway, NJ 08854-3910
908/844-2020

National Society to Prevent Blindness New York
Division
160 E 56th St, 8th Floor, New York, NY 10022
212/980-2020

National Society to Prevent Blindness North
Carolina Affiliate
1033 Wade Ave, Suite 126, Raleigh, NC 27605
919/832-2020

National Society to Prevent Blindness Ohio Affiliate
1500 W 3rd St, Suite 200
Columbus, OH 43212-2874
614/464-2020

Oklahoma Society to Prevent Blindness
6 NE 63rd St, Suite 150
Oklahoma City, OK 73105
405/848-7123

Puerto Rico Society for the Prevent Blindness
PO Box 3232, San Juan, PR 00904
809/722-3531

Rhode Island Society to Prevent Blindness
1800 17th Post Road, Warwick, RI 02886
401/738-1150

Tennessee Society to Prevent Blindness
95 White Bridge Road, Suite 513
Nashville, TN 37205
615/352-0450

Texas Society to Prevent Blindness
3211 W Dallas, Houston, TX 77019
713/526-2559

National Society to Prevent Blindness Utah Affiliate
661 South 200 East, Salt Lake City, UT 84111
801/524-2020

National Society to Prevent Blindness
Virginia Affiliate
3820 Augusta Ave, Richmond, VA 23230
804/355-0773

National Society to Prevent Blindness
Wisconsin Affiliate
759 N Milwaukee St, Milwaukee, WI 53202
414/765-0505

Blood

American Red Cross
17th and D Streets NW, Washington, DC 20006
202/737-8300

American Society of Hematology
6900 Grove Road, Thorofare, NJ 08086
609/845-0003

Blood Banks

American Association of Blood Banks
1117 N. 19th St., Arlington, VA 22209
703/528-8200

Board Certification in Blood Banking/
Transfusion Medicine
American Board of Pathology
5401 W. Kennedy Blvd., PO Box 25915
Tampa, FL 33622
813/286-2444

National Phlebotomy Association
2623 Bladensburgh Rd, N.E.
Washington, DC 20018
202/636-4515

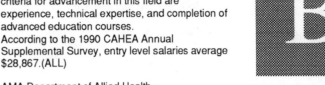

Blood Bank Technologist

History: In 1954, the first examination for blood bank technologists was administered by the American Society of Clinical Pathologists' Board of Registry. It is significant that both the examination and the process for approving blood bank schools were the result of a cooperative effort between the Board of Registry and the American Association of Blood Banks. Technologists working for five years in blood banking were eligible to take the examination.

After 1960, individuals could attend a 12-month educational program at an accredited school in lieu of the five year experience route. Levels of competency were established and the scope of knowledge pertinent to the field was prescribed to assure that the institutions would maintain acceptable standards of practice; would follow a curriculum that included all phases of blood bank technology, laboratory management, and transfusion services; and would support a faculty adequate to assume teaching responsibilities. As of 1988, 3,539 individuals have been certified as specialists in blood bank technology.

Because the number of programs had increased by 1969, Essentials were prepared by the Committee on Education of the American Association of Blood Banks and were adopted by the American Medical Association in 1971. Subsequently, the Essentials have undergone major revisions in 1977 and 1983, which were adopted by the AMA Council on Medical Education and the American Association of Blood Banks.

Occupational Description: Specialists in blood bank technology perform both routine and specialized tests in blood bank immunohematology in technical areas of the modern blood bank and perform transfusion services using the methodology that conforms to the Standards for Blood Banks and Transfusion Services of the American Association of Blood Banks.

Job Description: Specialists in blood bank technology demonstrate a superior level of technical proficiency and problem solving ability in such areas as:
- testing for blood group antigens, compatibility, and antibody identification;
- investigating abnormalities such as hemolytic diseases of the newborn, hemolytic anemias, and adverse responses to transfusion;
- supporting physicians in transfusion therapy, including patients with coagulopathies or candidates for homologous organ transplant;
- blood collection and processing, including selecting donors, drawing and typing blood, and performing pretransfusion tests to ensure the safety of the patient. Supervision, management and/or teaching comprise a considerable part of the responsibilities of the specialist in blood bank technology.

Employment Characteristics: Specialists in blood banking work in many types of facilities, including community blood centers, private hospital blood bank, university affiliated blood banks, transfusion services, and independent laboratories; they may also be part of a university faculty. Specialists may work some weekend and night duty, including emergency calls. Qualified specialists may advance to supervisory or administrative positions, or move into teaching or research activities. The criteria for advancement in this field are experience, technical expertise, and completion of advanced education courses.

According to the 1990 CAHEA Annual Supplemental Survey, entry level salaries average $28,867.(ALL)

AMA Department of Allied Health
312/464-4625

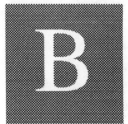

Blood Pressure

Contact local/state department of health for testing information or local heart association for consumer information

Citizens for the Treatment of High Blood Pressure, Inc.
888 17th Street, Suite 904, NW
Washington, DC 20006
202/466-4553

High Blood Pressure Information Center
120/80 National Institutes of Health
Bethesda, MD 20205
301/951-3260

Blood Tests

Contact local/state department of health for testing information

Book Donations
American Overseas Medical Aid Association
(medical books and journals)
4433 W. Montana St., Chicago, IL 60639
312/486-4809

Darien Book Aid Plan, Inc.
(books and journals)
1926 Post Rd., Darien, CT 06820
203/655-2777

The Foundation for Books to China
601 California St., San Francisco, CA 94108
415/392-1080

International Book Project, Inc.
(professional books and journals)
1440 Delaware Ave., Lexington, KY 40505
606/254-6771

Medical Books for China
13021 E Florence Ave.
Santa Fe Springs, CA 90670
213/946-8774

Books, Recommended

A Library for internists VII. Recommendations from the American College of Physicians. Ludmerer-KM. *Ann-Intern-Med.* 1991; 114(9): 811-32. (published in three year intervals)

Selected List of books and journals in allied health. Brandon AN, Hill DR. *Bull Med Lib Assoc.* 1992; 80(3): 223-239. (published each two years)

Selected List of books and journals for the small medical library. Brandon AN, Hill DR. *Bull Med Lib Assoc.* 1991; 79(2): 195-222. (published each two years)

Boxing

JAMA Theme Issue: Boxing
JAMA. 1986 May 9; 255(18)
Five articles discuss various medical aspects of boxing and its danger to the athlete. A clinical presentation of retinal detachment, a review of boxing and health listing 43 citations, comments of the liberty of choosing ones sport no matter how dangerous, a prototype program to help boxing evolve into a safer sport, and an editorial listing both the pros and cons against boxing make up this theme issue.

Brain Bank

Alzheimer's Disease and
Related Disorders Association
70 E. Lake St., Chicago, IL 60601
800/621-0379; 800/572-6037 (IL)

Brain Donors:
McLean Hospital Brain Bank, 115 Mill St.,
Belmont, MA 02178
617/855-2400

Brain Disorders, Pediatrics

National Brain Research Association
1439 Rhode Island Ave, N.W.
Washington, DC 20005
202/483-6272
(Also provides support groups for parents.)

Brain Injuries

National Institute of Neurological
Disorders and Stroke
900 Rockville Pike, Bethesda, MD 20892
301/496-5751

Brain Tumor

National Brain Tumor Foundation
323 Geary Street/Suite 510
San Francisco, CA 94102
415/296-0404

Association for Brain Tumor Research
3725 N. Talman Ave., Chicago, IL 60618
312/286-5571

Breast Cancer

National Alliance of Breast Cancer Organizations
1180 Ave. of the Americas, New York, NY 10036
212/719-0154

Y-Me Breast Cancer Support Program
18220 Harwood Ave, Homewood, IL 60430
708/799-8228
800/221-2141 (outside 708 area code)

Breast Feeding

La Leche League International
9616 Minneapolis Ave.
Franklin Park, IL 60131-8209
708/455-7730

Breast Implants

How doctors can participate in implant trials

Laurie Jones AMNews 5/4/92 p.58

Though details remain incomplete for the clinical trials under which silicone gel breast implants will now be available, one thing is sure, says FDA Chief David Kessler, MD.

"No one should think that we are saying it's business as usual."

For the first time ever in using implants, physicians will have to keep extensive documentation, remain in frequent contact with the manufacturer, and be conscious of Food and Drug Administration oversight.

Doctors who choose to participate in the clinical trials must first determine which study will be appropriate for their patients.

Physicians with patients who fulfill the "urgent need" criteria should contact an implant manufacturer as soon as possible to obtain necessary forms and participation details. These studies began in late April.

The FDA defines patients with an urgent need as: women with tissue expanders whose breast reconstruction following mastectomy was delayed by the moratorium; and women with silicone implants who need replacement or revision for medical reasons, such as rupture, gel leakage or severe contracture.

Doctors who take part in the urgent need studies are required to:
• Use a special consent form approved for this purpose, available from the device manufacturer.
• Certify on the consent form that the patient meets the criteria for one of the two groups of urgent need patients.
• Notify the manufacturers of all devices implanted and provide information needed for the patient registry.

The urgent need provision will be used until the "open availability" protocols begin sometime this summer. These studies will be open to all women who desire reconstruction and who have been certified by their doctor as being likely to get an unsatisfactory result from saline filled implants.

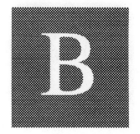

Once those studies are in place, limited "core" groups will be established for both augmentation and reconstruction patients. These studies will involve intensive research.

Only patients needed to answer the questions being investigated and only plastic surgeons designated by the manufacturers as clinical investigators will be able to take part in these core studies.

For both the open availability and core studies, physicians will be under supervision of a hospital Institutional Review Board.

In a recent letter to members, the American Society of Plastic and Reconstructive Surgeons recommended the following steps for Physicians to prepare:
• Learn about the Institution Review Board at the hospital at which you are affiliated. Talk to its director about the implant issue.
• Determine what forms are required for review.
• Make sure your curriculum vitae is up to date. Gather information about how many patients you have treated with implants over what period of time.

In the letter, ASPRS President Norman Cole, MD, urges doctors to keep in contact with patients who express interest in implants, as well as those who already have implants.

"It is vital that you do your part by continuing to respond promptly and compassionately to the concerns of every woman who calls your office," Dr. Cole Said.

No implant conclusion
FDA panel urges restrictions on silicone gel use

Laurie Jones AMNews 3/9/92 p.3+

After three grueling days of conflicting expert testimony and emotional pleas, thousands of documents and hours of tense discussion, an FDA advisory panel emerged with only one definite conclusion: No one knows if silicone gel breast implants are safe.

That conclusion frustrated both proponents and critics of the implants, many of whom were hoping for a definitive decision on the devices' safety.

But the committee decided there simply wasn't enough information to answer major questions, such as whether the implants are linked to various autoimmune diseases, as critics contend.

"At this point, we haven't seen concrete evidence of a cause-and-effect relationship, panel Chairwoman Elizabeth Connell, MD, said toward the end of the hearings.

Still, the committee found the anecdotal evidence, and the unknowns, troubling enough to raise serious doubts about the devices' long-term effects.

"I do not find the evidence convincing, but I do find it disturbing," said Jules Harris, MD, medical oncology director at Rush Presbyterian.

"The implants definitely need further evaluation," Dr. Connell said.

Thus came the recommendation: Leave silicone gel breast implants on the market, but under strict restrictions.

Women could get the implants only as part of a research protocol. Every woman who participates would be entered into a national registry for long-term monitoring.

All women who want the implants for reconstruction or to correct a disfigurement would qualify as research participants.

But only a limited number of those who want the devices for cosmetic purposes would be allowed to participate, The panel left the FDA to determine how the patients who want augmentation would be chosen.

The recommendation now goes to the FDA Commissioner David Kessler, MD, who has the final say. He said he would make a decision within 60 days. The voluntary moratorium on the use if silicone gel breast implants will remain in effect until that decision, he said.

The recommendation reflected the panel's struggle to balance the obligation to ensure that devices are safe and effective with the effort to meet a compelling public health need.

Many of the nine voting committee members said they viewed mastectomy patients' desire for reconstruction with implants as a legitimate public health need.

But other, non-voting, members expressed outrage at the panel's distinction between reconstruction and augmentation patients.

"I don't think it's legitimate to separate people in the basis of their reasons for the surgery," said Mary H. McGrath, MD, a non-voting panel member and professor of plastic surgery at George Washington University.

"This is a judgmental, paternalistic ruling on the legitimacy of cosmetic surgery, and that is nor our purpose here," Dr. McGrath said.

Silicone gel breast implants, which were introduced nearly 30 years ago, have not been regulated until now because they were on the market before Congress amended the Food, Drug and Cosmetic Act in 1976 to include medical devices.

But in recent years, there have been reports of numerous health problems said to be linked to the implants. Last year, the FDA required manufacturers to submit detailed implant safety data. The agency convened the advisory panel to review the data.

After hearings in November, the panel recommended leaving the implants on the market, but requiring manufacturers to significantly improve the way they collect safety data.

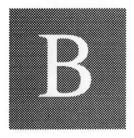

In early January, Dr. Kessler called for the moratorium after the agency received new information "that increases our concerns about safety."

That information included reports from rheumatologists who said they were seeing increasing numbers of autoimmune disorders among breast-implant patients. It also included internal memos and documents form Dow Corning Wright, the nation's leading maker of the implants. At the hearings in late February, Dow officials defended the company's record and testified that Dow studies as recent as 1990 "specifically targeted at immune response showed no systemic reaction."

But physicians testified that several studies in progress and increasing anecdotal evidence show a growing number of breast-implant patients with autoimmune disorders.

Frank Vasey, MD, of the University of South Florida College of Medicine told the panel that in a study to 50 women with breast implants, he found an unusually high rate of systemic lupus erythematosus.

Dr. Vasey said the patients improved dramatically when their implants were removed.

HHS estimates that between 300,000 and 1 million U.S. women have implants. Among the witnesses were nearly to dozen of them. Some, who said they had experienced no problems with their implants, pleaded with the committee to keep the devices on the market.

Barbara Quinn of Atlanta had a bilateral mastectomy in 1984 and got silicone gel implants which "restored my quality of life and my self-esteem."

"Because I've had breast cancer, all the women in my family are at high risk for breast cancer,: Quinn said. "If these implants aren't available, what about my daughter, my granddaughter, my six sisters? They can't have implants? Why should they be deprived of a normal life?"

Those with implants who had problems, ranging from hardening to ruptures to rheumatic illnesses, argued that alternatives such aa saline implants could be used more often.

In the end, the panel's recommendations raised more questions, some observers said.

"There's not a lot of detail there," said Norman Cole, MD, American Society of Plastic and Reconstructive Surgeons president.

"These studies would have to be terribly large to get meaningful data," said Cole. Attracting those large numbers may be difficult following the negative publicity about silicone gel implants, he said."

"But the important issue here is that silicone gel implants will continue to be available to patients - in a more structured way - but women haven't lost this option."

A Dow spokesman said the company had not decided whether to stay in the implant business. But even if it stops making implants, officials said the firm would carry out its planned safety studies.

Food and Drug Administration Implant Hotline
800/532-4440

Food and Drug Administration
Office of Device Evaluation
5600 Fishers Lane, Rockville, MD 20857
301/443-3170

Broadcasters, Physicians
National Association of Physician Broadcasters
515 N. State St., Chicago, IL 60610
312/464-5484

Bulimia
Anorexia Nervosa and Associated Disorders
Box 271, Highland Park, IL 60035
708/831-3438

Anorexia Nervosa and Related Eating Disorders
PO Box 5102, Eugene, OR 97405
503/344-1144

BASH (Bulimia Anorexia Self Help)
c/o Deaconess Hospital
6150 Oakland Avenue, St. Louis, MO 63139
800/762-3334
St. Louis area 314/768-3838 or 768-3292

Bureau of Health Professions
The Bureau provides national leadership in coordinating, evaluating, and supporting the development and utilization of the Nation's health personnel.

To accomplish this goal, the Bureau:
- serves as a focus for health care quality assurance activities, issues related to malpractice, and the operation of the National Practitioner Data Bank, and the Vaccine Injury Compensation Program;
- supports through grants health professions and nurse training institutions, targeting resources to areas of high national priority such as disease prevention, health promotion, bedside nursing, care of the elderly and HIV/AIDS;
- supports programs to increase the supply of primary care practitioners and to improve the distribution of health professionals;
- Develops, tests, and demonstrates new and improved approaches to the development and utilization of health personnel within various patterns of health care delivery and financing systems;
- provides leadership for promoting equity in access to health services and health careers for the disadvantaged;
- administers several loan programs supporting students training for careers in the health profession and nursing;
- funds regional centers to train faculty and practicing health professionals in the counseling, diagnosis, and management of HIV/AIDS infected individuals;

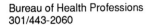

- collects and analyzes data and disseminates information on the characteristics and capacities of U.S. health training systems;
- assesses the Nation's health personnel force and forecasts supple and requirements; and
- in coordination with the Office of the Administrator Health Resources and Services Administration, serves as a focus for technical assistance activities in the international projects relevant to domestic health personnel problems. (USG)

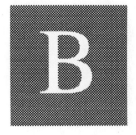

Bureau of Health Professions
301/443-2060

Burn Centers

Backus, K. Ed. *Medical and Health Information Directory* Gale Publishing Company, Detroit 1992-1993 ISSN 0749-9973; three volume set. Volume three, chapter 5 lists alphabetically by state the U.S. hospitals that provide specialized burn care services.

Burns

American Burn Association
c/o Shriners Burns Institute
202 Goodman St, Cincinnati, OH 45219
513/751-3900

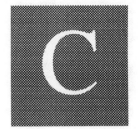

Cancer

American Cancer Society
1599 Clifton Rd, NE, Atlanta, GA 30329
404/320-3333, 800/227-2345

Cancer Information Clearinghouse, (NCI/OCC)
Bldg. 31, Rm. 10A18, 9000 Rockville Pike,
Bethesda, MD 21205
301/496-5583 - not for public inquiries, for health
professionals and health organizations only.

Candlelighters Childhood Cancer Foundation
1312 18th St, NW, Ste 200
Washington, D.C. 20036
202/659-5136, 800/366-2223

Insurance Problems
"Cancer Treatments Your Insurance
Should Cover"
Association of Community Cancer Centers
11600 Nebel St, Suite 201, Rockville, MD 20852
301/984-9496

National Cancer Institute
9000 Rockville Pike, Bethesda, MD 20892
301/496-5583
800/4CANCER (800/422-6237)

Sloan-Kettering Institute for Cancer Research
1275 York Ave., New York, NY 10021
212/639-2000

Cancer Research
*Contact the state or local office of the
American Cancer Society for a local
affiliate of the American Institute of
Cancer Research*

In general, this institution provides research
grants.
Health Professionals should contact:
Philanthropic Association of Virginia,
Council of Better Business Bureaus
1515 Wilson Blvd., Arlington, VA 22209
703/276-0133

Cancer Societies, Statewide
American Cancer Society Alabama Division
504 Brookwood Blvd, Homewood, AL 35209
205/879-2242

American Cancer Society Alaska Division
406 W Fireweed Lane, Suite 204
Anchorage, AK 99503
907/277-8696

American Cancer Society Arizona Division
2929 E Thomas Road, Phoenix, AZ 85016
602/224-0524

American Cancer Society Arkansas Division
901 N University, Little Rock, AR 72207
501/664-3480

American Cancer Society California Division
1710 Webster St, Oakland CA 94612
415/893-7900

American Cancer Society Colorado Division
2255 S Oneida, Denver, CO 80224
303/758-2030

American Cancer Society Connecticut Division
14 Village Lane, Wallingford, CT 06492
203/265-7161

American Cancer Society Delaware Division
92 Read's Way, New Castle, DE 19720
302/324-4227

American Cancer Society
District of Columbia Division
1825 Connecticut Ave, NW, Suite 315,
Washington, DC 20009
202/483-2600

American Cancer Society Florida Division
1001 S MacDill Ave, Tampa, FL 33629
813/253-0541

American Cancer Society Georgia Division
46 Fifth St, NE, Atlanta, GA 30308
404/892-0026

American Cancer Society Hawaii/Pacific Division
200 N Vineyard Blvd, Honolulu, HI 96817
808/531-1662

American Cancer Society Idaho Division
2676 Vista Ave, PO Box 5386, Boise, ID 83705
208/343-4609

American Cancer Society Illinois Division
77 E Monroe, Chicago, IL 60603
312/641-6150

American Cancer Society Indiana Division
8730 Commerce Park Place
Indianapolis, IN 46268
317/872-4432

American Cancer Society Iowa Division
8364 Hickman Road, Suite D
Des Moines, IA 50322
515/253-0147

American Cancer Society Kansas Division
1315 SW Arrowhead Road, Topeka, KS 66604
913/273-4114

American Cancer Society Kentucky Division
701 W Muhammad Ali Blvd, PO Box 1807,
Louisville, KY 40201-1807
502/584-6782

American Cancer Society Louisiana Division
837 Gravier St, Suite 700
New Orleans, LA 70112-1509
504/523-4188

American Cancer Society Maine Division
52 Federal St, Brunswick, ME 04011
207/729-3339

American Cancer Society Maryland Division
8219 Town Center Drive
White Marsh, MD 21162-0082
301/931-6868

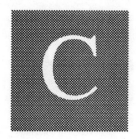

American Cancer Society Massachusetts Division
247 Commonwealth Ave, Boston, MA 02116
617/267-2650

American Cancer Society Michigan Division
1205 E Saginaw St, Lansing, MI 48906
517/371-2920

American Cancer Society Minnesota Division
3316 W 66th St, Minneapolis, MN 55435
612/925-2772

American Cancer Society Mississippi Division
1380 Livingston Lane, Jackson, MS 39213
601/362-8874

American Cancer Society Missouri Division
3322 American Ave, PO Box 1066
Jefferson City, MO 65102
314/893-4800

American Cancer Society Montana Division
313 N 32nd St, Suite 1, Billings, MT 59101
406/252-7111

American Cancer Society Nebraska Division
8502 W Center Road, Omaha, NE 68124-5255
402/393-5800

American Cancer Society Nevada Division
1325 E Harmon Ave, Las Vegas, NV 89119
702/798-6877

American Cancer Society New Hampshire Division
360 Route 101, Unit 501, Bedford, NH 03102-6800
603/472-8899

American Cancer Society New Jersey Division
2600 Route 1, CN 2201
North Brunswick, NJ 08902
908/297-8000

American Cancer Society New Mexico Division
5800 Lomas Blvd, NE, Albuquerque, NM 87110
505/260-2105

American Cancer Society New York State Division
6725 Lyons St, East Syracuse, NY 13057
315/437-7025

American Cancer Society Queens Division
112-25 Queens Blvd, Forest Hills, NY 11375
718/263-2224

American Cancer Society Long Island Division
145 Pidgeon Hill Road
Huntington Station, NY 11746
516/385-9100

American Cancer Society New York City Division
19 W 56th St, New York, NY 10019
212/586-8700

American Cancer Society Westchester Division
30 Glenn St, White Plains, NY 10603
914/949-4800

American Cancer Society North Carolina Division
11 S Boylan Ave, Suite 221, Raleigh, NC 27603
919/834-8463

American Cancer Society North Dakota Division
115 Roberts St, Fargo, ND 58102
701/232-1385

American Cancer Society Ohio Division
5555 Frantz Road, Dublin, OH 43017
614/889-9565

American Cancer Society Oklahoma Division
3000 United Founders Blvd
Suite 136, Oklahoma City, OK 73112
405/843-9888

American Cancer Society Oregon Division
0330 SW Curry, Portland, OR 97201
503/295-6422

American Cancer Society Pennsylvania Division
Route 422 Sipe Ave, PO Box 897
Hershey, PA 17033-0897
717/533-6144

American Cancer Society Philadelphia Division
1422 Chestnut St, 2nd Floor
Philadelphia, PA 19102
215/665-2900

American Cancer Society Puerto Rico Division
Calle Alverio, No. 577, Hato Rey, PR 00918
809/764-2295

American Cancer Society Rhode Island Division
400 Main St, Pawtucket, RI 02860
401/722-8480

American Cancer Society South Carolina Division
128 Stonemark Lane, Columbia, SC 29210
803/750-1693

American Cancer Society South Dakota Division
4101 Carnegie Place, Sioux Falls, SD 57106-2322
605/361-8277

American Cancer Society Tennessee Division
1315 8th Ave S, Nashville, TN 37203
615/255-1227

American Cancer Society Texas Division
2433 Ridgepoint Drive, Austin, TX 78754
512/928-2262

American Cancer Society Utah Division
610 E South Temple, Salt Lake City, UT 84102
801/322-0431

American Cancer Society Vermont Division
13 Loomis St, Drawer C, PO Box 1452,
Montpelier, VT 05601-1452
802/223-2348

American Cancer Society Virginia Division
4240 Park Place, Glen Allen, VA 23060
804/270-0142

American Cancer Society Washington Division
2120 1st Ave N, Seattle, WA 98109-1140
206/283-1152

American Cancer Society West Virginia Division
2428 Kanawha Blvd E, Charleston, WV 25311
304/344-3611

American Cancer Society Wisconsin Division
615 N Sherman Ave, Madison, WI 53704
608/249-0487

American Cancer Society Wyoming Division
2222 House Ave, Cheyenne, WY 82001
307/638-3331

Captioning

Captioned Films for the Deaf
Modern Talking Picture Service
5000 Park Street N., St. Petersburg, FL 33709
813/541-7571, 800/237-6213

National Captioning Institute, Inc.
5203 Leesburg Pike, Falls Church, VA 22041
703/998-2400

Cardiology

Cardiologist alternate title: heart specialist.
Diagnoses and treats diseases of heart disorders,
using medical instruments and equipment.
Studies diagnostic images and electrocardiograph
recordings to aid in making diagnoses. Prescribes
medications, and recommends dietary and activity
program, as indicated. Refers patient to Surgeon
specializing in cardiac cases when need for
corrective surgery is indicated. May engage in
research to study anatomy of and diseases
peculiar to heart.(DOT)

American College of Angiology
1044 Northern Blvd., Suite 103, Roslyn, NY 11576
516/484-6880

American College of Cardiology
9111 Old Georgetown Rd., Bethesda, MD 20814
301/897-5400

Board Certification in Cardiovascular Disease
American Board of Internal Medicine
3624 Market Street, Philadelphia, PA 19104
215/2431500, 800/441-ABIM (800/441-2246)

Learning to Hear

Neil Scheurich "Poetry and Medicine"
JAMA. 1992 Jul 1; 268(1): 39

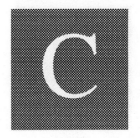

*Son, the stethoscope is a tool
connecting man to man, man
to world, for science is society.
Withdraw from cacophony into
the chamber of an interview.*

*Just as you might tear apart
the clouds at night to see
the burning stars, painfully bright,
so you hear the heart, the secret
of a body's architecture.*

*Auscultate - to the body's heartfelt
speech. A rhythm bound to vessel
bone and blood that voices huge
cries, echoed to mute whisperings
in the cleverness of a wrist.*

*Hearken - to the throb, the code
of earth's ancient persistence,
the soul of smile, of rage
and careless laughter, the slight
unsuspected continuum of life.*

*Listen - to that which speaks
just above and behind you
in the depths of restless time,
and yet to you alone
the axis of the spinning sky.*

Cardiopulmonary Resuscitation

A Historical Perspective: In the past thirty years,
since the introduction of modern techniques of
CPR, there have been dramatic advances in ECC
of victims of profound circulatory collapse and
cardiac arrest. These techniques have restored
the lives of many people when breathing has
ceased and the heart has stopped beating. For
those with spared neurological function and
treatable cardiopulmonary disease, prolonged and
vigorous life may ensue.

Sporadic accounts of attempted resuscitation are
recorded since antiquity[1,4,5] but until 1960
successful resuscitation was largely limited to
occasional victims of respiratory arrest.
Emergency thoracotomy with "open chest
massage" was described in the 1950s and was
often successful if definitive therapy was readily
available.[6] Electric reversal of ventricular
fibrillation by externally applied electrodes was
described in 1956.[7] The ability to reverse a fatal
arrhythmia without opening the chest challenged
the medical community to develop a method of
sustaining ventilation and circulation long enough
to bring the defibrillator to the patient's aid. In
1958 adequate rescue ventilation with
mouth-to-mouth technique was described.[8,9] In
1960 "closed-chest" compression was described,
ushering in the modern ere of CPR.[10] The
simplicity of this technique has led to its
widespread dissemination: "All that is needed are
two hands."[10] The interaction of closed-chest
compression with mouth-to-mouth ventilation was
developed as basic CPR, which offered the hope
for substantially reducing the nearly 1000 sudden
deaths that occurred each day in the United
States before the patients reached the hospital.

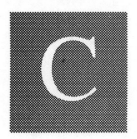

References:
1. Standards for cardiopulmonary resuscitation (CPR) and emergency cardiac care (ECC). JAMA.1974;227(suppl):833-68)
4. Safar P. History of cardiopulmonary-cerebral resuscitation. In: Kaye W, Bircherr N, eds. Cardiopulmonary Resuscitation. New York, NY: Churchill-Livingstone Inc; 1989:1-9
5. Paraskos JA. Biblical Accounts of resuscitation. J Hist Med Allied Sci. 1992;47: 310-21.
6. Stephenson HE Jr, Reid LC, Hinton JW. Some common denominators in 1200 cases of cardiac arrest. Ann Surg. 1953;137:731-44.
7. Zoll PM, Linenthal AJ, Gibson W, Paul MH, Norman LR. Termination of ventricular fibrillation in man by externally applied electric countershock. N Engl J Med. 1956;254:727-32.
8. Safar P, Escarraga L. Elam JO. A comparison of the mouth-to-mouth and mouth-to-airway methods of artificial respiration with the chest-pressure arm-lift method. N Engl J Med 1958;258:671-77.
9. Elam JO, Greene DG, Brown ES, Clements JA. Oxygen and carbon dioxide exchange and energy cost of expired air resuscitation. JAMA.1958;167:328-34.
10. Kouwenhoven WB, Jude JR, Knickerbocker GG. Closed-chest cardiac massage. JAMA.1960;173:1064-67. (JAMA. 1992 Oct 28:268(16))

Contact local heart association for CPR courses

JAMA Theme Issue: Emergency Cardiac Care (CPR) JAMA. 1992 Oct 28; 268(16) "The Guidelines for Cardiopulmonary Resuscitation and Emergency Cardiac Care" are printed here in nine detailed sections. A full listing of those individuals participating in the revision of these guidelines (see June 6, 1986 JAMA for previous version), editorials, conference news and book reviews round out this current treatment of the status of Emergency Cardiac Care.

"Standards and Guidelines for Cardiopulmonary Resuscitation and Emergency Care" available through:
American Heart Association,
2005 Hightower Dr., Garland, TX 75041
214/373-6300

Cardiovascular Technologist

History: In December 1981, the Council on Medical Education officially recognized cardiovascular technology as an allied health profession. Subsequently, organizations that had indicated an interest in sponsoring accreditation activities for the cardiovascular technologist were invited to appoint a representative to an ad hoc committee to develop Essentials. Interested individuals were also invited to join the committee.

The ad hoc committee on development of Essentials for the cardiovascular technologist held its first meeting on April 29, 1982 in Atlanta, Georgia. Twenty-one individuals attended the first meeting representing the following organizations: American College of Cardiology; American Medical Association; American Society of Echocardiography; American College of Radiology; American Registry of Diagnostic Medical Sonographers; Grossmont College, El Cajon, California; American Society of Radiologic Technologists; Society of Diagnostic Medical Sonographers; National Alliance of Cardiovascular Technologists; Society of Non-Invasive Vascular Technology; American College of Chest Physicians; American Cardiology Technologists Association; Santa Fe Community College, Gainesville, Florida; National Society for Cardiopulmonary Technology.

An initial draft of the proposed Essentials and Guidelines of an Accredited Educational Program in Cardiovascular Technology, was developed as a result of this meeting. Subsequent meetings were held to refine and polish the Essentials. In September 1983, the committee members reached agreement on the Essentials. The Joint Review Committee on Education in Cardiovascular Technology held its first meeting in November 1985 in preparation for its ongoing review of programs seeking accreditation in cardiovascular technology.

The following organizations have adopted the Essentials and sponsor the Joint Review Committee on Education in Cardiovascular Technology (JRC-CTV): American College of Cardiology, American College of Chest Physicians, American College of Radiology, American Institute of Ultrasound in Medicine, American Society of Echocardiography, National Society for Cardiovascular Technology/National Society for Pulmonary Technology (represents a merger of the American Cardiology Technologists Association, the National Alliance of Cardiovascular Technologists, and the National Society for Cardiopulmonary Technology), Society of Diagnostic Medical Sonographers, Society of Vascular Technology (formerly, the Society of Non-Invasive Vascular Technology), Society for Vascular Surgery/International Society for Cardiovascular Surgery.

Occupational Description: The cardiovascular technologist performs diagnostic examinations at the request or direction of a physician in one or more of the following three areas: (1) invasive cardiology; (2) noninvasive cardiology; and (3) noninvasive peripheral vascular study. Through subjective sampling and/or recording, the technologist creates an easily definable foundation of data from which a correct anatomic and physiologic diagnosis may be established for each patient.

Job Description: The cardiovascular technologist is qualified by specific technological education to perform various cardiovascular/peripheral vascular diagnostic procedures. The role of the cardiovascular technologist may include but is not limited to: (1) reviewing and/or recording pertinent patient history and supporting clinical data; (2) performing appropriate procedures and obtaining a record of anatomical, pathological and/or physiological data for interpretation by a physician; and (3) exercising discretion and judgment in the performance of cardiovascular diagnostic services

Employment Characteristics: Cardiovascular technologists may provide their services to patients in any medical setting, under the supervision of a doctor of medicine or osteopathy. The procedures performed by the cardiovascular technologist may be found in, but are not limited to, one of the following general settings: (1) invasive cardiovascular laboratories, including cardiac catheterization, blood gas and electrophysiology laboratories; (2) noninvasive

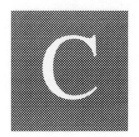

cardiovascular laboratories including echocardiography, exercise stress test and electrocardiography laboratories; and, (3) noninvasive peripheral vascular studies laboratories, including Doppler ultrasound, thermography and plethysmography laboratories. (ALL)

AMA Division of Allied Health
312/464-4634

National Society for Cardiovascular Technology
1133 15th St., NW, Suite 1000
Washington, DC 20005
202/293-5933

Careers, Medical (Physician)
How Wide is the Nonclinical Universe?

The short answer to that question is this: It's wide - and getting wider. Although the vast majority (79%) of today's physicians are involved in patient care, more than 111,000 are not.

What are all those nonclinicians doing? The AMA Physicians Career Resource has some ideas, gleaned from anecdotes offered by career consultants and search firms, and from the research of others. Career counselors report that physicians are finding nonclinical employment in the following fields, areas, and roles:

- Public relations. Many PR firms serve the field of medicine or its allied industries.
- Medical publishing - trade journals, books, abstracts, newsletters.
- Media consultants on medical issues. Appearing on radio and TV talk shows is an effective way for a physician to build his or her medical practice; some doctors, however, are able to make a full-time career out of medical education for the public.
- Copywriting for advertising agencies. Many ad agencies need people who can write copy that appeals to doctors and others in the medical community. The ad agencies' client include HMOs, private health care, pharmaceutical manufacturers, and so on.
- Heading up corporate medical departments.
- Consultant to law firms, insurance companies, and so on. Performed on a per diem basis or through a retainer arrangement, part-time consulting can be a low-risk of exploring other work environments and broadening one's network.
- Program analyst or policy planner. At a private foundation or for a government group, such as the National Institutes of Health.
- Investment banking. One physician/banker's job is to analyze companies that produce high-tech medical products. According to a career consultant, this is a hot area, one in which tremendous amounts of money can be made.
- Securities analysts. Physicians evaluate pharmaceutical firms or hospital chains for stock firms.
- Hospital administration/private health-care administration.
- Sales of medical equipment. As employees of large medical-wares suppliers, like Baxter, physicians sell very sophisticated technical equipment to other physicians.
- Sales of private health-care programs.
- Quality assurance. This is a good area for doctors who want to cut back on their schedules, because they can work at it part-time.
- Accreditation - being part of the team that evaluates hospitals.
- Peer-review panelists.
- Disability determination. A psychiatrist who works part-time for the federal government reviewing charts for people applying for disability benefits enjoys the flexible hours and "relaxing" work atmosphere. And if she ever decides to quit her regular full-time job, she knows she'll have at least some income while she's looking.
- Computer-system developers.
- Deans of medical schools.
- Staff physicians to advertising agencies. The physician's job is to watch for potential problems with the Food and Drug Administration (FDA) and offer advice on specific medical problems.
- Doctor-turned-writers. There are dozens of these, including the novelist/film-maker Michael Crichton and psychiatrists Robert Coles and Oliver Sacks.
- Real-estate developers. A lot of physicians are doing this, according to Chuck Woeppel of Jackson and Coker. They start by working with hospitals and see the opportunity to develop medical-office buildings and research facilities. Some start part-time and, when it grows large enough, jump into it full-time. "I would say that at every hospital in the country you'll find at least one of these people." For example, one physician has developed magnetic resonance imaging in several dozen locations, Woeppel said; another develops ophthalmological surgical centers around the country; yet another develops ENT surgical centers. And how much money is there to be made? "The average real-estate-developing physician, I would think, is definitely a millionaire," said Woeppel.

Speculation that many of today's dissatisfied physicians suffered as medical students or residents from a lack of good career information does exist. Martin D. Keller, MD, PhD, chairman of the Department of Preventive Medicine at Ohio State University, reports that the information medical students receive today about their career options is still woefully inadequate. "In residency, they're exposed to only a very narrow band of clinical specialties and to virtually nothing nonclinical," he told us. "This restricts their horizons terribly."

In response to this need, Keller and his colleague, T. Donald Rucker, PhD, published *Careers in Medicine*[1] in 1986, which included a study of nonclinical job titles. How wide was the nonclinical universe in 1986? Keller and Rucker unearthed more than 900 job titles - a number that has certainly risen in the ensuing years.

Their discoveries were somewhat expected: MDs working as executive VPs of quality control (in pharmaceutical manufacturing), associate deans of alumni affairs (in medical schools), directors of ethics advisory boards (at NIH), and health officers (for USAID) - and others were not: members of the U.S. House of Representatives, commanders in chief (for the Pacific Fleet), and mayors (of Coos Bay, Oregon). They also found numerous presidents (of a major oil company, a publishing company, the Flying Physicians Association, and baseball's American League). They even found a magician (part-time).

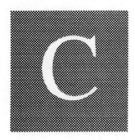

The recent rapid changes in medicine, and the many organizations that have sprung up around the nonclinical fields, have given Keller and his colleagues and idea. "Perhaps it's time for an offshoot of the American Board of Medical Specialties," he said recently, " - one that addresses the many nonclinical medical specialties. Perhaps an 'American Board of Nonclinical Medical Specialties'?"

Rucker and Keller did a multipage study on the diversity of the non-clinical options physicians have to choose from. The job titles, divided into 14 categories, "all...depict positions that differ significantly from those of traditional medical practice," Rucker and Keller note. Their search focused on jobs "where at least 80% of the physician's time was probably devoted to duties other than direct patient care."

Rucker and Keller compiled their information through a process Rucker describes as "haphazard incrementalism": for two and a half years he saved everything that crossed his desk that mentioned an MD in a nonclinical role. The sources included numerous periodicals, newsletters, directories, and related references. "Since the source material did not cover the entire universe, or purport to be representative," Rucker and Keller caution, "our examples should be approached as guideposts for career exploration and not as a road map that specifies every choice that may appear on your journey. Moreover, additional career options may be found as doctors create their own businesses and assume positions never held previously by a physician."

Rucker and Keller note the study's limitations, which include a bias toward executive positions and some duplications of titles with similar responsibilities. "In cases where minimum numbers could be established, a figure is reported as a suffix to the entry, viz., 'Publishing, Editor.'"

"Finally," they add, "certain positions may require special experience and/or additional training beyond the standard medical residency program"; for example, a dual doctorate (MD/PhD) may be required for some teaching or research positions, and "a master's degree in public health or business administration may be mandated by some employers."

References:
1. Rucker TD, Keller, MD, eds., Careers in Medicine: Traditional and Alternative Opportunities. Garrett Park MD: Garrett Park Press; 1986:223-245. Also see 1990 version. (BED adapted)

Leaving the Bedside: The Search for a Nonclinical Medical Career Chicago; American Medical Association; 1992. 118 pp.
ISBN 0-88870-464-6 OP392092AT.

Physician Executive Management Center
American Academy of Medical Directors
4830 W. Kennedy Blvd., Suite 648
Tampa, FL 33609
813/287-2000

Careers, Medical (Undergraduate)
Association of American Medical Colleges
2450 N Street, N.W., Washington, DC 20037
202/828-0400

National Association of Advisors for the Health Professions, Inc.
PO Box 5017-A, Champaign, IL 61825
217/333-0090

"200 Ways to Put Your Talent to Work in the Health Field"
National Health Council
350 Fifth Ave., New York, NY 10118
212/268-8900

"Medicine: a Chance to Make a Difference" or "Got that Healing Feeling" brochures available from the American Medical Association

Cataract
American Society of Cataract
and Refractive Surgery
3700 Pender Dr., Suite 108, Fairfax, VA 22030
703/591-2220

Census
U.S. Bureau of Census
Department of Commerce, Washington, DC 20033
301/763-5040

Centers for Disease Control and Prevention (CDC)
The Centers for Disease Control and Prevention, established as an operating health agency within the Public Health Service by the Secretary of Health, Education, and Welfare on July 1, 1973, is the Federal agency charged with protecting the public health of the Nation by providing leadership and direction in the prevention and control of diseases and other preventable conditions and responding to public health emergencies. It is composed of nine major operating components: Epidemiology Program Office, International Health Program Office, Public Health Practice Program Office, Center for Prevention Services, Center for Environmental Health and Injury Control, National Institute for Occupational Safety and Health, Center for Chronic Disease Prevention and Health Promotion, Center for Infectious Diseases, and the National Center for Health Statistics.

The Agency administers national programs for the prevention and control of communicable and vector-borne diseases and other preventable conditions. It develops and implements programs in chronic disease prevention and control, including consultation with State and local health departments. It develops and implements programs to deal with environmental health problems, including responding to environmental, chemical, and radiation emergencies.

The Agency directs and enforces foreign quarantine activities and regulations; provides consultation and assistance in upgrading the performance of public health and clinical laboratories; organizes and implements a National Health Promotion Program, including a nationwide program of research, information, and education in the field of smoking and health. It also collects, maintains, analyzes, and disseminates national data on health status and health services.

To ensure safe and healthful working conditions for all working conditions for all working people, occupational safety and health standards are developed, and research and other activities are carried out, through the National Health Institute for Occupational Safety and Health.

The Agency also provides consultation to other nations in the control of preventable diseases, and participates with national and international agencies in the eradication or control of communicable diseases and other preventable conditions.(USG)

Centers for Disease Control and Prevention
1600 Clifton Rd., NE, Atlanta, GA 30333
404/639-3311
Public Inquiry 404/639-3534

Center for Health Promotion and Education
Centers for Disease Control and Prevention,
Bldg. 1 South, Room SSB249
1600 Clifton Rd.,NE, Atlanta, GA 30333
404/639-3492; 404/639-3698

CDC Voice Information System and Disease
Information Hotline
404/332-4555
(Provides information on the Morbidity and Mortality Weekly Report and public health topics with an option to speak to a public health professional)

Cerebral Palsy
American Academy for Cerebral Palsy
and Developmental Medicine
1910 Byrd Avenue, PO Box 11086
Richmond, VA 23230
804/282-0036

United Cerebral Palsy Associations
7 Penn Plaza, New York, NY 10001
212/268-6655
800/USA-5UCP (800/872-5827)

CHAMPUS - Military Dependents Care
The Office of Civilian Health and Medical Program of the Uniformed Services (OCHAMPUS) was established as a field activity in 1974 under the policy guidance and operational direction of the Assistant Secretary of Defense (Health Affairs). The Office is responsible for administering a civilian health and medical care program for retirees and the spouses and dependent children of active duty, retired, and deceased service members. Also included are spouses and dependent children of totally disabled veterans. The Office also administers, for the Uniformed Services, a program for payment of emergency medical/dental services provided to active duty service members by civilian medical personnel.(USG)

Civilian Health and Medical Program
Office of CHAMPUS
Aurora, CO 80045-6900
303/361-1313

Office of Civilian Health and Medical Program of the Uniformed Services
Department of Defense, Denver, CO 80045.
303-361-8606

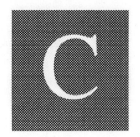

Charity
Evaluations of charitable groups:
National Charities Information Bureau
19 Union Square West, New York, NY 10003
212/929-6300

Chemotherapy
The treatment of infections of malignant diseases by drugs that act selectively on the cause of the disorder, but which may have substantial effects on normal tissue.(ENC)

Board Certification
American Board of Radiology
2301 W. Big Beaver Road, Suite 625
Troy, MI 48084
313/643-0300

Chemotherapy Foundation
183 Madison Ave, Room 403
New York, NY 10016
212/213-9292

Chest X-Ray

Contact local lung association or public health department

Child Abuse

Contact state department of Child and Family services for information on local programs and protective initiatives.

"AMA Diagnostic and Treatment Guidelines Concerning Child Abuse and Neglect" reflect literature as of March 1992 and are available from: American Medical Association
Department of Mental Health
312/464-5066

AMA diagnostic and treatment guidelines concerning child abuse and neglect. Council on Scientific Affairs. JAMA. 1985 Aug 9; 254(6): 796-800

Child maltreatment is a serious and pervasive problem. Every year, more than a million children in the United States are abused, and between 2,000 and 5,000 die as a result of their injuries. Physicians are in a unique position to detect child abuse and neglect and are mandated by law to report such cases. These guidelines were developed to assist primary care physicians in the identification and management of the various forms of child maltreatment. A brief historical introduction and specific information about vulnerable families and children are presented. The physical and behavioral diagnostic signs of physical abuse, physical neglect, sexual abuse, and emotional maltreatment are delineated. Information about specific techniques for interviewing the abused child and family, case management objectives, reporting requirements, and trends in treatment and prevention are also provided.

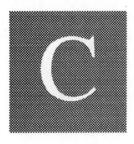

Clearinghouse on Child Abuse and Neglect
The Circle
8201 Greensboro Drive, McLean, VA 22102
703/821-2086

Child Help USA
(For calls expressing concern about & suspect of child abuse)
800/422-4453

National Child Abuse Hotline: Childhelps
PO Box 630, Hollywood, CA 90028
800/422-4453
(24-hour number)

National Coalition Against Domestic Violence
PO Box 34103, Washington, DC 20043-4103
202/638-6388
(For a listing of local safe houses and shelters)
800/333-SAFE (800/333-7233)

National Committee for Prevention of Child Abuse
332 S. Michigan Ave., Suite 950
Chicago, IL 60604
312/663-3520

National Council on Child Abuse
and Family Violence
1155 Connecticut Ave, NW
Washington, DC 20036
202/429-6695

Parents Anonymous Hotline
6733 S. Sepulveda Blvd, #270
Los Angeles, CA 90045
800/421-0353 800/352-0386(CA only)

Children, Hospitalized
Children in Hospitals
31 Wilshire Park, Needham, MA 02192
617/444-3877

Children and Youth Services, State Government Offices
Alabama Bureau of Family and Children's Services
64 N. Union St., Montgomery, AL 36130
205-242-9500

Alaska Division of Family and Youth Services
PO Box H, Juneau, AK 99811
907-465-3170

Arizona Children, Youth and Families
1717 W. Jefferson, Phoenix, AZ 85007
602-542-3981

Arkansas Children and Family Services
PO Box 1437, Little Rock, AR 72203
501-682-8770

California Office of Child Abuse Prevention
744 P St., MS 9-100, Sacramento, CA 95814
916-323-2888

Colorado Division of Family and Children's Service
1575 Sherman St., 2nd Fl., Denver, CO 80203
303-866-3672

Connecticut Department of Children
and Youth Services
170 Sigourney St., Hartford, CT 06105
203-566-3536

Delaware Department of Services for Children,
Youth and their Families
1825 Faulkland Rd., Wilmington, DE 19805
302-633-2500

District of Columbia Family Services Administration
First and I St., SW, Rm. 215
Washington, DC 20024
202-727-5947

Florida Children, Youth and Families
1317 Winewood, Building. 8, 3rd Fl.
Tallahassee, FL 32399
904-488-8762

Georgia Family and Children Services
878 Peachtree St., 4th Fl., Atlanta, GA 30309
404-894-6389

Hawaii Child Protective Services
810 Richards St., Ste. 400, Honolulu, HI 96813
808-548-6123

Idaho Division of Family and Children Services
450 W. State St., Boise, ID 83720
208-334-5700

Illinois Department of Children
and Family Services
406 E. Monroe, Springfield, IL 62701
217-785-2509
800/252-2873 (24-hour number to report child abuse)

Indiana Division of Families and Children
302 W. Washington, IGC-S, E414
Indianapolis, IN 46204
317-233-4451

Iowa Adult, Children and Family Services
Hoover State Office Building,
Des Moines, IA 50319
515-281-5521

Kansas Youth Services Social
and Rehabilitations Department
Smith-Wilson Building
300 SW Oakley, Topeka, KS 66606
913-296-3284

Kentucky Division of Family Services
275 E. Main St., Frankfort, KY 40601
502-564-6852

Louisiana Office of Community Services
PO Box 44367, Baton Rouge, LA 70804
504-342-4000

Maine Child and Family Services
State House Station #11, Augusta, ME 04333
207-289-5060

Maryland Child Welfare Services Office
300 W. Preston St., Baltimore, MD 04333
301-333-0208

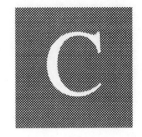

Massachusetts Department of Social Services
150 Causeway St., Boston, MA 02114
617-727-0900

Michigan Office of Children and Youth Services
300 S. Capitol, PO Box 30037, Lansing, MI 48909
517-373-4506

Minnesota Community Social Services Division
658 Cedar St., 4th Fl., St. Paul, MN 55155
612-297-2673

Mississippi Division of Family
and Children's Services
PO Box 352, Jackson, MS 39205
601-354-6661

Missouri Children's Services
Broadway Building, Box 88
Jefferson City, MO 65103
314-751-2882

Montana Department of Family Services
48 N. Last Chance Gulch, Helena, MT 59601
406-444-5902

Nebraska Division of Human Services
PO Box 95026, Lincoln, NE 68509
402-471-9308

Nevada Children and Family Services
505 E. King St., Carson City, NV 89710
702-687-4400

New Hampshire Children and Youth Services
Hazen Dr., Concord, NH 03301
603-271-4451

New Jersey Division of Economic Assistance
Quakerbridge Rd., CN 716, Trenton, NJ 08625
609-588-2361

New Mexico Children's Bureau
PO Box 2348 Santa Fe, NM 87504
505-827-8439

New York Department of Social Services
40 N. Pearl St., Albany, NY 12243
518-474-9475

North Carolina Division of Social Services
325 N. Salisbury St., Raleigh, NC 27603
919-733-3055

North Dakota Children and Family Services
State Capitol, Judicial Wing
600 E. Blvd., Bismarck, ND 58505
701-224-4811

Ohio Family and Children's Services Division
51 N. High St., 3rd Fl., Columbus, OH 43266
614-466-8783

Oklahoma Department of Human Services
PO Box 25352, Oklahoma City, OK 73125

Oregon Children's Services Division
198 Commercial St., SE Salem, OR 97310
503-378-4374

Pennsylvania Children, Youth and Families
PO Box 2675, Harrisburg, PA 17105
717-787-4756

Rhode Island Department of Children and Families
610 Mt. Pleasant Ave., Providence, RI 02908
401-861-6000

South Carolina Children and
Families Services Division
PO Box 1520, Columbia, SC 29202
803-734-5670

South Dakota Child Protection Services Division
Knelp Building, Pierre, SD 57501
605-773-3227

Tennessee Department of Human Services
111 Seventh Ave., N., Nashville, TN 37243
615-741-1820

Texas Department of Human Services
PO Box 149030, Austin, TX 78714
512-450-3080

Utah Division of Family Services
120 N. 200 W., 4th Fl., Salt Lake City, UT 84103
801-538-4004

Vermont Department of Social
and Rehabilitation Services
103 S. Main St., Osgood Building
Waterbury, VT 05671
802-241-2131

Virginia Department of Social Services
8007 Discovery Dr., Richmond, VA 23229
804-662-9236

Washington Children and Family Services Division
Office Building #2 M/S: OB-41
Olympia, WA 98504
206-586-8654

West Virginia Social Services Bureau
1900 Washington E., Building 6
Charleston, WV 25305
304-348-7980

Wisconsin Children Youth and Services
PO Box 7851, Madison, WI 53707
608-266-6946

Wyoming Division of Youth Services
Hathaway Building, 3rd Fl., Cheyenne, WY 82002
307-777-6095

American Samoa Child Abuse Commission
Pago Pago, AS 96799
684-633-4485

Guam Department of Public Health
and Social Services
PO Box 2816, Agana, GU 96910
671-734-7399

Northern Mariana Islands Youth Services Division
Office of the Governor, Saipan, MP 96950
670-322-9366

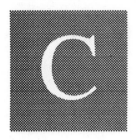

Puerto Rico Fernandez Juncos Station
PO Box 3349, Santurce, PR 00904
809-725-0753

U.S. Virgin Islands Department of Human Services
Barbel Plaza, S., St. Thomas, VI 00802
809-774-0930

Childbirth, Natural
American Society for Psychoprophylaxis in
Obstetrics (ASPO/Lamaze)
1840 Wilson Blvd./Suite 204, Arlington, VA 22201
703/524-7802

International Childbirth Education Association
(ICEA)
PO Box 20048, Minneapolis, MN 55420
612/854-8660

Children, Missing
Childfind Hotline
800/426-5678

Missing Child Hotline - National Center for Missing
and Exploited Children
800/843-5678 9 a.m.-Midnight

MEDWATCH
800/I-AM-LOST (800/426-5678)
(Sponsored by Wyeth Laboratories)

Children's Health
Association for the Care of Children's Health
3615 Wisconsin Ave., NW.
Washington, DC 20016
202/244-1801, 202/244-8922

Children's Defense Fund
122 C Street, NW., Suite 400
Washington, DC 20001
202/628-8787

National Institute of Child Health
and Human Development
9000 Rockville Pike, Bethesda, MD 20892
301/496-5133

Chiropractor
Alternate titles: Chiropractic; doctor, chiropractic
Diagnoses and treats musculoskeletal conditions
of spinal column and extremities to prevent
disease and correct body abnormalities believed
to be caused by interference with nervous system.
Examines patient to determine nature and extent
of disorder. Performs diagnostic procedures
including physical, neurologic, and orthopedic
examinations, laboratory tests, and other
procedures, using x-ray machine, proctoscope,
electrocardiograph, otoscope, and other
instruments and equipment. Manipulates spinal
column and other extremities to adjust, align, or
correct abnormalities caused by neurological and
kinetic articular dysfunction, Utilizes
supplementary measures, such as exercise, rest,
water, light, heat, and nutritional therapy. (DOT)

American Chiropractic Association
1701 Clarendon Blvd., Arlington, VA 22201
703/276-8800

JAMA Article of Note: Chiropractic decision and
General Counsel's statement. JAMA. 1988 Jan 1;
259(1): 81-3.

Chiropractic Assistant
Aids Chiropractor during physical examination of
patients, gives specified office treatments, and
keeps patient's records: Writes history of patient's
accident or illness, and shows patient to
examining room. Aids chiropractor in lifting and
turning patient under treatment. Gives
physiotherapy treatment, such as diathermy,
galvanics, or hydrotherapy, following directions of
chiropractor. Takes and records patient's
temperature and blood pressure, assists in x-ray
procedures, and gives first aid. Answers
telephone, schedules appointments, records
treatment information on patient's chart, and fills
out insurance forms. Prepares and mails patient's
bills. (DOT)

Chiropractic Schools

California
Cleveland Chiropractic College
590 N. Vermont Ave., Los Angeles, CA 90004
213-660-6166

Life Chiropractic College, West
2005 Via Barrett, PO Box 367
San Lorenzo, CA 94580
415-276-9013

Palmer College of Chiropractic, West
1095 Dunford Way, Sunnyvale, CA 94087
408-983-4000

Los Angeles College of Chiropractic
PO Box 1166, Whittier, CA 90609-1166
213-947-8755

Georgia
Life College
1269 Barclay Circle, Marietta, GA 30060
404-424-0554

Illinois
National College of Chiropractic
200 E. Roosevelt Rd., Lombard, IL 60148
708-629-2000

Iowa
Palmer College of Chiropractic
1000 Brady St., Davenport, IA 52803
319-326-9600

Minnesota
Northwestern College of Chiropractic
2501 W. 84th St., Bloomington, MN 55431
612-888-4777

Missouri
Logan College of Chiropractic
PO Box 1065, Chesterfield, MO 63006-1065
314-227-2100

Cleveland Chiropractic College
6401 Rockhill Rd., Kansas City, MO 64131
816-333-8230

New York
New York Chiropractic College
PO Box 167, Glen Head, NY 11545
516-626-2700

Orgeon
Western States Chiropractic College
2900 NE 132nd Ave., Portland, OR 97230
503-256-3180

Texas
Parker College of Chiropractic
2500 Walnut Hill Lane, Dallas, TX 75229
214-438-6932

Texas Chiropractic College
5912 Spenser Hwy., Pasadena, TX 77505
713-487-1170

Christian Medical Society
Christian Medical and Dental Society
1616 Gateway Blvd., PO Box 830689,
Richardson, TX 75083
214/783-8384

Chronic Fatigue
Chronic fatigue syndrome (CFS) is an illness
characterized by debilitating fatigue and several
flu-like symptoms such as pharyngitis, enlarged
lymph nodes, low-grade fever, muscle and joint
pains, headache, difficulty concentrating, and
exercise intolerance. The profound fatigue usually
comes on suddenly and persists throughout the
course of the illness. A small percentage of
physicians diagnose CFS in most or all patients
who complain to them about fatigue. (ALT)

Chronic Fatigue Immune Dysfunction
Syndrome Association
PO Box 220398, Charlotte, NC 28222-0398
704/362-2343

Chronic Fatigue Immune Dysfunction
Syndrome Society
PO Box 230108, Portland, OR 97223
503/684-5261

National Chronic Fatigue Association
3521 Broadway, Suite 222
Kansas City, MO 64111
816/931-4777
(Recorded message on publications--about 3
minutes long)

Cleft Palate
American Cleft Palate Educational Foundation
1218 Grandview Ave, Pittsburgh, PA 15211
800/242-5338

American Cleft Palate Association
1218 Grandview, Pittsburgh, PA 15211
412/481-1376

Cleveland Clinic
Cleveland Clinic Hospital
9500 Euclid Ave, Cleveland, OH 44195
216/444-2200

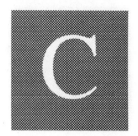

George Washington Crile 1864-1943
(JAMA. 1943 Jan 16; 121(3): 209)
cofounder of the Cleveland Clinic, died, January 7,
1943 at the Cleveland Clinic, aged 78, of subacute
bacterial endocarditis.

Dr. Crile was born in Chili, Ohio, Nov. 11, 1864.
He graduated at Ohio Northern University and in
1887 at the University of Wooster Medical
Department, Cleveland, now Western Reserve
University School of Medicine. Early in his career
Dr. Crile studied in Vienna, London and Paris. He
served at Wooster University first as lecturer and
demonstrator in histology and professor of the
principles and practice of surgery. He was
professor of clinical surgery at Western Reserve
University from 1900 to 1911 and professor of
surgery from 1911 to 1924. He was also director
of research at the Cleveland Clinic Foundation, of
which in 1921 he was a cofounder.

Research conducted by Dr. Crile included the
basic factors concerned in circulation, respiration,
blood chemistry and the body's source of energy.
He was perhaps first to make a direct blood
transfusion, performed in 1905.

Dr. Crile was awarded the Alvarenga prize by the
College of Physicians of Philadelphia in 1901, the
Cartwright prize by Columbia University in 1897
and 1903, the Senn prize by the American Medical
Association in 1898, the American Medicine medal
for service to humanity in 1914, the National
Institute Society Sciences medal in 1917 and the
Trimble Lecture medal in 1921. In 1925 the
Lannelongue International Medal of Surgery was
presented to him by the Societe internationale de
chirurgie de Paris, in 1931 the Cleveland medal
for public service and in 1940 the distinguished
service gold key of the American Congress of
Physical Therapy. He was a member of the
founders' group of the American Board of Surgery.
In 1923 he served as president of the American
Surgical Association.

A member of the board of regents of the American
College of Surgeons since 1913. Dr. Crile was
chairman of the board from 1917 to 1939 and
president of the college in 1916. In 1907 he was
Third Vice President of the American Medical
Association and chairman of its Section on
Surgery, 1910-1911. He was also an honorary or
corresponding fellow or member of many
American and European societies.

In 1898 Dr. Crile was brigade surgeon in the
volunteers with the rank of major, serving in Cuba
and Puerto Rico. He was a major in the Officers'
Reserve Corps, and professional director of the
U.S. Army Base Hospital number 4, Lakeside Unit
(British Expeditionary Force number 9) in service
in France for one year beginning May 1917,
subsequently serving as senior consultant in
surgical research, lieutenant colonel and in
November 1918 colonel. He was brigadier general
in the Medical Officers' Reserve Corps in 1921,
holding the same rank in the auxiliary reserve
corps since 1929. In 1919 he was awarded the
Distinguished Service Medal and in the same year
became an honorary member of the Military

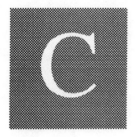

Division, third class, Companion of Bath (British). In 1922 he was made a Chevalier in the French Legion of Honor.

Dr. Crile was a prolific contributor to scientific literature. Among numerous articles and textbooks are Surgical Shock, 1897: Surgery of Respiratory System, 1899; Certain Problems Relating to Surgical Operations, 1901; On the Blood Pressure in Surgery, 1903; Hemorrhage and Transfusion, 1909; Anemia and Resuscitation, 1914; Anoci-Association (with Lower), 1914; second edition, Surgical Shock and the Shockless Operation Through Anoci-Association, 1920; Origin and Nature of the Emotions, 1915; A Mechanistic View of War and Peace, 1915; Man, an Adaptive Mechanism, 1916; the Kinetic Drive, 1916; the Fallacy of the German State Philosophy, 1918; A Physical Interpretation of Shock Exhaustion and Restoration, 1921; The Thyroid Gland (with others), 1922; Notes on Military Surgery, 1924; A Bipolar Theory of Living Processes, 1926; Problems in Surgery, 1928; Diagnoses and Treatment of Diseases of the Thyroid Gland (with others), 1932; Diseases Peculiar to Civilized Man,1934; The Phenomena of Life, 1936; the Surgical Treatment of Hypertension, 1938; and Intelligence, Power and Personality, 1941.

Dr Crile's contributions to experimental work through the years resulted in many improvements in surgery and medical practice. He traveled widely; his charm and his forceful personality marked him for leadership early in his career. The contributions of his active and curious mind are a lasting monument.

Clinical Investigation
American Society for Clinical Investigation
6900 Grove Rd., Thorofare, NJ 08086
609/848-1000

Clinical Laboratories
AMA Policy. Clinical Laboratory Improvement Act of 1988: It is the policy of the AMA to:

-continue and intensify its efforts to seek appropriate and reasonable modifications in the proposed rules for implementation of the CLIA 88;

-communicate to Congress and to HCFA the positive contribution of physician office laboratory testing to high quality, cost effective care so that through administrative revision of the regulations, clarification of Congressional intent and, if necessary, additional legislation, the negative impact of these proposed regulations on patient care and access can be eliminated;

-continue to work with Congress, HFCA, the Commission on Laboratory Assessment, and other medical and laboratory groups for the purposes of making the regulations for physicians' office laboratories reasonable, based on

scientific data, and responsive to the goal of improving access to quality services to patients;

-protest the reported high costs being considered for certification of laboratories and the limited number of laboratory categories proposed;

-encourage all components of the federation to express to HFCA and members of Congress their concerns about the effect of the proposed rules on access and cost of laboratory services; and

-protest the very limited list of waivered tests.

The Clinical Laboratory Improvement Amendments of 1988 (CLIA-88)
Janet Horan

Four years ago Congress passed the Clinical Laboratory Improvement Amendments of 1988 (CLIA-88) in response to reports in the lay press concerning deaths associated with misread pap smears. CLIA establishes the monitoring of all human clinical laboratory testing, no matter where testing is performed. The number of testing sites regulated is estimated by the Department of Health and Human Services (HSS) to be more than 200,000, over half of which are estimated to be physicians' offices, which were previously unregulated.

Two years ago, the Health Care Financing Administration (HCFA) published a proposed rule which, if finalized, would have been extremely unreasonable and expensive. In response to this proposal, the American Medical Association (AMA) spearheaded a campaign with the state and national medical specialty societies that generated an unprecedented 60,000 written comments on the regulations. As a result of these comments, a much more reasonable final regulatory scheme was published on February 28, 1992.

CLIA-88 applies to all testing of human specimens used in the diagnosis, prevention, or treatment of disease or health problems. This includes every testing entity, from physicians, who perform only basic tests for their patients, to hospitals and large clinical laboratories. The only exceptions are testing for forensic purposes, research labs that do not report patient results, employee drug testing programs, and facilities certified by the National Institute on Drug Abuse to perform only urine drug testing.

CLIA-88 is not a reimbursement regulation or a Medicare program. It applies to all clinical laboratory tests in the United States, whether or not they are reimbursed by Medicare. However, if only phlebotomy and/or collection of specimens (such as urine, culturettes, pap smears, or biopsy) are performed and specimens are transported to an approved laboratory, CLIA-88 does not apply to the "collecting" entity.

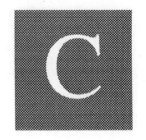

Clinical Laboratory Improvement Amendment
Public Law No. 101-578 enacted October 31, 1988

Contact CLIA Hotline or Regional HCFA Office for applications of the amendment within your state

CLIA Hotline
410/290-5850, 410/966-6802

Commission on Office Laboratory Assessment (COLA)
8701 Georgia Avenue, Suite 403B
Silver Spring, MD 20910
301/588-5882

Self-Instruction Manual for Today's Physician Office Laboratories
College of American Pathologists

Guide for conversion from conventional units to Systeme International (S.I.) Units (Catalog # 35-9-001-00)
American Society of Clinical Pathologists
2100 W. Harrison St., Chicago, IL 60612-3798
312/738-4890

JAMA Article of Note: S.I. (Systeme International) Units. JAMA. 1988 Jul 1; 260(1): 73-8

Clinics

Contact state or local Department of Health for Credentials on Free Clinics. Keep in mind that each state may vary as to what type of information they provide

Closing Your Medical Practice
Closing Checklist I (Advance Planning)

Recommended Steps to Take: Time Frame
Lease: At the beginning of next lease term:
Make arrangements for an "escape clause" to be written into your lease. Most landlords will agree to this with a six-month notice. If you cannot negotiate an escape clause, be sure you have the right to sublease your space.

Accounts Receivable: Two years before closing (or as soon as possible).
Consider asking for payment at the time of service charges. Begin aging your account receivable, if not presently done. Develop a polished mail and telephone collection program. Tighten up procedures for insurance filing. Be sure you have a tickler file established to follow up slow claims.

Employees: Approximately three months before closing (perhaps a bit longer, depending on employees' circumstances and the local job market).
Notify employees of your plans. Assist them in finding employment, if possible. Arrange for key person(s) to remain as long as you'll need them. Line up potential temporaries in the event people leave before your close. Be square with staff regarding overtime pay, unused sick leave, and vacation. Review your policy manual. Discuss the amount of vesting employees may have in pension plans and how funds are to be transferred.

Patients Records: Approximately three months before closing (or longer, based on circumstances) Identify patients that are active. Draft a notice to them of your plans. Mail local notice with an authorization to release records. Start processing transfers. Know your state regulations regarding patient access to records, patient access to records and retention requirements. Make arrangements for storage of remaining records, or microfilming. Draft a notice for the newspapers.

Equipment: Three months before closing. Explore sources available for sale and/or dispositions of office equipment and furniture. Have equipment appraised; placed ads in journals if your wish to sell. Consider donation if appraisals are low or you don't wish to bother trying to sell.

Closing Checklist II (To be attended to at or prior to closing):

• *Insurance:* Be Sure to Ask for Premium Refund! Office insurance, both personnel and contents, must be maintained until business is formally concluded. File final Unemployment return, cancel worker's compensation, office contents, and liability policies when premises are totally vacated, Keep any accounts receivable coverage until accounts are paid or turned over to a collector. Professional liability may be cancelled only if a physician plans to cease practicing entirely. If an MD has been covered under a "claims made" policy, arrange for "tail" coverage, and to keep all old policies easily accessible.

• *Accounts Payable Items:* Notify all suppliers and request final statements. Unopened containers may be returned . Notify utilities, including telephone, of the date service should be discontinued. Keep business checking account open for three months after closing, This would allow all bills to be paid. Deposits from patients and insurance payments may straggle in after that date, but can be deposited to a physician's personal account, so long as a record is kept. Check with an accountant for the most current information.

• Physician's Accountant Items:
File necessary final tax forms. Notify Keogh or corporate retirement plan of the intentions of the physician and his/her employees. Make arrangements for the retention of business and personnel records.

• Discontinue Magazine Subscriptions and Ask for Refund, or Notify Publishers of Your New Address.

• Write "Return to Sender" on All "Junk Mail."

• Notify Personal and/or Professional Associations.

• Leave a Forwarding Address with the Post Office.

• Send Personal Letters of Appreciation to Individuals Who Have Helped You in Your Career.

• Donate Books, Journals to a Medical Library.

• Dispose of Drugs According to DEA Instructions. Destroy All Unused Prescriptions Pads if You Are Discontinuing Practice.

• Securely Store All Diplomas, Licenses, Indications of Medical Membership.

• Give Some Thought to Keeping Your Answering Service Active for Anywhere Between Three

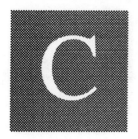

Months to a Year, Depending Upon Local Circumstances, Your Specialty and/or Patient population. Check with the Local Medical Society for an Advisory Opinion.
• Be sure to Advise Local Medical Society of the Location of Your Remaining Records.(CLO)

Cocaine
Cocaine Baby Helpline
800/327-BABE
Operated by Northwestern University Memorial Hospital-Chicago

Cocaine Baby Helpline
800/638-2229
National Association for Prenatal Addiction and Education

Cocaine Hotline
800/662-4357 (800/662-HELP)
Operated by the National Institute on Drug Abuse

Information about Cocaine
800/262-2463 (800/COCAINE)
Operated by Fair Oaks Hospital, Summit, NJ

National Clearinghouse for
Drug Abuse Information
PO Box 416, Kensington, MD 20795
301/443-6500

Cocaine Anonymous
312/202-8898

College Health
American College Health Association
1300 Piccard Drive, Suite 200
Rockville, MD 20850
301/963-1100

Colon Disease
Crohn's and Colitis Foundation
(Formerly National Foundation for
Ileitis and Colitis)
444 Park Ave. South, New York, NY 10016
212/685-3440 800/343-3637

Colon and Rectal Surgery
American Board of Colon and Rectal Surgery
8750 Telegraph Rd, Suite 410, Taylor, MI 48180
313/295-1740

American Society of Colon and Rectal Surgery
800 E. Northwest Highway, #1080
Palatine, IL 60067
708/359-9184

Competency Assurance
National Organization for Competency Assurance
1101 Connecticut Ave., NW
Washington D.C. 20036
202/857-1165

Complaints
Introduction: Physicians have long recognized that enforcement of their code of ethics is one of the fundamental responsibilities of the medical profession. As Principle II of the American Medical Association's Principles of Medical Ethics instructs, "A physician shall deal honestly with patients and colleagues, and strive to expose those physicians deficient in character or competence, or who engage in fraud or deception."

Enforcement of ethical guidelines has traditionally been conducted at several levels, including hospitals, county and state medical societies, and state licensing boards. Many state and county societies have met their responsibilities in this regard. Others have been deterred by the threat of expensive litigation. The purpose of this book is to provide direction to county and state medical societies for their enforcement activities, and by so doing increase the effectiveness of this essential form of professional self-regulation.

Following the procedures described herein will not eliminate the threat of litigation, but it should reduce the threat to an acceptable level of risk. The AMA will stand behind, and assist in the defense of, any medical society which follows these procedures in a good faith effort to enforce the AMA's Current Opinions and Principles of Medical Ethics.

This essay is not intended to preempt all other guidelines; the AMA recognizes that there are other acceptable approaches to enforcement.

General Considerations: A program to enforce professional conduct has both substantive and procedural components. That is, the program must include (1) standards for what constitutes professional misconduct and (2) guidelines for processing an allegation that professional misconduct has occurred.

Substantive Standards: Substantive standards for what constitutes professional misconduct must satisfy a number of criteria. First, they must be directly related to the purpose of ensuring competent, honest and lawful medical care and not act as unreasonable restraints on competition among physicians. Thus, for example, it is permissible to prohibit the alteration of a patient's medical records with fraudulent intent, the breaching of a professional confidence, or the practicing of medicine while impaired by alcohol, drugs, physical disability, or mental instability. On the other hand, it would not be permissible to prohibit all advertising of medical services by physicians.

The difference between appropriate ethical canons and inappropriate restraints on competition can be further illustrated by the following example. It would not be permissible for a medical society to issue a fee schedule for its members on the ground that price competition leads to deceptive advertising of prices. However, it would be permissible for a medical society to prohibit the deceptive advertising of prices.

Substantive standards must also meet a requirement of specificity. If a professional conduct standard is characterized by vague language, then it can be applied in an arbitrary fashion. For instance, it would not be permissible to require simply that a physician have the ability

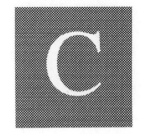

"to get along with others" since it is uncertain how such an ability would be determined. On the other hand, it probably would be acceptable to impose sanctions for an inability to work with professional colleagues such that patient care is compromised.

Substantive standards should cover the full range of potential misconduct, including those which are commonly the subject of complaints. For example, medical societies should process allegations of excessive fees, substandard care, sexual misconduct, discourteous service, improper withholding of medical records, and impairment by alcohol or other drug use. Other examples of appropriate substantive standards can be found in the AMA's ethics code and the standards for disciplinary action of state licensing boards.

Procedural Guidelines: Complaints against physicians that allege professional misconduct should be processed through two independent committees, a grievance committee and a disciplinary committee. The grievance committee screens, reviews, and/or refers complaints. In addition, it educates physicians and their patients about the professional obligations of physicians and decides whether disciplinary proceedings should be pursued.

When disciplinary proceedings are appropriate, they are conducted by a separate committee, the disciplinary committee. By maintaining the independence of the two committees, the disciplinary committee members undertake their responsibilities without any prior exposure to the case. This helps ensure that the ultimate judgment is rendered by an impartial decision maker.

The establishment of enforcement activities is an important public service, but such activities cannot succeed unless the public knows their existence and understands how to use them. The availability and the method of operation of the grievance and disciplinary committees should be continually publicized through appropriate channels of lay communication to the extent feasible. Concurrently, the profession should be kept informed of the committees' work by utilizing professional media such as medical journals, newsletters, secretary's letters and president's pages.

The cooperation of the members of the medical societies, both in serving as committee members and in subjecting themselves to the jurisdiction of the committees when charged with misconduct, is essential if the enforcement activities are to be a success. The committees cannot function effectively unless the committee members have the full and complete cooperation of all member-physicians. In order to help ensure cooperation, the society may define as a ground for discipline the failure of a physician to cooperate with the proceedings of grievance and disciplinary committees. In addition, if a physician does not respond to a complaint after receiving notice, then the committees should process the complaint on the basis of the information that is presented by the complainant and that is discovered in the process of the committees' review.

Jurisdiction: Ordinarily, a medical society can exercise jurisdiction over its members only.

However, it is in the interest of the public and the profession for patients to be able to pursue complaints against any physician. Consequently, non-member physicians should be encouraged to subject themselves to the jurisdiction of the committees. Some societies will accept a complaint against a non-member physician only if the non-member agrees to abide by the grievance and disciplinary procedures and to accept the decision of the grievance and disciplinary committees. In the absence of an agreement, these societies will refer the complaint to the state licensing board or another appropriate institution. Other societies will process a complaint against a non-member without the non-member's consent, although it may be difficult to do so without the non-member's cooperation.

Medical societies often ask non-member physicians to sign a consent form to demonstrate their willingness to abide by the grievance and disciplinary procedures. Other medical societies find a consent form unnecessary on the basis that non-member physicians demonstrate their willingness to cooperate by responding to the complaints against them. In some cases, the signing of a consent form may deter a non-member physician from pulling out of the process in midstream.

Bylaws/Rules And Regulations: All enforcement activities should be codified in the medical society's bylaws or the rules and regulations of the grievance and disciplinary committees to ensure that there is appropriate authority for the activities. Because amending bylaws is a cumbersome process, medical societies typically include much of the procedural information for grievance and disciplinary committees in the rules and regulations.

Some information should ordinarily be codified in the bylaws, including a statement of the authority of the grievance and disciplinary committees, the grounds for discipline, the size and general responsibilities of the committees, and the jurisdiction of the committees. Information that is not incorporated in the bylaws must still be provided to the medical society's membership, for example, in a policy manual.

Provisions for temporary committee members should be included for cases in which there is an insufficient number of committee members who qualify as impartial decision makers. Committee members will not meet the requirement of impartiality if they have prior involvement in the matter of if they have a conflict of interest.

Complaints: The handling of all complaints should include prompt acknowledgement, immediate review, impart hearings, and transmittal of the decisions up to those concerned.

Complaints may be filed by any person, professional or lay. While complaints are commonly filed by patients, they may also be filed by family or friends of patients or by colleagues of the physician. Ordinarily, complaints should be submitted in writing, and a simple form may be developed for the filing of complaints. The form should include places for the person making the complaint (the "complainant") to state: his/her name and address, the name and address of the physician against whom the complaint is being

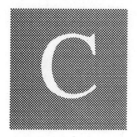

filed, the names and addresses of any other persons who have knowledge of the facts involved, and a brief description of the reasons why the complaint is being filed. In addition, the medical society should ask for permission from the complainant, or the patient if the complainant is not the patient, to review the medical records that are relevant to the complaint. If permission is not received, then the complainant should be informed that it may not be possible to process the complaint. It may be appropriate to require that the complainant's signature be notarized to limit the possibility of abuse of the complaint process and to ensure that there is authority for the release of the patient's medical records.

When it is not feasible for the complaint to be submitted in writing, some societies permit the complaint to be presented orally, and the society's staff prepares a verbatim transcript of the complaint. Other societies find that a requirement of a written complaint does not present problems. If the patient is impaired, for example, a family member of friend can prepare the complaint. Because of the difficulties with accepting oral complaints, it may make sense to take them only on the exceptional cases in which it is not reasonable to require a written complaint.

Once a complaint has been received, it should be acknowledged promptly. The complainant should be informed of the procedures that the medical society will follow in response to the complaint. A simple brochure may be printed for this purpose. In particular, the complainant should be given a sense of the time that may be required before the complaint can be resolved. If the complainant understands that the process may be a lengthy one, than a good deal of impatience, frustration and anger may be avoided.

In some cases, because of fear of reprisal, the complainant may desire that his/her name be kept confidential. If possible, a request for confidentiality should be honored. However, the complainant's desire for anonymity may conflict with the physician's right to confront or respond to any testimony or evidence that is used against him/her. While in some cases, the physician may not need to know who filed the complaint in order to respond to the charges, in other cases, the physician will need to know the name of the complainant. In such cases, the complainant should be notified that further proceedings may not be possible if the complainant is unwilling to have his/her name disclosed. (GRE adapted from)

Guidebook for Medical Society Grievance Committees and Disciplinary Committees Chicago; American Medical Association. 1991 36 pp. OP632891

Contact to Complain:
Advertisements on TV & Radio:
Federal Trade Commission
Sixth St. and Pennsylvania Ave., NW
Washington, DC 20580
202/326-2222

Advertisements in Newspapers:
Contact Regional Federal Trade Commission:

Clinics
Better Business Bureau
1515 Wilson Blvd., Arlington, VA 22209
202/276-0100
Contact local Better Business Bureau

Hospitals
Contact appropriate state or local hospital council

Physicians
Contact county or state medical society, not the American Medical Association.

Computers

American Association for Medical Systems and Informatics
1101 Connecticut Ave., NW Ste 700
Washington, DC 20036
202/857-1189

American Medical Informatics Association
4915 St. Elmo Ave, Suite 302
Bethesda, MD 20814
301/657-1291

Medical/Computer Journals:

"Computers and Medicine"
PO Box 36, Glencoe, IL 60022
708/446-3100
ISSN# 0163-0547

"M.D. Computing"
Springer-Verlag, 175 Fifth Ave.
New York, NY 10010
212/460-1500
ISSN 0724-6811

"Physicians and Computers"
Physicians Publications, Limited Partnership
2333 Waukegan Rd., Suite S-280
Bannockburn, IL 60015
ISSN# 708-940-8333

Consultants and Consulting Organizations

American Association of Healthcare Consultants
11208 Waples Mill Road, Suite 109
Fairfax, VA 22030
703/691-2242

Society of Medical-Dental Management Consultants (SMD)
7318 Raytown Road, Raytown, MO 64133
800/826-2264
In Missouri: 816/353-8488

Society of Professional Business Consultants (SPBC)
600 S. Federal St., Chicago, IL 60605
312/922-6222

Consumer Health Information Centers
Encourage Information Therapy

Katherine Lindner "A Piece of My Mind" JAMA.
1992 May 20; 267(19): 2592

About 8 years ago, all health professionals and the public had unrestricted access to the medical library where I was then employed, but patients were required to "ask their doctor" for information from the library. When patients themselves came in or called the library directly, many situations arose that required delicate handling and resulted in rather embarrassing situations. I would have to say, "Our policy requires that I consult with your physician. Sometimes he or she likes to help us select material for you. This arrangement can help you communicate better with your physician." Some patients who became perturbed by this policy might try sending a relative to the public library or might send their family member to get the materials from us later. We could give the materials to family members since they were "members of the public," but if we knew they were going to give the information to a patient, we had to explain and deal with the "doctor-approval policy."

As I became more distraught by the manner in which I had to handle patient requests for information, I began to investigate the ethics of restricting access to any information. The mandate to open medical libraries to health consumers has been with us since 1982, as stated in the President' Commission on Ethical Practices in Medicine. The Library Bill of Rights states that libraries should challenge censorship, and the American Library Association Statement of Professional Ethics states that librarians should protect each user's right to privacy.

The Office of Intellectual Freedom of the American Library Association also pointed out that there are state laws that guarantee confidentiality for library patrons (for example, New Jersey statute a:73-43.2 entitled "Confidentiality of Library Users' Records"). According to the administrators in the Intellectual Freedom Office, the policy of giving information to a patient only through his or her physician both breaches the patient's confidentiality and breaks the law by revealing the question to a third party, the physician.

The Medical Library Association has formulated standards for certain-sized hospital libraries recommending reference services to patients and the public. At the Medical Library Association's annual convention in Washington, DC, this week the membership will be voting to adopt the MLA Code of Ethics, which includes an ethical obligation "to advocate access to health information for all." There is a Consumer and Patient Health Information Section of the Medical Library Association with about 300 members, but there are still many medical libraries that are closed to consumers and many physicians who think it is inappropriate for health consumers to use them.

After becoming aware of the ethical standards and recommendations, the Englewood Hospital Library staff developed guidelines for providing information to patients and the public. We explain

that questions are kept confidential. We include a disclaimer letter with the material we send to health consumers at home or in the hospital. We state that we are nor recommending any particular treatment; that this material might not represent all that is available on the subject; that the information might not apply specifically to the patient's own condition; and that the material should be used to formulate questions for discussion with his or her physician.

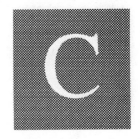

The following represent typical questions at our state-funded Regional Consumer Health Information Center. We received a phone call from a health consumer who wanted information on phrenic nerve paralysis secondary to the use of a Hickman catheter for chemotherapy. A man called whose wife was scheduled to have knee replacement surgery: "Can I stop in to pick up some information? She has to make up her mind." A public librarian called: "I have a patron who is interested in the latest research on amyotrophic lateral sclerosis." Consumers also request PDQ (Physician Data Query) computer searches on cancer treatment and protocols around the United States. Often a patient will find an alternative procedure or therapy in another area of the country, call the researcher, and ask for advice. Sometimes surgery is avoided; sometimes treatments are found that the patient's physician had not discussed. Some physicians wonder how we handle providing information on a disease with a probable fatal outcome. We always ask the person what he or she already knows. In 100% of the cases, the person already knew the prognosis and was presently looking for any new therapies.

Every scrap of information leading patients in the direction of discovering more about their disease becomes "information therapy." We have found that the physician-patient relationship is greatly enhanced when the physician says to the patient, "Go to the library, read about your disease, let me know what you find, and we'll discuss it." The process of finding information gives the patient a sense of control and empowerment. It is also a challenge for today's physicians to keep up with the great volume of medical literature by reading current journals, making information requests to libraries, and taking advantage of the new on-line and CD-ROM technologies that enable users to search MEDLINE from their office computers. All the information gathered by the patient and the physician is beneficial for continued care and treatment decisions.

Physicians and health professionals should continue on the path of sending their patients through the doors of medical libraries. Judging from the questions we librarians receive, there may be an information gap between what physicians are providing to patients and what patients want to know. Physicians can take advantage of consumer health library collections to build their own medical office resources. At the June 1991 meeting of the American Medical Association House of Delegates,, a resolution (No. 237) was proposed that encouraged hospitals and medical schools to make their libraries accessible for use by patients and their families. As the AMA Board of Trustees continues to study this resolution, we hope it will also encourage funding for consumer health resources and library staffing and medical school libraries.

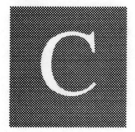

At a conference in June 1991, Dr. Bernie Siegel said, "The word patient means a submissive sufferer. If you have an illness, please just get the word uncooperative into your medical record. You do that and your statistics improve dramatically." We assume "uncooperative" means asking millions of questions, being persistent, examining one's own medical records, and so on. I am hoping that patients will get in their charts that they have "researched their disease [or procedure] in the medical library." Patients will be more satisfied with their care as they become more knowledgeable and participate in the decision-making process.

Center for Medical Consumers
237 Thompson St., New York, NY 10012
212/674-7105

Community Health Information Library
Hamady Health Sciences Library
Hurley Medical Center
One Hurley Plaza, Flint, MI 48502
313/257-9000

Consumer Health Information Network,
Mary Lou Himes Burton, 19 S. 22nd St.,
The College of Physicians of Philadelphia,
Philadelphia, PA 19103
215/561-6050

Consumer Information Center
Pueblo, CO 81009

Health Education Center
5th Avenue Pl., Ste 313
Pittsburgh, PA 15222-3099
412/392-3160

Health Library, Kaiser Permanente Medical Center
280 W. MacArthur Blvd., 12th floor
Oakland, CA 94611
415/428-6569

National Center for Health Education
30 East 29th Street, New York, NY 10016
212/689-1886

National Health Information Center
PO Box 1133, Washington, DC 20013-1133
800/336-4797

Office of Disease Prevention and Health Promotion
U.S. Department of Health and Human Services
800/336-4797, 301/565-4167

Consumer Health Protection

Contact local/state Dept. of Public Health
Consumer Protection Hotline:
Contact state Attorney General's office

Center for Science in the Public Interest
1501 16th Street, N.W., Washington, D.C. 20036
202/332/9110

Consumer Price Index
Bureau of Labor Statistics
441 G Street, N.W., Washington, DC 20212
202/523-1221

Consumer Product Safety
The Consumer Product Safety Commission protects the public against unreasonable risks of injury from consumer products; assists consumers in evaluating the comparative safety of consumer products; develops uniform safety standards for consumer products and minimizes conflicting State and local regulations; and promotes research and investigation into the causes and prevention of product-related deaths, illnesses and injuries.(USG)

Consumer Product Safety Commission
5401 Westbard Ave., Bethesda, MD 20207
800/638-2772, 301/492-6580
hearing impaired teletypewriter 800-638-8270

Contact Lens
Contact Lens Association of Ophthalmologists, Inc.
523 Decatur Street, Suite 1
New Orleans, LA 70130-1027
504/581-4000

Continuing Medical Education
Accreditation
Accreditation Council for Continuing Medical Education
PO Box 245, Lake Bluff, IL 60044
708/295-1490

Intrastate Accreditation:
Apply to state medical association.

Continuing Medical Education Learning Assessment Form (CLAF)
The CLAF is designed for use by a sponsor of continuing medical education courses to provide information about training in new procedures for which the physician will request new or expanded privileges. CLAF is not intended to document competency in a specific procedure. It is not designed for sponsors to use in all CME activities or for sponsors to use in CME courses on procedures that will not support a physician's request for a new or expanded hospital privileges. It may be useful to hospital credentialing committees as part of the evidence considered in their privileging decisions.

This form is available from:
The American Hospital Association or
The Continuing Medical Education Division of the American Medical Association.

Network for Continuing Medical Education
One Harmon Plaza, 7th Floor
Secaucus, NJ 07094
201/867-7600

Continuing Medical Education Opportunities
American Educational Institute
401 South Woodward Ave, #333
Birmingham, MI 48009
800/354-3507, FAX 313/433-0615

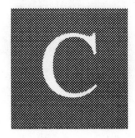

American Seminar Institute
PO Box 1400, Carbondale, CO 81623
800/446-5599, FAX 303/963-9112

Continuing Medical Education Directory 1992-1993
Chicago; American Medical Association 1992; 206
pp. ISBN 0-89970 5-057OP 412492AW

"Physicians' Travel and Meeting Guide"
a monthly publication that breaks down meeting
information by state, subject, sponsoring
organization, plus articles of travel interest.
PO Box 173306, Denver, CO 80217-3306
ISSN # 0745-4554
Subscriptions 800/637-6087

Cooley's Anemia
AHEPA Cooley's Anemia Foundation
1707 L St., NW, Washington, DC 20036
202/628-4974, 800/759-1515

Correctional Health Care
National Commission on Correctional Health Care
2105 N. Southport, Suite 200, Chicago, IL 60614
312/528-0818

County Medical Societies
List of County Medical Societies can be found in
Directory of Officials and Staff. American Medical
Association, Chicago, 1993. 164 pp.
ISBN 0-89970-529-4. OP311293

Credentialing
For Professional:
Data Bank (Information prior to 1990)
Federation of State Medical Boards
of the United States
6000 Western Place/Suite 707
Fort Worth, TX 76107
817/735-8445

National Physician Credentials Verification Service
AMA/Data Resource Development 800-677-6287

National Practitioner Data Bank
(Established under the Health Care Quality
Improvement Act)
UNISYS Corporation
8301 Greensboro Dr., Suite 1100
McLean, VA 22102
800/767-6732

For Public:
*American Medical Association Directory of
Physicians in the United States.* 33rd edition.
American Medical Association, Chicago. 1992.
4 volumes. ISBN 0-89970-523-5 OP390892.

Doctor Certification Line
American Board of Medical Specialties
800/776-2378 (information on board certification)

Critical Care
Board Certification
American Board of Anesthesiology
100 Constitution Plaza, Hartford, CT 06103
203/522-9857

American Board of Internal Medicine
U. City Science Ctr, 3624 Market St., Philadelphia,
PA 19104
215/243-1500
800/441-ABIM (800/441-2246)

American Board of Neurological Surgery
Smith Tower, Suite 2139, 6550 Fannin St.
Houston, TX 77030-2701
713/790-6015

American Board of Obstetrics and Gynecology
4225 Roosevelt Way, NE, Ste. 305
Seattle, WA 98105
206/547-4884

Pediatric Critical Care:
American Board of Pediatrics
111 Silver Cedar Ct., Chapel Hill, NC 27514
919/929-0461

Surgical Critical Care
American Board of Surgery
1617 John F. Kennedy Blvd., Ste. 860,
Philadelphia, PA 19103
215/568-4000

Society of Critical Care Medicine
8101 Kaiser Blvd, Anaheim, CA 92808-2214
714/282-6000

Cryosurgery
American College of Cryosurgery
1567 Maple Ave., Evanston, IL 60201
708/869-3954

Cults
Cult Hotline and Clinic
1651 Third Avenue, New York, NY 10028,
212/860-8533

Task Force on Cults
711 Third Avenue, 12th Floor
New York, NY 10017
212/983-4977

Current Procedural Terminology (CPT)
Coding Tips
Listed below are some general tips to ensure
accurate reporting of services performed by
physicians:
• Use current CPT Codes. CPT is updated
   annually; using an outdated code may delay the
   processing of the health insurance claims
   submitted.
• A Physician should update his superbill each
   year to correspond with the annual CPT code
   changes.
   The superbill should reflect the CPT codes for
   all the services an MD performs (e.g., all levels
   of service, common procedures).

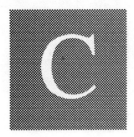

Allow ample space on the superbill to write in CPT and ICD-9 codes used infrequently, or to accommodate the use of modifiers.

ICD-9 Codes should be used at their highest level of specificity (e.g., assign the fifth digit subclassification code for those categories where it exists).
• Make sure the diagnoses and procedures performed match.
  The specific diagnosis/condition warranting each service should be included and linked to that service.
• Select the most specific CPT and ICD-9 code available to code the services documented by the physician.
  This may entail asking for clarification from the physician if the information/document is unclear or insufficient.
• Attend coding workshops to learn how to code effectively based on the latest information available.(CPT)

Many inquiries about the CPT process are received by the AMA e.g., how does a code get assigned for a service or a procedure performed by a physician? The following essay presents a brief history of the CPT which includes an overview of the CPT process.

How was CPT developed?: CPT was first developed and published by the American Medical Association (AMA) in 1966. This first edition was designed to serve as a method to cultivate the use of standard terms and descriptors for documentation of procedures in the medical record; to facilitate the communication of accurate information on procedures and services to agencies concerned with insurance claims; to provide the basis for a computer oriented system for the evaluation of operative procedures; and to contribute basic information for actuarial and statistical purposes.

The first edition of CPT was a preliminary document that included primarily surgical procedures, with limited sections on medicine, radiology and laboratory procedures. In 1970, the second edition was published and was presented as an expanded system of terms and codes for the designation of diagnostic and therapeutic procedures in surgery, medicine and the specialties. At this time, a five digit coding system was introduced, to replace the former four digit classification. Another significant change in the second edition was a listing of procedures relating to internal medicine.

In the mid to late 1970's, the third and fourth editions of CPT were introduced. The fourth edition, published in 1977, represented significant updates in medical technology. In this edition, a system of periodic updating was introduced to keep pace with the rapidly changing medical environment.

In 1983, CPT was adopted as part of the Health Care Financing Administration's (HCFA) Common Procedure Coding System (HCPCS). With this adoption, HCFA mandated the use of HCPCS for the reporting of services for Part B of the Medicare Program. By October 1986, HCFA had also required the use of HCPCS by State Medical

agencies for use in the Medical Management Information System. In July 1987, as part of the Omnibus Budget Reconciliation Act, HCFA mandated the use of CPT for reporting outpatient hospital surgical procedures.

Today, in addition to use in federal programs (Medicare and Medicaid), CPT is used extensively throughout the United States as the preferred system of coding and describing physicians' services.

Who maintains CPT?: The CPT Editorial Panel has the responsibility for the maintenance of CPT. This Panel is made up of twelve physicians, eight nominated by the AMA and one each nominated by the Blue Cross and Blue Shield Association, the Health Insurance Association of America, the Health Care Financing Administration and the American Hospital Association. This Panel of physicians has the authority to revise, update or modify CPT.

The American Medical Association provides staff support for the CPT Editorial Panel. The AMA appoints a staff secretary who is responsible for recording the minutes of the meetings and keeping records as are necessary for the work of the Panel.

Supporting the Editorial Panel in its work is the CPT Advisory Committee. The Advisory Committee is made up primarily of physicians nominated by the National Medical Specialty Societies represented in the AMA House of Delegates. The primary objectives are: 1) to serve as a resource to the Editorial Panel, by advising them on procedure coding and nomenclature as relevant to the member's specialty; 2) to provide documentation to staff and the Editorial Panel regarding the medical appropriateness of various medical and surgical procedures; and 3) to suggest revisions to CPT. Most of the work of the Advisory Committee is conducted through AMA Staff by letter and telephone. The Advisory Committee meets annually, to discuss items of mutual concern and to keep abreast of current issues in coding and nomenclature.

How are suggestions for changes to CPT reviewed?: A very specific pathway is followed when a suggestion is received for a revision of CPT, whether it be an addition or deletion of a code or modification of existing nomenclature.

First, AMA staff reviews all correspondence to evaluate coding suggestions. If it is determined that the question has already been addressed by the Panel, the requestor is informed of the Panel's interpretation. However, if it is determined that the request is a new issue or significant new information is received on an item that has been previously reviewed by the Panel, it is referred to the appropriate members of the Advisory Committee. If the advisors that have been contacted agree that no new code or revision is needed, then AMA staff responds to the requestor, providing information on how existing codes should be used to report the procedure.

However, if all advisors concur that a change should be made, or if two or more advisors disagree or give conflicting information, then the issue is referred to the Editorial Panel for resolution.

In addition to the Advisory Committee opinions, current medical periodicals and textbooks are used to provide up to date information about the procedure or service. Further data is also obtained about the efficacy and clinical utility of procedures from other sources like the AMA's Diagnostic and Therapeutic Technology Assessment Program (DATTA) and various other technology assessment panels.

Agenda materials for each Panel meeting are prepared by AMA staff. The topics for the agenda are gathered from several sources. Medical specialty societies, individual physicians, hospitals, third party payers and other interested parties may submit material for consideration by the Editorial Panel. Agenda materials are sent to Panel members at least 30 days in advance of each meeting. This gives each Panel member time to review the material and to confer with experts on each subject, as appropriate.

The CPT Editorial Panel meets quarterly and regularly faces complex problems associated with new and emerging technologies, as well as the difficulties encountered with outmoded procedures. The Panel addresses nearly 150 major topics a year, which typically involves over 2,000 votes on individual items.

The final meeting prior to publication of a new volume of CPT is held in August. For example, the August 1990 Panel meeting was the final meeting for changes to be made in CPT 1991.

How can I submit a suggestion for changes to CPT?: The effectiveness of CPT is dependent on constant updating to reflect changes in medical practice. This can only be accomplished through the interest and timely suggestions of practicing physicians, medical specialty societies, state medical associations and those who deal regularly with medical records. Accordingly, the AMA welcomes correspondence, inquiries and suggestions concerning old and new procedures.(CPT)

Current Procedural Terminology (CPT 1992), 4th ed., American Medical Association, Chicago. 1992
Book: ISBN 0-89970-443-3 OP054192
Floppy Disk: OP052491

Curriculum Vitae

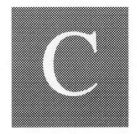

Outline for Physician Curriculum Vitae:
Name:
Address: (Home and office/hospital)
Telephone: (Home and office/hospital)
Certification and Licensure: (For example, Board Certified in Internal Medicine, September 1978; or Diplomate National Board of Medical Examiners, July 1978)
Education: (List in descending order, with most recent first, noting name of university, degree received, and dates)
Postgraduate Training: (List all training, such as internship, residency, and fellowships, with name of institution and dates)
Practice Experience: (List in descending order, with most recent first)
Professorial or Teaching Appointments:
Awards or Honors:
Professional Society Memberships:
Personal and Professional References: (Furnished on request)
Bibliography: (Presentations and publications)

Cystic Fibrosis

Cystic Fibrosis Foundation
6931 Arlington Road, Bethesda, MD 20814
800/344-4823, 301/951-4422

Cytotechnology

History: In the pioneer days of clinical pathology, it was the rare pathologist who did not have an assistant. These first technical "assistants," some of whom were trained by George N. Papanicolaou, MD, famed American anatomist and cytologist, were always the product of an apprentice type training. As their number and the number of "apprentice programs" grew, there was a need to certify that the "apprentices" had indeed learned their tasks well. The Board of Registry of the American Society of Clinical Pathologists (ASCP) offered the examination for the cytology technician for the first time in 1957.

Five years later, in 1962, the Essentials of an Acceptable School for the Cytotechnologists were developed by the Cytology Committee of the ASCP and the ASCP Board of Schools and were adopted by the House of Delegates of the AMA. Until 1975 representatives of the American Society of Clinical Pathologists served on the Cytotechnology Review Committee of the National Accrediting Agency for Clinical Laboratory Sciences (NAACLS), which replaced the ASCP Board of Schools in 1974. In 1975, the American Society of Cytology (ASC) was recognized as the organization which would collaborate with the AMA Council on Medical Education, and the ASC formed the Cytotechnology Programs Review Committee, which assumed the responsibilities formerly handled by NAACLS. In 1977 and 1983, the cytotechnology Essentials and Guidelines were revised and adopted by the AMA Council on Medical Education and the American Society of Cytology.

Occupational description: Cytology is the study of the structure and the function of cells. Cytotechnologists are trained medical laboratory technologists who work with pathologists to detect changes in body cells which may be important in the early diagnosis of cancer. This is done primarily with the microscope used to screen slide preparations of body cells for abnormalities in

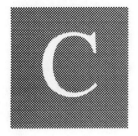

structure, indicating either benign or malignant conditions.

Job Description: Using special techniques, cytotechnologists prepare cellular samples for study under the microscope and assist in the diagnosis of disease by the examination of the samples. Cell specimens may be obtained form various body sites, such as the female reproductive tract, the oral cavity, the lung, or any body cavity shedding cells. Using the findings of cytotechnologists, the physician is then able in many instances to diagnose cancer long before it can be detected by other methods. Cytologic techniques can also be used to detect diseases involving hormonal abnormalities and other pathological disease processes. In recent years fine needles have been used to aspirate lesions, often deeply seated in the body, thus greatly enhancing the ability to diagnose tumors located in inaccessible sites.

Employment Characteristics: Most cytotechnologists work in hospitals or in private laboratories, while some prefer to work on research projects or to teach. Employment opportunities vary depending on geographic location, experience, and ability. The demand for trained cytotechnologists is high and is projected to remain high.

According to the 1990 CAHEA Annual Supplemental Survey, entry level salaries average $27,772. (ALL)

AMA Division of Allied Health
312/464-4625

American Society of Cytology
1015 Chestnut Street, Philadelphia, PA 19107
215/922-3880

Dalkon Shield

American College of Obstetricians and
Gynecologists
409 12th Street, S.W., Washington, DC 20024
202/638-5577

Dance Medicine

Center For Dance Medicine
41 E. 42nd Street, Room 200
New York, NY, 10017
212/661-8401

Dance Therapist. Plans, organizes, and leads
dance and body movement activities to improve
patients' mental outlooks and physical
well-beings: Observes and evaluates patient's
mental and physical disabilities to determine
dance and body movement treatment. Confers
with patient and medical personnel to develop
dance therapy program, Conducts individual and
group dances sessions to improve patient's
mental and physical well-being. Makes changes in
patient's program based on observation and
evaluation of progress. Attends and participates in
professional conferences and workshops to
enhance efficiency and knowledge.(DOT)

Dental

Dentist. Diagnoses and treats diseases, injuries,
and malformations of teeth and gums, and related
oral structures: Examines patient to determine
nature of condition, utilizing x rays, dental
instruments, and other diagnostic procedures.
Cleans, fills, extracts, and replaces teeth using
rotary and hand instruments, dental appliances,
medication, and surgical implements. Provides
preventive dental services to patient, such as
applications of fluoride and sealants to teeth, and
education in oral and dental hygiene. (DOT)

American Dental Association
211 E. Chicago Ave., Chicago, IL 60611
312/440-2500
Library open to public 8:30-5:00

Dental Assistant. Assists dentist during
examination and treatment of patients: Prepares
patient, sterilizes and disinfects instruments, sets
up instrument trays, prepares materials, and
assists dentist during dental procedures. Takes
and records medical and dental histories and vital
signs of patient. Exposes dental diagnostic x rays.
Makes preliminary impressions for study casts
and occlusal registrations for mounting study
casts. Pours, trims, and polishes study casts,
fabricates temporary restorations. Assists dentist
in management of medical and dental
emergencies. Instructs patients on oral hygiene
and plaque control programs. Provides
postoperative instructions prescribed by dentist.
Records treatment information in patient records.
Schedules appointments, prepares bills and
receives payment for dental services, completes
insurance forms, and maintains clerical records,
manually or using computer. May clean teeth,
using dental instruments. May apply protective
coating of fluoride to teeth. (DOT)

American Dental Assistants Association (ADAA)
919 N. Michigan Ave., Ste. 3400
Chicago, IL 60611
312-664-3327

Dental Hygienist. Performs dental prophylaxis:
Cleans calcareous deposits, accretions, and
stains from teeth and beneath margins of gums,
using dental instruments. Feels lymph nodes
under patient's chin to detect swelling or
tenderness that could indicate presence of oral
cancer. Feels and visually examines gums for
sores and signs of disease. Examines gums,
using probes, to locate periodontal recessed gums
and signs of gum disease. Applies fluorides and
other cavity preventing agents to arrest dental
decay. Charts conditions of decay and disease for
diagnosis and treatment by dentist. Exposes and
develops x-ray film. Makes impressions for study
casts. May remove sutures and dressings. May
administer local anesthetic agents. May place and
remove rubber dams, matrices, and temporary
restorations. May place, carve and finish amalgam
restorations. May remove excess cement from
coronal surfaces of teeth. May provide clinical
services and health education to improve and
maintain oral health of school children. May
conduct dental health clinics for community groups
to augment services of dentist.(DOT)

American Dental Hygienists Association (ADHA)
444 N. Michigan Ave., Suite 3400
Chicago, IL 60611
312-440-8929

National Institute of Dental Research
9000 Rockville Pike, Bethesda, MD 20892
301/496-4261

Dental Associations, Statewide

Alabama Dental Association
836 Washington Ave., Montgomery, AL 36104
205/265-1684

Alaska Dental Society
3400 Spenard Rd., Ste. 10, Anchorage, AK 99503
907- 277-4675

Arizona State Dental Association
4131 N. 36th St.,Phoenix, AZ 85018
602/957-4777

Arkansas State Dental Association
920 W. 2nd St., No. 204, Little Rock, AR 72201
501/372-3368

California Dental Association
PO Box 13749, Sacramento, CA 95853
916/443-0505

Colorado Dental Association
7535 E. Hampton Ave., Ste. 505
Denver, CO 80231
303/671-6600

Connecticut State Dental Association
62 Russ St., Hartford, CT 06106
203/278-5550

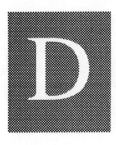

Delaware State Dental Society
1925 Lovering Ave., Wilmington, DE 19806
302/654-4335

District of Columbia Dental Society
502 C St. NE, Washington, DC 20002
202/547-7613

Florida Dental Association
3021 Swann Ave., Tampa, FL 33609
813/877-7597

Georgia Dental Association
2951 Flowers Rd. S., Ste. 112, Atlanta, GA 30341
404/458-6166

Hawaii Dental Association
1000 Bishop St., Ste. 805, Honolulu, HI 96813
808/536-2135

Idaho State Dental Association
1220 W. Hays, Boise, ID 83702
208/343-7543

Illinois State Dental Society
524 S. 5th St. PO Box 376, Springfield, IL 62705
217/525-1406

Indiana Dental Association
402 Jefferson Bldg. 1 Virginia Ave.
Indianapolis, IN 46204
317/634-2610

Iowa Dental Association
333 Insurance Exchange Bldg.
Des Moines, IA 50309
515/282-7250

Kansas Dental Association
5200 Huntoon, Topeka, KS 66604
913/272-7360

Kentucky Dental Association
1940 Princeton Dr. Louisville, KY 40205
502/459-5373

Louisiana Dental Association
3021 22nd St. Metairie, LA 70002
504/835-1612

Maine Dental Association
Association Dr. PO Box 215,
Manchester, ME 04351
207/622-7900

Maryland State Dental Association
6470 Dobbin Rd. Columbia, MD 21045
301/964-2880

Massachusetts Dental Society
83 Speen St. Natick, MA 01760
508/651-7511

Michigan Dental Association
230 N. Washington Sq., No. 208
Lansing, MI 48933
517/372-9070

Minnesota Dental Association
2236 Marshall Ave. St. Paul, MN 55104
612/646-7454

Mississippi Dental Association
2630 Ridgewood Rd. Jackson, MS 39216
601/982-0442

Missouri Dental Association
230 W. McCarty St. PO Box 1707
Jefferson City, MO 65102
314/634-3436

Montana Dental Association
PO Box 281 Helena, MT 59624
406/443-2061

Nebraska Dental Association
3120 O St., Lincoln, NE 68510
402/476-1704

Nevada Dental Association
6769 W. Charleston Blvd., No. D
Las Vegas, NV 89102
702/258-4230

New Hampshire Dental Society
PO Box 2229 Concord, NH 03301
603/225-5961

New Jersey Dental Association
1 Dental Plaza, North Brunswick, NJ 09802
201/821-9400

New Mexico Dental Association
3037 San Patricio NW, Albuquerque, NM 87107
505/345-9135

Dental Society of the State of New York
7 Elk St., Albany, NY 12207
518/465-0044

North Carolina Dental Society
PO Box 12047, Raleigh, NC 27605
919/832-1222

North Dakota Dental Association
419 Dakota Ave., Wahpeton, ND 58075
701/642-1881

Ohio Dental Association
1370 Dublin Rd.,Columbus, OH 43215
614/486-2700

Oklahoma Dental Association
629 W. Interstate 44, Service Rd.
Oklahoma City, OK 73118
405/ 848-8873

Oregon Dental Association
17898 SW McEwan Rd. Portland, OR 97224
503- 620-3230

Pennsylvania Dental Association
3501 N. Front St. PO Box 3341
Harrisburg, PA 17105
717/234-5941

Colegio de Cirujanos Dentistas de Puerto Rico
Avenue Domenech No. 200, Hato Rey, PR 00918
809/764-1969

Rhode Island Dental Association
200 Centerville Pl. Warwick, RI 02886
401/732-6833

South Carolina Dental Association
723 Queen St. Columbia, SC 29205
803/799-3649

South Dakota Dental Association
108 W. Dakota Ave. PO Box 1194
Pierre, SD 57501
605/224-9133

Tennessee Dental Association
2104 Sunset Pl. PO Box 120188
Nashville, TN 37212
615/383-8962

Texas Dental Association
1946 S. Interregional Hwy. Austin, TX 78704
512/443-3675

Utah Dental Association
1151 East 3900 South, Ste. B-160
Salt Lake City, UT 84124
801/ 261-5315

Vermont State Dental Society
132 Church St.,Burlington, VT 05401
802/864-0115

Virgin Islands Dental Association
4th St. Sugar Estate Road
Charlotte Amalie, VI 00802
809/774-1464

Virginia Dental Association
5006 Monument Ave., PO Box 6906
Richmond, VA 23230
804/358-4927

Washington State Dental Association
2033 6th Ave., No. 333, Seattle, WA 98121
206/448-1914

West Virginia Dental Association
300 Capitol St., No. 1002, Charleston, WV 25301
304/344-5246

Wisconsin Dental Association
633 W. Wisconsin Ave., Milwaukee, WI 53203
414/276-4520

Wyoming Dental Association
814 S. David, Casper, WY 82601
307/234-0777

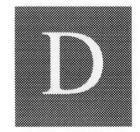

Dermatology

Dermatologist alternate titles: skin specialist.
Diagnoses and treats diseases of human skin:
Examines skin to determine nature of disease,
taking blood samples and smears for affected
areas, and performing other laboratory
procedures. Examines specimens under
microscope, and makes various chemical and
biological analyses and performs other tests to
identify disease-causing organisms or pathological
conditions. Prescribes and administers
medications, and applies superficial radiotherapy
and other localized treatments. Treats abscesses,
skin injuries, and other skin infections, and
surgically excises cutaneous malignancies, cysts,
birthmarks, and other growths. Treats scars, using
dermabrasion. (DOT)

American Academy of Dermatology
930 N. Meacham Road, PO Box 4014,
Schaumburg, IL 60168
708/330-0230, FAX 708/330-0050

American Board of Dermatology
Henry Ford Hospital, Detroit, MI 48202
313/876-2178

American Society for Dermatologic Surgery
930 N. Meacham Road, PO Box 4014,
Schaumburg, IL 60168
708/330-0230, FAX 708/330-0050
800/441-ASDS (800/441-2737)

D.E.B.R.A. of America, Inc.
(Dystrophic Epidermolysis Bullosa Research
Association)
141 Fifth Avenue, Suite 7-South
New York, NY 10010
212/995-2220

National Foundation for Ectodermal Dysplasia
108 N. First St., Suite 311, Mascoutah, IL 62258
618/566-2020

Society for Investigative Dermatology, Inc.
1001 Potrero St., Room 269, Bldg., 100
San Francisco, CA 94110
415/647-3992

Xeroderma Pigmentosum Registry
c/o Dept. of Pathology
Medical Science Bldg Room C 520
NJ Medical School,
185 South Orange Avenue
Newark, NJ 07103-2757
201/456-6255

Devices, Medical

Association for the Advancement
of Medical Instrumentation,
3330 Washington Blvd., Ste 400
Arlington, VA 22201
703/525-4890

For Health Care Professional to report malfunction:
USP 800/638-6725 (24 hour)
FDA 301/881-0256 (7:00 a.m. to 4:30 p.m. EST)

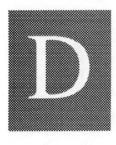

ECRI (to evaluate health care technology)
5200 Butler Pike, Plymouth Meeting, PA 19462
215/825-6700 or 6000

Health Industry Distributors Association
225 Reinekers Lane, #650, Alexandria, VA 22314
703/549-4432

Health Industry Manufacturers Association
1200 G Street, NW, Suite 400
Washington, DC 20005
202/783-8700

Medical Device Register: United States
and Canada:
Official Directory of Medical Suppliers. 1991.
2 vol., ISBN 0-942036-38-7
**international volume also available

Medical Device Register, Inc.
55 Washington Blvd, Stamford, CT 06901
203/348-6319

National Association of Medical
Equipment Suppliers
625 Slaters Lane, Suite 200, Alexandria, VA 22314
703/836-6263

Diabetes

American Diabetes Association
National Service Center, 1660 Duke St.,
Alexandria, VA 22314
703/549-1500 800/232-3472

National Diabetes Information Clearinghouse
Box NDIC, Bethesda, MD 20892
301/468-2162

Juvenile Diabetes Foundation
432 Park Ave., New York, NY 10016
800/223-1138
NY 212/889-7575

Diabetes Associations, Statewide

American Diabetes Association Alabama Affiliate
3 Office Park Circle, Suite 115
Birmingham, AL 35223
205/870-5172

American Diabetes Association Alaska Affiliate
4241 B St, Suite 102, Anchorage, AK 99503
907/563-6015

American Diabetes Association Arizona Affiliate
2328 W Royal Palm Road, Suite D, PO Box
37579, Phoenix, AZ 85069
602/995-1515

American Diabetes Association Arkansas Affiliate
11500 N Rodney Parham, Suite 19-20
Little Rock, AR 72212
501/221-7444

American Diabetes Association California Affiliate
10445 Old Placerville Road
Sacramento, CA 95827
916/369-0999

American Diabetes Association Colorado Affiliate
2450 S Downing St, Denver, CO 80210
303/778-7556

American Diabetes Association
Connecticut Affiliate
40 South St, West Hartford, CT 06110
203/953-4232

American Diabetes Association Delaware Affiliate
2713 Lancaster Ave, Wilmington, DE 19805
302/656-0030

American Diabetes Association District of
Columbia Affiliate
1211 Connecticut Ave, NW, No. 501
Washington, DC 20036
202/331-8303

American Diabetes Association Florida Affiliate
1101 N Lake Destiny Road, Suite 415
Maitland, FL 32751
407/660-1926

American Diabetes Association Georgia Affiliate
3783 Presidential Pkwy, Suite 102
Atlanta, GA 30340
404/454-8401

American Diabetes Association Hawaii Affiliate
510 S Beretania St, Honolulu, HI 96813
808/521-5677

American Diabetes Association Idaho Affiliate
1528 Vista Ave, Boise, ID 83705
208/342-2774

American Diabetes Association
Northern Illinois Affiliate
6 N Michigan Ave, Suite 1202, Chicago, IL 60602
312/346-1805

American Diabetes Association
Downstate Illinois Affiliate
2580 Federal Drive, Suite 403, Decatur, IL 62526
217/875-9011

American Diabetes Association Indiana Affiliate
222 S Downey Ave, Suite 320,
Indianapolis, IN 46219
317/352-9226

American Diabetes Association Iowa Affiliate
3829 71st St, Suite A, Marion, IA 50322
515/276-2237

American Diabetes Association Kansas Affiliate
3210 E Douglas, Wichita, KS 67208
316/684-6091

American Diabetes Association Kentucky Affiliate
745 W Main St, Suite 150, Louisville, KY 40202
502/589-3837

American Diabetes Association Louisiana Affiliate
9420 Lindale Ave, Suite B
Baton Rouge, LA 70815
504/927-7732

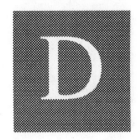

American Diabetes Association Maine Affiliate
9 Church St, PO Box 2208, Augusta, ME 04338
207/623-2232

American Diabetes Association Maryland Affiliate
2 Reservoir Circle, Suite 203
Baltimore, MD 21208
410/486-5515

American Diabetes Association
Massachusetts Affiliate
40 Speen St, Farmingham, MA 01701
508/879-1248

American Diabetes Association Michigan Affiliate
23100 Providence Drive, Suite 400
Southfield, MI 48075
313/552-0480

American Diabetes Association Minnesota Affiliate
715 Florida Ave S, Suite 307
Minneapolis, MN 55426
612/593-5333

American Diabetes Association Mississippi Affiliate
16 Northtown Drive, Suite 100
Jackson, MS 39211
601/957-7878

American Diabetes Association Missouri Affiliate
213 Adams St, PO Box 1674
Jefferson City, MO 65102
314/636-5552

American Diabetes Association Montana Affiliate
600 Central Plaza, Suite 201, Box 2411
Great Falls, MT 59403
406/761-0908

American Diabetes Association Nebraska Affiliate
2730 S 114th St, Omaha, NE 68144
402/333-5556

American Diabetes Association Nevada Affiliate
4045 S Spencer, Suite A-62
Las Vegas, NV 89119
702/369-9995

American Diabetes Association
New Hampshire Affiliate
104 Middle St, PO Box 595
Manchester, NH 03105
603/627-9579

American Diabetes Association
New Jersey Affiliate
312 N Adamsville Road, PO Box 6423,
Bridgewater, NJ 08807
908/725-7878

American Diabetes Association
New Mexico Affiliate
525 San Pedro NE, Suite 101
Albuquerque, NM 87108
505/266-5716

American Diabetes Association New York
Downstate Affiliate
505 8th Ave, New York, NY 10018
212/947-9707

American Diabetes Association New York
Upstate Affiliate
115 E Jefferson St, PO Box 1037
Syracuse, NY 13201
315/472-9111

American Diabetes Association
North Carolina Affiliate
2315-A Sunset Ave, Rocky Mount, NC 27804
919/937-4121

American Diabetes Association
North Dakota Affiliate
101 N Third St, Suite 400, Box 234, Grand Forks,
ND 58206-0234
701/746-4427

American Diabetes Association Ohio Affiliate
705-L Lakeview Plaza Blvd.
Worthington, OH 43085
614/436-1917

American Diabetes Association Oklahoma Affiliate
6465 S Yale Ave, Suite 519, Tulsa, OK 74136
918/492-3839

American Diabetes Association Oregon Affiliate
3607 SW Corbett St, Portland, OR 97201
503/228-0849

American Diabetes Association
Pennsylvania Affiliate
5020 Mechanicsburg, PA 17055
717/691-6170

American Diabetes Association
Puerto Rico Affiliate
Avenue Jesus T. Pineiro, 1161 Altos
Puerto Nuevo, PR 00920
809/793-1276

American Diabetes Association
Rhode Island Affiliate
250 Centerville Road, Warwick, RI 02886
401/738-5570

American Diabetes Association
South Carolina Affiliate
2838 Devine St, PO Box 50782
Columbia, SC 29250
803/799-4246

American Diabetes Association
South Dakota Affiliate
1524 W 20th St, PO Box 659
Sioux Falls, SD 57101
605/335-7670

American Diabetes Association Tennessee Affiliate
4004 Hillsboro Road, Suite B-216
Nashville, TN 37215
615/298-3066

American Diabetes Association Texas Affiliate
8140 N Mopac, Bldg 1, Suite 130
Austin, TX 78759
512/343-6981

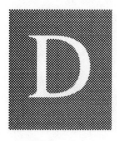

American Diabetes Association Utah Affiliate
643 East 400 South, Salt Lake City, UT 84102
801/363-3024

American Diabetes Association Vermont Affiliate
431 Pine St, Burlington, VT 05401
802/862-3882

American Diabetes Association Virginia Affiliate
404 8th St NE, Suite C, Charlottesville, VA 22901
804/293-4953

American Diabetes Association
Washington Affiliate
557 Roy St, LL, Seattle, WA 98103
206/282-4616

American Diabetes Association
West Virginia Affiliate
5625 MacCorkle, Kanawha City, WV 25364
304/925-6685

American Diabetes Association Wisconsin Affiliate
2949 N Mayfair Road, No. 306
Wauwatosa, WI 53222
414/778-5500

American Diabetes Association Wyoming Affiliate
2525 6th Ave, N, Billings, MT 59101
406/256-0616

Diagnostic and Statistical Manual of Mental Disorders (DSM III)

American Psychiatric Association
1400 K St., NW, Washington, DC 20005
202/682-6000

Diagnostic Medical Sonographer

History: In 1972, the American Society of Ultrasound Technical Specialists (ASUTS) appointed a committee to explore the mechanism of accreditation of educational programs for the ultrasound technical specialist through the American Medical Association (AMA) Council on Medical Education. In October 1973, members of ASUTS (now known as the Society of Diagnostic Medical Sonographers) met with a representative from the AMA Department of Health Manpower and initiated activities to receive formal recognition as occupation. One year later the occupation of diagnostic medical sonography received recognition by the AMA.

From 1974-79 the Essentials of an Accredited Educational Program for the Diagnostic Medical Sonographer were developed. Due to the multidisciplinary nature of diagnostic ultrasound, many interested medical and allied health organizations collaborated in drafting the Essentials, which were formally adopted by the following organizations: American College of Cardiology (withdrew as a sponsoring organization in 1983; resumed sponsorship in 1986,) American College of Radiology, American Institute of Ultrasound in Medicine, American Medical Association, American Society of Echocardiography, American Society of Radiologic Technologists, Society of Diagnostic Medical Sonographers, and Society of Nuclear Medicine (withdrew as a sponsoring organization in 1981). These organizations, with the exception

of the Society of Nuclear Medicine, currently sponsor the Joint Review Committee on Education in Diagnostic Medical Sonography. Educational programs were first accredited in January 1982.

Occupational Description: The diagnostic medical sonographer provides patient services, using diagnostic ultrasound under the supervision of a doctor of medicine or osteopathy responsible for the use of and interpretation of ultrasound procedures. The sonographer assists the physician in gathering sonographic data necessary to reach diagnostic decisions.

Job Description: The sonographer may provide patient services in a variety of medical settings in which the physician is responsible for the use and interpretation of ultrasound procedures. In assisting physicians in gathering sonographic data, the diagnostic medical sonographer is able to obtain, review, and integrate pertinent patient history and supporting clinical data to facilitate optimum diagnostic results; perform appropriate procedures and record anatomical pathological and/or physiological data for interpretation by a physician; record and process sonographic data and other pertinent observations made during the procedure for presentation to the interpreting physician; exercise discretion and judgment in the performance of sonographic services; provide patient education related to medical ultrasound; and promote principles of good health.

Employment Characteristics: Diagnostic medical sonographers may be employed in hospitals, clinics, private offices, and industry. There is also a need for suitably qualified educators, researchers, and administrators. The demand for sonographers continues to exceed the supply. The supply and demand ratio affects salaries, depending upon experience, job description, and geographical location.

According to the 1990 CAHEA Annual Supplemental Survey, entry level salaries average $26,538.

AMA Allied Health Department
312/464-4634

Dialysis Technician

Alternate titles: hemodialysis technician. Sets up and operates hemodialysis machine to provide dialysis treatment for patients with kidney failure: Attaches dialyzer and tubing to machine to assemble for use. Mixes dialysate, according to formula. Primes dialyzer with saline or heparinized solution to prepare machine for use. Transports patients to dialysis room and positions patient on lounge chair at hemodialysis machine. Takes and records patient's predialysis weight, temperature, blood pressure, pulse rate, and respiration rate. Explains dialysis procedure and operation of hemodialysis machine to patient before treatment to allay anxieties. Cleans area of access (fistula, graft, or catheter), using antiseptic solution. Connects hemodialysis machine to access in patient's forearm or catheter site to start blood circulating through dialyzer. Inspects equipment settings, including pressures conductivity (proportion of chemical to water), and temperature to ensure conformance to safety standards. Starts blood flow pump at prescribed rate. Inspect venous and arterial pressures as registered on equipment to ensure pressures are within

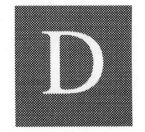

established limits. Calculates fluid removal or replacement to be achieved during dialysis procedure. Monitors patient for adverse reaction and hemodialysis machine for malfunction. Takes and record patient's postdialysis weight, temperature, blood pressure, pulse rate. May fabricate parts, such as cannulas, tubing, catheters, connectors, and fittings, using handtools. (DOT)

American Association of Nephrology
Nurses and Technicians
PO Box 56, North Woodbury Rd.
Pitman, NJ 08071
609/589-2187

Diet

Report of the Council on Scientific Affairs: Diet and Cancer: Where do matters stand?. Arch Intern Med 153(1) 1993 Jan 11. 50-6
During the past decade, the scientific literature base on the putative but elusive relationship between diet and cancer expanded enormously. Increased emphasis by funding agencies, fueled in turn by broadening public interest in the topic, led to this growth. The laboratory and epidemiologic research conducted in the past decade has shown that a simple solution does not exist. The key to the diet/cancer puzzle may lie in nutrient interactions and in individual response to dietary factors, determined in turn by genetic, physiologic and life-style factors. Given the rapid strides being made in furthering the understanding of the biochemistry and molecular biology of cancer, it may be possible to look forward to the day when optimal dietary and life-style guidelines can be tailored to a specific individualized basis.

Dietary fiber and health. Council on Scientific Affairs. JAMA. 1989 Jul 28; 262(4): 542-6
During the last 18 years, considerable research has been conducted on the role of dietary fiber in health and disease. Interest was stimulated by epidemiologic studies that associated a low intake of dietary fiber with the incidence of colon cancer, heart disease, diabetes, and other diseases and disorders. Dietary fiber is not a single substance. There are significant differences in the physiological effects of the various components of dietary fiber. A Recommended Dietary Allowance for dietary fiber has not been established. However, an adequate amount of dietary fiber can be obtained by choosing several servings daily from a variety of fiber-rich foods such as whole-grain breads and cereals, fruits, vegetables, legumes, and nuts.

JAMA Theme Issue: Cholesterol
JAMA. 1990 Dec. 19; 264(23)
This theme issue of JAMA presents several clinical articles discussing specific relationships of disease with and treatments for cholesterol problems. Two review articles, editorials, CDC reports, and various medical perspectives on Cholesterol round out what is printed here.

Dietitian, Clinical, alternate titles: dietitian, therapeutic. Plans therapeutic diets and implements preparation and service of meals for patients in hospital, clinic, or other health care facility: Consults with physician and other health care personnel to determine nutritional needs and diet restrictions, such as low fat or salt free, of patients. Formulates menus for therapeutic diets based on medical and physical condition of patients and integrates patient's menus with basic institutional menus. Inspects meals served for conformance to prescribed diets and for standards of palatability and appearance. Instructs patients and their families in nutritional principles, dietary plans, food selection, and preparation. May supervise activities of workers engaged in food. May teach nutrition and diet therapy to medical students and hospital personnel.(DOT)

American Dietetic Association
216 W. Jackson Blvd, Suite 800
Chicago, IL 60606
312/899-0040
Information line staffed by registered diatitians to answer nutritional questions:
800-366-1655

Diethylstilbestrol (DES)

DES Action-USA
c/o Long Island Jewish-Hillside Medical Center
New Hyde Park, NY 11040
516/775-3450

Legal turmoil over DES to continue
Manufacturer plans appeal

Richard Lewis AMNews 6/6/80

Eli Lilly and Co. will appeal court decisions in New York and California holding it liable for genital-tract abnormalities in the daughters of women who took diethylstilbestrol (DES) while pregnant.

The pharmaceutical firm is contesting a theory of joint liability in which the plaintiffs assert that all manufacturers of the allegedly carcinogenic drug are responsible for damages in proportion to their share of the market.

Product liability lawsuits are not unusual for any drug manufacturer, but the DES cases reveal the hidden snags in marketing a drug with unsuspected teratogenic effects that may not show up for years - or generations.

The DES claims are extraordinary because of the length of time that elapsed before the plaintiffs' injuries were discovered. Further, the plaintiffs are not the women who took the drug, but their children. Finally, Lilly has been directed to pay for damages that may have been caused by another manufacturer.

In the New York Supreme Court jury verdict last July, Lilly was told to pay $500,000 to 25-year-old Joyce Bichler, who charged that she contracted a rare form of vaginal cancer as a result of fetal exposure to DES.

As many as two million women took the drug, most during the 1950's, when many eminent clinicians considered the synthetic estrogen to be safe and effective for preventing miscarriages.

Although Bichler could not identify the specific brand of DES that caused her cancer, she named Lilly in the suit because it was an early and major manufacturer of DES.

Her attorneys - led by former New York state supreme court justice Leonard Finz - argued that the drug companies shared a common responsibility to test DES more thoroughly before putting it on the market.

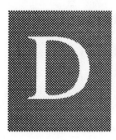

In a similar action, the California Supreme Court ruled March 20 that DES manufacturers could be ordered to pay damages according to their share of the market.

The 4-to-3 decision was a green light for two "DES daughters," Judith Sindell of Los Angeles and Maureen Rogers of Fontana, Calif., to proceed with their suits against Lilly and four other companies.

Like Bichler, the California women were unable to determine the source of the DES that their mothers took but they maintained that it was compounded from a common formula and that all the manufacturers knew or should have known that it could cause cancer.

The law generally requires plaintiffs to specify the manufacturers whose product caused the damages, but the California high court ruled that "...in an era of mass production and complex marketing methods, the traditional standard of negligence (is) insufficient to govern the obligations of the manufacturer to the consumer."

Raymond E. Rauch, senior counsel for Lilly, said that the decision amounts to a new theory of liability.

The decision "throws out all other theories of joint liability that have been advanced in other jurisdictions and adopts an entirely new liability based on market share.

"It makes some assumptions about market share that we believe are totally inaccurate, and doesn't recognize the problems that have been created by the opinion.

"We have petitioned for a re-hearing," Rauch told American Medical News.

In an interview, he added that the theory could be applied to other generic drugs and conceivably to other products that are interchangeable between manufacturers, including nails.

"If you step on a rusty nail you could sue the entire nail industry or pick out one nail manufacturer, if you can prove that he had a major share of the market, and make him pay the damages," the attorney said.

The Indianapolis-based company is currently a defendant in more than a hundred DES-related suits asking for a total of at least $3 billion in damages. Some claims have been settled out of court.

Plaintiffs contend that Lilly could have tested the drug on pregnant mice, sacrificed their offspring at the age of six months, operated on them surgically, and looked for cancer.

However, American pharmaceutical companies had tested the drug in clinical trial for nearly eight years before filing a new drug application with the Food and Drug Administration.

In the early 1950's, the FDA declared that DES was no longer a new drug, but was generally safe for the purposes it was being used for.

"From that time on, no one had to file a new drug application to market the drug. More than 200 companies began manufacturing DES and marketing it for the purpose of preventing accidents of pregnancy," according to Robert H. Furman, MD, vice president of corporate medical affairs for Lilly.

Lilly officials admit that they did not test the drug on pregnant mice. Had they done so, however, they still would not have found any inkling of the alleged carcinogenic effect, they contend.

"There is no animal model that would have flashed even a faint amber light...of caution that would make a company or any physician hesitant to use the drug for this purpose," according to Dr. Furman.

Toxicological studies still cannot convincingly demonstrates DES' alleged carcinogenicity, he said.

If the DES daughters are victorious in court, the drug company will have to pay a substantial portion of the losses form its own funds.

LLoyds of London and Home Insurance, New York, covered all of Lilly's liability until 1969, when Lilly decided to cut its costs by setting up a self-insurance program.

In 1976, the private carriers refused to continue coverage for the drug, and at present they neither concede nor deny that they are responsible for possible pay-out claimants.

"Technically they have reserved their rights so that coverage issues are currently unresolved," attorney Rauch said.

Study: DES daughters' cancer rate 1 in 1,000

AMNews 3/13/87 p.36

Genital cancer among the daughters of women who took the drug DES strikes only about 1 in 1,000 by their mid-30s, according to a recent study in the New England Journal of Medicine.

DES may be an incomplete carcinogen that does not in itself cause cancer, but may cause cancer when coupled with some other unknown factor, said an Associated Press report of the study, which was directed by Sandra Melnick, MD.

Recent findings confirm that the synthetic hormone DES, or diethylstilbestrol, which was prescribed to prevent miscarriage during the 1940s to the 1960s, can cause tumors called clear-cell adenocarcinoma of the vagina and cervix.

Physicians from the Registry on Hormonal Transplacental Carcinogenesis of the U. of Chicago studied 519 cases of the genital cancer reported through mid-1985, AP reported. The mothers of 60% of the patients had received DES during pregnancy, In another 12% of cases, the mothers had used other hormones or medications.

Some 91% of cases involving women exposed to DES were diagnosed when patients were 15 to 27 years of age. The study projected that one in

1,000 exposed women will develop the cancer by age 34.

"The rarity of the tumor suggests that diethylstilbestrol is an incomplete carcinogen," the study concluded.

Digestive Diseases
National Digestive Diseases Education and Information Clearinghouse
PO Box NODIC, Bethesda, MD 20892
301/468-6344

Disability Evaluation
Quality Care
One way in which a physician can provide high quality care is to assure that his or her opinion is substantiated by clear, concise and well-reasoned reports of initial impairment and follow-up treatment. The reports must contain sufficient information to allow a knowledgeable reviewer to understand the initial impairment, and the degree and speed of recovery. The physician must allot a sufficient amount of time to examine the patient thoroughly and to prepare such reports.

The following is an outline of the kinds of information that should be found on each report:

Medical Evaluation:
• A narrative history of the medical condition(s) with specific reference to onset and course of the condition, findings on previous examinations, treatment and responses to treatment.
• The results of the most recent clinical evaluation including any of the following which were obtained: physical examination findings, laboratory test results, electrocardiogram, x-rays, rehabilitation evaluation, other specific tests or diagnostic procedures, and, in the case of psychiatric disease, the results of mental status examination and psychological tests.
• Assessment of the current clinical status and plans for future treatment, rehabilitation and re-evaluation.
• Diagnoses and clinical impressions.
• Estimate of the expected date of full or partial recovery.

Analysis of the Findings:
• Explanation of the impact of the medical condition(s) on life activities.
• Narrative explanation of the medical basis for any conclusion that the medical condition has, or has not, become static or well stabilized.
• Narrative explanation of the medical basis for any conclusion that the individual is, or is not, likely to suffer sudden or subtle incapacitation as a result of the medical condition.
• Narrative explanation of the medical basis for any conclusion that the individual is, or is not, likely to suffer injury or harm or further medical impairment by engaging in activities of daily living or any other activity necessary to meet personal, social, occupational or legal demands.
• Narrative explanation of any conclusion that restrictions or accommodations are, or are not, warranted with respect to activities of daily living or any other activities required to meet personal, social, occupational or legal demands, and if they are, an explanation of the therapeutic or

risk avoiding value of the restrictions or accommodations.

If the examiner elects to use the American Medical Association's *Guide to the Evaluation of Permanent Impairment*, then the following should also be included in the report:

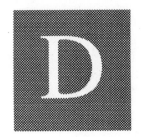

Comparison of the Results of Analysis with the Impairment Criteria:
• Description of specific clinical findings related to each impairment with reference to the relevance of the finding to the criteria of the chapter. Reference to the absence of, or inability to obtain, particular findings is essential.
• Comparison of the clinical findings with the criteria for the particular body system contained in the Guides.
• Explanation of the basis for each quantitative impairment rating with reference to the criteria.
• Summary list of all impairments with ratings.
• Combined "whole person" rating when more than one impairment is present.(WOR)

American Academy of Disability
Evaluating Physicians
PO Box 4313, Arlington Heights, IL 60006-4313
708/228-6095

"Disability Evaluation Under Social Security" available at local social security office or third party carrier for Medicare (Pub. #10089, November 1982)

Thirteen years elapsed between the publication of the first and second editions of the *Guides to the Evaluation of Permanent Impairment* (Guides). The third edition was published only four years after the second, yet was substantially revised. A number of trends accounted for this. First, the knowledge about impairment and how it is evaluated had developed rapidly. Major studies had appeared in the medical literature, and others had been commissioned by national organizations. Second, the growth of interest in impairments had been remarkable; conferences on this subject, which used to attract only a few, now are oversubscribed. Finally, expanded use of the Guides had increased the number of persons providing comments and suggestions and had provided comments and suggestions and had provided further impetus to revise the publication.(EVL)

Engelberg, AL. *Guides to the Evaluation of Permanent Impairment* 3rd ed. Revised Chicago. American Medical Association, 1990.
ISBN 0-89970-433-6. OP25490

National Association of Disability Examiners
3299 K Street, NW, 7th Floor
Washington, D.C. 20007
202/965-1544

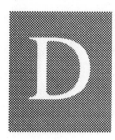

Disabled Physicians

AMA Policy: Provisions for Physicians with Handicaps: The AMA encourages all medical schools, residency programs, state licensing boards, and medical specialty boards to establish written policies governing the education, licensure and certification of physicians with handicaps, and to establish procedures for the examination of physicians with handicaps.

American Society of Handicapped Physicians
105 Morris Drive, Bastrop, LA 71220
318/281-4436

Department of Veteran Affairs, Technology Information Center
Rm 237, 810 Vermont Ave NW
Washington DC 20420
202/233-5524

Disaster Medical Care

American Red Cross
17th and D Streets, NW, Washington, DC 20006
202/737-8300

Medecins Sans Frontieres
(Doctors Without Borders)
8, rue St. Sabin, F-75544 Paris Cedex 11, France
1 40212929

New York Office:
30 Rockefeller Plaza, Suite 5425
New York, NY 10112
212/649-5961

Diving

Undersea and Hyperbaric Medical Society, Inc.
9650 Rockville Pike, Bethesda, MD 20814
301/571-1818

DAN (Divers Alert Network)
Hall Laboratory for Environmental Science
Duke University Medical Center
Durham, NC 27710
919/684-8111

Doctor's Day, National

Observed March 30

US (Officially) Honors Physicians With First 'National Doctors' Day

Andrew Skolnick, JAMA. 1991 March 6; 265(9): 1069

This national observance is authorized by Congress and the President. In signing the proclamation, President George Bush noted that the March 30 special day honors physicians for what he and Congress call their "invaluable contributions" to the welfare of the nation.

Actually, Doctors' Day began 58 years ago when Eudora B. Almond of the Barrow County (Ga.) Medical Society Auxiliary suggested that her auxiliary set aside March 30 to recognize the contributions of local physicians. March 30 was selected because it was on that day in 1842 that Crawford W. Long, MD, a Georgian, became the first physician to use ether anesthesia in surgery.

Well Received

The Barrow County auxiliary immediately approved the suggestion. Members agreed that this could be an "observance demanding some act of kindness, gift, or tribute in remembrance of the doctors."

The idea quickly gained wider acceptance. Doctors' Day became a regional observance on March 30, 1935, when the Souther Medical Association Auxiliary, Birmingham, Ala, adopted a similar resolution.

Since then, an increasing number of communities have used this day to express appreciation for the care physicians have provided the sick, for the advances they have made in medical knowledge, and for their leadership in improving public health. In fact, through the nationwide network of medical auxiliaries, Doctors' Day became a national project long before Congress and the President established it as a national day, say Norma Skoglund, Roseburg, Ore, president of the American Medical Association Auxiliary.

Cards, Flowers, and More

Those observing that first Doctors' Day in 1933 did so by mailing cards to the doctors (and their spouses) of Winder, Ga, and by placing flowers on the graves of deceased physician. Since then, Doctors' Day has been celebrated in many communities across the country by diverse activities that include the donation of medical equipment and furniture to hospitals and nursing homes, delivering meals to the elderly, blood donation drives, health fairs, the awarding of scholarships for studies in health-related fields, and numerous other generous acts, Skoglund says.

Sometimes, physicians are the recipients of needed services, as on Doctors' Day in 1988, when Greensboro, NC, auxiliary arranged for the busy physicians themselves to receive free physical examinations from colleagues. Since 1935, the traditional tribute for physicians on Doctors' Day, however, has been a gift of red carnations.

For each annual Doctors' Day, the American Medical Association Auxiliary is urging its members to honor their physicians by supporting medical education through contributions to the AMA Education and Research Foundation.

"From the rural doctor to the most highly trained specialist, physicians touch the lives of almost every person in the community. We must promote this caring, involved image to our fellow citizens," says Roberta Barnett, president of the Southern Medical Association Auxiliary.

"On Doctors' Day, it's important for auxiliary members to become involved in community service projects on a local basis," she adds. "Our involvement shows the public that physicians are interested in and contribute to their local communities."

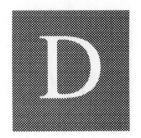

"The AMA auxiliary has a national clearinghouse for medical auxiliary programs," say Skoglund. "We have a catalog that lists more than 800 projects developed by auxiliaries. Approximately 30 of these are projects by which communities can recognize the contributions of their physicians."

Do-Not-Resuscitate Orders

Guidelines for Appropriate Use of Do-Not-Resuscitate Orders. Council on Ethical and Judicial Affairs, American Medical Association. JAMA. 1991 April 10; 265(14): 1868-71

Cardiopulmonary resuscitation (CPR) is routinely used on hospitalized patients who suffer cardiac or respiratory arrest. Consent to administer CPR is presumed since the patient is incapable at the moment of arrest of communicating his or her treatment preference, and failure to act immediately is certain to result in the patient's death. Two exceptions to the presumption favoring CPR have been recognized, however. First, a patient may express in advance his or her preference that CPR be withheld. If the patient is incapable of expressing a preference, the decision to forgo resuscitation may be made by the patient's family or other surrogate decision maker. Second, CPR may be withheld if, in the judgement of the treating physician, an attempt to resuscitate the patient would be futile. In December 1987, the American Medical Association's Council on Ethical and Judicial Affairs issued a series of guidelines to assist hospital medical staffs in formulating appropriate resuscitation policies. The Council's position on the appropriate use of CPR and do-not-resuscitate orders is updated in this report.

Domestic Violence

Violence

George D. Lundberg, Roxanne K. Young, Annette Flanagin, C. Everett Koop.

Murder. Arson. Drive-by-shooting. Rioting. Rape. Mugging. Stabbing. Wilding. Suicide. Assault. Incest. Spouse, Partner, Child, Elder Abuse.

A picture of American society is emerging, and it is at once both horrifying and numbing. So much so that we have been unable to stop it. We have become a society at war with itself, a nation at the mercy of a savage beast - violence.

Many of us have long recognized violence as a devastating social and public health problem. But even more of us have allowed ignorance, fear, powerlessness, and other problems that divert our attention to keep us from doing anything to resolve the problem. Certainly if violence were caused by a virus, we would have found its treatment and prevention long ago.

In an attempt to increase public and professional attention to violence, the editors of JAMA, American Medical News, and the American Medical Association's nine specialty journals published numerous articles on violence between January and June 1992. The best of these articles, which are collected in this Compendium, include epidemiologic studies, clinical research, government reports, case descriptions, and commentaries on a wide range of violence, from firearm homicide to abuse of children and pregnant women.

For this Compendium, we define violence as any human action resulting in injury or abuse, generally of the interpersonal variety, rather than that resulting from war or natural disasters. A pervasive, deceptive force, such violence destroys the basic, human foundation of our society and is best characterized with numbers: Homicide is the third leading cause of death among 15-to 24- year olds and the leading cause of death among 15-to 24-year old black males. The homicide rates for children and adolescents have more than doubled in the last 30 years.
- More than 1.5 million individuals in our country are victims of assault each year, and more than 650,000 women are victims of rape.
- 1.8 million women are beaten by their male partners each year, and 8% to 11% of pregnant women report being physically assaulted during pregnancy.
- Two to four million of our children were abused or neglected in 1991, and more than 1 million elderly were mistreated last year.

These statistics, although alarming, are probably underestimations. There is no denying that violence in America is a public health emergency - demanding immediate attention and corrective action.

These data paint a grotesque of a society steeped in violence, with such ubiquity and prevalence as to be seemingly accepted as inevitable. The authors and editors of this Compendium do not accept this situation as inevitable. No civilized society should be so permeated by firearm assault, homicide, rape, and child abuse. The situation is unacceptable. Prior solutions have not succeeded. New approaches are required.

We must demand unprecedented support for additional research into the causes, prevention, and treatments, for both victims and perpetrators, of all forms of violence. We need to recognize and treat violence as more than just a social aberrancy - it is a social disease. We need to educate everyone - physicians, nurses, other health professionals, students, politicians, and the public at large - about what is now known and what can now be done to address this emergency.(VIO)

Batterers Anonymous
1269 N. E. St., San Bernardino, CA 92405
714/355-1100

National Coalition Against Domestic Violence
PO Box 34103, Washington, DC 20043-4103
202/638-6388
--(For a listing of local safe houses and shelters)
800/333-SAFE (800/333-7233)
--(Telecommunication Device for the
Hearing Impaired)
800/873-6363

National Council on Child Abuse
and Family Violence
1155 Connecticut Ave, NW
Washington, DC 20036
202/429-6695

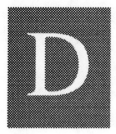

Violence against Women. Relevance for medical practitioners. Council on Scientific Affairs, American Medical Association. JAMA. 1992 Jun 17; 267(23): 3184-9

Evidence collected over the last 20 years indicates that physical and sexual violence against women is an enormous problem. Much of this violence is perpetrated by women's intimate partners or in relationships that would presumably carry some protective aura (eg, father-daughter, boyfriend-girlfriend). This violence carries with it both short- and long-term sequelae for women and affects both their physical and psychological well-being. The high prevalence of violence against women brings them into regular contact with physicians; at least one in five women seen in emergency departments has symptoms relating to abuse. However, physicians frequently treat the injuries only symptomatically or fail to recognize the injuries as abuse. Even when recognized, physicians are often without resources to address the needs of abused women. This report documents the extent of violence against women and suggests a path that the physician community might take to address the needs of victims.

Resources for abused women and their doctors

Janice Perrone AMNews 1/6/1992 p.17.

Once a battered woman decides that she wants to do something about her situation, how can her physician help?

"Unless the doctor is knowledgeable, the best thing would be direct her to a crisis line or hot line.

"Such a program should be able to help her sort out what to do and what help is available," said Diana Onley-Campbell, former executive for the Denver-based National Coalition Against Domestic Violence, a network or organizations that provide services for battered women.

Organization that can provide your patients with shelter, information or counseling include:
• The National Domestic Violence Hotline: (800) 333-SAFE. It's a 24-hour-a-day resource to help victims find local shelters. Counselors speak English and Spanish. The telecommunications device for the deaf number is (800) 873-6363.
• Local domestic violence shelters and statewide domestic violence programs also should be listed in your phone in your phone book. They can help victims with housing, information about their legal rights, welfare applications and counseling, including peer groups and counseling for children. Many programs offer these services free. Phone callers may remain anonymous, and many of these programs operate 24 hours a day.
• The National Woman Abuse Prevention Center publishes fact sheets on domestic violence, a quarterly newsletter and a series of seven brochures, including "Helping the Battered Woman" and "Domestic Violence, Understanding a Community Problem." Some of the material is translated into Spanish and Polish. For ordering information, contact the project: 1112 16th St. N.W., Suite 920, Washington, D.C. 20036; (202) 857-0216.

The AMA is also distributing several of these brochures to community locations and physician offices. For free copies, call (312) 464-4444.
• The Michigan Coalition Against Domestic Violence has brochures and other materials that physicians can distribute to women patients. Single copies are free. All the materials may be reproduced, but physicians can order multiple copies of some items from the coalition. (There is a charge for multiple copies.) The coalition also provides physicians with information on how best to use these materials. For information write the coalition: PO Box 463100, Mount Clemens, Mich. 48046; (313) 954-1180.
• The American College of Obstetrics and Gynecologists publishes "The Abused Woman," which is directed at patients and includes a discussion of risk factors for family violence, its relationship to child abuse, violence during pregnancy and how to get help if you're a victim. To obtain free single copies, call (202) 863-2518. To order in bulk, call (800) 762-ACOG. A pack of 50 is $14. Janice Perrone

National Woman Abuse Prevention Project
2000 P Street, NW, Suite 508
Washington, DC 20036
202/337-6070

JAMA Article: Elder abuse and neglect. Council on Scientific Affairs. JAMA. 1987 Feb 20; 257(7): 966-71

Estimates of elder abuse approximate 10% of Americans over 65 years of age; obtaining accurate incidence and prevalence figures is complicated by factors including denial by both the victim and perpetrator and minimalization of complaints by health professionals. Broad agreement exists in categorizing elder abuse as physical, psychological, and financial and/or material, despite lack of uniformity in definitions. Systematic scientific investigation provides limited knowledge about the causes of elder abuse. Most experts, however, believe that family problems and conflict are a major precipitating factor. Preliminary hypotheses for elder abuse include dependency, lack of close family ties, family violence, lack of financial resources, psychopathology in the abuser, lack of community support, and certain factors that may precipitate abuse in institutional settings. This report presents potential indicators of physical and psychological abuse, along with classification of elderly individuals at high risk, to assist the health professional in identification and prevention of elder abuse.

Diagnosing elder abuse: Guidelines for physicians

Roberta Gerry AMNews 12/14/92 p.2

• When examining an elderly patient, routinely ask questions directly related to abuse or neglect.
• If answers confirm abuse, follow up to learn how and when it occurs and who is responsible.
• Examine the patient thoroughly and document findings, including patient's statements, behavior and appearance.
• Be aware that abuse may be physical, psychological, financial or material, or any combination of these.
• When assessing for mistreatment, consider the patient's safety, emotional health and functional

status, social and financial resources, and the frequency, severity and intent of the abuse.
- Be aware that in institutions, elder abuse may be perpetrated by a staff member, another patient, an intruder or a visitor.
- Note that many states require physicians to report suspected elder abuse and neglect to a designated state agency. Failure to do so can make doctors liable.
- Keep, thorough, well documented medical records and photographs. These provide concrete evidence and may be crucial in any legal case.
- Your duty to report suspected abuse supersedes doctor-patient confidentiality issues, most experts say.

National Institute of Mental Health
Anti-Social and Violent Behavior Branch, DBAS, Parklawn Building, Room 18-105
5600 Fishers Lane, Rockville, MD 20857
301/443-3728

Donations, Books
American Overseas Medical Aid Association
(medical books and journals)
4433 W. Montana St., Chicago, IL 60639
312/486-4809

Darien Book Aid Plan, Inc.
(books and journals)
1926 Post Rd., Darien, CT 06820
203/655-2777

The Foundation for Books to China
601 California St., San Francisco, CA 94108
415/392-1080

International Book Project, Inc.
(professional books and journals),
1440 Delaware Ave., Lexington, KY 40505
606/254-6771

Medical Books for China
13021 E Florence Ave.
Santa Fe Springs, CA 90670
213/946-8774

Donations, Medical Supplies
American Near East Refuge Aid, Inc.
(pharmaceutical and medical supplies)
1522 K St. NW, #202, Washington, DC 20005
202/347-2558

American Overseas Medical Aid Association
(surgical and diagnostic equipment, pharmaceutical)
4433 W. Montana St., Chicago, IL 60639
312/486-4809

Catholic Medical Mission Board, Inc.
(pharmaceutical and medical equipment)
10 W. 17th St., New York, NY 10011
212/242-7757

Direct Relief International
(pharmaceutical, medical equipment and supplies)
PO Box 30820, Santa Barbara, CA 93130
805/687-3694

Focus, Inc.
(ophthalmologic supplies)
Department of Ophthalmology, Loyola University Medical Center
2160 S. First Ave., Maywood, IL 60153
708/216-9408

Interchurch Medical Assistance, Inc.
(pharmaceutical and hospital supplies)
PO Box 429, New Windsor, MD 21776
301/635-6474

Pan American Development Foundation
(medical equipment and supplies)
1889 F St., NW, Washington, DC 20006
202/789-3969

Plenty
(medical equipment and supplies, pharmaceutical)
The Farm, 156 Drakes Ln.
Summertown, TN 38483

Rescue Now
(medical equipment and supplies, pharmaceutical)
870 Market St., Rm. 1050
San Francisco, CA 94102
415/894-6365

World Medical Relief, Inc.
(pharmaceutical, medical equipment and supplies)
11745 Twelfth St., Detroit, MI 48206
313/866-5322

World Opportunities International
(medical supplies)
1415 N. Cahuangua Blvd., Hollywood, CA 90028
213/466-7187

Drug Abuse
American Council for Drug Education
5820 Hubbard Dr., Rockville, MD 20852
301/984-5700

Office of Drug Control Policy
Executive Office of the President
Washington, DC 20500
202/467-9800

Drug and Alcohol Hotline Information and Referral Service
800/252-6465

National Clearinghouse for Drug Abuse Information
PO Box 416, Kensington, MD 20795
301/468-2600

National Federation of Parents for Drug-Free Youth
800/554-KIDS

National Institute on Drug Abuse
800/843-4971 (hotline to assist medical departments of business and industry in establishing programs to deal with drug-related problems in work force)

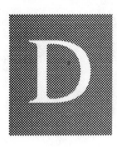

National Institute on Drug Abuse
800/662-HELP
(treatment and referral hotline)

"National Directory of Alcoholism, Drug Abuse
Treatment Programs"
Available from U.S. Journal of
Drug and Alcohol Dependence
1721 Blount Rd., Suite 1
Pompano Beach, FL 33069
800/851-9100

Pregnancy and drug abuse
800/327-BABE (800-327-2223) or
800/638-BABY (800-638-2229)

Drug Enforcement Administration (DEA)

The Drug Enforcement Administration (DEA) is
the lead Federal agency in enforcing narcotics
and controlled substances laws and regulations. It
was created in July 1973, by Reorganization Plan
No. 2 of 1973 (5 U.S.C. app.), which merged four
separate drug law enforcement agencies.

DEA's responsibilities include:
• investigation of major narcotic violators who
  operate at interstate and international levels;
• seizure and forfeiture of assets derived from,
  traceable to, or intended to be used for illicit
  drug trafficking;
• enforcement of regulations governing the legal
  manufacture, distribution, and dispensing of
  controlled substances;
• management of a national narcotics intelligence
  system;
• coordination with Federal, State, and local law
  enforcement authorities and cooperation with
  counterpart agencies abroad; and
• training, scientific research, and information
  exchange in support of drug traffic prevention
  and control. (USG)

U.S. Dept. of Justice
Drug Enforcement Administration,
600-700 Army-Navy Dr., Arlington, VA 22202
202/307-1000

Public Affairs Section
Drug Enforcement Administration
Department of Justice, Washington, DC 20537
202-307-7977

Physician can obtain a registration
number by calling:
202/254-8255 or 8259 is this at the above office?

Drug Information

Drug Evaluations Series: Annual or Subscription
American Medical Association, Chicago.
Annual:1993. ISBN 0-89970-498-0 / OP025592CL
2202 pp.
Subscription:1993. ISBN 0-89970-490-5 /
NR000117CL
Three volume set; updated quarterly

Drug Information Association
PO Box 3113, Maple Glen, PA 19002
215/628-2288

"Patient Medication Instruction Sheets" (PMI)
Information sheets by the USPC on particular
drugs, available at two educational levels,
prepared especially for the consumer.

USP DI System 11th edition, 1991; USPC,
Rockville, MD
3 vol in 4 pieces ISBN 0913595519 Updated by
"USP DI Update." USPC publications available
from:

United States Pharmacopeial Convention (USPC)
Order Department
PO Box 5367, Twinbrook Station
Rockville, MD 20851
301/881-0666
800/227-8772 (Visa and Mastercard orders only)

Physicians' Desk Reference
Medical Economics Co.
5 Paragon Drive, PO Box 430
Montvale, NJ 07645-1742
201/358-7200
800/922-0937; 800/624-0472 (NJ only)

Drug Program, Indigent

Report listing pharmaceutical companies and the
prescription drugs they provide for the needy. May
be requested in writing from:
Senate Special Committee on Aging, Room G-31,
Dirksen Senate Office building
Washington D.C. 20510-6400.

A program to aid physician's in locating drug
companies offering free prescription drugs to
indigent patients. The directory and hot line for this
information is for use of physician's only:
For the directory, please write:
1992 Directory of Prescription Drug Indigent
Programs,
PMA, 1100 15th St., NW.
Washington D.C., 20005
Hot line: 800/762-4636 or locally, 202/393-5200

***Contact your state Department of Aging for
local programs.***

Drug Testing

Guidelines: American College of
Occupational Medicine
55 W. Seegers Road, Arlington Heights, IL 60005
708/228-6850

College of American Pathologists
325 Waukegan Road, Northfield, IL 60095
708/446-8800

JAMA Article of Note: The Efficacy of
preemployment drug screening for marijuana and
cocaine in predicting employment outcome.
Zwerling, C., Ryan, J.,Orav, E.J.
JAMA.1990 Nov 28;264(20):2639-43.
(see also JAMA.1985 April 26).

Scientific issues in drug testing. Council on Scientific Affairs. JAMA. 1987 Jun 12; 257(22): 3110-4

Testing for drugs in biologic fluids, especially urine, is a practice that has become widespread. The technology of testing for drugs in urine has greatly improved in recent years. Inexpensive screening techniques are not sufficiently accurate for forensic testing standards, which must be met when a person's employment or reputation may be affected by results. This is particularly a concern during screening of a population in which the prevalence of drug use is very low, in which the predictive value of a positive result would be quite low. Physicians should be aware that results from drug testing can yield accurate evidence of prior exposure to drugs, but they do not provide information about patterns of drug use, about abuse of or dependence on drugs, or about mental or physical impairments that may result from drug use.

Drunk Driving

Waste

George D. Lundberg "A Piece of My Mind" JAMA. 1986 Sept 19; 256(11): 1493

He was the best pathology resident I had ever known, before or since that day nine years ago. And that includes hundreds of residents at seven institutions where I have had direct responsibility. He has entered medical school later in life than most, having first become a cytotechnologist, thus acquiring a skill that helped him work his way through medical school. Only three months into his internship, he made a pathology presentation to medical grand rounds at the largest teaching hospital in the United States and received a standing ovation from the usually cynical crowd. In addition to excelling in every standard rotation in anatomic and clinical pathology, he ran a major course in general and systemic pathology for 150 sophomore pharmacy students as an add-on to his second-year residency duties.

He was also an exceptional human being on a personal level. I remember a softball game at a fund-raising Medical Olympics where he made a spectacular catch in centerfield. His wife was a flight attendant, so even though he was a resident they were able to take long trips from time to time. He told me that the thing he liked best was fly-fishing for trout in New Zealand lakes at high altitudes.

When I left to become a departmental chair, I tried hard to recruit him. Despite the fact that he was still in training, he was first on the list of those people I wanted most to bring along from my prior institution to help revitalize my new organization.

The last time I saw him was at a national professional meeting in Las Vegas in 1977, where I took him to dinner to continue my efforts to recruit him. He was grappling with the common problem of whether he should stay in academia, which he loved, or go into private practice with its more immediate tangible rewards, especially since he had by then a number of children to support as well. Obviously, he had many professional opportunities.

The next time I heard about him, he was dead. While he was going home from work one evening, an oncoming car swerved over the center divider and smashed his small sports car head on. An

embankment to his right had prevented any evasive action. The next morning in the medical examiner's office his resident colleague did not even recognize him, so severely was he damaged. Both the driver and the passenger in the offending car were drunk. But Lynn was a devout Mormon. He had recently told me that he had never tasted a drop of alcohol in his life.

Mothers Against Drunk Driving
PO Box 541688, Dallas, TX 75354-1688
214/744-6233

National Commission Against Drunk Driving
114 Connecticut Ave. NW, Suite 804, Washington, DC 20036
202/452-0130

National Safety Council
1121 Spring Lake Drive, Itasca, IL 60143-3201
708/285-1121 (brochure available)

Dyslexia

Orton Dyslexia Society
724 York Road, Baltimore, MD 21204
800/ABCD-123 (800-222-3123)
301/296-0232 (in MD)

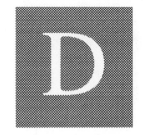

Easter Seals

The National Easter Seal Society
70 E. Lake Street, Chicago, IL 60601
312/726-6200

Echocardiography

American Society of Echocardiography
1100 Raleigh Building,
5 West Hargett St., Raleigh, NC 27601
919/787-5181

Echocardiograph Technician

Alternate titles: diagnostic cardiac sonographer.
Produces two-dimensional ultrasonic recordings
and Doppler flow analyses of heart and related
structures, using ultrasound equipment, for use by
physician in diagnosis of heart disease and study
of heart: Explain procedures to patient to obtain
cooperation and reduce anxieties of patient.
Attaches electrodes to patient's chest to monitor
heart rhythm and connects electrodes to leads of
ultrasound equipment. Adjusts equipment controls
according to physician's orders and areas of heart
to be examined. Keys patient information into
computer keyboard on equipment to record
information on video cassette and strip printout of
test. Starts ultrasound equipment that produces
images of real time tomographic cardiac anatomy,
and adjusts equipment to obtain quality images.
Moves transducer, by hand, over patient's heart
areas, observes ultrasound display screen, and
listens to Doppler signals to acquire data for
measurement of blood flow velocities. Prints
pictures of graphic analysis recordings and
removes video cassette for permanent record of
internal examination. Measures heart wall
thicknesses and chamber sizes recorded on strip
printout, using calipers and ruler, or keys
commands into video tape, and compares
measurement to standard norms to identify
abnormalities in heart. Measures blood flow
velocities and calculates data, such as cardiac
physiology and valve areas for evaluation of
cardiac function by physician. Reviews test results
with interpreting physician. (DOT)

Electrocardiograph Technicians

Alternate titles: ecg technician; ekg technician.
Produces recordings of electromotive variations
on patient's heart muscle, using
electrocardiograph (ECG), to provide data for
diagnosis of heart ailments: Attaches electrodes
to chest, arms, and legs of patient. Connects
electrodes leads to electrocardiograph and starts
machine. Moves electrodes along specified area
of chest to produce electrocardiogram that
records electromotive variations occurring in
different areas of heart muscle. Monitors
electrocardiogram for abnormal patterns. Keys
information into machine or marks tracing to
indicate positions of chest electrodes.
Replenishes supply of paper and ink in machine
and reports malfunctions. Edits and forwards final
test results to attending physician for analysis and
interpretation. May attach electrodes of Holter
monitor (electrocardiograph) to patient to record
data over extended period of time. (DOT)

National Society for Cardiovascular
Technology/Pulmonary Technology
1133 15th St, NW, Ste 1000, Washington, DC
20005 202/293-5933

Ecology

Citizens for a Better Environment
Reference Center
33 E. Congress Pkwy, Ste 523, Chicago, IL 60605
312/939-1530

Pesticides and Related Medical Treatment Hotline
EPA Hotline 800/858-7378

National Institute of Environmental
Health Sciences
PO Box 12233 Research Triangle Park
NC 27709
919/541-3345

Educational Commission for Foreign Medical Graduates

Educational Commission for Foreign Medical
Graduates (ECFMG)
3624 Market St., Philadelphia, PA 19104
215/386-5900

Electroencephalography

Alternate titles: eeg technologist. Measures
electrical activity of brain waves, using
electroencephalograph (EEG) instrument, and
conducts evoked potential response tests for use
in diagnosis of brain and nervous system
disorders: Measures patient's head and other
body parts, using tape measure, and marks points
where electrodes are to be placed. Attaches
electrodes to predetermined locations, and verifies
functioning of electrodes and recording
instrument. Operates recording instruments (EEG
and evoked potentials) and supplemental
equipment and chooses settings for optimal
viewing of nervous system. Records montage
(electrode combination) and instrument settings,
and observes and notes patient's behavior during
test. Conducts visual, auditory, and
somatosensory evoked potential response tests to
measure latency of response to stimuli. Writes
technical reports summarizing test results to assist
physician in diagnosis of brain disorders. May
perform other physiological tests, such as
electrocardiogram, electrooculogram, and
ambulatory electroencephalogram. May perform
video monitoring of patient's actions during test.
May monitor patient during surgery, using EEG or
evoked potential instrument. May supervise other
technologists and be known as Chief
Electroencephalographic Technologist. (DOT)

American Medical Electroencephalographic Assn.
850 Elm Grove Rd., Elm Grove, WI 53122
414/797-7800

Electromyography

Alternate titles: emg technician. Measures
electrical activity in peripheral nerves, using
electromyograph (EMG) instrument, for use by
physician in diagnosing neuromuscular disorders:
Explains procedures to patient to obtain
cooperation and relieve anxieties during test.
Rubs electrode paste on patient's skin to ensure
contact of electrodes. Attaches surface recording
electrodes to extremity in which activity is being
measured to detect electrical impulse. Attaches
electrodes to electrode cables or leads connected
to EMG instrument and selects nerve conduction
mode on EMG. Operates EMG instrument to

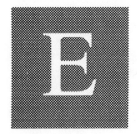

record electrical activity in peripheral nerves. Presses button on manually held surface stimulator electrode to deliver pulse and send electrical charge along peripheral nerve. Monitors response on oscilloscope and presses button to record nerve conduction velocity. Measures and records time and distance between stimulus and response, manually or using computer, and calculates velocity of electrical impulse in peripheral nerve. Removes electrodes from patient upon conclusion of test and cleans electrode paste from skin, using alcohol and cotton. (DOT

American Association of Electromyography and Electrodiagnosis Brackenridge Skyway Plaza 21 2nd St, NW, Ste 306, Rochester, MN 55902 507/288-0100

Electroneurodiagnostic Technologist

History: The background of AMA involvement in the evaluation and accreditation and educational programs in electroencephalographic (EEG) technology began in 1972 with the recognition as an allied health profession by the AMA Council on Health Manpower. Subsequently, AMA staff worked with representatives of the professional organizations representing this clinical discipline to develop a draft of the Essentials of an Accredited Educational Program for the Electroencephalographic Technologist.

In 1973, representatives of the American EEG Society, the American Medical EEG Association, and the American Society of Electroneurodiagnostic Technologists (then the American Society of EEG Technologists) presented statements supporting the Essentials. These organizations and the AMA House of Delegates then considered and adopted the Essentials for entry educational programs for the electroencephalographic technologist.

The Joint Review Committee on Education in Electroencephalographic Technology was established and held its initial meeting in September 1973. In 1988, the name of the committee was changed to the Joint Review Committee on Education in Electroneurodiagnostic Technology. This Review body is composed of eight members - four members appointed by the American Electroencephalographic Association. Meetings are held twice annually. The committee develops recommendations on accreditation status of programs which are subsequently forwarded to the Committee on Allied Health Education and Accreditation for final action. Essentials were revised in 1980 and again 1987, Evoked Potentials (EP) techniques were included in Essentials for programs desiring recognition in both EEG and EP.

Occupational Description: Electoneurodiagnostic technology is the scientific field devoted to recording and studying the electrical activity of the brain. Electroneurodiagnostic technologists possess the knowledge, attributes, and skills to obtain interpretable recording of patients' nervous system function. They work in collaboration with the electroencephalographer.

Job Description: The electroneurodiagnostic technologist is skilled in the following function: communicating with patient, family, and other health care personnel: taking and abstracting histories; applying adequate recording electrodes and using EEG and EP techniques; documenting the clinical condition of patients; understanding and employing the optimal utilization of EEG and EP equipment. Among other duties, the electroneurodiagnostic technologist also understands the interface between EEG and EP equipment and other electrophysiological devices; recognizes and understands EEG and EP activity displayed; manages medical emergencies in the laboratory; and prepared a descriptive report of recorded activity for the electroencephalographer. The responsibilities of the technologist may also include laboratory management and the supervision of the EEG technicians.

Employment Characteristics: Although electroneurodiagnostic personnel work primarily in the neurology departments of hospitals, many work in private offices of neurologists and neurosurgeons. Growth in employment in the profession is expected to be greater than the average for all occupations due to the increased use of EEG and EP in surgery and in diagnosing and monitoring patients with brain disease. Technologists generally work a 40-hour week.

According to the 1990 CAHEA Annual Supplemental Survey, entry level salaries average $20,573.

AMA Department of Allied Health 312/464-4625

Emergency Medical Technician--Paramedic

History: The development of educational standards for the EMT-Paramedic began with a forum for representatives of over 30 professional organizations and agencies called by the American Medical Association in May 1976. In the following month an ad hoc task force formulated an initial draft of standards - Essentials - for the education and training of the EMT-Paramedic and submitted it to participants of the May forum for review and comment. A second draft was then prepared and distributed for consideration at a forum held in Boston in November 1976. A third draft of the proposed Essentials, which resulted from that meeting, was distributed widely in March 1977 to the organizations which had contributed to their original development, to recognized educators of EMT-Paramedics, and to others who had been identified as having an interest in this project. In September, another mailing was made to all potential sponsors of the proposed accreditation program to determine if and when then their organizations would have a formal position on the proposal. By the end of 1977, seven organizations had given notice of their interest in becoming sponsors of a national accreditation program for EMT-Paramedic education, These organizations included the American College of Emergency Physicians, American Heart Association, American Psychiatric Association, American Society of Anesthesiologists, National Association of Emergency Medical Technicians, and National Registry of Emergency Medical Technicians.

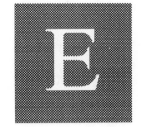

The fifth draft of the proposed Essentials was distributed widely to national organizations, educators, and others for final review and comment during July 1978. The AMA Council on Medical Education held public hearings on the proposed standards for EMT-Paramedic education during August. On the basis of this review, the Council adopted the proposed Essentials on behalf of the American Medical Association in September 1978. During the next six months the Essentials were adopted by the American College of Emergency Physicians, the American College of Surgeons, the American Psychiatric Association, the American Society of Anesthesiologists, the National Association of Emergency Medical Technicians, and the National Registry of Emergency Medical Technicians.

Beginning in February 1978, these same organizations recommended establishing an ad hoc task force to develop the necessary policies, procedures, and documents to enable implementation of the proposed accreditation effort. In April 1979 this task force became known as the Joint Review Committee on Educational Programs for the Emergency Medical Technician-Paramedic. The first educational programs were accredited by CAHEA in January 1982.

Occupational Description: Emergency medical technician-paramedics (EMT-paramedics), working under the direction of a physician (often through radio communication), recognize, assess, and manage medical emergencies of acutely ill or injured patients in pre-hospital care settings. EMT-paramedics work principally in advanced life support units and ambulance services which are under medical supervision and direction.

Job Description: EMT-paramedics are competent in recognizing a medical emergency, in assessing the situation, and in managing the emergency care. This includes the ability to recognize the patient's condition and to initiate appropriate invasive and non-invasive treatments for a variety of surgical and medical emergencies, including airway and respiratory problems, cardiac dysrhythmias and standstills, and psychological crises. In addition, EMT-paramedics are able to assess the response of the patient to the treatment received and to modify that therapy as required through the direction of a designated physician or other authorized individuals.

EMT-paramedics maintain written records and dictate details relating to a patient's emergency care and a description of the incident which led to that care. They also direct the maintenance and preparation of emergency care equipment and supplies, as well as direct and coordinate the transport of patients. EMT-paramedics are responsible for exercising personal judgment when communication failures interrupt contact with medical direction or, in cases of immediate life threatening conditions, when such care has been specifically authorized in advance.

Employment Characteristics: Variations in geographic, sociologic, and economic factors impact on emergency medical services and subsequently on the type of practice engaged in by EMT-paramedics. Some EMT-paramedics are employed by community fire and police departments and have related responsibilities in those fields, or they serve as community volunteers. Not only are these individuals being employed in the pre-hospital phase of acute care provided by fire departments, police departments, public services, and private purveyors, but there is also an increased demand for their skills in hospital emergency departments and private industry.

According to the 1990 CAHEA Annual Supplemental Survey, entry level salaries average $20,799.

AMA Allied Health Department 312/464-4634

National Association of Emergency
Medical Technicians
9140 Ward Parkway, Kansas City, MO 64114
816/444-3500

National Registry of Emergency
Medical Technicians
PO Box 29233, Columbus, OH 43229
614/888-4484

Emergency Medicine
American Board of Emergency Medicine
200 Woodland Pass, Suite D, Lansing, MI 48823
517/332-4800

American College of Emergency Physicians
PO Box 619911, Dallas, TX 75261-9911
214/550-0911

Wilderness Medical Society
PO Box 397
Point Reyes Station, CA 94956 415/663-9107

Employee Assistance Programs
Beth Bengston, The AMA Reporter 9/1989

A major change has occurred in corporate America since the middle 1900s. [In the past, employers dealt with employees' personal problems in various ways. The problems were ignored or covered up, or if they affected one's work employees might have been disciplined or fired.] Today, more and more companies are concerned with helping troubled employees regain their health and productivity rather than using discipline alone.

A major tool employers use to accomplish this is the implementation of Employee Assistance Programs (EAPs). An EAP is a confidential, professional way to help employees tackle personal problems. Most current EAPs are considered "broadbrush" programs, because they help employees deal with a wide range of problems, including job stress, single parenting, financial, or legal problems, including job stress, single parenting, financial or legal problems, marital and family relations, alcohol and drug dependency, emotional problems, gambling addiction, and eating disorders. More and more emphasis is being place on problem prevention and on catching problems early, before they become crises.

Employee Assistance Programs have experienced phenomenal growth in the U.S. in the past 40 years. Their scope has also changed dramatically,

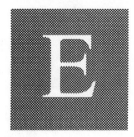

from a focus mainly on alcohol and drug problems to a more comprehensive approach. Interestingly, the initial EAP boom coincided with the AMA recognizing, and the public beginning to accept, alcoholism as a disease rather than a personal deficiency. There were fewer than 100 EAPs operating in 1950, compared to [approximately 6000 in 1989.]

How Do EAPs Work?

Through an EAP, employees can obtain private personal assistance for any kind of personal problem from a trained professional. Typically, an EAP is a starting point to help people help themselves. Some EAPs are internal - staffed and run by counselors who are employed by the company - but many employers use an independent professional assistance agency to implement an EAP.

The Process begins when an employee voluntarily calls the EAP. The next stop is professional assessment of his or her situation. Sometimes the problem cam be resolved in just a few sessions with the EAP professional. Other cases may call for further specialized help. In these situations, the client is referred by the EAP to an outside resource - a hospital program, a counselor, an agency, or a self-help group specializing in the individual's particular problem. The EAP counselor then stays in touch with the client to see how he or she is progressing and to offer support and encouragement. Clients are recommended to follow through with the program, but have the option to leave or re-enter it at any time.

Confidentiality

Confidentiality and privacy are essential elements of any EAP. Counselors are required to maintain a client's privacy and confidentiality within strict State and Federal guidelines, and there are stiff penalties for a person who wrongfully discloses confidential information. Information from the EAP cannot be released to anyone without the client's written permission, except in rare cases of extreme danger to self or others, or in cases of unreported child abuse.

EAPs away from the worksite are conducive to a great degree of confidentiality - employees can meet a counselor after working hours, away from coworkers and manager. In some cases an independent auditor is used to evaluate the EAP and ensure that employee confidentiality is maintained.

Management Training

Since managing a problem employee can be fraught with uncertainty, an ongoing management education and training function is part of most EAPs. This training is invaluable to supervisors. It's crucial that a supervisor know how to talk with an employee and encourage him or her to contact the EAP.

This type of discussion between a manager and employee does not hinder confidentiality since participation in the EAP is voluntary - the employee alone is responsible for calling the EAP, seeing the counselor and following through with the prescribed course. A counselor can disclose no information to the manager or anyone else at the workplace unless the employee consents. Job security and promotional opportunities are based on work performance and attendance, and are not affected by participation or non-participation in the EAP.

The success of any EAP hinges on the employees who utilize it. For a program to be effective, employees must understand it, know how it works, and feel comfortable using it. To encourage this, most employers conduct employee orientation sessions. Situations where an EAP may help, how the procedure works, how confidentiality is maintained, and who is eligible to participate are generally discussed. The orientation is also an important time for employees to ask questions about the program.

The Employee/Employer Partnership

An employee assistance program is obviously meant to benefit employees, but the employer also comes out a winner. By helping the employee, the company also benefits as the employee becomes more productive. Studies have shown decreased absenteeism and accidents, lower turnover, better morale, and greater job satisfaction after the introduction of an EAP.

Employee Assistance Professionals Association
4601 N Fairfax Drive, Suite 1001
Arlington, VA 22203
703/522-6272

Employee Assistance Society of North America
2728 Phillips, Berkely, MI 48072
313/545-3888

Endocrinology
Endocrine Society 9650 Rockville Pike
Bethesda, MD 20814
301/571-1802

Board Certification in Endocrinology
and Metabolism:
American Board of Internal Medicine
3624 Market Street, Philadelphia, PA 19104
215/243-1500 /800/441-ABIM/(800/441-2246)

Board Certification in Reproductive Endocrinology
American Board of Obstetrics and Gynecology
4225 Roosevelt Way, NE, Suite 305
Seattle, WA 98105
206/547-4884

Endodontist

Examines, diagnoses, and treats diseases of nerve, pulp, and other dental tissues affecting vitality of teeth: Examines teeth, gums, and related tissues to determine condition, using dental instruments, x ray, and other diagnostic equipment. Diagnoses condition and plans treatment. Treats exposure of pulp by pulp capping or removal of pulp from pulp chamber and root canal, using dental instruments. Performs partial or total removal of pulp, using surgical instruments. Treats infected root canal and related tissues, and fills pulp chamber and canal with endodontic materials. Removes pathologic tissue at apex of tooth, surgically. Reinserts teeth that have been knocked out of mouth by accident. Bleaches discolored teeth to restore natural color. (DOT)

Endometriosis

Endometriosis is a condition in which fragments of the endometrium (lining of the uterus) are found in other parts of (or on organs within) the pelvic cavity.

Incidence and Cause

Endometriosis is most prevalent between 25 and 40 and is a common cause of infertility. About 10 to 15 percent of infertility patients have endometriosis and about 30 to 40 percent of women suffering from endometriosis are infertile.

The exact cause of endometriosis is uncertain, but in some cases it is thought to occur because fragments of the endometrium that are shed during menstruation do not leave the body with the menstrual flow. Instead, they travel up the fallopian tubes and into the pelvic cavity. There, they may adhere to and grow on any of the pelvic organs.

These displaced patches of endometrium continue to respond to the menstrual cycle as if they were still inside the uterus, so each month they bleed. This blood cannot escape, however, and causes the formation of slowly growing cysts from the size of a pinhead to the size of a grapefruit. The growth and swelling of the cysts are responsible for much of the pain associated with endometriosis.

Symptoms and Signs

The symptoms of endometriosis vary widely, with abnormal or heavy menstrual bleeding being most common. There may be severe abdominal and/or lower back pain during menstruation, which is often most severe toward the end of a period. Other possible symptoms include dyspareunia and digestive tract symptoms such as diarrhea, constipation, or painful defecation. Rectal bleeding that happens only at the time of the menses may occur. In some cases, however, endometriosis causes no symptoms.(ENC)

Endometriosis Association
8585 N. 76th Pl, Milwaukee, WI 53223
800/992-ENDO (800/992-3636)
414/355-2200 (in WI)

Environmental Protection Agency (EPA)

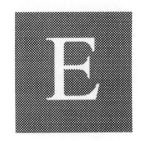

The Environmental Protection Agency protects and enhances our environment today and for future generations to the fullest extent possible under the laws enacted by Congress. The Agency's mission is to control and abate pollution in the areas of air, water, solid waste, pesticides, radiation, and toxic substances. Its mandate is to mount an integrated, coordinated attack on environmental pollution in cooperation with State and local government.

The Environmental Protection Agency was established in the executive branch as independent agency pursuant to Reorganization Plan No. 3 of 1970 (5 U.S.C. app.), effective December 2, 1970.

The Environmental Protection Agency was created to permit coordinated and effective government action on behalf of the environment. It endeavors to abate and control pollution systematically, by proper integration of a variety of research, monitoring, standard setting, and enforcement activities. As a complement to its other activities, the Agency coordinates and supports research and antipollution activities by State and local governments, private and public groups, individuals, and educational institutions. It also reinforces efforts among other Federal agencies with respect to the impact of their operations on the environment, and it is specifically charged with publishing its determinations when those hold that a proposal is unsatisfactory from the standpoint of public health or welfare or environmental quality. In all, the Environmental Protection Agency is designed to serve as the public's advocate for a livable environment.(USG)

Environmental Protection Agency 401 M St, SW, Rm 211B, Washington, DC 20460
Public Information 202/382-2080

Environmental Health

American Academy of Environmental Medicine
PO Box 16106, Denver, CO 80216
303/622-9755

Citizens for a Better Environment
Reference Center,
33 E. Congress Pkwy, Ste 523, Chicago, IL 60605
312/939-1530

National Institute of Environmental
Health Sciences
PO Box 12233 Research Triangle Park
NC 27709
919/541-3345

Pesticides and Related Medical Treatment/Hotline
EPA Hotline 800/858-7378

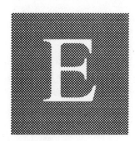

Epilepsy

American Epilepsy Society
179 Allyn St., Suite 304, Hartford, CT 06103
203/232-4825

Epilepsy Foundation of America
4351 Garden City Dr., Ste. 406
Landover, MD 20785 301/459-3700

Epilepsy Information Line 800/332-1000

Ethics

Principles of Medical Ethics

Preamble:

The medical profession has long subscribed to a body of ethical statements developed primarily for the benefit of the patient. As a member of this profession, a physician must recognize responsibility not only to patients, but also to society, to other health professionals, and to self. The following Principles adopted by the American Medical Association are not laws, but standards of conduct which define the essentials of honorable behavior for the physician.

I. A physician shall be dedicated to providing competent medical service with compassion and respect.

II. A physician shall deal honestly with patients and colleagues, and strive to expose those physicians deficient in character or competence, or who engage in fraud or deception.

III. A physician shall respect the law and also recognize a responsibility to seek changes in those requirements which are contrary to the best interests of the patients.

IV. A physician shall respect the rights of patients, of colleagues, and of other health professionals, and shall safeguard patient confidences within the constraints of the law.

V. A physician shall continue to study, apply and advance scientific knowledge, make relevant information available to patients, colleagues, and the public, obtain consultation, and use the talents of other health professionals when indicated.

VI. A physician shall, in the provision of appropriate patient care, except in emergencies, be free to choose whom to serve, with whom to associate, and the environment in which to provide medical services.

VII. A physician shall recognize a responsibility to participate in activities contributing to an improved community.

Current Opinions of the Council on Ethical and Judicial Affairs of the American Medical Association: including the Principles of Medical Ethics and the Rules of the Council for Ethical and Judicial Affairs" OP632290 /ISBN 0-89970-406-9

Hastings Center
255 Elm Road, Briarcliff Manor, NY 10510
914/762-8500

Joseph and Rose Kennedy Institute of Ethics
National Reference Center for Bioethics Literature
Georgetown University
Washington, DC 20057
800/MED-ETHX (800-633-3849)

Equipment, Medical

Association for the Advancement of Medical Instrumentation
3330 Washington Blvd., Ste 400
Arlington, VA 22201 703/525-4890

For Health Care Professional to
report malfunction:
U.S. Pharmacopeial Convention 800/638-6725
(24 hour)
Food and Drug Administration 301/881-0256
(7:00 a.m. to 4:30 p.m. EST)

ECRI (to evaluate health care technology)
5200 Butler Pike, Plymouth Meeting, PA 19462
215/825-6700 or 6000

Health Industry Distributors Association
225 Reinekers Lane, #650, Alexandria, VA 22314
703/549-4432

Health Industry Manufacturers Association
1200 G Street, NW, Suite 400, Washington, DC
20005 202/783-8700

National Association of Medical
Equipment Suppliers
625 Slaters Lane, Suite 200
Alexandria, VA 22314
703/836-6263

Ethnic Physicians Associations

Association of American Indian Physicians
10015 S. Pennsylvania
Oklahoma City, OK 73159
405/692-1202

National Medical Association (African-American)
1012 Tenth Street, NW, Washington, DC 20001
202/347-1895

Asian-American Medical Society (Only for Indiana)
8695 Connecticut, Suite D, Merrillville, IN 46410
219/769-1124

Chinese American Medical Society
185 S. Orange Avenue, Newark, NJ 07103
201/456-5006

Colombian Medical Association
PO Box 857, Northbrook, IL 60065-0857

Haitian Medical Association Abroad
608 Ogden Avenue, Teaneck, NJ 07666
201/836-2199

California Hispanic-American Medical Association
1020 S. Arroyo Parkway, Suite 200
Pasadena, CA 91066 818/799-5456

American Association of Physicians of India
PO 4370, Flint, MI 48504
313/767-4946

Islamic Medical Association
4121 S. Fairview Avenue, Suite 203, Downers
Grove, IL 60515 708/852-2122

Italian American Medical Association
1127 Wilshire Blvd, Los Angeles, CA 90017
213/481-0896

Association of Pakistani Physicians
4121 Fairview Avenue, Suite L2, Downers Grove,
IL 60515-2236 708/968-8585

Association of Philippine Physicians in America
10004 Kennerly Road, Ste 280B
St. Louis, MO 63128 314/872-8345

Association of Philippine Surgeons in America
2147 Old Greenbrier Road
Chesapeake, VA 23320
804/424-5485

National Medical and Dental Association (Polish)
459 W. Water Street, Elmira, NY 14905
607/733-7503

American Russian Medical and Dental Society
6221 Wilshire Boulevard, #607
Los Angeles, CA 90048 213/933-0711

Turkish American Physicians Association
175 Jericho Turnpike, Suite 312
Syosset, NY 11791
516/921-1223

Virchow-Pirquet Medical Society
515 Madison Avenue, Room 1720
New York, NY 10022
212/734-0682

Euthanasia
"It's Over, Debbie"

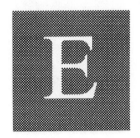

Name Withheld By Request "A Piece of My Mind"
JAMA. 1988 Jan 8; 259(2): 272

The call came in the middle of the night. As a gynecology resident rotating through a large private hospital, I had come to detest telephone calls, because invariably I would be up for several hours and would not feel good the next day. However, duty called, so I answered the phone. A nurse informed me that a patient was having difficulty getting rest, could I please see her. She was on 3 North. That was the gynecologic-oncology unit, not my usual duty station. As I trudged along, bumping sleepily against walls and corners and not believing I was up again, I tried to imagine what I might find at the end of my walk. Maybe an elderly woman with an anxiety reaction, or perhaps something particularly horrible.

I grabbed the chart from the nurses' station on my way to the patient's room, and the nurse gave me some hurried details: a 20-year-old girl named Debbie was dying of ovarian cancer. She was having unrelenting vomiting apparently as the result of an alcohol drip administered for sedation. Hmmm, I thought. Very sad. As I approached the room I could hear loud, labored breathing. I entered and saw an emaciated, dark-haired woman who appeared much older than 20. She was receiving nasal oxygen, had an IV, and was sitting in bed suffering from what was obviously severe air hunger. The chart noted her weight at 80 pounds. A second woman, also dark-haired but of middle age, stood at her right, holding her hand. Both looked up as I entered. The room seemed filled with the patient's desperate effort to survive. Her eyes were hollow, and she had suprasternal and intercostal retractions with her rapid inspiration. She had not eaten or slept in two days. She had not responded to chemotherapy and was being given supportive care only. It was a gallows scene, a cruel mockery of her youth and unfulfilled potential. Her only words to me were, "Let's get this over with."

I retreated with my thoughts to the nurses' station. The patient was tired and needed rest. I could not give her health, but I could give her rest. I asked the nurse to draw 20 mg of morphine sulfate into a syringe. Enough, I thought, to do the job. I took the syringe into the room and told the two women I was going to give Debbie something that would let her rest and say good-bye. Debbie looked at the syringe, than laid her head on the pillow with her eyes open, watching what was left of the world. I injected the morphine intravenously and watched to see if my calculations on its effect would be correct. Within seconds her breathing slowed to a normal rate, her eyes closed, and her features softened as she seemed restful at last. The older woman stroked the hair of the now-sleeping patient. I waited for the inevitable next effect of depressing the respiratory drive. With clocklike certainty, within four minutes the breathing rate slowed even more, then became irregular, then ceased. The dark-haired woman stood erect and seemed relieved.

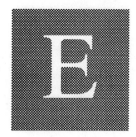

Letters to the Editor:
JAMA. 1988 Apr 8; 259(14): 2095

• To the Editor
I was deeply impressed by the article entitled, "It's Over, Debbie." I would like to expend my most enthusiastic congratulations to the author for having the courage to submit this account. Faced with a similar situation as a resident some years ago, the morphine approach seemed to be the obvious situation. But I just didn't have the strength to relive a young man's suffering in view of the possible repercussions of such an action. It is encouraging to learn that at least one of us risked his career to relieve the suffering of another.
Charles B. Clark, MD

• To the Editor
I am outraged by the action of the physician in this case who served as jury, judge, and executioner of this young patient, and I believe that the vast majority of physicians feel the same way. I also strongly protest JAMA's publication of this article. It casts the medical profession in a very unfavorable light. Is it any wonder that most polls in recent years have shown that physicians are not held in as high esteem as they used to be?
John G. Manesis, MD

Dr. Kevorkian calls for a new discipline - providing euthanasia

Diane M. Gianelli AMNews 2/10/92 p.3

While a grand jury weighs possible murder charges against him for his role in the deaths of two Michigan women, Jack Kevorkian, MD, again finds himself in the limelight.

This, time the man who proudly calls himself "Dr. Death" has taken to the pages of the American Journal of Forensic Psychiatry to outline his proposal for a new medical specialty of euthanasia practitioners.

This specialty would be called "obitiatry," the practice "medicide" and the practitioners " obitiatrist".

The article is accompanied by commentaries from more than a dozen psychiatrists and psychologists. While many praised Dr. Kevorkian's actions in sparking professional debate over euthanasia and physician-assisted suicide, most decried his methods and proposals.

Dr. Kevorkian is the 63-year-old retired Royal Oak, Mich., pathologist who won notoriety in the summer of 1990 for his role in helping an Oregon woman kill herself with his "self-execution" machine.

Last fall, he acknowledged assisting in the suicides of two Michigan women. The local county medical examiner ruled those deaths homicides and a grand jury has been convened to determine whether to recommend criminal charges, which could range up to murder (AMN, Jan. 13). He was charged with murder in the 1990 case, but the charge was later dismissed.

While Dr. Kevorkian might be viewed as one of the nation's most radical proponents of active euthanasia, his cause is not without supporters.

A bitterly fought proposal to legalize euthanasia failed narrowly in Washington state last November. Similar efforts are now under way in California, where supporters are gathering signatures in hopes of putting the issue before voters there. Other states will soon face the issue as well - either in the form of legislation or initiatives.

In his 41-page journal article, Dr. Kevorkian says he envisions his specialty to be like others, in that practitioners - all physicians - would undergo residencies, board certification and the like. He says "pioneers" such as himself would pass on the tools of the trade.

Dr. Kevorkian says euthanasia and physician-assisted suicide have historically been viewed as "ethical" services, "widely practiced by physicians and endorsed by almost all segments of society" in ancient Greece. He blames "inflexible and harshly punitive" Western Judeo-Christian principles for the current backlash against euthanasia.

He compares today's physicians who obey laws against euthanasia with Nazi Physicians who "were guilty of obeying obviously immoral laws, dictated by their own peculiar National-Socialist 'religion,' which compelled them to do to or for patients what they should not even have thought about doing."

Dr. Kevorkian sees medicine as a strictly secular endeavor and says medical ethics should be entirely separate from religious ethics. As an example, he says a Catholic doctor should be prepared to provide an atheistic woman with an abortion without suffering religious qualms. He acknowledges that those who oppose euthanasia frequently do so because they fear abuse. His plan, he says, is fail-safe.

Dr. Kevorkian proposes that the nation's first obitiatry model begin in his home state of Michigan, which he has divided into 11 zones with one central headquarters.

Requests for medicide would be sent to this headquarters, in writing, by a patients' personal physician. The headquarters' secretary would call a obitiatrist, who would meet with the patient, his or her family and doctor. At least five obitiatrists would be involved in each case, two of whom would actually perform the euthanasia. The other three would confirm the patient's diagnosis, provide a psychiatric evaluation and perform other ancillary services.

Dr. Kevorkian says the patient should also see a social worker and have the opportunity to consult with a representative of the clergy.

To flesh out his proposal, Dr. Kevorkian's article includes a euthanasia scenario featuring a cast of hypothetical characters. These include a Wanda Endittal, the patient requesting medically assisted suicide; Flo N. and Justin Tiers as her parents; Drs. Will B. Reddy, Les Payne and Shelby Dunne as obiatrists; and Lotte Goode and Sy Keyes as psychiatric obiatrists.

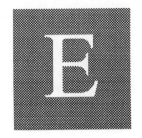

Many of those commenting on Dr. Kervorkian's proposal agreed that he has furthered public debate on the issue. But most questioned some of his basic premises, as well as the bulk of his proposal.

Navy psychiatrist Kenneth Karols, MD, PhD, called the article "thought-provoking in the extreme," but dismissed the bureaucracy Dr. Kervorkian proposed as "truly horrifying."

"If such a monster were created, it would probably kill its clients through frustration and boredom," he wrote.

Douglas Anderson, MD, a New York clinical and forensic psychiatrist wrote a spirited rebuttal that took a swipe at some of Dr. Kervorkian's witticisms.

Dr. Anderson suggested calling the obiatrist an "assisted suicide specialist" or ASS. He also suggested that "headquarters" sounded to officious, instead recommending "suicide sites" or SS. "This might be particulary appropriate for sites which offer the 'lethal gas' option."

Dr. Anderson noted that Dr. Kevorkian's specialty would certainly save taxpayers a lot of money now being spent on medical research.

"At a stroke, Dr. Kevorkian has discovered the means to end the pain and suffering of all but the most masochistic of patients. So we shall no longer need to fund any more research into cancer, AIDS, multiple sclerosis, or cerebral palsy. Just think of it: no more telethons!" he wrote.

Ronald Shlensky, MD, a Santa Barbara, Calif., psychiatrist and attorney, said Dr. Kevorkian's proposal neglected those most in need of physician assisted deaths: the "senile living dead."

"These ghosts of our parents occupy our nursing homes, aggravate their loved ones and consume precious resources...The time has come when growing emphasis on relief of human suffering, rather than only the preservation of life, is appropriate and meaningful as a medical undertaking," he said.

Jay B. Cohn, MD, PhD. of Long Beach, Calif., said he was a firm believer in self-determination and that "if a patient was wants to kill himself, and he is mentally competent enough to make the decision...the means are there. It's not really that hard and one can do it without a doctor's assistance."

Seattle psychiatrist Dr. D.J. Bonnington, MD, rejected Dr. Kevorkian's premise outright. "No matter what rationalization he uses to assist a patient in suicide, regardless of the checks and balances he meticulously spells out, physician-assisted suicide remains an immoral and unethical act unbecoming the physician."

He recommended that more attention be given to the treatment of depressed patients in the form of antidepressants, narcotics and psychotherapy. "Proper handling of the depression can have a salutary effect upon the pain and suffering that Dr. Kevorkian wishes to treat with suicide."

Dr. Bonnington also warned that "elderly patients in nursing homes can be subtly influenced by the staff to request suicide if such becomes the law. Running out of money would present a real threat since it could mean running out of life."

And he took issue with Dr. Kevorkian's assertion that the personal and professional ethics of the physician should be entirely separate.

"The physician had moral values long before he donned the cloak of physicianhood," Dr. Bonnington wrote.

Choice in Dying
250 W. 57th St. Rm. 831, New York, NY 10107
212/246-0493 800/248-2122

Hemlock Society
PO Box 11830, Eugene, OR 97440-3900
503/342-5748

Executives (Medical)

Director, Dental Services Administers dental program in hospital and directs departmental activities in accordance with accepted national standards and administrative policies: Confers with hospital administrators to formulate policies and recommend procedural changes. Establishes training program to advance knowledge and clinical skill levels of resident dentists studying for dental specializations. Implements procedures for hiring of professional staff and approves hiring and promotion of staff members. Establishes work schedules and assigns staff members to duty stations to maximize efficient use of staff. Observes and assists staff members at work to ensure safe and ethical practices and to solve problems and demonstrate techniques. Confers with hospital administrator to submit budget and statistical reports used to justify expenditures for equipment, supplies, and personnel. (DOT)

Adminstrator, Health Care Facility Directs adminstration of hospital, nursing home, or other health care facility within authority of governing board: Administers fiscal operations, such as budget planning, accounting, and establishing rates for health care services. Directs hiring and training of personnel. Negotiates for improvement of and additions to buildings and equipment. Directs and coordinates activities of medical, nursing, and administrative staffs and services. Develops policies and procedures for various establishment activities. May represent establishment at community meetings and promote programs through various news media. May develop or expand programs or services for scientific research, preventive medicine, medical and vocational rehabilitation, and community health and welfare promotion. May be designated according to type of health care facility as Hospital Administrator (medical ser.) or Nursing Home Adminstrator (medical ser.). (DOT)

Director, Pharmacy Services Directs and coordinates, through subordinate supervisory personnel, activities and functions of hospital pharmacy: Plan and implements procedures in hospital pharmacy according to hospital policies, and legal requirements. Directs pharmacy personnel programs, such as hiring, training, and intern programs. Confers with computer personnel to develop computer programs for pharmacy

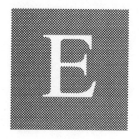

information management systems, patient and department charge systems, and inventory control. Analyzes records to indicate prescribing trends and excessive usage. Prepares pharmacy budget and department reports required by hospital administrators. Attends staff meetings to advise and inform hospital medical staff of drug applications and characteristics, Observes pharmacy personnel at work and develops quality assurance techniques to ensure safe, legal, and ethical practices. Oversees preparation and dispensation of experimental drugs. (DOT)

American Association of Medical
Society Executives
515 N. State, Chicago, IL 60610
312/464-2555

American College of Healthcare Executives
840 N. Lake Shore Dr., Chicago, IL 60611
312/943-0544

American College of Physician Executives
(previously American Academy
of Medical Directors)
4830 West Kennedy Blvd., Suite 648
Tampa, FL 33609 813/287-2000

American Medical Directors Association
10480 Little Patuxent Pkwy, Suite 760,
Columbia, MD 21044
301/740-9743

Medical Group Management Association
1355 S. Colorado Blvd., Denver, CO 80222
303/799-1111

National Association of Health
Services Executives
1101 14th Street, N.W./10th Floor
Washington, DC 20005
202/289-1029

Exercise

Aerobics and Fitness Association of America
15250 Ventura Blvd, Ste 310,
Sherman Oaks, CA 91403
800/445-5950

Aquatic Exercise Association
PO Box 497, Port Washington, WI 53074
414/284-3416

National Fitness Foundation
2250 E. Imperial Hwy., Suite 412,
El Segundo, CA 90245
213/640-0145

President's Council on Physical Fitness and
Sports 450 5th St. NW, Suite 7103,
Washington, DC 20001
202/272-3421

Exercise Physiology

American Physiological Society
9650 Rockville Pike, Bethesda, MD 20014
301/530-7164

Exercise Physiologist develops, implements, and coordinates exercise programs and administers medical tests, under physician's supervision, to program participants to promote physical fitness: Explains program and test procedures to participant. Interviews participant to obtain vital statistics and medical history and records information. Records heart activity, using electrocardiograph (EKG) machine, while participant undergoes stress test on treadmill, under physician's supervision. Measures oxygen consumption and lung functioning, using spirometer. Measures amount of fat in body, using such equipment as hydrostatic scale, skinfold calipers, and tape measure, to assess body composition. Performs routine laboratory test of blood samples for cholesterol level and glucose tolerance, or interprets test results. Schedules other examinations and tests, such as a physical examination, chest x-ray, and urinalysis.

Records, test data in patient's chart or enters data into computer. Writes initial and follow-up exercise prescriptions for participants, following physician's recommendation, specifying equipment, such as treadmill, track, or bike. Demonstrates correct use of exercise equipment and exercise routines. Conducts individual and group aerobic, strength, and flexibility exercises. Observes participants during exercise for signs of stress. Teaches behavior modification classes, such as stress management, weight control, and related subjects. Orders material and supplies and calibrates equipment. May supervise work activities of other staff members. (DOT)

National Dance Association
1900 Association Drive, Reston, VA 22091
703/476-3436

Exhibits, Health Care

Health Care Exhibitors Association
5775 Peachtree, Building D, Suite 500
Atlanta, GA 30342
404/252-3663

Eyes

Eye Bank Association of America
1511 K St. NW, Suite 830, Washington, DC 20005
202/638-4280

National Eye Institute,
Office of Scientific Reporting Building 31
Room 6A32,
Bethesda, MD 20892 (free brochures)

National Eye Care Project (for needy)
800/222-EYES

National Eye Research Foundation
910 Skokie Blvd., Suite 207A
Northbrook, IL 60062
708/564-4652

Familial Polyposis

Familial Polyposis Registry
Department of Colorectal Surgery, Cleveland
Clinic Foundation
9500 Euclid Avenue, Cleveland, OH 44195-5044
216/444-6470

Family Practice

Family Practitioner - alternate titles: family
physician Provides comprehensive medical
services for members of family, regardless of age
or sex, on continuing basis: Examines patients,
using medical instruments and equipment. Elicits
and records information about patient's medical
history. Orders or executes various tests,
analyses, and diagnostic images to provide
information on patient's condition. Analyzes
reports and findings of tests and examination, and
diagnoses condition of patient. Administers or
prescribes treatments and medications. Promotes
health by advising patients concerning diet,
hygiene, and methods for prevention of disease.
Inoculates and vaccinates patients to immunize
patients from communicable diseases. Provides
prenatal care to pregnant women, delivers babies,
and provides postnatal care to mothers and
infants. Performs surgical procedures
commensurate with surgical competency. Refers
patients to medical specialist for consultant
services when necessary for patient's well-being.
(DOT)

American Board of Family Practice
2228 Young Dr., Lexington, KY 40505
606/269-5626

American Academy of Family Physicians
8880 Ward Parkway, Kansas City, MO 64114
816/333-9700

Federal Licensure Exam (Flex Exam)

(Exam administered by individual
state licensing boards)
Federation of State Medical Boards of the United
States, Inc.
6000 Western Place/Suite 707
Ft. Worth, TX 76107-4618
817/735-8445

Federal Trade Commission (FTC)

Federal Trade Commission
Pennsylvania Ave at Sixth St, NW
Washington, DC 20580
202/326-2222

The purpose of the Federal Trade Commission is
expressed in the Federal Trade Commission Act
(15 U.S.C. 41-51) and the Clayton Act (15 U.S.C.
12), both passed in 1914 and both successively
amended in the years that have followed. The
Federal Trade Commission Act prohibits the use
in commerce of "unfair methods of competition"
and "unfair or deceptive acts or practices." The
Clayton Act outlaws specific practices recognized
as instruments of monopoly. As administrative
agency, acting quasi-judicially and
quasi-legislatively, the Commission was
established to deal with trade practices on a
continuing and corrective basis. It has no authority
to punish; its function is to "prevent," through

cease-and-desist orders and other means, those
practices condemned by the law of Federal trade
regulation; however, court-ordered civil penalties
up to $10,000 may be obtained for each violation
of a Commission order or trade regulation rule.
(USG)

Fertility

American Fertility Society
2140 11th Avenue South, Suite 200
Birmingham, AL 35205-2800
205/933-8494

Fertility Research Foundation
1430 Second Ave., Suite 103
New York, NY 10021
212/744-5500

Resolve, Inc.
PO Box 474, Belmont, MA 02178
617/484-2424

JAMA Theme Issue: Human Reproduction.
JAMA. 1986 Jan 3; 255(1)
Various aspects of human reproduction are
presented here. Letters regarding DES, and
smoking, sex and pregnancy are reproduced.
Fully developed articles include those on maternal
mortality and urban sex education, comments and
editorials on related and independent subjects,
plus discussions of contraception and artificial
insemination communicate some of the thoughts
of the profession in the mid-eighties.

Fetal Tissue

Medical Application of Fetal Tissue
Transplantation. Council on Scientific Affairs and
Council on Ethical and Judicial Affairs.
JAMA. 1990 Jan 26; 263(4): 565-70
Fetal tissue transplantation has been attempted for a limited
number of clinical disorders, including Parkinson's disease,
diabetes, immunodeficiency disorders, and several metabolic
disorders. Fetal tissue has intrinsic properties--ability to
differentiate into multiple cell types, growth and proliferative
ability, growth factor production, and reduced antigenicity--that
make it attractive for transplantation research. At this time the
results from fetal tissue grafts for Parkinson's disease and
diabetes have not demonstrated significant long-term clinical
benefit to patients with these disorders. Further research will
be necessary to determine the potential value of fetal tissue
transplantation. For these clinical investigations to proceed,
specific ethical guidelines are needed to ensure that fetal
tissue derived from elective abortions is used in a morally
acceptable manner. These guidelines should separate, to the
greatest extent possible, the decision by a woman to have an
abortion from her consent to donate the postmortem tissue for
transplantation purposes. Such ethical guidelines are offered
in this report.

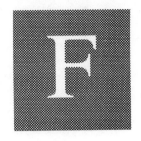

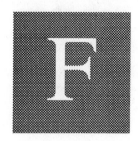

Fifth Pathway

AMA Policy: Fifth Pathway: *(1) The AMA believes that the Fifth Pathway is fulfilling its purpose of improving the education of U.S. FMGs who have completed the program and has served to help maintain standards for licensure in those jurisdiction which would have been politically pressed to lower them to accommodate these students without additional education. (2) To reaffirm the intent of the Fifth Pathway policy, namely to provide an alternative route of entry graduate medical education for qualified students studying abroad who are not eligible through the ECFMG route, the policy should be revised to ask the sponsoring medical schools to establish more stringent requirements for admission to and successful completion of a Fifth Pathway program. (3) The AMA supports the principle that any existing or proposed alternative programs conducted by U.S. medical schools to facilitate entry of U.S. citizens studying in foreign medical schools into U.S. programs should assure that those who complete such programs are reasonably comparable to the school's regularly enrolled and graduated students.*

Food and Drug Administration (FDA)

The name **Food and Drug Administration** was first provided by the Agriculture Appropriation Act of 1931 (46 Stat. 392), although similar law enforcement functions had been in existence under different organizational titles since January 1, 1907, when the Food and Drug Act of 1906 (21 U.S.C. 1-15) became effective. The Food and Drug Administration's activities are directed toward protecting the health of the Nation against impure and unsafe foods, drugs and cosmetics, and other potential hazards. (USG)

Office of Consumer Affairs, Public Inquiries
5600 Fishers Lane, Rockville, MD 20857
301/443-3170
Breast Implant Hotline 800/532-4440

Foreign Medical Schools

Educational Commission for
Foreign Medical Graduates
3624 Market St, Philadelphia, PA 19104
215/386-5900

World Directory of Medical Schools, 6th ed. World Health Organization, Geneva. 1988. pp. 311.
ISBN 92-4-150008-5
WHO Publications USA, 49 Sheridan Ave.,
Albany, NY 12210
518/436-9686

Directory of Medical Schools Worldwide, 5th edition. US Directory Service, Miami. 1991 pp. 178. ISBN 0-916524-41-8
US Directory Service, 655 NW 128 St.
Miami, FL 33168
305-769-1700

Forensic Medicine

American Board of Forensic Psychiatry
1211 Cathedral St., Baltimore, MD 21201
301/539-0872

International Reference Organization in Forensic Medicine and Sciences
c/o Dr. William G. Eckert
PO Box 8282 Wichita, KS 67208
316/685-7612

Milton Helpern Institute of Forensic Medicine
520 First Ave., New York, NY 10016
212/340-0102

National Association of Medical Examiners
1402 S. Grand Blvd., St. Louis, MO 63104
314/577-8298

Foster Care

Foster Parents Plan, Inc.
155 Plan Way, Warwick, RI 02886
800/556-7918

Contact state office of Children and Family Services for foster care options.

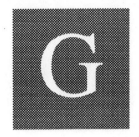

Gastroenterology

American College of Gastroenterology
4222 King St, Alexandria, VA 22302
703/549-4440

American Gastroenterological Association
6900 Grove Rd., Thorofare, NJ 08086
609/848-9218

American Society for Gastrointestinal Endoscopy
13 Elm St., Manchester, MA 01944
508/526-8330

For information and standards on laparoscopic
cholecystectomy contact:
Society of American Gastrointestinal
Endoscopic Surgeons
1271 Stoner Ave, Los Angeles, CA 90025
213/479-3249

Gaucher Disease

National Gaucher Foundation
1424 K Street, NW, 4th Floor,
Washington, DC 20005
202/393-2777

General Practitioner

Alternate titles: physician, general practice
Diagnoses and treats variety of diseases and
injuries in general practice: Examines patients,
using medical instruments and equipment. Orders
or executes various tests, analyses, and
diagnostic images to provide information on
patient's condition. Analyzes reports and findings
of tests and of examination, and diagnoses
condition. Administers or prescribes treatments
and drugs. Inoculates and vaccinates patients to
immunize patients from communicable diseases.
Advises patients concerning diet, hygiene, and
methods for prevention of disease. Provides
prenatal care to mother and infant. Reports births,
deaths, and outbreak of contagious diseases to
governmental authorities. Refers patients to
medical specialist or other practitioner for
specialized treatment. Performs minor surgery.
May make house and emergency calls to attend
to patients unable to visit office or clinic. May
conduct physical examinations to provide
information needed for admission to school,
consideration for jobs, or eligibility for insurance
coverage. May provide care for passengers and
crew aboard ship and be designated Ship's
Doctor. (DOT)

Genetics

Genetics Society of America
9650 Rockville Pike, Bethesda, MD 20814
301/571-1825

National Center for Human Genome Research
The Center advises the Director of NIH and senior
staff on all aspects of genomic analysis;
coordinates the integration, review, and planning
of genomic analysis; formulates research goals
and long-range plans with the guidance of the NIH
Program Advisory Committee on Complex
Genomes; serves as a focal point for coordination
with NIH and will be the HHS point of contact for
Federal interagency coordination, collaboration
with industry and academia, and international
cooperation; fosters, conducts, supports, and
administers research and research training
programs directed at promoting the growth and
quality of research relating to mapping and
sequencing of complex genomes through: (a)
research grants, contracts, and cooperative
agreements with institutions and individuals, (b)
individual and institutional research training
awards, (c) promotion of closer interaction with
other bases of genomic analysis research, and (d)
collection and dissemination of research findings
in these areas. The Center develops plans for the
centralized, systematic-targeted effort to create
detailed maps of the genomes of organisms;
sponsors scientific meetings and symposia to
promote progress through information sharing;
and fosters national and international information
exchanges with industry and academia concerning
research on complex genomes.(USG)

Genetic Syndromes

Charcot-Marie-Tooth International
Charcot-Marie Tooth is also known as Peroneal
Muscular Atrophy/Heredity Motor
and Sensory Neuropathy)
One Springbank Drive, St. Catharines, Ontario,
Canada L25 2K1
416/687-3630

Cornelia De Lange Syndrome Foundation
c/o Julie Mairano, 60 Dyer Ave.,
Collinsville, CT 06022
800/223-8355

Cri Du Chat Syndrome Society
11609 Oakmont, Overland Park, KS 66210
913/469-8900

National **Down's Syndrome** Society
141 5th Ave., New York, NY 10010
212/460-9330
800/221-4602 (Hotline)

Fragile X Foundation
PO Box 300233, Denver, CO 80220
800/835-2246, ext.58
The Fragile X Syndrome is an inherited defect of
the X chromosome that causes mental
retardation. Fragile X syndrome is the most
common cause of mental retardation in males
after Down's syndrome.

The disorder occurs within families according to
an X-linked recessive pattern of inheritance.
Although males are mainly affected, women are
able to carry the genetic defect responsible for the
disorder and pass it on to some of their daughters,
who in turn become carriers of the defect.

Approximately one in 1,500 men is affected by the
condition; one in 1,000 women is a carrier. In
addition to being mentally retarded, affected
males are generally tall, physically strong, have a
prominent nose, and jaw, increased ear length,
large testicles, and are prone to epileptic seizures.
About one third of female carriers show some
degree of intellectual impairment.

There is no treatment for the condition. If a woman
has a history of the syndrome in her family, it is
useful to seek genetic counseling regarding the
risk of a child being affected.(ENC)

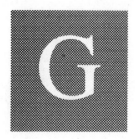

Friedreich's Ataxia Group in America
PO Box 11116, Oakland CA 94611
415/655-0833
Friedreich's Ataxia is a very rare inherited disease in which degeneration of nerve fibers in the spinal cord causes ataxia (loss of coordinated movement and balance). The disease is the result of a genetic defect, usually of the autosomal recessive type. It affects about two people per 100,000.

Symptoms first appear in late childhood or adolescence. The main symptoms are unsteadiness when walking, clumsy hand movements, slurred speech, and rapid, involuntary eye movements. In many cases there are also abnormalities of bone structure and alignment.

There is as yet no cure for the disease. Once it has developed, it becomes progressively more severe, and, within 10 years of onset, more than half the sufferers are confined to wheelchairs. IF cardiomyopathy (heart muscle disease) develops, it may contribute to an early death. People who have blood relatives with Friedreich's ataxia should seek genetic counseling before starting a family.(ENC)

National **Marfan** Foundation
382 Main Street, Port Washington, NY 11050
516/883-8712

Meniere's Disease
EAR Foundation
200 Church Street, Box 111, Nashville, TN 37236
615/329-7809

Spina Bifida Association of America
1700 Rockville Pike, Ste., Rockville, MD 20852
800/621-3141; 301/770-7222
A congenital defect in which part of one (or more) vertebrae fails to develop completely, leaving a portion of the spinal cord exposed. Spina bifida can occur anywhere on the spine but is most common in the lower back. The severity of the condition depends on how much nerve tissue is exposed.(ENC)

National **Tay Sach's** and Allied
Diseases Association
385 Elliot St., Newton, MA 02164
617/964-5508
A serious inherited brain disorder that results in very early death. Tay-Sachs disease was formerly known as amaurotic family idiocy.

Tay-Sachs disease is caused by a deficiency of hexosaminidase, a certain enzyme (a protein essential for regulating chemical reactions in the body). Deficiency results in a buildup of a harmful substance in the brain. The disease is most common among Ashkenazi Jews. The incidence in this group is around one in 2,500, which is 100 time higher than in any other ethnic group. The gene for Tay-Sachs disease is recessive and an Ashkenazi Jew has a one in 25 chance of carrying it. If two carriers marry, there is a one in four chance that they will have an affected child.

Signs of the illness, which appear during the first six months of life, are blindness, dementia, deafness, seizures, and paralysis. An exaggerated startle response to sound is an early sign. Symptoms progress rapidly and the affected child usually dies before age 3.(ENC)

Geriatrics

Aging and Caring

Paul E. Ruskin, MD "A Piece of My Mind" JAMA. 1983 Nov 11; 250(18): 2440

I was invited to present a lecture to a class of graduate nurses who were studying the "Psychosocial Aspects of Aging." I started my lecture with the following case presentation:

The patient is a white female who appears her reported age. She neither speaks nor comprehends the spoken word. Sometimes she babbles incoherently for on end. She is disoriented about person, place, and time. She does, however, seem to recognize her own name. I have worked with her for the past six months, but she still does not recognize me.

She shows complete disregard for her physical appearance and makes no effort whatsoever to assist in her own care. She must be fed, bathed, and clothed by others. Because she is edentulous, her food must be pureed, and because she is incontinent of both urine and stool, she must be changed and bathed often. Her shirt is generally soiled from incessant drooling. She does not walk. Her sleep pattern is erratic. Often she wakens in the middle of the night, and her screaming awakens others.

Most of the time she is very friendly and happy. However, several times a day she gets quite agitated without apparent cause. Then she screams loudly until someone comes to comfort her.

After the case presentation, I asked the nurses how they would feel about taking care of a patient such as the one described. They used words such as "frustrated," "hopeless," "depressed," and "annoyed" to describe how they would feel.

When I stated that I enjoyed taking care of her and that I thought they would, too, the class looked at me in disbelief. I then passed around a picture of the patient: my 6-month-old daughter.

After the laughter had subsided, I asked why it was so much more difficult to care for a 90-year-old than a 6-month-old with identical symptoms. We all agreed that it is physically easier to take care of a helpless baby weighing 15 pounds than a helpless adult weighing 100, but the answer seemed to go deeper than this.

The infant, we all agreed, represents new life, hope, and almost infinite potential. The demented senior citizen, on the other hand, represents the end of life, with little potential for growth.

We need to change our perspective. The aged patient is just as lovable as the child. Those who are ending their lives in the helplessness of old age deserve the same and attention as those who are beginning their lives in the helplessness of infancy.
American Geriatrics Society
770 Lexington, New York, NY 10021
212/308-1414

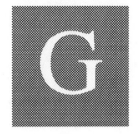

Board Certification
American Board of Family Practice
2228 Young Dr., Lexington, KY 40505
606/269-5626

American Board of Internal Medicine
3624 Market Street, Philadelphia, PA 19104
215/243-1500
800/441-ABIM (800/441-2246)

Gerontological Society of America
1275 K. St., NW, Ste 350, Washington, DC 20005
202/842-1275

Gifts to Physicians from Industry
Annotated Guidelines of Gifts to
Physicians from Industry:
Council on Ethical and Judicial Affairs
American Medical Association, Chicago, Illinois
Final Version: Issued October 9, 1991

On December 3, 1990, the Council on Ethical and
Judicial Affairs issued its guidelines on gifts to
physicians from industry. Since then, the Council
has received numerous requests for
interpretations of the guidelines. In order to
facilitate application of the guidelines, the Council
has developed the following annotated version
that includes representative questions about the
guidelines:

General Questions:
• *When do the interpretations take effect?*
The guidelines and interpretations are in full
force. However, the interpretations do not apply
retroactively to programs that have been
planned in a good faith that they complied with
the guidelines.
• *Do the guidelines apply only to pharmaceutical,
device, and equipment manufacturers?*
"Industry" includes all "proprietary health-related
entities that might create a conflict of interest,"
as recommended by the American Academy of
Family Physicians.

***Guideline One. Any gifts accepted by physicians
individually should primarily entail a benefit to
patients and should not be of substantial value.
Accordingly, textbooks, modest meals and other
gifts are appropriate if they serve a genuine
educational function. Cash payments should not
be accepted.***

a. *May physicians accept gram stain test kits,
stethoscopes or other diagnostic equipment?*
Diagnostic equipment primarily benefits the
patient.Hence, such gifts are permissible as long
as they are not of substantial value. In considering
the value of the gift, the relevant measure is not
the cost to the company of providing the gift.
Rather, the relevant measure is the cost to the
physician if he purchased the gift on the open
market.

b. *May companies invite physicians to a dinner
with a speaker and donate $100 to a charity or
medical school on behalf of the physician?*
There are positive aspects to the proposal. The
donations would be used for a worthy cause, and
the physicians would receive important
information about patient care. There is a direct
personal benefit to the physician as well, however.

An organization that is important to the physician -
and one that the physician might have ordinarily
felt obligated to make a contribution to - receives
financial support as a result of the physician's
decision to attend the meeting. On balance,
physicians should make their own judgment about
these inducements. If the charity is predetermined
without the physician's input, there would seem to
be little problem with the arrangement.

c. *May contributions to a professional society's
general fund be accepted from industry?*
The guidelines are designed to deal with gifts from
industry which affect, or could appear to affect, the
judgment of individual practicing physicians. In
general, a professional society should make its
own judgment about gifts from industry to the
society itself.

d. *When companies invite physicians to a dinner
with a speaker, what are the relevant guidelines?*
First, the dinner must be a modest meal. Second,
the guideline does allow gifts that primarily benefit
patients and that are not of substantial value.
Accordingly, textbooks and other gifts that
primarily benefit patient care and that have a value
to the physician in the general range of $100 are
permissible.

e. *May physicians accept vouchers that reimburse
them for uncompensated care they have provided?*
No. Such a voucher would result directly in
increased income for the physician.

f. *May physicians accumulate "points" by
attending several educational or promotional
meetings and then choose a gift from a catalogue
of educational options?*
This guideline permits gifts only if they are not of
substantial value. If accumulation of points would
result in physicians receiving a substantial gift by
combining insubstantial gifts over a relatively short
period of time, it would be inappropriate.

g. *May physicians accept gift certificates for
educational materials when attending promotional
or educational events?*
The Council views gift certificates as a grey area
which is not per se prohibited by the guidelines.
Medical text books are explicitly approved as gifts
under the guidelines. A gift certificate for
educational materials, i.e., for the selection by the
physician from an exclusively medical text book
catalogue, would not seem to be materially
different. The issue is whether the gift certificate
gives the recipient such control as to make the
certificate similar to cash. As with charitable
donations, pre-selection by the sponsor removes
any question. It is up to the individual physician to
make the final judgment.

***Guideline Two. Individual gifts of minimal value
are permissible as long as the gifts are related to
the physician's work (e.g., pens and notepads).***

***Guideline Three. Subsidies to underwrite the
costs of continuing medical education
conferences or professional meetings can
contribute to the improvement of patient care
and therefore are permissible. Since the giving
of a subsidy directly to a physician by a
company's sales representative may create a
relationship which could influence the use of the***

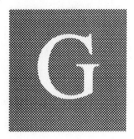

company's products, any subsidy should be accepted by the conference's sponsor who in turn can use the money to reduce the conference's registration fee. Payments to defray the costs of a conference should not be accepted directly from the company by the physicians attending the conference.

a. *Are conference subsidies from the educational division of a company covered by the guidelines?*
Yes. When the Council says "any subsidy," it would not matter whether the subsidy comes from the sales division, the educational division or some other section of the company.

b. *May a company or its intermediary send physicians a check or voucher to offset the registration fee at a specific conference or a conference of the physician's choice.*
Physicians should not directly accept checks or certificates which would be used to offset registration fees. The gift of a reduced registration should be made across the board and through the accredited sponsor.

Guideline Four. Subsidies from industry should not be accepted directly or indirectly to pay for the costs of travel, lodging or other personal expenses of physicians attending conferences or meetings, nor should subsidies be accepted to compensate for the physicians' time. Subsidies for hospitality should not be accepted outside of modest meals or social events held as a part of a conference or meeting. It is appropriate for faculty at conferences or meetings to accept reasonable honoraria and to accept reimbursement for reasonable travel, lodging and meal expenses. It is also appropriate for consultants who provide genuine services to receive reasonable compensation and to accept reimbursement for reasonable travel, lodging and meal expenses. Token consulting or advisory arrangements cannot be used to justify compensating physicians for their time or their travel, lodging and other out-of-pocket expenses.

a. *If a company invites physicians to visit its facilities for a tour or to become educated about one of its products, may the company pay travel expenses and honoraria?*
This question has come up in the context of a rehabilitation facility that wants physicians to know of its existence so that they may refer their patients to the facility. It has also come up in the context of surgical device or equipment manufacturers who want physicians to become familiar with their products.
In general, travel expenses should not be reimbursed, nor should honoraria be paid for the visiting physician's time since the presentations are analogous to a pharmaceutical company's educational or promotional meetings. The Council recognizes that medical devices, equipment and other technologies may require, in some circumstances, special evaluation or training in proper usage that can not practicably be provided except on site. Medical specialties are in a better position to advise physicians regarding the appropriateness of reimbursement with regard to these trips. In cases where the company insists on such visits as a means of protection from

liability for improper usage, physicians and their specialties should make the judgment. In no case would honoraria be appropriate and any travel expenses should be only those strictly necessary.

b. *If the company invites physicians to visit its facilities for review and comment on a product, to discuss their independent research projects or to explore the potential for collaborative research, may the company pay travel expenses and honorarium?*
If the physician is providing genuine services, reasonable compensation for time and travel expenses can be given. However, token advisory or consulting arrangements cannot be used to justify compensation.

c. *May a company hold a sweepstakes for physicians in which five entrants receive a trip to the Virgin Islands or airfare to the medical meeting of their choice?*
No. The use of a sweepstakes or raffle to deliver a gift does not affect the permissibility of the gift. Since the sweepstakes is not open to the public, the guidelines apply in full force.

d. *If a company convenes a group of physicians to recruit clinical investigators or convenes a group of clinical investigators for a meeting to discuss their results, may the company pay for their travel expenses?*
Expenses may be paid if the meetings serve a genuine research purpose. One guide to their propriety would be whether the NIH conducts similar meetings when it sponsors multi-center clinical trials. When travel subsidies are acceptable, the guidelines emphasize that they be used to pay only for "reasonable" expenses. The reasonableness of expenses would depend on a number of considerations. For example, meetings are likely to be problematic if overseas locations are used for exclusively domestic investigators. It would be inappropriate to pay for recreation or entertainment beyond the kind of modest hospitality described in this guideline.

e. *How can a physician tell whether there is a "genuine research purpose?"*
A number of factors can be considered. Signs that a genuine research purpose exists include the facts that there are (1) a valid study protocol, (2) recruitment of physicians with appropriate qualifications or expertise, and (3) recruitment of an appropriate number of physicians in light of the number of study participants needed for statistical evaluation.

f. *May a company compensate physicians for their time and travel expenses when they participate in focus groups?*
Yes. As long as the focus groups serve a genuine and exclusive research purpose and are not used for promotional purposes, physicians may be compensated for time and travel expenses. The number of physicians used in a particular focus group or in multiple focus groups should be an appropriate size to accomplish the research purpose, but no larger.

g. *Do the restrictions on travel, lodging and meals apply to educational programs run by medical schools, professional societies or other accredited organizations which are funded by industry, or do they apply only to programs developed and run by industry?*

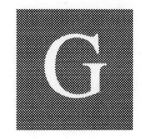

The restrictions apply to all conferences or meetings which are funded by industry. The Council drew no distinction on the basis of the organizer of the conference or meeting. The Council felt that the gift of travel expenses is too substantial even when the conference is run by a non-industry sponsor. (Industry includes all "proprietary health-related entities that might create a conflict of interest" as recommended by the American Academy of Family Physicians.)

h. *May company funds be used for travel expenses and honoraria of bona fide faculty at educational meetings?*
This guideline draws a distinction between attendees and faculty. As was stated, "[i]t is appropriate for faculty at conferences or meetings to accept reasonable honoraria and to accept reimbursement for reasonable travel, lodging, and meal expenses."
Companies need to be mindful of the guidelines of the Accreditation Council on Continuing Medical Education. According to those guidelines, "[f]unds from a commercial source should be in the form of an educational grant made payable to the CME sponsor for the support of programming."

i. *May travel expenses be reimbursed for physicians presenting a poster or a "free paper" at a scientific conference?*
Reimbursement may be accepted only by a bona fide faculty. The presentation of a poster or a free paper does not by itself qualify a person as a member of the conference faculty for purposes of these guidelines.

j. *When a professional association schedules a long-range planning meeting, is it appropriate for industry to subsidize the travel expenses of the meeting participants?*
The guidelines are designed to deal with gifts from industry which affect, or could appear to affect, the judgment of individual practicing physicians. In general, a professional society should make its own judgment about gifts from industry to the society itself.

k. *May continuing medical education conference be held in the Bahamas, Europe or South America?*
There are no restrictions on the location of conferences as long as the attendees are paying their own travel expenses.

l. *May travel expenses be accepted by physicians who are being trained as speakers or faculty for educational conferences and meetings?*
In general, no. If a physician is presenting as independent expert at a CME event both the training and its reimbursement raise questions about independence. In addition, the training is a gift because the physician's role is generally more analogous to that of an attendee than a participant. Speaker training sessions can be distinguished from meetings (See 4b) with leading researchers, sponsored by a company, designed primarily for an exchange of information about important developments or treatments, including the sponsor's own research, for which reimbursement for travel may be appropriate.

m. *What kinds of social events during conferences and meetings may be subsidized by industry?*

Social events should satisfy three criteria. First, the value of the event to the physician should be modest. Second, the event should facilitate discussion among attendees and/or discussion between attendees and faculty. Third, the educational part of the conference should account for a substantial majority of the total time accounted for by the educational activities and social events together. Events that would be viewed (as in the succeeding question) as lavish or expensive should be avoided. But modest social activities that are not elaborate or unusual are permissible, e.g., inexpensive boat rides, barbecues, entertainment that draws on the local performers. In general, any such events which are a part of the conference program should be open to all registrants.

n. *May a company rent an expensive entertainment complex for an evening during a medical conference and invite the physician attending the conference?*
No. The guidelines permit only modest hospitality.

o. *If physicians attending a conference engage in interactive exchange, may their travel expenses be paid by industry?*
No. Mere interactive exchange would not constitute genuine consulting services.

p. *If a company schedules a conference and provides meals for the attendees that fall within the guidelines, may the company also pay the costs of the meals for spouses?*
If a meal falls within the guidelines, then the physician's spouse may be included.

q. *May companies donate funds to sponsor a professional society's charity golf tournament?*
Yes. But it is sensible if physicians who play in the tournament make some contribution themselves to the event.

r. *If a company invites a group of consultants to a meeting and a consultant brings a spouse, may the company pay the costs of lodging or meals of the spouse? Does it matter if the meal is part of the program for the consultants?*
Since the costs of having a spouse share a hotel room or join a modest meal are nominal, it is permissible for the company to subsidize those costs. However, if the total subsidies become substantial, then they become unacceptable.

Guideline Five. Scholarship or other special funds to permit medical students, residents and fellows to attend carefully selected educational conferences may be permissible as long as the selection of students, residents or fellows who will receive the funds is made by the academic or training institution.

a. *When a company subsidizes the travel expenses of residents to an appropriately selected conference, may the residents receive the subsidy directly from the company?*
Funds for scholarships or other special funds should be given to the academic departments or the accredited sponsor of the conference. The disbursement of funds can then be made by the departments or the conference sponsor.

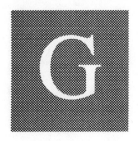

Guideline Six. No gifts should be accepted if there are strings attached. For example, physicians should not accept gifts which are given in relation to the physician's prescribing practices. In addition, when companies underwrite medical conferences or lectures other than their own, responsibility for and control over the selection of content, faculty, educational methods and materials should belong to the organizers of the conferences or lectures.

a. May companies send their top prescribers, purchasers, or referrers on cruises?
No. There can be no link between prescribing or referring patterns and gifts. In addition, travel expenses, including cruises, are not permissible.

b. May the funding company itself develop the complete educational program that is sponsored by an accredited continuing medical education sponsor?
No. the funding company may finance the development of the program through its grant to the sponsor, but the accredited sponsor must have responsibility and control over the content and faculty of conferences, meetings, or lectures. Neither the funding company nor an independent consulting firm should develop the complete educational program for approval by the accredited sponsor.

c. How much input may a funding company have in the development of a conference, meeting, or lectures?

Contact the Accreditation Council on Continuing Medical Education for guidelines on commercial support of continuing medical education.

JAMA Article of Note: Gifts to Physicians from Industry. Opinion of the Council on Ethical and Judicial Affairs. JAMA. 1991 Jan. 23/30; 265(4): 501

Government Printing Office

Government Printing Office
North Capitol and H Streets, NW
Washington, DC 20401
Publication orders and inquiries
202/783-3238
Information
202/275-3648

Bookstores

U.S. Government Printing Office Bookstore
710 N Capitol St, NW, Washington, DC 20401
202/512-0132 or 1510 H St, NW
Washington, DC 20005
202/653-5075

Alabama
U.S. Government Bookstore, O'Neill Bldg
2021 Third Ave, N, Birmingham, AL 35203
205/731-1056

California
U.S. Government Bookstore, ARCO Plaza,
C-Level
505 S Flower St, Los Angeles, CA 90071
213/239-9844

U.S. Government Bookstore,
Room 1023, Federal Bldg
450 Golden Gate Ave, San Francisco, CA 94102
415/252-5334

Colorado-
U.S. Government Bookstore,
Room 117, Federal Bldg
1961 Stout St, Denver, CO 80294
303/844-3964

U.S. Government Bookstore, World Savings Bldg
720 N Main St, Pueblo, CO 81003
719/544-3142

Florida
U.S. Government Bookstore
100 W Bay St, Suite 100, Jacksonville, FL 32202
904/353-0569

Georgia
U.S. Government Bookstore
275 Peachtree St, NE
Room 100, PO Box 56445, Atlanta, GA 30343
404/331-6947

Illinois
U.S. Government Bookstore,
One Congress Center
401 S State St, Suite 124, Chicago, IL 60605
312/353-5133

Marylandl
U.S. Government Printing Office
Warehouse Sales Outlet
8660 Cherry Lane, Laurel, MD 20707
301/953-7974, 301/792-0262

Massachusetts
U.S. Government Bookstore
Thomas P. O'Neill Bldg
Room 169, 10 Causeway St, Boston, MA 02222
617/720-4180

Michigan
U.S. Government Bookstore
Suite 160, Federal Bldg
477 Michigan Ave, Detroit, MI 48226
313/226-7816

Missouri
U.S. Government Bookstore, 120 Bannister Mall
5600 E Bannister Road, Kansas City, MO 64137
816/765-2256

New York
U.S. Government Bookstore
Room 110, Federal Bldg
26 Federal Plaza, New York, NY 10278
212/264-3825

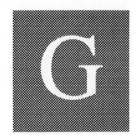

Ohio
U.S. Government Bookstore
Room 1653, Federal Bldg
1240 E 9th St, Cleveland, OH 44199
216/522-4922

U.S. Government Bookstore
Room 207, Federal Bldg
200 N High St, Columbus, OH 43215
614/469-6956

Oregon
1305 SW First Ave, Portland, OR 97201-5801
503/221-6217

Pennsylvania
U.S. Government Bookstore, Robert Morris Bldg
100 North 17th St, Philadelphia, PA 19103
215/597-0677

U.S. Government Bookstore
Room 118, Federal Bldg
1000 Liberty Ave, Pittsburgh, PA 15222
412/644-2721

Texas
U.S. Government Bookstore
Room IC46, Federal Bldg
1100 Commerce St, Dallas, TX 75242
214/767-0076

U.S. Government Bookstore, Texas Crude Bldg
801 Travis St, Suite 120, Houston, TX 77002
713/228-1187

Washington
U.S. Government Bookstore
Room 194, Federal Bldg
915 Second Ave, Seattle, WA 98174
206/553-4270

Wisconsin
Room 190, Federal Bldg
517 E Wisconsin Ave, Milwaukee, WI 53202
414/297-1304

Graduate Medical Education

Accreditation Council on
Graduate Medical Education
515 N. state St, Chicago, IL 60610
312/464-5000, x4920

AMA-FREIDA (3 1/2" Disk)
"AMA Fellowship & Residency Electronic
Interactive Database Access"
ISBN 0-89970-439-5\OP411691
AMA-FREIDA (5 1/4" Disk)

"AMA Fellowship & Residency Electronic
Interactive Database Access"
ISBN 0-89970-439-5\OP411791

AMA-FREIDA Database Hotline
312/464-5000, x4886

Council on Graduate Medical Education (COGME)
Bureau of Health Professions
Department of Health and Human Services
5600 Fishers Lane, Rockville, MD 20850
301/443-6190, 301/443-6326

Fellowships:

FREIDA (Fellowship and Residency Electronic
Interactive Database Access) Hotline
312/464-5000, x4886

Certification of subspecialty programs
Internal Medicine, Pathology, and Pediatrics will
be listed in the "Directory of Graduate Medical
Education Programs" also part of the FREIDA
program

No formal list exists, contact the specialty societies

For Internal Medicine:
National Study for Internal Medicine Manpower
Center for Health Administration
University of Chicago
1101 E. 58th St., Chicago, IL 60637
312/702-7753

*Directory of Graduate Medical Education
Programs.* American Medical Association,
Chicago. Annual. 1992/93 ed. 771 pp.
ISBN 0-89970-463-8/ISSN 0892-0109/OP
OP416792.

Grammar - Dial A Grammarian
Auburn University
205/844-5749

Grammar Hotline, Eastern Illinois University
217/581-5929

Grammar Hotline, Illinois State University
309/438-2345

Grammarline, Illinois Valley Community College
815/224-2720

Grammarphone, Triton College
708/456-0300

Purdue University
317/494-3723

Write Line, Oakton Community College
708/635-1948

Grief
The Compassionate Friends
PO Box 3696, Oak Brook, IL 60522-3696
708/990-0010

Grief Education Institute
2422 South Downing St., Denver, CO 80210
303/759-6048

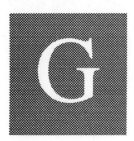

Group Practice

More doctors joining more group practices

Mike Mitka AMNews 10/5/90 p.16

Medical groups continue to be a growing practice option being selected by physicians, and managed care apparently is spurring the relationship.

As of 1988 (the last year data were available), there were 16,579 group practices with 115,628 physicians. Both are huge increases since 1965, when there were 4,289 groups with 28,381 doctors, according to the AMA's newly released 1990 *Medical Groups in the U.S.* (Please see current *Medical Groups in the U.S.* for current numbers.

The survey also found that 30% of all physicians now practice in groups, compared with 11% in 1965.

AMA Group Practice Manager Penny Havlicek, who ran the survey, said physicians should expect the number of groups to continue growing because of managing care.

"This is something we're going to keep seeing in the future," she said. "Given the managed care environment, groups become attractive to physicians because they can better represent them. There's power in numbers."

The survey found that 50% of groups contract with one or more health maintenance organizations, 20% do business with HMOs on a referral basis, 8% of all groups are organized to provide services to an HMO, and 15% of average annual group revenue comes from HMOs. As for preferred provider organizations, 56% of all groups contract with one or more, and 15% of average annual revenue is derived from PPOs, the survey said.

Single-specialty groups, as a proportion of groups, have increased from 50% to 71%, the survey said. On average, the number of physicians per single-specialty group is six, while the number per multispecialty group is 24.

Havlicek noted the smaller size of single-specialty groups as a reason why they are increasingly popular.

"Maybe the single-specialty groups combine the attractive features of group practices with solo practices," Havlicek said.

"There's other physicians you can rely on when you are on vacation, but at the same time there isn't the overwhelming bureaucracy you have to deal with that is associated with big groups."

Another set of findings highlighted by the survey centered on group ownership and control. The survey found that 71% of groups are organized as professional corporations and 16% are partnerships with 71% of a group's physicians being owners.

For the majority of groups, a committee of doctors rather than administrators determines group practice policy concerning the evaluation of therapeutic equipment (62%), evaluation of diagnostic equipment (61%), physician hours (57%), hiring and firing physicians (56%), and fee setting (51%).

Other findings of the survey were:
- The Average number of physicians per group is 10, with 50% of all groups reporting only three or four doctors.
- The 118 largest groups, while less than 1% of all groups, represent about 25% of all group doctors.

The survey was conducted by mail and telephone. Of the 19,372 eligible groups, 17,339 responded.

American Group Practice Association
1422 Duke St., Alexandria, VA 22314
703/838-0033

Medical Group Management Association
1355 S. Colorado Blvd., Denver, CO 80222
303/799-1111

Growth

Human Growth Foundation
4720 Montgomery Lane, Bethesda, MD 20814
301/656-7540

Gynecology

Gynecologist: Diagnoses and treats diseases and disorders of female genital, urinary, and rectal organs: Examines patient to determine medical problem, utilizing physical findings, diagnostic images, laboratory test results, and patient's statements as diagnostic aids. Discusses problem with patient, and prescribes medication and exercise or hygiene regimen, or performs surgery as needed to correct malfunctions or remove diseased organ. May care for throughout pregnancy and deliver babies.(DOT)

American Board of Obstetrics and Gynecology
4225 Roosevelt Way, NE, Suite 305
Seattle, WA 98105
206/547-4884

American College of Obstetricians
and Gynecologists (ACOG)
409 12th St., SW
Washington, DC 20024-2188
202/638-5577

American Association of
Gynecologic Laparoscopists
13021 E. Florence Ave.
Santa Fe Springs, CA 90670
213/946-8774

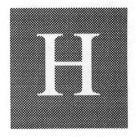

Hair Loss
American Hair Loss Council
4500 S. Broadway, Tyler, TX 75703
214/581-8717

National Alopecia Areata Foundation
714 C Street, Suite 216, San Rafael, CA 94901
415/456-4644

Hand Surgery
American Association for Hand Surgery
435 N. Michigan Ave, Chicago, IL 60611
312/644-0828

American Society for Surgery of the Hand
3025 S. Parker Road, Aurora, CO 80014
303/755-4588

Board Certification:
American Board of Orthopaedic Surgery
737 N. Michigan Ave., Suite 1150
Chicago, IL 60611
312/664-9444

American Board of Plastic Surgery
7 Penn Center, Suite 400
1635 Market St., Philadelphia, PA 19103
215/587-9322

American Board of Surgery
1617 John F. Kennedy Blvd., Ste. 860,
Philadelphia, PA 19103
215/568-4000

Handicapped
Americans with Disabilities Act
Pub Law No.101-336 enacted on July 26, 1990

Department of Justice
Tenth St and Constitution Ave, NW
Washington, DC 20530
202/514-0301

Architectural and Transportation Barriers
Compliance Board
1331 F St., NW, Ste. 1000
Washington, DC., 20004-1111
202-272-5434/800/872-2253(800-USA-ABLE)

Mobility International
(Assistance to handicapped people
when traveling)
228 Borough High St, London, SEI 1JX
England
71 4035688

Mobility International, U.S.A.
(North American affiliate of Mobility International)
PO Box 3551, Eugene, OR 97403
503/343-1284

National Foundation of Dentistry
for the Handicapped
1600 Stout Street, Suite 1420, Denver, CO 80202
303/573-0264

National Information Center for Handicapped
Children and Youth
PO Box 1492, Washington, DC 20013

Handicapped Physicians
American Society of Handicapped Physicians
105 Morris Drive, Bastrop, LA 71220
318/281-4436

Department of Veteran Affairs, Technology
Information Center
Rm 237, 810 Vermont Ave NW
Washington DC 20420
202/233-5524

Head Injury
National Head Injury Foundation
333 Turnpike Rd., Southborough, MA 01772
508/485-9950

Headaches
American Association for the
Study of the Headache
PO Box 5136, San Clemente, CA 92672
714/498-1846
800/255-ACHE (800/255-2243)

National Headache Foundation
(formerly National Migraine Foundation)
5252 N. Western Ave., Chicago, IL 60625
312/878-7715 .
800/843-2256; 800/523-8858 (IL only)

Health Administration
Association of University Programs
in Health Administration
1911 N. Fort Myer Dr., Suite 503
Arlington, VA 22209
703/524-5500

Health and Human Services, Dept. of
The Department of Health and Human Services is
the Cabinet-level department of the Federal
executive branch most concerned with people and
most involved with the Nation's human concerns.
In one way or another - whether it is mailing out
social security checks or making health services
more widely available - HHS touches the lives of
more Americans than any other Federal agency. It
is literally a department of people serving people,
from newborn infants to our most elderly citizens.
(USG)

Department of Health and Human Services
200 Independence Avenue, SW
Washington, DC 20201
202/245-6296

Health Associations
American Council on Science and Health
1995 Broadway, New York, NY 10023
212/362-7044

Catholic Health Association
4455 Woodson Rd., St. Louis, MO 63134
314/427-2500

Group Health Association of America
1129 20th St. NW, #600, Washington, DC 20036
202/778-3200

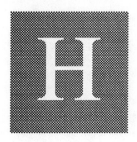

National Health Council
350 Fifth Ave., Suite 1118
New York, NY 10018-6765
212/268-8900

Health Care Financing Administration (HCFA)

The Health Care Financing Administration (HCFA) was established by the Secretary's reorganization of March 8, 1977, as a principal operating component of the Department. It places under one Administration the oversight of the Medicare and Medicaid Programs and related Federal medical care quality control staffs.

Medicare. The Medicare Program is a Federal health insurance program for persons over 65 years of age and certain disabled persons. It is funded through social security contributions, premiums, and general revenue. The Administration develops and implements policies related to program recipients, the providers of services such as hospitals, nursing homes, physicians, and contractors who process claims. It also coordinates with the States to develop departmental programs, activities, and organizations that are closely related to the Medicare Program.

Medicaid. The Medicaid Program, through grants to States, provides medical services to the needy and the medically needy. The Administration is responsible for working with the States to develop approaches toward meeting the needs of those who cannot afford adequate medical care.

The Medicare/Medicaid Programs include a quality assurance focal point to carry out the quality assurance provisions of the Medicare and Medicaid Programs; the development and implementation of health and safety standards for providers of care in Federal health programs; and the implementation of the End Stage Renal Disease Program and the Professional Review provisions.

For further information, contact the Administrator, Health Care Financing Administration, Department of Health and Human Services, 200 Independence Avenue SW., Washington DC 20201. Phone, 301-966-3000.(USG)

For the Health Care Financing Administration statement of organization, see the *Federal Register* of March 25, 1991, 56 FR 2374

Health Care Financing Administration (HCFA)
Baltimore, MD 21207
202/245-6726

Regional HCFA Offices:

Region I – (CT, ME, MA, NH, RI, VT)
JFK Federal Building, Room 1211
Boston, MA 02203
617/565-1322

Region II – (NJ, NY, PR, VI)
26 Federal Plaza, Room 3821
New York, NY 10278
212/264-1121

Region III – (DE, DC, MD, PA, VA, WV)
3535 Market Street, P.O Box 7760, Philadelphia, PA 19101
215/596-6571

Region IV – (AL, FL, GA, KY, MS, NC, SC, TN)
101 Marietta Tower, Suite 601
Atlanta, GA 30323
404/841-2361

Region V – (IL, IN, MI, OH, WI)
105 West Adams St, 15th Floor
Chicago, IL 60603-6201
312/353-9804

Region VI – (AR, LA, NM, OK, TX)
1200 Main Tower Building, Room 1935, Dallas, TX 75202
214/767-6301

Region VII – (IA, KS, MO, NE)
601 E. 12th St, Room 242
Kansas City, MO 64106
816/426-2408

Region VIII – (CO, MT, ND, SD, UT, WY)
1961 Stout St, Room 1185
Denver, CO 80294
303/844-4721

Region IX – (AZ, CA, HI, NV, US Pacific Islands)
75 Hawthorne St, 4th Floor
San Francisco, CA 94105
415/744-3679

Region X – (AK, ID, OR, WA)
2201 Sixth Ave, Mail Stop RX-42
Seattle, WA 98121
206/553-0511

Healthcare Financial Management Association
2 Westbrook Corp., Ste 700
Westchester, IL 60154
708/531-9600

Health Council

American Council on Science and Health
1995 Broadway, New York, NY 10023
212/362-7044

National Health Council
350 Fifth Ave., Suite 1118
New York, NY 10018-6765
212/268-8900

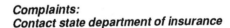

Health Fraud
Advertisements on TV & Radio
Federal Trade Commission
Sixth St. and Pennsylvania Ave. NW
Washington, DC 20580
202/326-2222

Advertisements in Newspapers:
Better Business Bureau
4200 Wilson Blvd., Arlington, VA 22203
202/276-0100

Zwicky, J. *Reader's Guide to Alternative Health Methods.* Chicago: American Medical Association, 1993. 348 pp. ISBN 0-89970-525-1. OP313792.

Hafner, Arthur W. *Guide to the American Medical Association Historical Health Fraud and Alternative Medicine Collection.* Chicago; American Medical Association,1992. 215 pp. ISBN 0-89970-441-7. OP310492.

National Council Against Health Fraud
PO Box 1276, Loma Linda, CA 92354
714/824-4690

Health Maintenance Organizations

A health maintenance organization (HMO) is an organized system of health care delivery available to persons in an enrolled group who reside in a specific geographic area. The HMO provides a specific set of health care benefits to its members including the services of physicians and other health care professionals, as well as those of inpatient and outpatient facilities. The HMO member/enrollee pays a preset monthly fee, regardless of actual services used.

How HMO's Evolved: In his 1971 health message to Congress, President Richard M. Nixon focused on prepaid medical practices, which had become known as HMOs, as the centerpiece of national health policy. Two years elapsed before passage of the Health Maintenance Act of 1973 (PL93-222). Federal funds in the form of loans and grants were used by individual HMOs for two or three years of initial study and development.

An integral part of the Health Maintenance Act of 1973 concerned federal HMO qualification. For an HMO to qualify for federal financial support it must have been deemed financially viable and able to supply certain health services to its members. These included diagnostic and therapeutic services, inpatient hospital services, short-term rehabilitation services, emergency services, mental health care services for alcohol or drug abuse, home health care, family planning, and preventive health care. No HMO could offer lower-priced contracts with benefits less than those specified and obtain federal qualification. An additional provision in the law that gave added impetus to the growth of HMOs was the stipulation that all employers with more than 25 workers must offer their employees the opportunity to enroll in a federally qualified HMO if one was available in their geographic area. This was the "dual choice option" provision.

Continued federal commitment to the HMO concept included 1976 and 1978 legislation that eased existing regulations to encourage HMO growth. The 1976 amendment waived the 1973

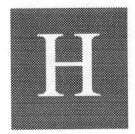

requirement in which physicians were to devote at least one-half of their practice to the HMO for three years. The legislation also repealed the thirty day open enrollment periods for smaller, newly developed HMOs and allowed the HMOs to deny enrollment or delay coverage to persons institutionalized with chronic illness or permanent injury. Mandatory dual choice option regulation was also reiterated in the new legislation. These changes removed many of the barriers that had limited HMO growth.

In 1978, the federal government passed legislation to provide further financial assistance to HMOs. The amendment extended HMO program authorization for three years, increased the maximum dollar limit for initial development grants, and raised loan guarantees from one to two million dollars. Although the 1978 amendment increased federal financing for HMOs, the legislation also established strict financial reporting guidelines and enrollment practices.

A new era of HMO development began with the Reagan Administration, which viewed the HMO approach as a way to encourage competition in the health care marketplace while reducing federal government involvement. In the 1980s, the Reagan Administration slowly removed federal assistance to HMOs. Thus, an increasing number of new and existing HMOs became for-profit entities. Growing national concern with health care costs, the increased role of for-profit health care, and wider public acceptance of prepaid health care delivery are among the factors that have accelerated recent HMO growth. (HDS)

Complaints:
Contact state department of insurance

American Medical Care and Review Association
1227 25th St, NW, Suite 610
Washington, DC 20037
202/728-0506

Group Health Association of America
1129 20th Street, NW, Suite 600
Washington, DC 20036
202/778-3200

Health Resources and Services Administration
Bureau of Health Maintenance Organizations
and Resources
5600 Fishers Lane, Rm 903, Rockville, MD 20857
401/966-0474

HMOs - Medicare

In recent years HMOs have expanded their markets to include the Medicare population. Prior to 1972, Medicare paid HMOs for Part B care on either a fee-for-service or capitation basis, but Part A* care was paid for directly by the government program. However, with the enactment of the Social Security Amendments of 1972 (PL 9-603), capitation reimbursement to HMOs for both Part A and Part B services provided to Medicare beneficiaries was allowed for the first time, Under the new legislation, capitation-based reimbursement could be made either on the basis of the existing "reasonable cost" or on a new risk-sharing basis.

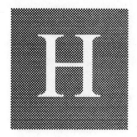

Under a "reasonable cost" contract, the HMO was paid a monthly capitation fee for each Medicare beneficiary enrolled. At the end of the contract year, the HMO was required to calculate the reasonable cost of services actually provided. The costs were compared with the capitation payments adjustments were made to increase or decrease payments to the HMO.

Under a risk-sharing approach, the HMOs reasonable costs were compared at the end of the year with a federally established statistic called the adjusted average per capita cost (AAPCC). The AAPCC was calculated as the estimated costs that would have been charged to Medicare had the HMO enrollees been treated by non-HMO providers. If the reasonable costs were less than the AAPCC, the HMO could retain up to 50 percent of the savings. However, if costs exceeded the AAPCC, the HMO absorbed the entire loss.

Both of these reimbursement mechanisms proved unacceptable since most HMOs operate on the basis of a prospective budget that does not involve year-end reconciliation of costs and capitation payments. Thus, incentives created through risk-sharing contracts were often considered inadequate because the HMO could not obtain full benefits of savings achieved. Similarly, the cost-based HMOs were penalized for cost-conscious behavior because reimbursement decreased as the reasonable cost per Medicare enrollee decreased. In addition, in 1976 Medicare added a further restriction that only federally-qualified HMOs could be eligible to enter into contracts with Medicare.

Many of these limitations on Medicare-HMO relationships grew out of congressional concerns that HMOs, operating under their traditional economic incentives, might underserve the elderly and avoid sicker Medicare beneficiaries. To encourage Medicare beneficiary participation on HMOs, the Health Care Financing Administration (HCFA) instituted demonstration projects to test various risk-based reimbursement methodologies in 1978. Although final fiscal evaluations of these demonstrations were not complete, preliminary results were used in creating new HMO regulations. (HDS)

Note: Medicare Part A covers inpatient hospital care and post-hospital stays in skilled nursing facilities. Medicare Part B covers physicians' services, hospital outpatient care, and some other non-hospital care.)

For HMOs that accept Medicare recipients: Contact regional Health Care Financing Administration office

Health Professional Shortage Areas
Financial Assistance and Education Programs to Encourage Care to the Underserved. Barzansky, B., Jonas, H.S. JAMA. 1992 Sept 2; 268(9): 1089

Concerns about the adequacy of physician supply in certain areas of the US have been raised,[1] and there are data to support the existence of shortages.[2,3] For more than two decades, attempts have been made at the federal and state levels to correct the geographic imbalance in physician supply. In general, corrective actions tied to medical education have been of two kinds: financial support to educational programs or the sites where educational experienced offered, and direct financial assistance to medical students in return for service to defined populations. Most often, the goal of both kinds of programs is to increase the number of primary care providers practicing in areas of need.

Financial Support to Educational Programs or Sites:
In 1971, the federal government began supporting primary care physician training through Title VII of the Public Health Service Act. At about the same time, Congress passed legislation to support the creation of Area Health Education Centers (AHECs). AHECs function to enhance the level of care to underserved populations and to provide sites of training for physicians and other health professionals.[4] In fiscal year 1989, the AHEC program was modified to add Health Education and Training Centers, which support regions and populations with acute and longstanding shortages of health personnel.[5]

With the passage of the Health Professions Education Assistance Act of 1963 (Pub L No. 88-129), medical schools began to receive federal aid to support expansion of their class sizes. In 1976, an amendment to this legislation (Pub L No. 94-484) tied this support, in part, to expanding primary care residency positions.[6] While capitation was successful in its primary objective - increasing the total number of physicians graduated - less clear was the specific impact on the supply of primary care physicians and the availability of care to the underserved[1].

States also participated in the expansion of medical education during the 1960s and 1970s. Of the 39 medical schools organized between 1960 and 1979, 30 were publicly supported and nine were private.[7] Many of these schools were founded with a mission of serving their regions and producing practitioners for the state (Politzer et al[1] and Liaison Committee on Medical Education Annual Medical Questionnaire, Part II, 1992, data kept at American Medical Association, Chicago, Ill).

Financial Assistance Programs: The federal mechanisms for providing financial support to physicians-in-training has been through the National Health Service, both of which currently have scholarship and loan repayment programs tied to eventual service in areas of need. The level of support for all these programs has varied over the years. For example, the National Health Service Corps program decreased sharply from 2339 new scholarships to medical students in 1978-1979 to 25 in 1986-1987.[8] The availability of scholarships has increased in recent years, to a total of 400 for all health professions in 1992-1993.

Sixteen states have one or more types of financial assistance programs tied to service in rural shortage areas for set periods of time. These include a direct scholarship or loan programs and loan repayment programs.[9] The programs often are managed through state rural health offices. For more information about federal or state financial assistance programs tied to service in shortage areas, contact the American Medical

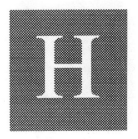

Association Division of Undergraduate Medical Education.

References:
1. Politzer R, Harris D, Gaston M, Mullan F. "Primary care physician supply and the medically underserved."JAMA. 1991 Jul 3;266(1):104-109.
2. Kindig D, Movassaghi H. The adequacy of physician supply in small rural counties. Health Aff. 1989;8:63-76.
3. Kindig D, Movassaghi H, Dunham N, Zwick D, Taylor C. Trends in physician availability in 10 urban areas from 1963 to 1980. Inquiry. 1987;24:136-146.
4. Cranford C. Linking medical education and training to rural America: the rural Arkansas AHEC program (1991) (testimony before the Special Senate Committee on Aging).
5. The Health Education and Training Centers (HECT) of the National AHEC Program. San Francisco: The California AHEC System; 1991.
6. Scofield J. New and Expanded Medical Schools, Mid-Century to the 1980s. San Francisco, Calif: Jossey-Bass Inc; 1984.
7. "Medical schools in the United States." JAMA.1991 Aug 21;266(7):1007-1011. Appendix II.
8. AAMC Data Book (January 1992). Washington, DC: Association of American Medical Colleges; 1992.
9. McCloskey A, Luehrs J. State Initiatives to Improve Rural Health Care. Washington, DC: National Governors' Association; 1990.

List of primary health manpower shortage areas
published periodically in the *Federal Register*. See *Federal Register*. 1990 June 29, 55(126): 27010-85

Summary: This notice provides two lists. The first is a list of all areas, population groups, or facilities designated as primary medical care health manpower shortage areas (HMSAs) as of December 31, 1989. Second is a list of previously-designated primary medical care HMSAs that have been found to no longer meet the HMSA criteria and are therefore being withdrawn from the HMSA list. HMSAs are designated or withdrawn by the Secretary of Health and Human Services (HHS) under the authority of section 332 of the Public Health Service Act.

Supplementary Information:
Section 332 of the Public Health Service Act provides that the Secretary of Health and Human Services shall designate health manpower shortage areas based on criteria established by regulation. Health manpower shortage areas (HMSAs) are defined in section 332 to include (1) urban and rural geographic areas, (2) population groups, and (3) facilities with shortages of health manpower. Section 332 further requires that the Secretary publish a list of the designated geographic areas, population groups, and facilities. The list of areas is to be reviewed at least annually and revised as necessary. The Health Resources and Services Administration's Bureau of Health Care Delivery and Assistance has the responsibility for designated and updating these HMSAs.
Public or nonprofit entities in (or with a demonstrated interest in) these HMSAs are eligible to apply for assignment of National Health Service Corps (NHSC) personnel to provide health services in, or to, the areas or populations involved. These HMSAs are also eligible

obligated-service areas for certain Public Health Service scholarship, loan repayment, and traineeship programs; entities located therein are eligible to apply for (or receive preference for) certain Public Health Service grant programs; physicians delivering services in non-metropolitan HMSAs may be eligible for increased Medicare reimbursement; and nurse practitioners and physician's assistants serving Rural Health Clinics in HMSAs are eligible for Medicaid or Medicare reimbursement.

Bureau of Health Care Delivery and Assistance
Office of Shortage Design, Parklawn Building, Room 8-47,
5600 Fishers Lane, Rockville, MD 20857
301/443-6932

Marder, WD. *Physician Supply and Utilization by Specialty: Trends and Projections.* Chicago, American Medical Association, 1988 135pp. ISBN 0-89970-315-1. OP193788

Health Officials
Association of State and Territorial Health Officials
6728 Old McLean Village Dr, McLean, VA 22101
703/556-9222

Health Policy
National Governor's Association
Health Policy Group
444 N. Capitol St., Ste 250
Washington, DC 20001
202/624-5344

Health Services
Accrediting Commission on Education for Health Services Administration
1911 N. Fort Myer Drive, Suite 503
Arlington, VA 22209
703/524-0511

U.S. National Center for Health Services Research
5600 Fisher Lane, Room 1812
Rockville, MD 20857
301/443-4100

Health System Agencies
Federation of American Health Systems
1111 19th St. NW, Suite 402
Washington, DC 20036
202/833-3090

Administrative Offices:
1405 N. Pierce, No. 311, Little Rock, AR 72207
501/661-9555

Hearing Impaired
American Deafness and Rehabilitation Association
PO Box 55369, Little Rock, AR 72225
501/375-6643

American Hearing Research Foundation
55 E. Washington, Suite 2022, Chicago, IL 60602
312/726-9670

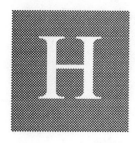

American Speech-Language-Hearing Association
10801 Rockville Pike, Rockville, MD 20852
301/897-5700
800/638-8255 (800/638-TALK)

Captioned Films for the Deaf
800/237-6213

Deafness Research Foundation
9 E. 38th St., 7th Floor, New York, NY 10016
800/535-3323

Gallaudet College (Deaf Education)
800 Florida Avenue, NE, Washington, DC 20002
800/672-6720

Hearing Helpline
800/424-8576

International Hearing Dog Inc.
5901 E. 89th Ave., Henderson, CO 80640
303/287-3277

National Captioning Institute
5203 Leesburg Pike, Falls Church, VA 22014
703/998-2400 (Voice/TDD)

National Hearing Aid Society
20361 Middlebelt, Livonia, MI 48152
800/521-5247

Occupational Hearing Service
PO Box 1880, Media, PA 19063
800/222-3277

SHHH (Self Help for Hard of Hearing People, Inc)
7800 Wisconsin Avenue, Bethesda, MD 20814
301/657-2248

TDD (Telecommunication Device for the Deaf)
800/325-0778

TRIPOD (Information for families
with deaf children)
PO Box 19429, Springfield, IL 62794-9429
217/785-9304
800/352-8888

Heart Associations, Statewide

American Heart Association Alabama Affiliate
1449 Medical Park Dr, Birmingham, AL 35213
205/592-7100

American Heart Association Alaska Affiliate
2330 E 42nd Ave, Anchorage, AK 99508
907/563-3111

American Heart Association Arizona Affiliate
1550 E Meadowbrook, Phoenix, AZ 85014
602/277-4846

American Heart Association Arkansas Affiliate
909 W 2nd St, Little Rock, AR 72201
501/375-9148

American Heart Association Greater
Los Angeles Affiliate
3550 Wilshire Blvd, 5th Fl, Los Angeles, CA 90010
213/385-4231

American Heart Association California Affiliate
805 Burlway Rd, Burlingame, CA 94010-1795
415/342-5522

American Heart Association of Colorado
1280 S Parker Rd, Denver, CO 80231
303/369-5433

American Heart Association Connecticut Affiliate
5 Brookside Dr, Wallingford, CT 06492
203/294-0088

American Heart Association of Delaware
4C Trolley Sq, Delaware Ave & DuPont St,
Wilmington, DE 19806
302/654-5269

American Heart Association
Nation's Capitol Affiliate
2233 Wisconsin Ave, NW, Washington, DC 20007
202/337-6400

American Heart Association Florida Affiliate
1213 16th St N, St. Petersburg, FL 33705-1092
813/894-7400

American Heart Association Georgia Affiliate
1685 Terrell Mill Road, Marietta, GA 30067
404/952-1316

American Heart Association Hawaii Affiliate
245 N Kukui St, Honolulu, HI 96817
808/538-7021

American Heart Association of Idaho
3295 Elder St, Suite 140, Boise, ID 83705
208/384-5066

American Heart Association
of Metropolitan Chicago
20 N Wacker Drive, Chicago, IL 60606
312/346-4675

American Heart Association Illinois Affiliate
1181 N Dirksen Pkwy, Springfield, IL 62708
217/525-1350

American Heart Association Indiana Affiliate
8645 Guion Road, Suite H, Indianapolis, IN 46268
317/876-4850

American Heart Association Iowa Affiliate
1111 9th St, Suite 280, Des Moines, IA 50314
515/224-3278

American Heart Association Kansas Affiliate
5375 SW 7th St, Topeka, KS 66606
913/272-7056

American Heart Association Kentucky Affiliate
207 Speed Bldg, Louisville, KY 40202
502/587-8641

American Heart Association of Louisiana
105 Campus Dr E, Destrehan, LA 70047
504/764-8711

American Heart Association Maine Affiliate
20 Winter St, Augusta, ME 04330
207/623-8432

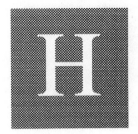

American Heart Association Maryland Affiliate
415 N. Charles St, Baltimore, MD 21203
301/685-7074

American Heart Association
Massachusetts Affiliate
33 4th Ave, Needham Heights, MA 02194
617/449-5931

American Heart Association of Michigan
16310 W 12 Mile Road, Lathrup Village, MI 48076
313/557-9500

American Heart Association Minnesota Affiliate
4701 W 77th St, Minneapolis, MN 55435
612/835-3300

American Heart Association Mississippi Affiliate
4830 E McWillie Circle, Jackson, MS 39236
601/981-4721

American Heart Association Missouri Affiliate
105 E Ash, Suite 2, Columbia, MO 65205
314/442-3193

American Heart Association Montana Affiliate
510 1st Ave N, No. 4, Great Falls, MT 59401
406/452-2362

American Heart Association Nebraska Affiliate
3624 Farnam, Omaha, NE 68131
402/346-0771

American Heart Association Nevada Affiliate
3355 Spring Mountain Road, Suite 4
Las Vegas, NV 89102
702/367-6490

American Heart Association
New Hampshire Affiliate
309 Pine St, Manchester, NH 03103
603/669-5833

American Heart Association New Jersey Affiliate
2550 Route 1, North Brunswick, NJ 08902
201/821-2610

American Heart Association New Mexico Affiliate
1330 San Pedro NE, Suite 105
Albuquerque, NM 87110
505/268-3711

American Heart Association New York City Affiliate
205 E 42nd St, New York, NY 10017
212/661-5335

American Heart Association New York State
Affiliate
100 N Concourse, North Syracuse, NY 13212
315/454-8166

American Heart Association North Carolina Affiliate
300 Silver Cedar Court, Chapel Hill, NC 27515
919/968-4453

American Heart Association Dakota Affiliate
1005 12th Ave, SE, Jamestown, ND 58401
701/252-5122

American Heart Association
Northeast Ohio Affiliate
1689 E 115th St, Cleveland, OH 44106
216/791-7500

American Heart Association Ohio Affiliate
5455 N High St, Columbus, OH 43214
614/848-6676

American Heart Association Oklahoma Affiliate
2915 N Classen, Suite 220
Oklahoma City, OK 73136
405/521-9838

American Heart Association Oregon Affiliate
1425 NE Irving, No. 100
Portland, OR 97232-4201
503/233-0100

American Heart Association Southeastern
Pennsylvania Affiliate
121 S Broad St, Philadelphia, PA 19107
215/735-3865

American Heart Association Pennsylvania Affiliate
Pennsboro Center, 1019 Mumma Road
PO Box 8835, Camp Hill, PA 17011-8835
717/975-4800

Puerto Rico Heart Association
Cabo Alverio 554, Hato Rey, PR 00918
809/751-6595

American Heart Association Rhode Island Affiliate
40 Broad St, Pawtucket, RI 02860
401/728-5300

American Heart Association
South Carolina Affiliate
400 Percival Road, Columbia, SC 29206
803/738-9540

American Heart Association Dakota Affiliate
1005 12th Ave, SE, Jamestown, ND 58401
701/252-5122

American Heart Association Tennessee Affiliate
1200 Division St, Suite 201, Nashville, TN 37203
615/726-0108

American Heart Association Texas Affiliate
1700 Rutherford Lane, Austin, TX 78754
512/836-7220

American Heart Association Utah Affiliate
645 East 400 South, Salt Lake City, UT 84102
801/322-5601

American Heart Association Vermont Affiliate
12 Hurricane Lane, Williston, VT 05495
802/878-7700

American Heart Association Virginia Affiliate
4217 Park Place Court, Glen Allen, VA 23060
804/747-8334

American Heart Association Washington Affiliate
4414 Woodland Park Ave N, Seattle, WA 98103
206/632-6881

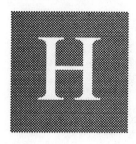

American Heart Association West Virginia Affiliate
211 35th St SE, Charleston, WV 25304
304/346-5381

American Heart Association Wisconsin Affiliate
795 N. Van Buren St, Milwaukee, WI 53202
414/271-9999

American Heart Association of Wyoming
1320 Hugur Ave, Cheyenne, WY 82001
307/632-1746

Heart Disease
American Heart Association
7320 Greenville Ave., Dallas, TX 75231
214/373-6300

American College of Angiology
1044 Northern Blvd., Suite 103, Roslyn, NY 11576
516/484-6880

American College of Cardiology
9111 Old Georgetown Rd., Bethesda, MD 20814
301/897-5400

Board Certification in Cardiovascular Disease:
American Board of Internal Medicine
3624 Market Street, Philadelphia, PA 19104
215/243-1500 800/441-ABIM (800/441-2246)

National Heart, Lung and Blood Institute
9000 Rockville Pike, Bethesda, MD 20892
301/496-4236

Contact local Heart Association for patient information and local programs.

Height-Weight Tables
For Adults:
Metropolitan Life Insurance Co.
Attn: Health and Safety Education Dept.--16W
1 Madison Ave., New York, NY 10010
212/578-2211

Heimlich Maneuver Poster
Card/chart single copies free
Employers Insurance of Wausau
Wausau, WI 5440l

Hematology
American Society of Hematology
1101 Constitution Ave, NW, Suite 700,
Washington, DC 20036
202/857-1118

Board Certification in Hematology:
American Board of Internal Medicine
3624 Market St., Philadelphia, PA 19104
215/243-1500
800/441-ABIM (800/441-2246)

American Board of Pathology
5401 W. Kennedy Blvd., PO Box 25915
Tampa, FL 33622
813/286-2444

Hemochromatosis
Hemochromatosis Research Foundation, Inc.
PO Box 8569, Albany, NY 12208
518/489-0972

Hemophilia
National Hemophilia Foundation
The Soho Bldg., 110 Green St., Rm. 406
New York, NY 10012
212/219-8180

Hippocrates [460?-377? B.C.]

The Oath

I swear by Apollo the Physician, and Aesculapius, and health, and all-heal and all the Gods and Goddesses, that, according to my ability and judgement, I will keep this oath and stipulation:

To reckon him who taught me this art equally dear to me as my parents, to share my substance with him, and relieve his necessities if required; to regard his offspring as on the same footing with my own brothers, and to teach them this art, if they shall wish to learn it, without fee or stipulation; and that by precept, lecture, and every other mode of instruction, I will impart a knowledge of the Art to my own sons, and those of my teachers, and to disciples bound by a stipulation and oath according to the law of medicine, but to none others.

I will follow that method of treatment which, according to my ability and judgement, I consider for the benefit of my patients, and abstain from whatever is deleterious and mischievous. I will give no deadly medicine to any one if asked, nor suggest any such counsel; furthermore, I will not give to a woman an instrument to produce abortion.

With Purity and with Holiness I will pass my life and practice my Art. I will not cut a person who is suffering with a stone, but will leave this to be done by men who are practitioners of this work. Into whatever houses I enter I will go into them for the benefit of the sick and will abstain from every voluntary act of mischief and corruption; and further from the seduction of females or males, bond or free.

Whatever, in connexion with my professional practice, or not in connexion with it, I may see or hear in the lives of men which ought not to be spoken abroad I will not divulge, as reckoning that all such should be kept secret.

While I continue to keep this oath unviolated may it be granted to me to enjoy life and the practice of the art, respected by all men at all times but should I trespass and violate this oath, may the reverse be my lot.

Histologic Technology

Occupational Description: Physicians, usually pathologists, and other scientists specializing in biological sciences or related clinical areas, such as chemistry, work in partnership with medical laboratory workers to analyze blood, tissues, and fluids from humans (and sometimes animals), using a variety of precision instruments. The results of these tests are used to detect and diagnose disease and other abnormalities.

The main responsibility of the histologic technician/technologist in the clinical laboratory is preparing sections of body tissue for examination by a pathologist. This includes the preparation of tissue specimens of human and animal origin for diagnostic, research, or teaching purposes. Tissue sections prepared by the histologic technician/technologist for a variety of disease entities enable the pathologist to diagnose body dysfunction and malignancy.

Job Description: Histotechnicians process sections of body tissue by fixation, dehydration, embedding, sectioning, decalcification, microincineration, mounting, and routine and special staining. Histotechnologists perform all the functions of the histotechnician as well as the more complex procedures for processing tissues. They identify tissue structures, cell components, and their staining characteristics, and relate them to physiological functions; implement and test new techniques and procedures; make judgements concerning the results of quality control measures; and institute proper procedures to maintain accuracy and precision. Histotechnologists apply the principles of management and supervision when they function as section supervisors and of educational methodology when they teach students. (Histologic technologist programs are designated in the program listing with an asterisk.)

Employment Characteristics: Most histologic technicians /technologists work in hospital laboratories, averaging a 40-hour week. Salaries vary depending on the employer and geographic location.

AMA Department of Allied Health
312/464-4625

History of Medicine

Bibliography of the History of Medicine.
Bethesda, MD
National Library of Medicine. For sale by the GPO. Annual: series begun 1965.
ISSN 0067-7280

The *Bibliography of the History of Medicine* focuses on the history of Medicine and its related sciences, professional and institutions. The general history and philosophy of science have been admitted only sparingly. All chronological periods and geographic areas are covered. Journal articles, monographs, and analytical entries for symposia, congresses, and similar composite publications, as well as historical chapters in general monographs, are included.(BIB)

American Association for the History of Medicine
Arthur J. Viseltear, PhD, Yale School of Medicine
333 Cedar St., New Haven, CT 06510
203/785-4338

HIV, HIV Infection and Disease

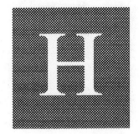

The Stages of HIV Infection: a
Predictable Progressive Disease

Donald S. Burke, MD and Robert R. Redfield, MD

The first of the human immunodeficiency viruses, HIV-1, was identified in 1984 and the second, HIV-2, in the following year. Identification of HIV as the etiological agent responsible for the underlying immunosuppression in AIDS allowed for the discovery and development of the first antiretroviral agent, zidovudine (also known as azidothymidine or AZT). At present, a number of other antiretroviral agents are in clinical trials. The recent report of AZT's efficacy in asymptomatic HIV-infected patients has been estimated to be of potential value for approximately 600,000 patients in the United States. This, and the promise of additional therapies for HIV-infected patients, raises the question as to whom in the future will provide care for the increasing number of treatable patients. As pointed out by Surgeon General C.E. Koop in the Introduction to this book, [HIV Infection and Disease, 1989] the present case load of 1.5 million infected Americans cannot be handled by a limited number of specialists. What then of the future?

HIV disease, not just AIDS (the final preterminal phase of HIV-infection), is a very complex problem both medically and socially. A number of ethical, legal and psychological issues are intertwined with this devastating disease, complicating patient management in a way not encountered by the physicians in other diseases. It is difficult enough for physicians and other health care workers to keep abreast of the burgeoning scientific literature; an intense commitment is needed, but time is not always available.(HIV)

What is AIDS? "AIDS," the Acquired Immunodeficiency Syndrome, was originally defined by the U.S. Centers for Disease Control (CDC) as a disease, at least moderately predictive of a defect in cell-mediated immunity, occurring in a person with no known cause for diminished resistance to that disease. Kaposi's sarcoma (KS) and Pneumocystis carinii pneumonia (PCP) were the most frequently recognized clinical manifestations of the immunodeficiency syndrome.

It is now known that the syndrome "AIDS" is simply the end-stage manifestation of a prolonged, chronic erosion of the immune system caused by the Human Immunodeficiency Virus (HIV). The clinical manifestations of disease in any given individual are largely due to a reactivation and/or uncontrolled proliferation of microorganisms or neoplasms that are normally held in check by the intact human immune system.

Two related but distinct types of HIV have been isolated and characterized, HIV-1 and HIV-2. All but a few of the HIV infections in the United States are HIV-1. At present HIV-2 is largely confined to Western Africa. The clinical disease associated with HIV-1 is well recognized. However, the clinical spectrum of disease associated with HIV-2 remains to be clarified.

The original syndrome-defined categorization "AIDS" was a brilliantly effective epidemiological tool: by 1985 the major modes of transmission

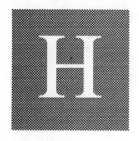

had been elucidated and the etiologic retrovirus HIV had been isolated and characterized. Over the ensuing years the relationship between HIV infection of "AIDS" has become clear. In 1987, the CDC published a revised definition of "AIDS" and the current definition is evolving. "AIDS" is an aggregate of preterminal manifestations of a predictable, progressive loss of immune competence caused by HIV. In the remainder of this essay the outdated syndrome-defined term "AIDS" will not be used; the omission is intentional. Instead, the term "late stage HIV infection" will be used to emphasize the concept that HIV causes a spectrum of disease.

Optimal medical management of HIV infection, as with all medical conditions, requires two fundamental steps. First, an accurate diagnosis must be established, and second, the extent of target organ damage must be precisely measured. Armed with this information, the knowledgeable physician can offer improvements in the quality and duration of life to his or her HIV-infected patient. Although HIV disease is not (at present) curable, it is most certainly treatable.

Diagnosis of HIV Infection: While there are many legal and ethical concerns about the use of HIV tests, physicians must clearly understand that willful ignorance of the possibility of HIV infection is a disservice to the patient. A diagnosis of HIV should be no more avoided than would be a diagnosis of diabetes or cancer.

Some physicians hold that it is unnecessary to obtain laboratory confirmation of a diagnosis of HIV in a patient with obvious clinical manifestation of disease. While this may be true, the same might be said about the necessity of obtaining a hematocrit in a patient with clinical signs of profound anemia, or of obtaining an electrocardiogram in a patient with an "obvious" myocardial infarction. We believe that a specific etiologic diagnosis should be sought in every case of suspected HIV infection. Rarely, other diseases such as lymphoma or HTLV-1 infection may present as an acquired immune deficiency. The careful physician confirms his or her clinical diagnosis with appropriate laboratory tests, even in patients with "pathognomonic" late stage illness.

More importantly, patients with early or asymptomatic HIV infections will have few or no clinically evident signs of HIV. In these cases, laboratory tests for HIV must be performed if an early diagnosis is to be established.

History of the HIV-1 Epidemic in the United States:

- C.B. 1976 Beginning of silent HIV-1 epidemic
- C.B. 1979 Initial sporadic cases of PCP and KS
- 1981 Epidemic nature of disease recognized
- 1982 The concept of "AIDS" developed
- 1984 Causative retrovirus HIV-1 isolated and characterized
- 1985 HIV-1 blood tests licensed
  1987 Antiretroviral drug zidovudine (AZT) approved
- 1988 President's Commission report issued (HIV)

Rapoza, N. Ed. *HIV Infection and Disease: Monographs for Physicians and Other Health Care Workers* (16 monographs in one volume) Chicago; American Medical Association. 1989. 202pp. ISBN 0-89970-376-3. OP014690

Holistic Medicine

A form of therapy aimed at treating the whole person - body and mind - not just the part or parts in which symptoms occur. A holistic approach is claimed to be emphasized by practitioners of alternative medicine, such as homeopathists, acupuncturists, and herbalists. (ENC)

American Holistic Medical Association
4101 Lake Boone Trail, Suite 201
Raleigh, NC 27607
919/787-5146

Chelation therapy is performed by intravenous administration of a synthetic amino acid called ethylenediamine tetraacetic acid (EDTA), along with several vitamins and other substances. A course of treatment consists of 20 to 50 intravenous infusions. Chelation therapy is heavily promoted as an alternative to coronary bypass surgery. Many proponents have claimed that EDTA works as a "chemical roto-rooter," pulling calcium out of atherosclerotic plaques. However, most proponents now claim that the procedure works by pulling toxic metals out of the body, thereby reducing the formation of free radicals and enabling areas of atherosclerosis to heal. There is no scientific evidence that either of these mechanisms exists or that chelation therapy is effective against atherosclerosis. Chelation therapy is also claimed to be effective against kidney and heart disease, arthritis, Parkinson's disease, emphysema, multiple sclerosis, gangrene, psoriasis, and many other serious conditions. However, no controlled trial has shown that chelation therapy can help any of these conditions, and manufacturers of EDTA do not list them as appropriate for EDTA treatment. (ALT)

AMA Policy. Chelation Therapy: (1) There is no scientific documentation that the use of chelation therapy is effective in the treatment of cardiovascular disease, atherosclerosis, rheumatoid arthritis, and cancer. (2) If chelation therapy is to be considered a useful medical treatment for anything other than heavy metal poisoning, hypercalcemia or digitalis toxicity, it is the responsibility of its proponents to conduct properly controlled scientific studies, to adhere to FDA guidelines for drug investigation, and to disseminate study results in the usually accepted channels.

Home Births

Informed Homebirth/Informed Birth and Parenting
PO Box 3675, Ann Arbor, MI 48106
313/662-6857

Position on Homebirth:
American College of Obstetricians and Gynecologists
409 12th St., SW, Washington, DC 20024
202/638-5577

Home Health Care

House Calls

Ronald F. Galloway, MD "A Piece of My Mind"
JAMA. 1991 Aug 14; 266(6): 786

The first time I saw him, Mr. Henry was standing in front of a mirror, his back to the door of his hospital room, tinkering with his electric razor and fixing to shave. I called his name; he turned, put down his razor, smiled, and reached out to grasp my hand. He was tall, skinny as a rail, a bit stoop-shouldered, but he moved about pretty spryly.

As a thoracic surgeon, I had been asked to see Mr. Henry regarding a possible resection for a lemon-sized tumor in his left lung. He was 80 years old at the time. I had already seen his chest film and reviewed his chart and was, I admit, trying to think of a gentle way to explain to him that, at his age, he would not likely do well after major chest surgery. My preconceived notion was reinforced by the fact that he had been admitted with a proved diagnosis of carcinoma of the prostate. However, his smile and his firm handshake cut through that preconception, so I explained to him all the ifs, ands, and buts of a pulmonary lobectomy and informed him that his attending urologist planned a total orchiectomy at the same sitting. At the end of my detailed talk I paused and asked for question. He had only one: "When do we do this?" I told him. He smiled again and said, "I'm ready."

Mr. Henry tolerated both surgical procedures well, had no complications, and soon went. At his follow-up visit at my office a few weeks later, I learned that his wife's health was poor, that he didn't drive a car especially well, and that his coming to my office for checkups was difficult at best. So, I told him that on occasion I drive to the South Carolina coast and that his town was on the way. I offered to stop by to visit him from time to time. He seemed surprised but obviously appreciative that I would volunteer to do this.

Some weeks later I drove through that small town, followed his directions to its outskirts, and found the house trailer on concrete blocks that Mr. and Mrs. Henry called home. The yard was well kept - a small, neat garden decorated one corner. I hadn't called for an "appointment" but had presumed that his wife's poor health kept Mr. Henry close to home. I knocked on the door and was greeted by Mr. Henry with a smile as big as all outdoors and his special warm handshake. I examined him, noted that he was doing quite well, and spent a while just visiting with them both. As I left, felt absolutely wonderful.

I've returned to the Henrys several times since that first encounter. They seemed to enjoy my visits, and each trip has been an unqualified blessing for me.

It has occurred to me that I could, if I wished, file a claim with Medicare for reimbursement for these 72-mile (144 miles round-trip) "house calls." But, the thought of the hassle the Medicare people would give me and the probability that they wouldn't believe I made the 72-mile house calls in the first place have deterred me. Then, too, the frozen boiled peanuts Mr. Henry gave me on one trip, the tomatoes he promised me this summer, the pride he takes in showing me his garden, the look in his eyes when I appear at his door, and my personal "hands-on" knowledge that he continues to do well are worth far more than any amount I might be able to argue out of Medicare.

And there's no deductible to meet.

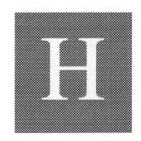

Contact local medical society for referrals to physicians who make house calls.

Educating physicians in home health care. Council on Scientific Affairs and Council on Medical Education. [corrected] [published erratum appears in JAMA. 1991 May 8; 265(18): 2340] JAMA. 1991 Feb 13; 265(6): 769-71
A growing proportion of health care, especially long-term care, should best and most appropriately be provided in the home setting. Physicians have largely remained on the periphery of this reemerging area of health care. Yet if home health care is to reach its full potential, physicians must fulfill their essential role as members of the home health team. Direct physician input and participation are needed to ensure that home health care is safe and medically appropriate. Physician involvement will enhance the supervision of medical care in the home, and physicians' expertise is also much needed for home health care quality assurance and clinical research. Role models and training experiences must be developed for new physicians so that they can integrate home health care skills and values into their future practices. Although most of the usual physician objections to home health care involvement can be addressed by education, the problem of inadequate reimbursement is substantive and must be addressed by policy change.

American Federation of Home Health Agencies
1320 Fenwick Lane, Suite 100
Silver Spring, MD 20910
301/588-1454

Joint Commission on Accreditation
of Healthcare Organizations
Home Care Project
One Renaissance Blvd.
Oakbrook Terrace, IL 60181
708/916-5741

National Association for Home Care
519 C St. NE, Washington, DC 20002
202/547-7424

National Association of Private
Geriatric Care Managers
1315 Talbott Tower, Dayton, OH 45402
513/222-2621

Guidelines for the Medical Management of the Home-Care Patient, American Medical Association Home Care Advisory Panel, Arch Fam Med: 1993(2) 1993 Feb; 194-206.
Increasing numbers of patients of all ages are receiving needed health care services in non-institutional settings. Acute, subacute, rehabilitative, preventive, long-term, and hospice services are provided in the home under the physician's supervision. The safe and appropriate treatment of these patients involves the physician in a team effort as most home care is provided by nurses, other allied health professionals, and family members. The guidelines cover such areas as the role of the physician; the physician-patient

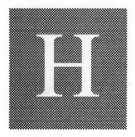

relationship; the elements of medical management in home care, including the evaluation/assessment process, the selection of the interdisciplinary team, and the development of the care plan; patient's rights and responsibilities; the coordination of care; and the use of community resources.

The Role of the Physician in Home Care :

There is no place like home for providing a familiar, supportive environment for healing, This is a concept embraced by patients but not fully accepted by physicians. Seeing patients at home can be a very rewarding experience for physicians and is very much appreciated by patients. It allows physicians to expand their role as advisors and educators both to their patients and to other health care professionals. Home care also allows patients to be more active participants in the treatment process.

The separation of the practice of medicine from the home setting is a relatively recent phenomenon. During the nineteenth and early twentieth centuries, the home visit was an intrinsic part of the physician practice. As medical treatment became more invasive and more technologically bound to services available only in the medical office or hospital, caring for patients in the home was viewed by many in the medical profession as inefficient and inadequate. Gradually, physicians abdicated home care to nursing and the physician house call became a rare event.

Today, changes in medical technology and a broader understanding of the pathology of disease, disability, and convalescence have expanded the scope and desirability of medically supervised home treatment. The patient's plea to go home sooner or the family's search for an alternative to the nursing home for frail relatives has also stimulated physician interest and involvement in home care and formal home health care services. An estimated 46 percent of family care practitioners spend part of their week doing home care, and a growing number of physicians are becoming more active in the delivery and management of home healthcare services.

Incorporating Home Care into A Practice:
If a physician chooses to include home care in his or her practice, what do patients expect? First, home care is as much a matter of style as it is didactic content. Yes, it is necessary to understand the clinical aspects of home treatment, the durable medical equipment (DME) and other modalities that make up home care. This can be learned. Experienced home care nurses, for example, are a valuable source of information on how to care for decubiti in the home without resorting to hospitalization or on what simple maneuvers may help the patient with impaired mobility.

Beyond these techniques, however, there must be a special commitment to the patient. A commitment to look at disease from the patient's perspective and to seek solutions that go beyond traditionally conceived medical intervention and demonstrate a concerned, compassionate, competent response. This does not imply expertise in all areas of home care, but it does require that the physician actively investigate who on the home team can get the answers. It does not imply that the physician will resolve all

problems, but that he or she will consider the social, psychological, and cultural context of a patient's life in devising care plans and will help mobilize the necessary resources to implement those plans.

Home care is different than hospital or office-based practice. The home environment is a place of enormous emotional significance to the patient. It is a place where the physician is the patient's guest in contrast to the patient being a captive in the hospital or a visitor in the doctor's office. Because of the more intimate relationship established with the patient and family in the home setting, it is inevitable that the physician's whole approach to treatment will be more humane. It is important to note that this is indeed a two-way street. An implicit part of this is a more humane treatment of the doctor by the patient. We become more complete human beings to each other.

More and more doctors are recognizing the advantages of incorporating home care into their practices. Some of these advantages are
- good public relations and community image for the physician - especially for new practices;
- the enhancement of physician-patient relationships, allowing physicians to express their commitment to the health and well-being of their patients beyond the walls of their office or hospital;
- the timely identification and management of medical care and other health concerns, reducing the incidence of emergent situations and complications;
- an enhancement of practice efficiency, allowing the physician to draw upon the talents and skills of specially trained home care providers and to respond effectively to the "quicker and sicker" discharge attributed to Medicare's DRG system;
- the opportunity to work with other health care professionals and share knowledge on the resolution of illness and disability
- the ability to tailor treatment and care plans to a broader spectrum of patient needs by understanding the home environment and the patient's ability to perform activities of daily living in the face of illness and disability;
- the opportunity to educate patients and their families in self care and health promotion activities; and most basic of all,
- the ability to practice good medicine.

"Home care is an enhancement of care, not a compromise of care."
R Lawrence, H. Bernstein, MD (HOM)

Physician Guide to Home Health Care. Chicago; American Medical Association. 1989; 63 pp. ISBN 0-89970-3-429. OP055989

Homeless
The Quality of Mercy

Ralph Crawshaw, MD "A Piece of My Mind"
JAMA. 1991 Aug 7; 266(5): 614-15

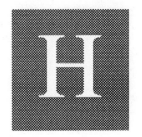

Travel has a way of stretching the mind. The stretch comes not from travel's immediate reward, the inevitable myriad new sights, smells, and sounds, but with experiencing first-hand how others do differently what we have believed to be the right and only way.

Not all travelers know that their ultimate destination is a wider view of themselves, that personal questions arise whose answers will not be found in guidebooks. We exert our sharpest powers of curiosity only when our mind is its own, wondering, reflecting, contemplating. At its best, travel proves a healthy convalescence from life's routine, a time when quickened imagination nurtures a revaluing of self.

A recent trip my wife and I made to Venice is a case in point. We love that city without automobiles; that city free of the imprint and coercion of machines, except of course, the vaporetto, that humble, rocking beast of burden, more like a tamed hippopotamus than a ferryboat, created to bear a full crowd of human beings not very far not very fast. Venice, all walks and water byways, is and remains a monument to human dimensions.

We stayed at the Hotel La Fenice et des Artistes, in a third-floor room overlooking the small piazza of the Theatro Fenice. Naturally, jet lag haunted us the first few days, leaving us wakeful while the rest of Venice slept. On the first night, about 3AM, I heard a noise coming through the window, not the cooing of sleepy Venetian pigeons, but a strange scraping sound. Rising, I looked out. The single streetlight, suspended on a cable across the piazza, cast a distinct ring of light. At first I was unable to make out the source of the noise. Only as my eyes grew accustomed to the surrounding darkness did I discern a strange sight.

Across the way crouched a small woman, all but overwhelmed by her ill-fitting coat. To all appearances she met the US definition of a bag lady. Hunched down, she noiselessly picked through a plastic bag. With great care, she regularly brought forth spoonfuls of some unknown material, which she deposited into a ring of tin cans surrounding her. The scraping noise came as she cleaned the spoon against the side of each can.

As my eyes fully accommodated, I could see, sitting in a wider ring beyond the tin cans, an attentive pride - small, perhaps feral house cats of indeterminate origin. Once the lady finished her ritual with the tin cans, the cats moved in, the largest ones first, and set to eating with gusto. While they ate she remained in the center of the circle, only to interrupt her vigil as now and then she scurried to fill an empty tin or deliver an additional can to a hesitant visitor beyond the range of light: a cat too shy to join the dinner party.

During our entire stay in Venice the scraping began punctually at 3AM. Each night we watched from our window, and the only other person to share the scene a carabiniere, who once,

apparently on his rounds, sauntered through the piazza. He hardly glanced at the cat lady, while her attention never strayed from her wards. Without a word or sign of recognition, he passed into the night. For all I know she is busy every night, ladling out portions to Venice's homeless cats.

Like it or not, my mind was stretched. What was I looking at? When I asked others, their answers varied little. "Madness," they would say, and then regale me with a tale or two of grate-sleeping, homeless bag ladies defying the limits of common sense by defecating on a street corner or badgering peaceful passersby.

Nor was science of much help in understanding what I had seen. In its Christmas edition, *New Scientist* carried an article about England's 6 million disease-ridden, spraying, caterwauling feral cats who "needed" to be trapped and neutered.* Even this dispassionate account contributed to my mind stretching as it reported how a "devoted member of the public" has for the last 20 years been giving breakfast every day before dawn to cats in Regent's Park, London. Is there a syndrome of cat-feeding madness, or, I found myself asking, had I witnessed an act of mercy?

But feelings, particularly when they identify an action, need to be more than named; they need to be made real. What more is meant by the mercy than a passing recognition of goodness. The word mercy hardly finds a place in the parlance of medical scientists. We may know charity, for many of us give at the office. But what is mercy? It neither has pity's sterile distance and faint aroma of disdain, nor joins compassion's impulsive rush to embrace the afflicted. No, mercy, while appearing to hesitate, pauses to judge carefully both the near and far anguish, the responsibility for and innocence of wrong. Despite the dictates of reasonable justice, mercy accepts what is as it is, redeeming the insignificant other with solace and support; support that touches with gentle fingers and soft words the body, mind, and heart of suffering. Therein lies the meaning. Mercy is considered intimacy with despair.

One need not look far to see there is precious little mercy, either strained or dropping like a gentle rain, for homeless cats or human beings. I know, for recently, I joined a fellowship in my city attempting to establish an infirmary for the homeless. Like the people who claim Our Lady of the Cats is mad, a bank official, when offered an opportunity to help fill the need of the homeless, replied, "Our organization is doing everything it can to distance itself from the problem."

In contrast, when the local medical society was asked for help with homeless human beings, 60 local physicians volunteered. Yet you cannot help but wonder what is thought of these doctors. Are they mad for not distancing themselves from human suffering? What ware we to think when we hear these doctors scraping their medical cabinets clean for a circle of nameless sick?

Much as my pupils dilated in the darkness of the Venetian night, my mind expanded to the somber question, Are doctors mad for serving the homeless? Long ago, while traveling on the Red Arrow Express to Leningrad, I shared a compartment with a Russian physician. We could

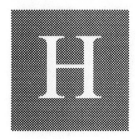

converse because he was as fluent in English as I was clumsy in Russian. We talked intimately as travelers do when they discover their compatibility uncompromised by threat of continuing responsibilities. He illustrated his concern for understanding the difficult position of a physician during wartime by recounting his conflicting feelings while treating wounded Nazi soldiers captured shortly after the had murdered a schoolroom of children by throwing them down a well. My companion paused and from his depth witnessed, "Compassion is not a concept. It is an experience."

The memory led me to reflect on Charity's three daughters: Compassion, the impulsive one, the youngest, spontaneous, and direct; Pity, who stands apart and points; and Mercy, the oldest, who seeks no truce with sorrow. Mercy illuminates the question of madness in charitable doctors, though hesitant, perhaps reserved, she carefully measures the distance between her heart and the other's pain, always considering her part in what transpires. Only then does Mercy act to sweep up the anguish as substance from which to fashion forgiveness. With judgement fulfilled, Mercy extends both mind and heart in the balm of forgiveness, laying on the spirit of life, a willing merger with souls in despair.

My colleagues who volunteered to care for the homeless know, perhaps not as well as Our Lady of the Cats, that only as we experience mercy do we live as merciful people. They infuse our profession with mercy, though they may appear mad to a world that judges by direct returns, be it commercial profit or military victory. Anticipating another stretching, my mind has me searching for a land where Our Lady of the Merciful can be found in the darkness before dawn, feeding value-less, spirit-starved feral souls.

*Young S. The kindest cut. New Scientist. December 22/29, 1990:81.

Health care needs of homeless and runaway youths. Council on Scientific Affairs. JAMA. 1989 Sept 8; 262(10): 1358-61
Large numbers of homeless adolescents can be found in this country, with estimates of their numbers ranging from 500,000 to more than 2 million. Some are runaways while others are involuntarily without shelter, often having been forced out of their homes. Most receive no help from social service agencies and their lack of skills forces them into a marginal existence, leaving them vulnerable to abuse and victimization. Health problems are numerous and health care is generally inadequate for several reasons, including a lack of treatment facilities, the behavior of the adolescents themselves, the ability of providers to deal with such youths, and the questionable legal status of homeless adolescents. The Council on Scientific Affairs urges that reliable and up-to-date data on the extent of homelessness among adolescents and the nature of their needs be generated and that guidelines for the medical care of such youths be developed.

Contact local Travelers and Immigrant Aid

National Coalition for the Homeless
1439 Rhode Island Ave., Washington, DC 20005
202/265-2371

Homeopathic Medicine
A system of alternative medicine that seeks to treat patients by administering small doses of medicines that would bring on symptoms similar to those of the patient in a healthy person. For example, the homeopathic treatment for diarrhea would be a minuscule amount of a laxative. (ENC)
National Center for Homeopathy

801 North Fairfax St, Suite 306
Alexandria, VA 22314
703/548-7790

Hormone
National Hormone and Pituitary Program
210 West Fayette St., Suite 501-9,
Baltimore, MD 21201
301/328-2746

Hospice
Accreditation:
Joint Commission on Accreditation
of Healthcare Organizations
One Renaissance Blvd.
Oakbrook Terrace, IL 60181
708/916-5741

Children's Hospice International
1101 King Street, Suite 131, Alexandria, VA 22314
703/684-0330

Hospice Education Institute
PO Box 713, 5 Essex Square, Suite 3-B
Essex, CT 06426
800/331-1620

National Hospice Organization
1901 N. Moore St., Suite 901, Arlington, VA 22209
703/243-5900

Hospital
American Hospital Association
840 N. Lake Shore Dr., Chicago, IL 60611
312/280-6000
Hospital Data 312/280-6589
Library 312/280-6263
Order Dept. 312/280-6030
Statistics Center 312/280-6521

Accreditation Manual for Hospitals, Vol 1
(AMH-Vol 1) Joint Commission on Accreditation of Healthcare Organizations, Oakbrook, IL.
Annual: 1993: 253 pp. ISBN 0-86688-272-3

Contact for Questions regarding:
Accreditation:
Joint Commission on Accreditation of Healthcare Organizations (to check on hospital's accreditation standing)

Charges
Contact state/local cost containment council

Complaints, in general
Contact local/state health care council or department of public health

Complaints about fees
American Hospital Association 312/280-6000

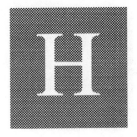

Hospital Management Companies:
Federation of American Health Systems
1405 N. Pierce, #311, Little Rock, AR 72207
501/661-9555

Hospital Medical Staff:
National Association of Medical Staff Services
500 N. Michigan, Suite 1400, Chicago, IL 60611
312/661-1700

Public information:
"Tips on Choosing a Hospital,"
(Send $.25 and stamped self-addressed
envelope to)
Council of Better Business Bureaus
1515 Wilson Blvd., Arlington, VA 22209

Booklet on how to identify problems in
hospital bills:
Emergency Medicine Alliance
800-553-0735

Hospital Associations, Statewide

Alabama Hospital Association
500 N East Blvd, PO Box 17059
Montgomery, AL 36193
205/272-8781

Health Association of Alaska
319 Seward St, Juneau, AK 99801
907/586-1790

Arizona Hospital Association
2411 W 14th St, Suite 410
Tempe, AZ 85281-6943
602/968-1083

Arkansas Hospital Association
419 Natural Resources Drive
Little Rock, AR 72205
501/224-7878

California Association of Hospitals
and Health Systems
1201 K St, Suite 800, PO Box 1100
Sacramento, CA 95814
916/443-7401

Colorado Hospital Association
2140 S Holly St, Denver, CO 80222
303/758-1630

Connecticut Hospital Association
110 Barnes Road, PO Box 90
Wallingford, CT 06492
203/265-7611

Association of Delaware Hospitals
1280 S Governors Ave, PO Box 471
Dover, DE 19901
302/674-2853

District of Columbia Hospital Association
1250 I St, NW, Suite 700, Washington, DC 20005
202/682-1581

Florida Hospital Association
307 Park Lake Circle, PO Box 531107
Orlando, FL 32853-1107
407/841-6230

Georgia Hospital Association
North by Northwest Office Park, Atlanta, GA 30339
404/955-0324

Healthcare Association of Hawaii
932 Ward Ave, Suite 430, Honolulu, HI 96814
808/521-8961

Idaho Hospital Association
6520 Norwood Drive, PO Box 8927
Boise, ID 83707-2927
208/377-2211

Illinois Hospital Association
1151 E Warrenville Road, PO Box 3015,
Naperville, IL 60566
708/505-7777

Indiana Hospital Association
One American Square, PO Box 82063,
Indianapolis, IN 46282
317/633-4870

Iowa Hospital Association
100 E Grand Ave, Des Moines, IA 50309
515/288-1955

Kansas Hospital Association
1263 Topeka Ave, PO Box 2308
Topeka, KS 66601
913/233-7436

Kentucky Hospital Association
1302 Clear Spring Trace, PO Box 24163,
Louisville, KY 40224
502/426-6220

Louisiana Hospital Association
9521 Brookline Ave, PO Box 80720
Baton Rouge, LA 70898-0720
504/928-0026

Maine Hospital Association
160 Capitol St, Augusta, ME 04330
207/622-4794

Maryland Hospital Association
1301 York Road, Suite 800
Lutherville, MD 21093-6087
301/321-6200

Massachusetts Hospital Association
5 New England Executive Park
Burlington, MA 01803
617/272-8000

Michigan Hospital Association
6215 W Saint Joseph Highway, Lansing, MI 48917
517/323-3443

Minnesota Hospital Association
2221 University Ave, SE, Suite 425
Minneapolis, MN 55414-3085
612/331-5571

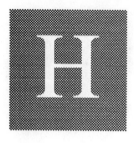

Mississippi Hospital Association
6425 Lakeover Road, Jackson, MS 39213
601/982-3251

Missouri Hospital Association
4713 Highway 50 W, PO Box 60
Jefferson City, MO 65102
314/893-3700

Montana Hospital Association
1720 9th Ave, PO Box 5119, Helena, MT 59601
406/442-1911

Nebraska Hospital Association
1640 L St, Suite D, PO Box 94833
Lincoln, NE 68508-2509
402/476-0141

Nevada Hospital Association
4600 Kietzke Lane, Suite A-108, Reno, NV 89502
702/827-0184

New Hampshire Hospital Association
125 Airport Road, Concord, NH 03301-5388
603/225-0900

New Jersey Hospital Association
746-760 Alexander Road, CN-1
Princeton, NJ 08543-0001
609/275-4000

New Mexico Hospital Association
2625 Pennsylvania NE, Suite 2000
PO Box 36090, Albuquerque, NM 87176
505/889-3393

Hospital Association of New York State
74 N Pearl St, Albany, NY 12207
518/434-7600

North Carolina Hospital Association
112 Cox Ave, PO Box 10937, Raleigh, NC 27605
919/832-9550

North Dakota Hospital Association
919 S 7th St, Bismark, ND 58504
701/224-9732

Ohio Hospital Association
21 W Broad St, Columbus, OH 43215
614/221-7614

Oklahoma Hospital Association
4000 Lincoln Blvd, Oklahoma City, OK 73105
405/427-9537

Oregon Association of Hospitals
4000 Kruse Way Place
Bldg 2, Suite 100, Lake Oswego, OR 97035-2543
503/636-2204

Hospital Association of Pennsylvania
4750 Lindle Road, PO Box 8600
Harrisburg, PA 17105-8600
717/564-9200

Puerto Rico Hospital Association
Villa Nevarez Professional Center
Rio Piedras, PR 00927
809/764-0290

Hospital Association of Rhode Island
345 Blackstone Blvd, 2nd Floor, PO Box 9627
Providence, RI 02940
401/421-7100

South Carolina Hospital Association
101 Medical Circle, PO Box 6009
West Columbia, SC 29171-6009
803/796-3080

South Dakota Hospital Association
3708 Brooks Place, Suite 1, Sioux Falls, SD 57106
605/361-2281

Tennessee Hospital Association
500 Interstate Blvd S, Nashville, TN 37210
615/256-8240

Texas Hospital Association
6225 US Highway, 290 E, PO Box 15587
Austin, TX 78761-5587
512/465-1000

Utah Hospital Association
515 S 7th E, Suite 2-D, Salt Lake City, UT 84102
801/364-1515

Vermont Hospital Association
148 Main St, Montpelier, VT 05602
802/223-3464

Virginia Hospital Association
PO Box 31394, Richmond, VA 23294
804/747-8600

Washington State Hospital Association
190 Queen Anne Ave N, Seattle, WA 98109
206/281-7211

West Virginia Hospital Association
3422 Pennsylvania Ave, Charleston, WV 25302
304/345-9842

Wisconsin Hospital Association
5721 Odana Road, Madison, WI 53719-1289
608/274-1820

Wyoming Hospital Association
2015 S. Greeley Highway, PO Box 5539,
Cheyenne, WY 82003
307/632-9344

Huntington's Disease
Huntington's Disease Society of America
140 W. 22nd Street, 6th Floor
New York, NY 10011
212/242-1968 or 800/345-4372

Hypertension
Abnormally high blood pressure (the pressure of
blood in the main arteries). Blood pressure goes
up as a normal response to stress and physical
activity. However, a person with hypertension has
a high blood pressure at rest.

Hypertension is usually defined as a resting blood
pressure greater than 140 mm Hg (systolic)/90
mm Hg (diastolic). However, an elderly person
normally has blood pressure readings above these
values because blood pressure increases with

age. Young children usually have blood pressure readings well below these values.

Causes: The majority of people have no obvious cause for their elevated blood pressure; in such cases it is called essential hypertension. However, in about percent of patients, a definite cause can be found, including various disorders of the kidney, certain disorders of the adrenal glands, and coarctation of the aorta.

Tobacco smoking and obesity significantly increase the risk of hypertension. Hypertension sometimes develops in women who are taking the birth-control pill.

Symptoms and Complications: Hypertension usually causes no symptoms and generally goes undiscovered until detected by a physician during the course of a routine physical examination.

Possible complications of untreated hypertension include stroke, heart failure, kidney damage, and retinopathy (damage to the retina at the back of the eye). Severe hypertension may cause confusion and seizures.

Treatment: Mild hypertension may respond to weight reduction and a reduction in personal stress. Smokers should stop smoking and heavy drinkers should drastically reduce their consumption of alcohol. Restriction of salt intake is sometimes recommended.

If these measures have no effect, antihypertensive drugs, may be prescribed. Occasionally, in severe cases, admission to the hospital for investigation of the cause, emergency treatment, and bed rest are required. (ENC)

Citizens for the Treatment of High Blood Pressure
888 17th St., N.W./Suite 904
Washington, DC 20006
202/466-4553

National High Blood Pressure Education Program:
National Institutes of Health, Bethesda, MD 20014
301/496-1051
Free publications:
High Blood Pressure 120/80
National Institutes of Health, Bethesda, MD 20014

Hypnosis
American Society of Clinical Hypnosis
2250 E. Devon Ave., Suite 336
Des Plaines, IL 60018
708/297-3317

Hypnotherapist induces hypnotic state in client to increase motivation or alter behavior patterns: Consults with client to determine nature of problem. Prepares client to enter hypnotic state by explaining how hypnosis works and what client will experience. Tests subject to determine degree of physical and emotional suggestibility. Induces hypnotic state in client, using individualized methods and techniques of hypnosis based on interpretation of test results and analysis of client's problem. May train client in self-hypnosis conditioning. (DOT)

Hypoglycemia
National Hypoglycemia Association
PO Box 120, Ridgewood, NJ 07451

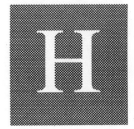

Identification Cards (Emergency)

Medic Alert Foundation
PO Box 1009, 2323 Colorado, Turlock, CA 95380
209/668-3333

Medical information on microfilm
National Safety Council
1121 Spring Lake Drive, Itasca, IL 60143-3201
708/285-1121

Immunization Guides

Contact state/local public health department

Children
American Academy of Pediatrics
141 Northwest Point Blvd.
Elk Grove Village, IL 60007
708/228-5005\ 800/433-9016

International travel
"Vaccination Requirements and Health Advice for
International Travel," (Brochure)
World Health Organization - Geneva
WHO Publications Center USA
49 Sheridan Ave., Albany, NY 12210
518/436-9686

Blair, F. Ed. *Countries of the World: and their
Leaders Yearbook.* Gale Research Inc., Detroit,
MI. Annual. ISSN # 0196-2809.
See Vol 2, section intitled "Foreign Travel: Health
Information."
May be available in many public libraries.

Immunology

American Association of Immunologists
9650 Rockville Pike, Bethesda, MD 20814
301/530-7178

American Board of Allergy and Immunology
3624 Market St., Philadelphia, PA 19104
215/349-9466

Impaired Physician

Licensure and Discipline
*AMA Policy 1. Impairment: (a) Impairment
should be reported to the hospital's
in-house impairment program, if available,
or if the type of impairment is not normally
addressed by an impairment program, e.g.,
extreme fatigue and emotional distress,
then the chief of an appropriate clinical
service, the chief of staff of the hospital, or
other appropriate supervisor (e.g., the chief
resident) should be alerted. (b) If a report
cannot be made through the usual hospital
channels, then a report should be made to
an external impaired physician program.
Such programs typically would be
operated by the local medical societies or
state licensing boards. (c) Physicians in
office-based practices who do not have the
clinical privileges at an area hospital
should be reported directly to an impaired*

*physician program. (d) If reporting to an
individual or program which would
facilitate the entrance of the impaired
physician into an impaired physician
program cannot be accomplished, then the
impaired physician should be reported
directly to the state licensing board.*

JAMA Theme Issue: Impaired Physicians
JAMA. 1987 Jun 5;2 57(21)
The inability of a person to perform to their fullest
potential due to a physical or chemical impairment
is a serious problem. JAMA looked at this issue
and how it affects physicians in depth in this 1987
issue. Original contributions to this effort discuss
alcohol-use patterns through medical school,
several programs combating the problem,
alcoholic women in medicine and medical
education on substance abuse. Editorials included
discuss physician suicide, and the relationship of
physical impairment to the experience of medical
school, among others.

Impaired Physician Program
Talbott Recovery Center
5448 Yorktown Drive, Atlanta, GA 30349
404/994-0185

International Doctors in Alcoholics Anonymous
7250 France Ave S, Suite 400 C, Minneapolis, MN
55435
612/835-4421

What is Impairment?

*In general terms, impairment exists when physical
or mental illness and/or drug or alcohol abuse
interfere with family, social, or work life.*

The American Medical Association has
operationally defined the impaired physician as
one who is unable to practice medicine with
reasonable skill and safety because of mental
illness or excessive use or abuse of drugs,
including alcohol.

Actual diagnosis of impairment must be made by
professionals because the problem can exist in
many different forms. For example, in some
cases, mental illness may be the underlying cause
of substance abuse. Alcoholism is the most
common cause of impairment though many
people become addicted to other drugs. Some
people may combine the use of alcohol with other
drugs.

The following are some of the most commonly
used substances that can cause impairment.

Alcohol - The use of alcohol is the number one
drug problem. Alcohol is considered a drug
because it dramatically affects the central nervous
system, producing slowed reflexes and
drowsiness. It is the major psychoactive chemical
ingredient in wines, beers, and distilled beverages
such as scotch, gin, and vodka.

Depressants - As prescription drugs, depressants
are used for the relief of anxiety, irritability, and
tension, and for the treatment of insomnia. In
excessive amounts, they produce a state of
intoxication similar to alcohol, including impaired
judgment, slurred speech, and loss of motor

coordination. Among the more commonly used depressants are antianxiety drugs such as the benzodiazepines (which include Valium and Librium) and barbiturates (such as Nembutal, Seconal, and Amytal). Barbiturates can be highly addictive and especially dangerous when mixed with alcohol, a practice which sometimes can cause accidental death.

Narcotics - As prescription drugs, narcotics are the most effective agents known for the relief of intense pain. Narcotics tend to induce pinpoint pupils and reduced vision, drowsiness, decreased physical activity, and constipation. Larger doses may induce sleep, but there is an increased possibility of nausea, vomiting, and respiratory depression, the major toxic effect of these drugs. Except in cases of acute intoxication, there is no loss of motor coordination or slurred speech as in the case of depressants. Narcotics include opium, morphine, codeine, heroin, and meperidine (Demerol).

Stimulants - These drugs stimulate the central nervous system, causing the user to feel stronger, more decisive, and to experience a rush of exhilaration, wakefulness, and loss of appetite. Stimulants include amphetamines, such as Dexedrine and Benzedrine, which have been prescribed for the treatment of obesity and narcolepsy. One of the more commonly abused stimulants is methamphetamine or "speed." Cocaine, also considered a stimulant, is commonly regarded as a "status" recreational drug and produces intense euphoria. Early signs of stimulant use include repetitive grinding of the teeth, performing a task repeatedly, suspiciousness, and paranoia.

The Impaired Physician

Physicians are no different from other people in experiencing the difficulties in life that can lead to impairment. And, in fact, the characteristics physicians often develop to adapt to the extreme stresses involved in the training and practice of medicine may put them at special risk for the problem.

Risks for Impairment - The process of training physicians can be like an endurance test. The demands for the profession are so great that trainees may feel overworked and overstressed. To succeed, medical students and residents may become obsessed with work, self-sacrificing, highly competitive, and outwardly unemotional.

Medical school and residency often create an environment with intense competition for grades, excessive workloads, pressure to learn "everything," a continual pervasive for perfection, and fear of failure, which is a particularly pervasive problem. Medical students and residents may be afraid of flunking out, not keeping up with the workload, failing board exams, or making an incorrect diagnosis.

Sleep deprivation is one of the most debilitating aspects of medical students may stay up all night to study and residents can be up all night treating patients while on call. Residents may be overwhelmed by the stress of making their own decisions about patients during the middle of the night. Yet they are afraid to ask for help from peers, because it will appear that they are unable

to handle the pressure. Residents may also feel further debilitation from the pressure to perform competently without having had any sleep the night before.

These intense pressures on medical students and residents leave them with little time or energy for personal relationships or other life-enriching experiences, a factor that alienates them from society.

Once physicians begin to practice, stresses and behavior patterns tend to stay much the same. Excessive time demands still exist or may increase, with pressures to keep up with patient care and with new technology and medical advances. Physicians feel required to suppress emotions toward their patients and to distance themselves from death. They also continue to feel pressure over whether they have provided the proper treatment for difficult cases.

In addition to these continual stresses, other frustrations occur for physicians after they begin practice. During the training years, physicians may have dreamed about the independence they would have. Yet once in practice, many become disillusioned when they find that the independence does not really exist, particularly today with constraints from the government and third-party payers.

As in the training years, the marriages and family lives of physicians may be adversely affected by the demands of the medical profession. Too little time at home may make it difficult for them to maintain successful relationships with family members. This may be especially true for those physicians who are compelled to use time at home to do paperwork or catch up on their reading of medical journals. The promises of what can be bought with the money that results from the physician's hard work will not replace the love and involvement family members want and need.

When physicians bring home the autocratic sense of authority that is often used in the office, family members may resent being treated like patients and being told what to do. Physicians may also strain marital relations in other ways. They may postpone or cancel family outings and vacations due to work demands or expect spouses to handle all household problems because of their concerns with the medical practice.

A lack of fulfillment may develop in physicians who have been in practice for some time. Physicians go into practice with the ideals of saving lives and making great contributions to the community and sometimes it is difficult for them to accept the everyday, routine work that is a part of a medical practice. These physicians may start to question whether all of the hard work has been worth it and may feel a sense of emptiness and failure.

The demands of medical practice cause physicians to experience numerous pressures throughout their careers and to deny many of the human needs for social and family interaction. These pressures and deprivations can cause anger, anxiety, fear, and stress - factors that may lead to mental illness, and/or drug and alcohol abuse in some physicians.

The psychiatric disorders that lead to impairment most often involve depressive illnesses. While depression alone can cause impairment in physicians, it can often lead to further impairment through alcohol and/or drug abuse.

Alcohol or drug abuse may have begun as early as the training years as a way to cope with the stress. Physicians are especially at risk for drug abuse - and not just because of their easy access to drugs. As medical students, they are trained to use medication to solve patients' problems and they may come to view drugs as an easy and appropriate way to solve their own problems as well. Also, because of their medical training, physicians may feel that they are knowledgeable enough to control drug use without becoming addicted.

Coping Mechanisms

Obviously, all physicians suffer from stresses that can potentially lead to impairment. Yet not all physicians become impaired. If depends on how the stresses affect them. If physicians are aware of the inherent risks of impairment in the medical profession and employ certain coping mechanisms, the pressures are less likely to result in impairment.

Due to an increased awareness of the risks for impairment, many medical schools and residency training programs are offering workshops, seminars, and support groups to help trainees learn to cope with stress, improve and maintain their personal communication skills, and manage their practices. By learning these skills in the training years, students and residents can avoid developing the counterproductive coping mechanism (such as alcohol or drugs) that may lead to impairment.

Some of the coping mechanisms recommended for all physicians include:
- establishing good communications and intimacy with spouses, children, and friends so that a solid support system can be established for coping with life's pressures;
- leaving medical concerns at the office or hospital so that physicians can experience quality time with family and friends;
- ensuring successful family interactions by taking 30 minutes to decompress from office pressure before getting involved in situations at home;
- learning to manage time and define goals so that physicians can be involved with one activity without worrying about other responsibilities;
- cultivating outside interests or hobbies that are fun, not work, so that medicine does not become so all-consuming;
- taking care of personal health by getting plenty of exercise, eating properly, and avoiding excess use of alcohol, tobacco, and caffeine. (SPI)

Indigent Health Care

Contact county/state board of health.

Industrial Health
American Industrial Health Council
1330 Connecticut Ave. NW
Washington, D.C. 20036
202/659-0060

American Industrial Hygiene Association
345 White Pond Drive, Akron, OH 44321
216/873-2442

Industry, Health
Health Industry Distributors Association
1701 Pennsylvania Ave. NW, Suite 470,
Washington, DC 20006
202/659-0050

Health Industry Manufacturers Association
1200 G Street, NW, Suite 400
Washington, DC 20005
202/783-8700

Medical and Health Care Marketplace Guide. 7th ed. International Biomedical Information Services, Inc, Philadelphia, 1991. ISBN 0-926700-04-9
800/223-2030

Infectious Diseases
National Foundation for Infectious Diseases
4733 Bethesda Ave., Suite 750
Bethesda, MD 20814
301/656-0003

Board Certification
American Board of Internal Medicine
3624 Market St., Philadelphia, PA 19104
215/243-1500, 800/441-ABIM (800/441-2246)

Board Certification in Pediatric Infectious Disease
American Board of Pediatrics
111 Silver Cedar Court, Chapel Hill, NC 27514
919/929-0461

Informed Consent
***AMA Policy.* Informed Consent and Decision-Making in Health Care*:
1) Health care professionals should inform patients or their surrogates of their clinical impression or diagnosis; alternative treatments and consequences of treatments, including the consequence of no treatment; and recommendations for treatment. Full disclosure is appropriate in all cases, except in rare situations in which such information would, in the opinion of the health care professional, cause serious harm to the patient.
(2) Individuals should, at their own option, provide instructions regarding their wishes in the event of their incapacity. Individuals may also wish to designate a surrogate decision-maker. When a patient is incapable of making health care decision, such decisions should be made by a surrogate acting

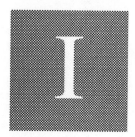

pursuant to the previously expressed wishes of the patient, and when such wishes are not known or ascertainable, the surrogate should act in the best interests of the patient.

(3) A patient's health record should include sufficient information for another health care professional to assess previous treatment, to ensure continuity of care, and to avoid unnecessary or inappropriate tests or therapy.

(4) Conflicts between a patient's right to privacy and a third party's need to know should be resolved in favor of patient privacy, except where that would result in serious health hazard or harm to the patient or others.

(5) Holders of health record information should be held responsible for reasonable for security measures through respective licensing laws. Third parties that are granted access to patient health care information should be held responsible for reasonable security measures and should be subject to sanctions when confidentiality is breached.

(6) A patient should have access to the information in his or her health record, except for that information which, in the opinion of the health care professional, would cause harm to the patient or to other people.

(7) Disclosures of health information about a patient to a third party may only be made upon consent by the patient or the patient's lawfully authorized nominee, except in those cases in which the third party has a legal or predetermined right to gain access to such information.

Injury
National Injury Information Clearinghouse
5401 Westbard Ave., Room 625
Bethesda, MD 20207
301/492-6424

Insurance, Health
Alliance of American Insurers
1501 Woodfield Road, Suite 400
Schaumburg, IL 60123
708/330-8500

American Insurance Agency
1130 Conecticut Ave, NW, Suite 1000,
Washington, DC 20036
202/828-7100

Health Insurance Claim Form

The Health Insurance Claim Form 1500 was revised early in 1992. The required date for use of the new form for Medicare was May 1, 1992. Many other carriers have not set a required date for implementation of the new forms. Any questions regarding the use of the new 1500 form should be directed to a local Medicare carrier office.

The **major changes** to the new form are discussed in this article.

Format

The format has been revised to accommodate additional information. This change was made to reduce the number of attachments that may be required on some claims. The format was changed significantly enough to affect computer systems. If your claim form is computerized, contact the software vendor to change the format of the 1500 form.

OCR Red Scannable Ink
The revised form is printed in Optical Character Recognition (OCR) red scannable ink. The red scannable ink is mandated by Medicare. The reason for change in ink is that Medicare and other third party payors are now scanning the information into their computer system instead of using manual entry. Photocopies of the form cannot be sent to Medicare or other payors requiring OCR ink. For best results, use OCR scannable forms for all claims.

Place of Service Codes
The place of service codes and definitions have been revised and expanded.

Codes Definitions
00-10 (Unassigned)

11 Office
Location, other than a hospital, Skilled Nursing Facility (SNF), Military Treatment Facility, Community Health Center, State or Local Public Health Clinic or Intermediate Care Facility (ICF), where the health professional routinely provides health examinations, diagnosis and treatment of illness or injury on an ambulatory basis.

12 Patient's Home
Location, other than a hospital or other facility, where the patient receives care in a private residence.

13-20 (Unassigned)

21 Inpatient Hospital
A facility, other than psychiatric, which primarily provides diagnostic, therapeutic (both surgical and nonsurgical) and rehabilitation services by, or under, the supervision of physicians to patients admitted for a variety of medical conditions.

22 Outpatient Hospital
A portion of a hospital which provides diagnostic, therapeutic (both surgical and nonsurgical), and rehabilitation services to sick or injured persons who do not require hospitalization or institutionalization.

23 Emergency Room - Hospital
A portion of a hospital where emergency diagnosis and treatment of illness or injury is provided.

24 Ambulatory Surgical Center
A freestanding facility, other than a physician's office, where surgical and diagnostic services are provided on an ambulatory basis.

25 Birthing Center
A facility, other than a hospital's maternity facilities or a physician's office, which provides a setting for labor, delivery and immediate port-partum care as well as immediate care of newborn infants.

26 Military Treatment Facility
A medical facility operated by one or more of the Uniformed Services. Military Treatment Facility (MTS) also refers to certain former U.S. Public Health Service (USPHS) facilities now designated as Uniformed Service Treatment Facilities (USTF).

27-30 (Unassigned)

31 Skilled Nursing Facility
A facility which primarily provides inpatient skilled nursing care and related services to patients who require medical, nursing, or rehabilitative services but does not provide the level of care or treatment available in a hospital.

32 Nursing Facility
A facility which primarily provides to residents skilled nursing care and related services for the rehabilitation of injured, disabled, or sick persons, or, on a regular basis, health-related care services above the level of custodial care to other than mentally retarded individuals.

33 Custodial Care Facility
A facility which provides room, board and other personal assistance services, generally on a long-term basis, and which does not include a medical component.

34 Hospice
A facility, other than a patient's home, in which palliative and supportive care for terminally ill patients and their families are provided.

35-40 (Unassigned)

41 Ambulance-Land
A land vehicle specifically designed, equipped and staffed for lifesaving and transporting the sick or injured.

42 Ambulance-Air or Water
An air or water vehicle specifically designed, equipped and staffed for lifesaving and transporting the sick or injured.

43-50 (Unassigned)

51 Inpatient Psychiatric Facility
A facility that provides inpatient psychiatric services for the diagnosis and treatment of mental illness on a 24-hour basis, by or under the supervision of a physician.

52 Psychiatric Facility Partial Hospitalization
A facility for the diagnosis and treatment of mental illness that provides a planned therapeutic program for patients who do not require full-time hospitalization, but who need broader programs than are possible from outpatient visits in a hospital-based or hospital-affiliated facility.

53 Community Mental Health Center
A facility that provides comprehensive mental health services on an ambulatory basis primarily to individuals residing or employed in a defined area.

54 Intermediate Care Facility/Mentally Retarded
A facility which primarily provides health-related care and services above the level of custodial care to mentally retarded individuals but does not provide the level of care or treatment available in a hospital or SNF.

55 Residential Substance Abuse Treatment Facility
A facility which provides treatment for substance (alcohol and drug) abuse to live-in residents who do not require acute medical care. Services include individual and group therapy and counseling, family counseling, laboratory tests, drugs and supplies, psychological testing, and room and board.

56 Psychiatric Residential Treatment Center
A facility or distinct part of a facility for psychiatric care which provides a total 24-hour therapeutically planned and professionally staffed group living and learning environment.

57-60 (Unassigned)

61 Comprehensive Inpatient Rehabilitation Facility
A facility that provides comprehensive rehabilitation services under the supervision of a physician to out-patients with physical disabilities. Services include physical therapy, occupational therapy, and speech pathology services.

62 Comprehensive Outpatient Rehabilitation Facility
A facility that provides comprehensive rehabilitation services under the supervision of a physician to outpatients with physical disabilities. Services include physical therapy, occupational therapy, and speech pathology services.

63-64 (Unassigned)

65 End Stage Renal Disease Treatment Facility
A facility other than a hospital which provides dialysis treatment, maintenance and/or training to patients or care givers on an ambulatory or home-care basis.

66-70 (Unassigned)

71 State or Local Public Health Clinic

72 Rural Health Clinic
A certified facility which is located in a rural medically underserved area that provides ambulatory primary medical care under the general direction of a physician.

73-80 (Unassigned)

81 Independent Laboratory
A laboratory certified to perform diagnostic and/or clinical tests independent of an institution or a physician's office.

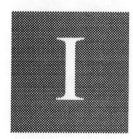

82-98 (Unassigned)

99 Other Unlisted Facility
Other service facilities not identified above.

Editor's Note: The definitions for several of these place of service terms may differ from those found in CPT 1992. The process used to revise the claim form is different than the CPT revision process.

UPIN Number
In field 17B you will be required to report the Unique Physician Identification Number (UPIN) of the referring physician. This field is used to track providers referring patients.

HCPCS/CPT Codes
When reporting HCPCS and/or CPT codes, the narrative description is no longer required. This was done to save space and eliminate narrative descriptions which are not used when processing claims.

Required for Local Use
There are several areas on the revised form to indicate specific information that may be required for your local carrier. Contact your local third party payors to determine if information will be required in any of these fields.

Bar Code/No Bar Code
The bar code is used by many third party payors and local Medicare offices for microfilming and tracking claim forms. HCFA does not mandate the use of a bar-coded form but many local Medicare offices request them. Please contact your local carriers to determine which form you will need prior to placing an order. (CPT)

Complaints
Contact state department of insurance

Fraud:
National Healthcare Anti-Fraud Association
1255 23rd St., NW/Suite 800
Washington, DC 20037
202/659-5955

Health Insurance Association of America
1025 Connecticut Ave, NW, 12th Floor,
Washington, DC 20036
202/223-7780

Insurance Information Institute
110 William St, New York, NY 10036
212/669-9200

National Insurance Consumer Hotline
(Sponsored by the insurance industry, can answer questions about life, health, home, or auto insurance)
800/942-4242

"Understanding and Choosing
your Health Insurance":
American Society of Internal Medicine
1101 Vermont Ave, Suite 500
Washington, DC 20005-3547
202/289-1700

Insurance Departments, Statewide

Alabama Insurance Department
135 S. Union St, Montgomery, AL 36130
205/269-3550

Alaska Division of Insurance
Commerce & Economic Development Department
PO Box D, Juneau, AK 99811
907/465-2515

Arizona Department of Insurance
3030 N Third St, Room 1100, Phoenix, AZ 85012
602/255-5400

Arkansas Insurance Department
400 University Tower Bldg, Little Rock, AR 72204
501/686-2900

California Department of Insurance
770 L St, Suite 1120, Sacramento, CA 95814
916/445-5544

Colorado Division of Insurance
Department of Regulatory Agencies
303 W Colfax Ave, 5th Floor, Denver, CO 80204
303/866-3201

Connecticut Department of Insurance
PO Box 816, Hartford, CT 06142
203/297-3802

District of Columbia
Insurance Administration, Consumer &
Regulatory Affairs
613 C St, NW, Room 600, Washington, DC 20001
202/727-8000

Delaware Department of Insurance
The Green, Dover, DE 19901
302/739-4251

Florida Department of Insurance
State Capitol, PL 11, Tallahassee, FL 32399
904/922-3100

Georgia Office of the Insurance Commissioner
704 W Tower, 2 M.L. King, Jr., Drive
Atlanta, GA 30334
404/656-2056

Hawaii Division of Insurance
Commerce & Consumer Affairs Department
1010 Richards St, Honolulu, HI 96813
808/586-2790

Idaho Department of Insurance
500 S 10th, Boise, ID 83720
208/334-2250

Illinois Department of Insurance
320 W Washington St, 4th Floor
Springfield, IL 62767
217/782-4515

Indiana Department of Insurance
311 W Washington St, Suite 300
Indianapolis, IN 46204
317/232-2406

Iowa Insurance Division
Department of Commerce
Lucas State Office Bldg, Des Moines, IA 50319
515/281-5705

Kansas Insurance Department
420 SW Ninth St, Topeka, KS 66612
913/296-3071

Kentucky Department of Insurance
Public Protection & Regulation Cabinet
229 W Main St, Frankfort, KY 40601
502/564-6027

Louisiana Department of Insurance
PO Box 94214, Baton Rouge, LA 70804
504/342-5900

Maine Bureau of Insurance
Professional & Financial Regulations
State House Station #34, Augusta, ME 04333
207/582-8707

Maryland Division of Insurance
Licensing & Regulation Department
501 Saint Paul St, Baltimore, MD 21202
410/333-2520

Massachusetts Division of Insurance
Executive Office of Consumer Affairs
280 Friend St, Boston, MA 02114
617/727-7189

Michigan Commissioner of Insurance
Licensing & Regulation Department
611 W Ottawa, PO Box 30220, Lansing, MI 48909
517/373-9273

Minnesota Department of Commerce
133 E Seventh St, Saint Paul, MN 55101
612/296-4026

Missouri Division of Insurance
Department of Economic Development
Truman Bldg, Box 690, Jefferson City, MO 65102
314/751-4126

Mississippi Department of Insurance
1804 Sillers Bldg, Jackson, MS 39201
601/359-3569

Montana Insurance Division
Office of the State Auditor
Mitchell Bldg, Helena, MT 59620
406/444-2040

Nebraska Department of Insurance
The Terminal Bldg, 941 O St, Suite 400,
Lincoln, NE 68508
402/471-2201

Nevada Insurance Division
Department of Commerce
1665 Hot Springs Road, Carson City, NV 89710
702/687-4270

New Hampshire Insurance Department
169 Manchester St, Concord, NH 03301
603/271-2261

New Jersey Department of Insurance
20 W State St, CN 325, Trenton, NJ 08625
609/633-7667

New Mexico Department of Insurance
PERA Bldg, Room 428, Santa Fe, NM 87503
505/827-4297

New York Insurance Department
Empire State Plaza, Agency Bldg #1
Albany, NY 12257
518/474-4550

North Carolina Department of Insurance
430 N Salisbury St, Raleigh, NC 27603
919/733-7343

North Dakota Insurance Department
State Capitol, 5th Floor
600 East Blvd, Bismarck, ND 58505
701/224-2440

Ohio Department of Insurance
2100 Stella Court, Columbus, OH 43266
614/644-2651

Oklahoma Insurance Department
408 Will Rogers Bldg, Oklahoma City, OK 73105
405/521-2828

Oregon Department of Insurance and Finance
21 Labor & Industries Bldg, Salem, OR 97310
503/378-4120

Pennsylvania Insurance Department
Strawberry Square, 13th Floor
Harrisburg, PA 17120
717/787-6835

Rhode Island Department of Business Regulation
233 Richmond St, Suite 233
Providence, RI 02903
401/277-2223

South Carolina Department of Insurance
1612 Marion St, Columbia, SC 29201
803/737-6117

South Dakota Division of Insurance
Commerce & Regulations Department
910 Sioux, State Capitol, Pierre, SD 57501
605/773-3563

Tennessee Department of
Commerce and Insurance
500 James Robertson Parkway
Nashville, TN 37243
615/741-2241

Texas Board of Insurance
1110 San Jacinto Blvd, Austin, TX 78701
512/463-6464

Utah State Insurance Department
3110 State Office Bldg, Salt Lake City, UT 84114
801/538-3800

Vermont Department of Banking and Insurance
120 State St, Montpelier, VT 05602
802/828-3301

Virginia State Corporation Commission
1220 Bank St, 13th Floor, Richmond, VA 23219
804/786-3603

Washington Office of the Insurance Commissioner
Insurance Bldg, M/S: AQ-21, Olympia, WA 98504
206/753-7301

West Virginia Division of Insurance
2100 Washington St, E, Charleston, WV 25305
304/348-3394

Wisconsin Office of the Commissioner
of Insurance
123 W Washington Ave, PO Box 7873
Madison, WI 53707
608/266-3585

Wyoming Insurance Department
Herschler Bldg, Cheyenne, WY 82002
307/777-7401

American Samoa Insurance Commissioner
Office of the Governor, Pago Pago, AS 96799
684/633-4116

Guam Department of Revenue and Taxation
855 W Marine Drive, Agana, GU 96910
671/477-5144

Northern Mariana Islands Commerce
and Labor Department
Office of the Governor, Saipan, MP 96950
670/322-8711

Puerto Rico Insurance Commission
PO Box 8330, Santurce, PR 00910
809/722-8686

U.S. Virgin Islands
Lieutenant Governor
7 & 8 King St, Kongens Gade
St. Thomas, VI 00802
809/774-2991

Internal Medicine

American Board of Internal Medicine
3624 Market Street, Philadelphia, PA 19104
215/243-1500
800/441-ABIM (800/441-2246)

American Society of Internal Medicine
1101 Vermont Ave. NW, Suite 500
Washington D.C. 20005
202/289-1700

Internist alternate titles: internal medicine
specialist. Diagnoses and treats diseases and
injuries of human internal organ systems:
Examines patient for symptoms or congenital
disorders and determines nature and extent of
injury or disorder, referring to diagnostic images
and tests, and using medical instruments and
equipment. Prescribes medication and
recommends dietary and activity program, as
indicated by diagnosis. Refers patient to medical
specialist when indicated. (DOT)

International Classification of Diseases (ICD-9-CM)

The *International Classification of Diseases, 9th
Revision, Clinical Modification (ICD-9-CM)* is
based on the official version of the World Health
Organization's 9th Revision, *International
Classification of Diseases (ICD-9)*. *ICD-9* is
designed for the classification of morbidity and
mortality information for statistical purposes, and
for the indexing of hospital records by disease and
operations, for data storage and retrieval. The
historical background of the *International
Classification of Diseases* may be found in the
Introduction to ICD-09*(see below).

The concept of extending the *International
Classification of Diseases* for use in hospital
indexing was originally developed in response to a
need for a more efficient basis for storage and
retrieval of diagnostic data. In 1950, the U.S.
Public Health Service and the Veterans
Administration began independent tests of the
International Classification of Diseases for hospital
indexing purposes. In the following year, the
Columbia Presbyterian Medical Center in New
York City adopted the *International Classification
of Diseases*, 6th Revision, with some
modifications for use in its medical record
department. A few years later, the Commission on
Professional and Hospital Activities adopted the
International Classification of Diseases for use in
hospitals participating in the Professional Activity
Study.

The problem of adapting *ICD* for indexing hospital
records was taken up by the U.S. National
Committee on Vital and Health Statistics through
its subcommittee on hospital statistics. The
subcommittee reviewed the modifications made by
the various users of *ICD* and proposed that
Uniform changes be made. This was done by a
small working party.

In view of the growing interest in the use of the
International Classification of Diseases for hospital
indexing, a study was undertaken in 1956 by the
American Hospital Association and the American
Medical Record Association (the American
Association of Medical Record Librarians) of the
relative efficiencies of coding systems for
diagnostic indexing. This study indicated that the
International Classification of Diseases provided a
suitable and efficient framework for indexing
hospital records. The major users of the
International Classification of Diseases for hospital
indexing purposes then consolidated their
experiences and an adaptation was first published
in December 1959. A revision was issued in 1962
and the first "Classification of Operations and
Treatments" was included.

In 1966, the international conference for the
revision of the *International Classification of
Diseases* noted that the 8th revision of *ICD* has
been constructed with hospital indexing in mind
and considered that the revised classification
would be suitable, in itself, for hospital use in
some countries. However, it was recognized that
the basic classification might provide inadequate
detail for diagnostic indexing in other countries. A
group of consultants was asked to study the 8th
revision of *ICD* (*ICD*-8) for applicability to various
users in the United States. This group
recommended that further detail be provided for
coding of hospital and morbidity data. The

American Hospital Association was requested to develop the needed adaptation proposals. This was done by advisory committee (the Advisory Committee to the Central Office on ICDA). In 1968 the United States Public Health Service published the product, *Eighth Revision International Classification of Diseases, Adapted for Use in the United States* (PHS publication 1693). This became commonly known as ICDA-8, and beginning in 1968 it served as the basis for coding diagnostic data for both official morbidity and mortality statistics in the United States.

*Manual of the International Classification of Diseases, Injuries, and Causes of Death, World Health Organization, Geneva, Switzerland, 1977.

Other Adaptations

In 1968, the Commission on Professional and Hospital Activities (CPHA) of Ann Arbor, Michigan, published the Hospital Adaptation of ICDA (H-ICDA) based on both the original ICD-8 and ICDA-8. In 1973, CPHA published a revision of H-*ICD*A, referred to as H-*ICD*A-2. Hospitals throughout the United State have been divided in their usage of these classifications. Effective January 1979, *ICD*-9-CM provides a single classification intended primarily for use in the United States replacing these earlier related but somewhat dissimilar classifications.

ICD-9-CM Background

In February 1977, A Steering Committee was convened by the National Center for Health Statistics to provide advice and counsel to the development of a clinical modification of the *ICD*-9.

The organizations represented on the Steering Committee included:

American Association of Health Data Systems
American Hospital Association
American Medical Record Association
Association for Health Records
Council on Clinical Classifications
Health Care Financing Administration, Department of Health and Human Services
WHO Center for Classification of Diseases for North America, sponsored by the National Center for Health Statistics, Department of Health and Human Services

The Council on Clinical Classifications is sponsored by:
American Academy of Pediatrics
American College of Obstetricians and Gynecologists
American College of Physicians
American College of Surgeons
American Psychiatric Association
Commission on Professional and Hospital Activities

The Steering Committee met periodically in 1977. Clinical guidance and technical output were provided by Task Forces on Classification from the Council on Clinical Classification's sponsoring organizations.

ICD-9-CM is a clinical modification of the World Health Organizations's *International Classification of Diseases, 9th Revision (ICD-9)*. The term "clinical" is used to emphasize the modification's intent: to serve as a useful tool in the area of classification of morbidity data for indexing of medical records, medical care review, and ambulatory and other medical care programs, as well as for basic health statistics. To describe the clinical picture of the patient, the codes must be more precise than those needed only for statistical groupings and trend analysis.

The Procedure Classification

An important new development occurred with the publication of *ICD*-9; a Classification of Procedures in Medicine. Heretofore, procedure classification had not been a part of *ICD*, but were published with the adaptations to it produced in the United States.

The *ICD*-9 Classification of Procedures in Medicine is published separately from the disease classification in a series of supplementary documents called fascicles. Each fascicle contains a classification of modes of therapy, surgery, radiology, laboratory, and other diagnostic procedures. The decision to publish each fascicle as a unique document was made in order to permit its revision on a separate schedule from the disease classification. Primary input to Fascicle V, "Surgical Procedures," came from the United States whose adaptations of *ICD* had contained a procedure classification since 1962. This experience was invaluable in constructing a classification to permit analysis of health care services in hospitals and primary care settings.

The *ICD*-9-CM Procedure Classification is a modification of WHO's Fascicle V, "Surgical Procedures," and is published as Volume 3 of *ICD*-9-CM. It contains both a Tabular List and an Alphabetic Index. Greater detail has been added to the *ICD*-9-CM Procedure Classification necessitating expansion of the codes from three to four digits. Approximately 90% of the rubrics refer to surgical procedures with the remaining 10% accounting for other investigative and therapeutic procedures.

Specifications for the Procedure Classification

1. The *ICD-9-CM* Procedure Classification is published in its own volume containing both a Tabular List and an Alphabetic Index.

2. The classification is a modification of Fascicle V "Surgical Procedures" of the *ICD-9* Classification of Procedures in Medicine, working from the draft dated Geneva, 30 September-6 October 1975, and labeled WHO/ICD-9/Rev. Conf. 75.4.

3. All three-digit rubrics in the range 01-86 are maintained as they appear in Fascicle V, whenever feasible.

4. Nonsurgical procedures are aggregated from the surgical procedures and confined to the rubrics 87-99, whenever feasible.

5. Selected detail contained in the remaining fascicles of the *ICD-9* Classification of Procedures in Medicine is accommodated where possible.

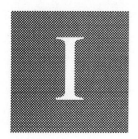

6. The structure of the classification is based on anatomy rather than surgical specialty.

7. The *ICD-9*-cm Procedure Classification is numeric only, i.e., no alphabetic characters are used.

8. The classification is based on a two-digit structure with two decimal digits where necessary.

9. Compatibility with the ICD-09 Classification of Procedures in Medicine was not maintained when a different axis was deemed more clinically appropriate.

Guidance in the Use of *ICD-9-CM*

To code accurately, it is necessary to have a working knowledge of medical terminology and to understand the characteristics, terminology and conventions of the *ICD-9-CM.* Transforming verbal descriptions of diseases, injuries, conditions, and procedures into numerical designations (coding) is a complex activity and should not be undertaken without proper training.

Originally coding was accomplished to provide access to medical records by diagnoses and operations through retrieval for medical research, education, and administration. Medical codes today are utilized to facilitate payment of health services, to evaluate utilization patterns, and to study the appropriateness of health care costs. Coding provides the bases for epidemiological studies and research into the quality of health care.

Coding must be performed correctly and consistently to produced meaningful statistics to aid in the planning for the health needs of the nation.

Questions regarding the use and interpretation of the International Classification of Diseases, 9th Revision, Clinical Modification can be directed to any of the organizations listed below.(ICD)

Questions regarding specific codes or new codes: American Hospital Association Center for ICD-9 Chicago, IL 60611 312/280-6430

World Health Organization Collaborating Center for Classification of Diseases in North America National Center for Health Statistics Department of Health and Human Services 3700 East-West Highway Hyattsville, Maryland 20782

Office of Research, Demonstrations, and Statistics Health Care Financing Administration Department of Health and Human Services 330 Independence Avenue, SW HHS Building Washington, D.C. 20201

International Classification of Diseases, 9th Revision, Clinical Modification (*ICD-9-CM*), Vols. 1 and 2. National Center for Health Statistics. 1989. ISBN 0-685-40119-7

International Health

American College of International Physicians
5530 Wisconsin Ave, Ste. 1149
Washington, DC 20815
301/986-8741

National Council for International Health
1701 K St., NW, Suite 600, Washington, DC 20006
202/833-5900

Project Hope, People-to-People Health Foundation
Project Hope Health Sciences
Millwood, VA 22646
800/544-HOPE (800/544-4673) 703/837-2100

International Medical Graduates, Physicians, Schools, etc.

AMA Policy. Foreign Medical Graduates: The AMA supports the following principles, based on recommendations of the Ad Hoc Committee on Foreign Medical Graduates (FMGs): 1 The AMA encourages American specialty boards to adjust certification procedures to FMGs returning to their home countries. This does not suggest that FMGs should be awarded certificates on the basis of lower standards, but that requisites such as post-qualifying practice in the U.S. should be adapted to FMG diplomates returning home.

(2.) The AMA supports the practice of U.S. teaching hospitals and foreign medical educational institutions entering into appropriate relationships directed toward providing clinical educational experiences for advanced medical students who have completed the equivalent of U.S. core clinical clerkships. Policies governing the accreditation of U.S. medical education programs specify that core clinical training be provided by the parent medical school; consequently, the AMA strongly objects to the practice of substituting clinical experiences provided by U.S. institutions for core clinical curriculum of foreign medical schools. Moreover, it strongly disapproves of the placement of any medical school undergraduate students in hospitals and other medical care delivery facilities which lack educational resources and experience for supervised teaching of clinical medicine.

(3) The AMA urges the ECFMG to evaluate current for determining the proficiency of alien FMGs in the use of English.
(4) The AMA recognizes that certain state and local medical societies have provided English language training programs to FMGs and encourages other medical societies, in areas where there are concentrations of FMGs needing such training, to consider providing it. Medical societies in areas where there are a few FMGs are encouraged to recommend appropriate language programs to FMGs in need of them.

American College of International Physicians
711 Second St, NE, Suite 200
Washington, DC 20002
202/544-7498

Educational Commission for Foreign
Medical Graduates
3624 Market St, Philadelphia, PA 19104
215/386-5900

Iron Overload

Iron Overload Diseases Association
224 Datura St., Ste 911
W. Palm Beach, FL 33401
407/659-5616

Kidney Disease
Disorders of the Kidney

The kidneys are susceptible to a wide range of disorders. However, only one normal kidney is needed for good health, so disease is rarely life-threatening unless it affects both kidneys and has reached an advanced stage.

Hypertension.(high blood pressure) can be both a cause and effect of kidney damage. Other effects of serious disease or damage include the nephrotic syndrome (in which large amounts of protein are lost in the urine and fluid collects in body tissues) and acute or chronic renal failure.

Congenital and Genetic Disorders. Congenital abnormalities of the kidneys are fairly common. In horseshoe kidney, the two kidneys are joined at their base. Some people are born with one kidney missing, both kidney on one side, or a kidney that is partially duplicated and gives rise to two ureters (duplex kidney). These conditions seldom cause problems. In rare cases, a baby is born with kidneys that are so underdeveloped that they are barely functional.

Polycystic disease of the kidneys is a serious inherited disorder in which multiple cysts develop on both kidneys. In Fanconi's syndrome and renal tubular acidosis (which are rare), there are subtle abnormalities in the functioning of the kidney tubules, so that certain substances are inappropriately lost in the urine.

Impaired Blood Supply. Various diseases may cause damage to, or lead to obstruction of, the small blood vessels within the kidneys, impairing blood flow. Diabetes mellitus and hemolytic-uremic syndrome are examples. In physiological shock, blood pressure and flow through the kidneys are seriously reduced; this can cause a type of damage known as acute tubular necrosis. The larger blood vessels in the kidney may be affected by periarteritis nodosa and systemic lupus erythematosus. In rare cases, there is a defect of the renal artery supplying a kidney, which may lead to hypertension and tissue damage.

Autoimmune Disorders. Glomerulonephritis refers to an important group of autoimmune disorders in which the glomerular filtering units of the kidneys become inflamed. It sometimes develops after infection with streptococcal bacteria.

Tumors. Benign kidney tumors are rare. They may cause hematuria (blood in the urine), although most cause no symptoms. Malignant tumors are also rare. Renal cell carcinoma, the most common type, occurs mostly in adults over 40; nephroblastoma (Wilms' tumor) affects mainly children under four.

Metabolic Disorders. Kidney stones are common in middle age. They are usually caused by excessive concentrations of various substances (such as calcium) or lack of inhibitors of crystallization in the urine. In hyperuricemia, there is a tendency for uric acid stones to form.

Infection. Infection of a kidney is called pyelonephritis. An important predisposing factor is obstruction of the flow of urine through the urinary tract, leading to stagnation and subsequent infection spreading up from the bladder. The cause of the obstruction may be a congenital defect of the kidney or ureter, a kidney, or ureteral stone, a bladder tumor, or, in a man, enlargement of the prostate gland.

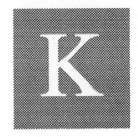

Drugs. Allergic reactions to certain drugs can cause an acute kidney disease, with most of the damage affecting the kidney tubules. Other drugs may directly damage the kidneys if taken in large amounts for prolonged periods. For example, renal failure can develop after many years of taking excessive amounts of analgesics. Some potent antibiotics can damage the kidney tubules, producing acute tubular necrosis.

Other Disorders. Hydronephrosis refers to a kidney swollen with urine as a result of obstruction further down the urinary tract. In the crush syndrome, kidney function is disrupted by proteins (released into the blood from severely damaged muscles) that block the filtering mechanisms.

Investigation. Kidney disorders are investigated by kidney imaging techniques such as ultrasound scanning, intravenous or retrograde pyelography, angiography, and CT scanning; by renal biopsy (removal of a small amount of tissue for analysis); by blood tests; and by kidney function tests, such as urinalysis.(ENC)

American Association of Kidney Patients
1 Davis Blvd., Ste LL1, Tampa, FL 33606
813/251-0725

American Kidney Fund
6110 Executive Blvd, Suite 1010
Rockville, MD 20852
800/638-8299
(in Maryland: 800/492-8361; in DC: 301/881-3052)

American Society of Nephrology
1101 Connecticut Ave, NW
Washington, DC 20036
202/857-1190

National Institute of Diabetes, Digestive and Kidney Disease
9000 Rockville Pike, Bethesda, MD 20892
301/496-3583

National Kidney Foundation
30 E. 33rd St., New York, NY 10016
212/889-2210, 800/622-9010

Renal Physicians Association
1101 Vermont Avenue, NW, Ste 500
Washington, DC 20005
202/898-1562

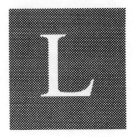

Language
American Speech-Language-Hearing Association
10801 Rockville Pike, Rockville, MD 20852
301/897-5700
800/638-8255 - for referrals

Laryngology
American Laryngological Association
203 Lathrop St., Ste 500, Pittsburgh, PA 15213
412/647-2110

American Laryngological, Rhinological and
Otological Society
(Also called: The Triological Society)
PO Box 155, Bethesda Church Road, East
Greenville, PA 18041
215/679-7180

Laser
American Society for Laser Medicine and Surgery
2404 Stewart Square, Wausau, WI 54401
715/845-9283

Laser argon photo coagulation
American Academy of Ophthalmology
415/561-8500

Legal Affairs
American Bar Association
750 N. Lake Shore Drive, Chicago, IL 60611
312/988-5000

Alabama State Bar
415 Dexter Ave, PO Box 671
Montgomery, AL 36101
205/269-1515

Alaska Bar Association
PO Box 100279, Anchorage, AL 99510
907/272-7469

State Bar of Arizona
363 N 1st Ave, Phoenix, AZ 85003-1580
602/252-4804

Arkansas Bar Association
Arkansas Bar Center
400 W Markham St, Little Rock, AK 72201
501/375-4605, 800/482-9406

The State Bar of California--Los Angeles
1230 W Third St, Los Angeles, CA 90017
213/482-8220

The State Bar of California--Sacramento
Suite 315, 1100 Eleventh St.
Sacramento, CA 95814
916/444-2762

The State Bar of California--San Francisco
555 Franklin St, San Francisco, CA 94102
415/561-8200

The Colorado Bar Association
Suite 950, 1900 Grant St, Denver, CO 80203-4309
303/860-1112, 800/332-6736

Connecticut Bar Association
101 Corporate Place, Rocky Hill, CT 06067
203/721-0025

Delaware State Bar Association
820 N French St, Wilmington, DE 19801
302/658-5278

The District of Columbia Bar
6th Floor, 1707 L St NW
Washington, DC 20036-4202
202/331-3883

The Florida Bar
650 Apalachee Parkway
Tallahassee, FL 32399-2300
904/861-3600

State Bar of Georgia
800 The Hurt Bldg, 50 Hurt Plaza
Atlanta, GA 30303
404/527-8700

Hawaii State Bar Association
PH-One, 1136 Union Mall, Honolulu, HI 96810
808/537-1868

Idaho State Bar
204 W State St, PO Box 895
Boise, ID 83701-0895
208/342-8956

Illinois State Bar Association
Illinois Bar Center, 424 S 2nd St.
Springfield, IL 62701
217/525-1760, 800/252-8908

Illinois State Bar Association--
Chicago Regional Office
Suite 900, 20 S Clark St, Chicago, IL 60603-1802
312/726-8775

Indiana State Bar Association
Indiana Bar Center, 230 E Ohio St.
Indianapolis, IN 46204
317/639-5465

Iowa State Bar Association
1101 Fleming Bldg, Des Moines, IA 50309-4098
515/243-3179

Kansas Bar Association
1200 Harrison St, PO Box 1037
Topeka, KS 66601-1037
913/234-5696

Kentucky Bar Association
Kentucky Bar Center
W Main at Kentucky River
Frankfort, KY 40601-1883
502/564-3795

Louisiana State Bar Association
601 Saint Charles Ave, New Orleans, LA 70130
504/566-1600

Maine State Bar Association
124 State St, PO Box 788
Augusta, ME 04332-0788
207/622-7523

Maryland State Bar Association, Inc
520 W Fayette St, Baltimore, MD 21201
410/685-7878

Massachusetts Bar Association
20 West St, Boston, MA 02111-1218
617/542-3602

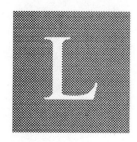

State Bar of Michigan
306 Townsend St, Lansing, MI 48933-2083
517/372-9030, Ext 3027

Minnesota State Bar Association
403 Minnesota Bar Center
430 Marquette Ave, Minneapolis, MN 55401
612/333-1183, 800/292-4152

Mississippi State Bar
PO Box 2168, Jackson, MS 39225-2168
601/948-4471

The Missouri Bar
The Missouri Bar Center
326 Monroe St, PO Box 119
Jefferson City, MO 65102
314/635-4128

State Bar of Montana
Suite 2A, 46 N Last Chance Gulch
PO Box 577, Helena, MT 59624-0577
406/442-7660

Nebraska State Bar Association
2nd Floor, 635 S 14th St, PO Box 81809
Lincoln, NE 68501-1809
402/475-7091

State Bar of Nevada
295 Holcomb Ave, Suite 2, Reno, NV 89502-1085
702/329-4100

New Hampshire Bar Association
112 Pleasant St, Concord, NH 03301
603/224-6942

The New Jersey State Bar Association
New Jersey Law Center
One Constitution Square
New Brunswick, NJ 08901-1500
908/249-5000

State Bar of New Mexico
121 Tijeras NE, Springer Square
PO Box 25883, Albuquerque, NM 87125
505/842-6132, 800/876-6227

New York State Bar Association
One Elk St, Albany, NY 12207
518/463-3200

The North Carolina State Bar
North Carolina State Bar Bldg
208 Fayetteville Street Mall, PO Box 25908,
Raleigh, NC 27611
919/828-4620

State Bar Association of North Dakota
Suite 101, 515 1/2 E Broadway, PO Box 2136,
Bismarck, ND 58502
701/255-1404, 800/472-2685

Ohio State Bar Association
33 W Eleventh Ave, Columbus, OH 43201
614/487-2050, 800/282-6556

Oklahoma Bar Association
1901 N Lincoln Blvd, PO Box 53036
State Capitol Station, Oklahoma City, OK 73152
405/524-2365, 800/522-8065

Oregon State Bar Association
5200 SW Meadows Road
PO Box 1689, Lake Oswego, OR 97035-0889
503/620-0222

Pennsylvania Bar Association
100 South St, PO Box 186, Harrisburg, PA 17108
717/238-6715

Rhode Island Bar Association
115 Cedar St, Providence, RI 02903
401/421-5740

South Carolina Bar
950 Taylor St, PO Box 608
Columbia, SC 29202-0608
803/799-6653

State Bar of South Dakota
222 E Capitol, Pierre, SD 57501
605/224-7554

Tennessee Bar Association
3622 West End Ave, Nashville, TN 37205
615/383-7421

State Bar of Texas
1414 Colorado, PO Box 12487
Capitol Station, Austin, TX 78711
512/463-1463

Utah State Bar
Utah Law & Justice Center
645 S 200 E, Salt Lake City, UT 84111
801/531-9077

Vermont Bar Association
PO Box 100, Montpelier, VT 05601
802/223-2020

Virginia State Bar
Suite 1000, Ross Bldg, 801 E Main St.
Richmond, VA 23219
804/786-2061

Washington State Bar Association
500 Westin Bldg, 2001 6th Ave.
Seattle, WA 98121-2599
206/448-0441

The West Virginia State Bar
State Capitol, Charleston, WV 25305
304/348-2456

State Bar of Wisconsin
402 W Wilson St, PO Box 7158
Madison, WI 53707-7158
608/257-3838

Wyoming State Bar
500 Randall Ave, PO Box 109
Cheyenne, WY 82003-0109
307/632-9061

American College of Legal Medicine
(persons with both law and medical degrees)
611 E. Wells St., Milwaukee, WI 53202
414/276-1881
800/433-9137

American Society of Law and Medicine
765 Commonwealth Ave., 16th Floor
Boston, MA 02215
617/262-4990

National Health Lawyers Association
1620 I St., NW, Suite 900, Washington, DC 20006
202/833-1100

Leprosy

American Leprosy Foundation
(Leonard Wood Memorial)
11600 Nebel St., Suite 210, Rockville, MD 20852
301/984-1336

American Leprosy Missions
One Broadway, Elmwood Park, NJ 07407
201/794-8650
800/543-3131

Leukemia

Leukemia Society of America, Inc.
733 Third Ave., New York, NY 10017
212/573-8484

National Leukemia Association
585 Stewart Ave., Ste. 536
Garden City, NY 11530
516/222-1944

Libraries, Medical Regional
National Network of Libraries of Medicine

The purpose of the National Network of Libraries of Medicine (NN/LM) is to provide health science practitioners, investigators, educators, and administrators in the United States with timely, convenient access to biomedical and health care information resources.

The Network is administered by the National Library of Medicine. It consists of eight Regional Medical Libraries (major institutions under contract with the National Library of Medicine), 131 Resource Libraries (primarily at Medical Schools), and some 3,300 Primary Access Libraries (primarily at hospitals). The Regional Medical Libraries administer and coordinate services in the Network's eight geographic regions.

New programs focus on reaching health professionals in rural, inner city, and other areas who do not have access to medical library resources. The goal is to make them aware of the services that Network libraries can provide. Other important Network programs include the interlibrary lending of more than two million journal articles, books and other published materials each year; reference services; training and consultation; and online access to MEDLINE and other databases made available by the National Library of Medicine.

Three of the Regional Medical Libraries have been designated Online Centers, to conduct National Library of Medicine online training classes and coordinate online services in several regions.

For general Network information contact the National Library of Medicine.

For more information about specific network programs in a region, call the appropriate Regional Medical Library at their direct dial or call 1-800-338-7657.

The following is a list of Regional Medical Libraries and the areas served by each.

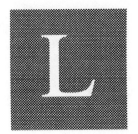

Middle Atlantic Region - Region 1
New York Academy of Medicine
2 East 103rd Street, New York, NY 10029
212-876-8763/FAX 212-534-7042

States served: DE, NJ, NY, PA
ONLINE Center for Regions 1,2 and 8

Southeastern/Atlantic Region - Region 2
University of Maryland at Baltimore
Health Science Library
111 South Greene Street,
Baltimore, MD 21201-1583
301-328-2855/FAX 301-328-0099

States served:
AL,FL,GA,MD,MS,NC,SC,TN,VA,WV, District of Columbia, Puerto Rico and the U.S. Virgin Islands

Greater Midwest Region - Region 3
University of Illinois at Chicago
Library of the Health Sciences
PO Box 7509, Chicago, IL 60680
312-996-2464/FAX 312-996-2226

States served: IA,IL,IN,KY,MI,MN,ND,OH,SD,WI

Midcontinental Region - Region 4
University of Nebraska Medical Center
Leon S. McGoogan Library of Medicine
600 South 42nd Street, Omaha, NB 68198-6706
402-559-4326/FAX 402-559-5498

States served: CO,KS,MO,NE,UT,WY
ONLINE Center for Regions 3, 4 and 5

South Central Region - Region 5
Houston Academy of Medicine-
Texas Medical Center Library
1133 M.D. Anderson Blvd, Houston, TX 77030
713-790-7053/FAX 713-790-7030

States served: AR,LA,NM,OK,TX

Pacific Northwest Region - Region 6
University of Washington
Health Sciences Center Library, SB-55
Seattle, WA 98195
206-543-8262/FAX 206-543-2469

States served: AK,IS,MT,OR,WA

Pacific Southwest Region - Region 7
University of California at Los Angeles
Louise Darling Biomedical Library
10833 Le Conte Ave.
Los Angeles, CA 90024-1798
310-825-1200/800-338-7657/FAX 310-825-5389

States served: AZ,CA,HA,NV, and U.S. Territories in the Pacific Basin
ONLINE Center for Regions 6 and 7

New England Region - Region 8
University of Connecticut Health Center
Lyman Maynard Stowe Library
263 Farmington Ave., Farmington, CT 06034-4003
203-679-4500/FAX 203-679-4046

States served: CT,ME,MA,NH,RI,VT

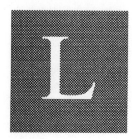

Resource Libraries by Region

Region 1

New Jersey
University of Medicine and Dentistry of New Jersey
George F. Smith Library of the Health Sciences
30 12th Ave., Newark, NJ 07103-2706
201-456-4358

New York
Columbia University Libraries
Butler Library, Room 313
535 W. 114th St., New York, NY 10027
212-305-3692

State University of New York at Buffalo
University Libraries
433 Capen Hall, Buffalo, NY 14260
716-831-3900

SUNY Health Science Center at Syracuse, Health
Science Library
766 Irving Ave., Syracuse, NY 13210
315-464-4581

New York Academy of Medicine Library
Two E. 103rd St., New York, NY 10029-5293
212-876-0375 (for librarians)
212-876-8200 ex. 321 (for general)

Pennsylvania
University of Pennsylvania
Biomedical Library/Johnson Pavillion
36th and Hamilton Walk, Philadelphia, PA
19104-6060
215-898-5817

University of Pittsburgh
Maurice and Laura Falk Library
of the Health Sciences
Scaife Hall, Second Floor, Pittsburg, PA 15261
412-648-8824

Region 2

Alabama
University of Alabama at Birmingham
Lister Hill Library of the Health Sciences
UAB Station, Birmingham, AL 35294
250/934-5460

University of South Alabama Biomedical Library
Mobile, AL 36688
205-460-7043

District of Columbia
George Washington University Medical Center
Himmelfarb Health Sciences Library
2300 Eye St., NW, Washington, DC 20037
202-994-3528

Howard University, Health Sciences Library
PO Box 553, Washington, DC 20059
202-806-6433

Georgetown University Medical Center Dahlgren
Memorial Library
3900 Reservoir Rd., NW
Washington, DC 20007
202-687-1187

Florida
University of South Florida, Health Sciences
Center Library
12901 Bruce B. Downs Blvd.
Tampa, FL 33612-4799
813-974-2399

University of Florida,
Health Sciences Center Library
Box J-206, JHMHC, Gainsville, FL 32610-0206
904-392-4016

University of Miami School Library
Louis Calder Memorial Library
PO Box 016950, Miami, FL 33101
305-547-6441

Georgia
Emory University, Health Sciences Center Library
1462 Clifton Rd., NE, Atlanta, GA 30322
404-727-5820

Medical College of Georgia
Robert B. Greenblatt, M.D. Library
Augusta, GA 30912-4400
404-721-3441

Morehouse School of Medicine Multi-Media Center
720 Westview Dr. SW, Atlanta, GA 30310-1495
404-752-1531

Mercer University School of Medicine
Medical Library, Macon, GA, 31207
912-752-2515

Maryland
University of Maryland at Baltimore
Health Sciences Library
111 S. Greene St., Baltimore, MD 21201
410-328-7545

William H. Welch Medical Library
1900 E. Monument St., Baltimore, MD 21205-2113
410-955-2702

Mississippi
University of Mississippi Medical Center
Rowland Medical Library
2500 North State St., Jackson, MS 39216-4505
601-984-1290

North Carolina
Bowman Gray School of Medicine
Wake Forest University, Coy C. Carpenter Library
Medical Center Blvd.
Winston-Salem, NC 27157-1069
919-684-2092

Duke University Medical Center Library
S.G. Mudd Building
Box 3702 Medical Center
Durham, NC 27710-3702
919-684-2092

University of North Carolina at Chapel Hill
Health Sciences Library, CB# 7585
Chapel Hill, NC 27599-7585
919-966-2111

East Carolina University Health Sciences Library
Brody Medical Sciences Building
Greenville, NC 27858-4354
919-551-2212

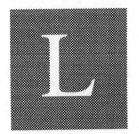

Puerto Rico
University of Puerto Rico,
Medical Sciences Campus Library
G.PO Box 5067
San Juan, PR 00936
809-758-8199

South Carolina
Medical University of South Carolina Library
171 Ashley Ave., Charleston, SC 29425-3001
803-792-2374

University of South Carolina
School of Medicine Library
Columbia, SC 29208
803-733-3344

Tennessee
East Tennessee State University
Department of Learning Resources
Medical Library
PO Box 23290A, Johnson City, TN 37614
615-929-6252

Meharry Medical College Library
1005 D.B. Todd Blvd., Nashville, TN 37208-3599
615-327-6728

University of Tennessee, Memphis,
Health Sciences Library
877 Madison Ave., Memphis, TN 38163
901-528-5638

Vanderbilt University Medical Center Library
Nashville, TN 37232-2340
615-322-2299

Virginia
Eastern Virginia Medical School,
Moorman Memorial Library
PO Box 1980, Norfolk, VA 23501
804-446-5841

Virginia Commonwealth University,
Tomkins-McCaw Library
Box 582, 509 N. 12th St.
Richmond, VA 23298-0582

Unversity of Virginia,
Claude Moore Health Sciences Library
Box 234, UVA Health Sciences Center
Charlottesville, VA 22908
804-924-5464

West Virginia
West Virginia University Health Sciences Library
Basic Sciences Building, Morgantown, WV 26506
304-293-3832

Region 3
note: interlibrary loan (InterLibrary Loan) number
is a library contact ONLY.

Illinois
American Dental Association
Bureau of Library Services
211 E. Chicago Ave, Chicago, IL 60611
312-440-2642
312-440-2653 (InterLibrary Loan)

Chicago College of Osteopathic Medicine,
Alumni Memorial Library
555 W. 31st St., Downers Grove, IL 60515
708-5156185/FAX 708-515-6195
708-515-6176 (InterLibrary Loan)

John Crerar Library of the University of Chicago
5730 S. Ellis, Chicago, IL 60637
312-702-7715/FAX 312-702-3022
312-702-7031 (InterLibrary Loan)

Loyola University of Chicago,
Loyola Medical Center Library
2160 S. First Ave., Maywood, IL 60153
708-216-9192 (InterLibrary Loan)

Northwestern University
Galter Health Sciences Library
303 E. Chicago Ave., Chicago, IL 60611
312-503-8133/FAX 312-908-8028
312-503-1908 (InterLibrary Loan)

Southern Illinois University School
of Medicine Library
801 N. Rutledge St.
PO Box 19231, Springfield, IL 62708
217-782-2658/FAX 217-782-7503
217-782-2658/217-785-2124 (InterLibrary Loan)

University of the Health Sciences Library,
Chicago Medical School
3333 Green Bay Rd., North Chicago, IL
708-578-3242/FAX 708-578-3401
708-578-3000 ex.648 (InterLibrary Loan)

University of Illinois at Chicago
Library of the Health Sciences
PO Box 7509, Chicago, IL 60680
312-996-8974/FAX 312-996-1899
312-996-8991 (InterLibrary Loan)

Indiana
Indiana University, Ruth Lilly Library
975 W. Walnut St., Indianapolis, IN 46202-5121
317-274-7182/FAX 317-274-2088
317-274-7184 (InterLibrary Loan)

Iowa
University of Iowa,
Hardin Library for the Health Sciences
Iowa City, IA 52242
319-335-9871/FAX 319-335-9897
319-335-9874 (InterLibrary Loan)

Kentucky
University of Kentucky, Medical Center Library
800 Rose St., Lexington, KY 40536-0084
606-233-5726/FAX 606-258-1040
606-233-6514 (InterLibrary Loan)

University of Louisville
Kornhauser Health Sciences Library
Lexington, KY 40292
502-588-5771
502-588-5769 (InterLibrary Loan)

Michigan
Michigan State University Library
East Lansing, MI 48824-1048
517-355-2344/FAX 517-353-9806
517-355-7641 (InterLibrary Loan)

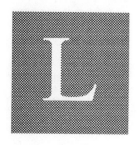

University of Michigan
Alfred Taubman Medical Library
1135 E. Catherine St., Ann Arbor, MI 48109-0726
313-764-1210/FAX 313-763-1473
313-763-6407 (InterLibrary Loan)

Wayne State University, Shiffman Medical Library
4325 Brush St., Detroit, MI 48201
313-577-1088/FAX 313-577-0706
313-577-1100 (InterLibrary Loan)

Minnesota
Mayo Foundation Medical Library
200 First St., SW, Rochester, MN 55905
507-284-2061/FAX 507-284-2215
507-284-2042 (InterLibrary Loan)

University of Minnesota, Bio-Medical Library
Diehl Hall, 505 Essex St. SE
Minneapolis, MN 55455
612-626-0998/FAX 612-626-3824
612-626-2969 (InterLibrary Loan)

University of Minnesota, Duluth
Health Sciences Library
215 Health Science Library
Ten University Dr., Duluth, MN 55812
218-726-8587/FAX 218-726-6205
218-726-8585/8589 (InterLibrary Loan)

North Dakota
University of North Dakota
Harley E. French Library of the Health Sciences
Grand Forks, ND 58202-9002
701-777-3993/FAX 701-772-0405
701-777-2606 (InterLibrary Loan)

Ohio
Cleveland Health Sciences Library
11000 Euclid Ave., Cleveland, OH 44106
216-368-6420/3644 (InterLibrary Loan)

Medical College of Ohio at Toledo
Raymond H. Mulford Library 3000 Arlington Ave.
PO Box 10008, Toledo, OH 43699-0008
419-381-4223/FAX 419-382-8842
419-381-4215/3406 (InterLibrary Loan)

Northeastern Ohio University College of Medicine
Oliver Ocasek Regional Medical
Information Center
4209 SR 44, PO Box 95, Rootstown, OH 44272
216-325-2511/FAX 216-325-0522
216-325-2511, ext 530 (InterLibrary Loan)

Ohio State University
John A. Prior Health Sciences Library
376 W. 10th Ave., Columbus, OH 43210-1240
614-292-4851/FAX 614-292-5717
614-292-4894 (InterLibrary Loan)

Ohio University Alden Health Science Library
Athens, OH 45701-2978
614-593-2680/FAX 614-593-4693
614-593-2690/2691 (LL)

State Library of Ohio
65 South Front St., Columbus, OH 432266-0334
614-644-7061/FAX 614-466-3584
614-644-6956 (InterLibrary Loan)

University of Cincinnati, Health Sciences Library
231 Bethesda Ave., Cincinnati, OH 45267-0574
513-558-5627
513-558-4637 (InterLibrary Loan)

Wright State University
Fordham Health Sciences Library
PO Box 927
Dayton, OH 45410-0927
513-873-2266/FAX 513-879-2675
513-873-4110 (InterLibrary Loan)

South Dakota
University of South Dakota
Lommen Health Sciences Library
School of Medicine, Vermillon, SD 57069-2390
605-677-5347/FAX 605-677-5124

Wisconsin
Medical College of Wisconsin Libraries
8701 Watertown Plank Rd., Milwaukee, WI 53226
414-257-8249
414-257-8460 (InterLibrary Loan)

University of Wisconsin
Center for Health Science Libraries
1305 Linden Dr., Madison, WI 53706
608-262-2371
608-262-6524 (InterLibrary Loan)

Region 4

Colorado
Denison Memorial Library
University of Colorado Health Science Center
4200 East Ninth Ave., Denver, CO 80262
303-270-5125/FAX 303-270-7227

Kansas
The Archie R. Dykes Library
of the Health Sciences
University of Kansas Medical Center
2100 West 39th St., Kansas City, KS 66103
913-588-7166/1-800-332-4193 (KS only)/FAX
913-588-7304

Missouri
J. Otto Lottes Health Sciences Library
University of Missouri-Columbia
Health Sciences Center, Columbia, MO 65212
314-882-6141/FAX 314-882-5574

Washington University School of Medicine Library
660 South Euclid Ave., St. Louis, MO 63110
314-362-7081/FAX 314-362-9862

St. Louis University Medical Center Library
1401 South Grand Blvd., St. Louis MO 63104
314-577-8607/FAX 314-772-1307

Nebraska
Creighton University Health Sciences Library
2500 California Ave., Omaha, NE 68178
402-280-5108/FAX 402-280-5134

McGoogan Library of Medicine
University of Nebraska Medical Center
600 S. 42nd St., Omaha, NE 68198-6705
402-559-6221/FAX 402-559-5498

Utah
Spenser S. Eccles Health Sciences Library
University of Utah, Salt Lake City, UT 84112
801-581-8771/FAX 801-581-3632

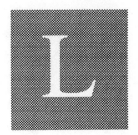

Wyoming
Science and Technology Library
University of Wyoming
University Station Box 3262
Laramie, WY 82071
307-766-6203/FAX 307-766-3611

Region 5

Arkansas
University of Arkansas for Medical Sciences
Library - Slot 586
4301 West Markham Ave., Little Rock, AR 77205
501-686-5980/FAX 501-686-6745

Louisiana
Louisiana State University - Medical Center Library
433 Bolivar St., New Orleans, LA 70112-2882
504-568-6100/FAX 504-568-7720

Louisiana State University - Medical Center Library
PO Box 33932, Shreveport, LA 71130
318-674-5445/FAX 318-674-5442

Tulane Medical Center
Rudolph Matas Medical Library
1430 Tulane Ave., New Orleans, LA 70112
504-588-5155/FAX 504-587-7417

New Mexico
University of New Mexico Medical Center Library
North Campus, Albuquerque, NM 87131
505-277-2311/FAX 505-277-5350

Oklahoma
Oklahoma College of Osetopathic Medicine and
Surgery - Medical Library
1111 W. 17th St., Tulsa, OK 74107
918-582-1972/FAX 918-582-6316

University of Oklahoma College of Medicine,
Tulsa, Library
2808 South Sheridan, Tulsa, OK 74129
918-582-1972/FAX 918-582-6316

University of Oklahoma Health Science Center
Robert M. Bird Health Sciences Library
PO Box 26901, Oklahoma City, OK 73190
405-271-2285/FAX 405-271-3297

Texas
Texas A&M University
Medical Sciences Library
College Station, TX 77843
409-845-7427/FAX 409-845-7493

University of Texas Health Sciences Center at
San Antonio
Dolph Brisco Library
7703 Floyd Curl Drive, San Antonio, TX 78284
512-567-2400/FAX 512-567-2490

Texas College of Osteopathic Medicine
Health Sciences Library
3500 Camp Bowie, Fort Worth, TX 76107
817-735-2380/FAX 817-735-2283

University of Texas Medical Branch Moody
Medical Library
Ninth and Market Street
Galveston, TX 77555-1035
409-772-2371/FAX 409-765-9852

Houston Academy of Medicine
Texas Medical Center Library
1133 M.D. Anderson Blvd., Houston, TX 77030
713-795-4200/FAX 713-790-7052

University of Texas Southwestern Medical Center
at Dallas - Library
5323 Harry Hines Blvd., Dallas, TX 75235-9049
214-688-3368/FAX 214-688-3277

Texas Tech University Health Sciences Center
Library of the Health Sciences
3601 4th St., Lubbock, TX 79430
806-743-2203/FAX 806-743-2218

Region 6

Oregon Health Science University Library
3181 SW Sam Jackson Park Road
PO Box 573, Portland, OR 97207-0573
503-494-8026/FAX 503-494-5241

Region 7

Arizona
University of Arizona,
Arizona Health Sciences Center Library
1501 N. Campbell Ave., 1501 N. Campbell Ave.,
Tucson, AZ 85724
602-626-2831/FAX 602-626-2831

California
University of California, Davis,
Carlson Health Sciences Library
Davis, CA 95616
916-752-1214/FAX 916-752-4718

University of California, Irvine, Biomedical Library
PO Box 19556, Irvine, CA 92712
714-856-5212/FAX 714-856-8095

University of California, San Diego
Biomedical Library C-075B
La Jolla, CA 92093
619/534-3253/FAX 619-534-3308

Loma Linda University
Del E. Webb Memorial Library
Anderson and University Streets
Loma Linda, CA 92350
714-824-4581/FAX 714-824-4188

University of Southern California
Norris Medical Library
2003 Zonal Ave., Los Angeles, CA 90033
213-342-1116/FAX 213-221-1235

University of Southern California
Dental Library; DEN 201
University Park-MC 0641
Los Angeles, CA 90089-0641
213-740-6476/Fax 213-748-8565

University of California, Irvine
Medical Center Library
101 City Drive South, Orange, CA 92668
714/456-5585

University of California, Davis
Medical Center Library
4301 X Street, Room 1005
Sacramento, CA 95817
916-734-3529/FAX 916-734-7418

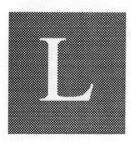

University of California, San Diego
Medical Center Library
225 Dickinson St., San Diego, CA 92103
619/543-6520

University of California, San Francisco Library
513 Parnassus Ave., Ste. 257
San Francisco, CA 94143-0840
415/476-8293/FAX 415/476-7946

Stanford University Medical Center
Lane Medical Library
Stanford, CA 94305-5323
415-723-6831/FAX 415-725-7471

Hawaii
Hawaii Medical Library
1221 Punchbowl St., Honolulu, HI 96813
808-536-9302/FAX 808-524-6956

Nevada
University of Nevada-Reno, Savitt Medical Library
School of Medicine, Reno, NV 89557-0046
702-784-6533/FAX 702-784-4529

Region 8

Connecticut
University of Connecticut Health Center
Lyman Maynard Stowe Library
PO Box 4003, Farmington, CT 06034-4003
203-679-2547/FAX 203-679-4046

Yale University
Harvey Cushing/John Hay Whitney Medical Library
333 Cedar Street, PO Box 3333
New Haven, CT 06510
203-785-5352/FAX203-785-4369

Maine
Veteran's Administration Medical Center Learning
Resource Service
Togus, ME 04330
207-623-8411 x5625/FAX 207-623-5766

Massachusetts
Boston College O'Neill Library
O'Neill 410, Chestnut Hill, MA 02167
617-552-4489/FAX 617-552-2600

Boston University School of Medicine Alumni
Medical Library
80 E. Concord St., L-12, Boston, MA 02118
617-638-4230/FAX 617-638-4233

Harvard Medical School
The Francis A. Countway Library of Medicine
10 Shattuck St., Boston, MA 02115
617-432-2142/FAX 617-432-0693

Massachusetts College of Pharmacy and Allied
Health Sciences
Sheppard Library
179 Longwood Ave., Boston, MA 02115
617-732-2808/FAX 617-278-1566

Tufts University Health Sciences Library
145 Harrison Ave., Boston, MA 02111
617-956-6708/FAX 617-350-8039

University of Massachusetts Medical Center
Lamar Soutter Medical School Library
55 Lake Avenue North, Worcester, MA 01655
508-856-2206/FAX 508-856-5899

New Hampshire
Dartmouth College Dana Biomedical Library
Hanover, NH 03755
603-650-1622/FAX 603-650-1354

Rhode Island
Brown University Sciences Library
Box I, Providence, RI 02912
401-863-3334/FAX401-863-2753

Vermont
University of Vermont
Charles A. Dana Medical Library
Health Science Complex, Burlington, VT 05405
802-656-2200/FAX 802-863-1136

Libraries, National

National Agricultural Library
Agriculture Department
10301 Baltimore Blvd., Beltsville, MD 20705
301/504-5719

National Library of Medicine

The Library, which serves as the Nation's chief
medical information source, is authorized to
provide medical library services and on-line
bibliographic searching capabilities, such as
MEDLINE, TOXLINE, and others, to public and
private agencies and organizations, institutions,
and individuals. It is responsible for the
development and management of a Biomedical
Communications Network, applying advanced
technology to the improvement of biomedical
communications, and operates a computer-based
toxicology information system for the scientific
community, industry, and other Federal agencies.
Through its National Center for Biotechnology
Information, the Library has a leadership role in
development new information technologies to aid
in the understanding of the molecular processes
that control health and disease. In addition, the
Library acquires and makes available for
distribution audiovisual instruction material, and
develops prototype audiovisual communication
programs for the health educational community.
Through grants and contracts, the Library
administers programs of assistance to the Nation's
medical libraries that include support of a Regional
Medical Library network, research in the field of
medical library science, establishment and
improvement of the basic library resources, and
supporting biomedical scientific publications of a
nonprofit nature. (USG).

National Library of Medicine
8600 Rockville Pike, Bethesda, MD 20894
General Information 301/496-6095
MEDLINE 800/638-8480

United States Library of Congress
101 Independence Ave, SE
Washington, DC 20540
202/287-5000
For information on tours, exhibits 800/334-4465

Library Associations

Billings, John Shaw (1840?-1913)
JAMA. 1913 March 15; 60(11): 846

John Shaw Billings, M.D. lieutenant-colonel U.S. Army, retired. Curator of the Army Medical Museum and Library for many years, the Index Catalogue of which will stand as a lasting monument to his industry and genius; died in the New York Hospital, March 11, from pneumonia, aged 73.

He was born in Switzerland County, Ind., and was graduated from the Medical College of Ohio, Cincinnati, in 1860. He also has had conferred on him the honorary degree of LL.D. the University of Munich in 1889 and by Dublin University in 1892 and the degree of D.C.L. by the University of Oxford in 1889.

After serving for a year as demonstrator in anatomy in his alma mater, he entered the United States Army as assistant surgeon, April 16, 1862; was made captain and assistant surgeon four years later; after 10 years was promoted to major and surgeon, and June 6, 1894, was made lieutenant-colonel and deputy surgeon-general and was retired from the Army at his own request, after more than thirty years service, Oct. 1, 1895. In 1869 he was ordered to the Surgeon-General's office, Washington, where he had charge of the organization of the Veteran Reserve Corps; of matters pertaining to contract surgeons and of all property and disbursing accounts until 1885, when he was placed in charge of the Library of the Surgeon-General's office, serving in this capacity until 1893, when he was appointed curator of the Army Medical Museum and Library. He was placed in charge of the division of vital and social statistics of the tenth and eleventh censuses. In 1870 Dr. Billings was engaged in the reorganization of the United States Marine Hospital Service and from 1879 to 1882 served as vice-president of the National Board of Health.

His contributions to the medical literature were numerous and varied, the best known being the Index Catalogue of the Library of the Surgeon-General's Office and the National Medical Dictionary. He was professor of hygiene in the University of Pennsylvania and director of its laboratory of hygiene from 1893 to 1896, when he accepted the directorship of the New York Public Library, Astor, Lenox and Tilden Foundations, holding this position until his death.

Dr. Billings survived his co-worker, Dr. Robert Fletcher, by only four months. His work as an administrative officer and as a bibliographer is unique in the history of American medicine.

Keeping Up With the Literature

by Howard J. Bennett, MD "A Piece of My Mind"
JAMA.1992 Feb. 19;267(7):920

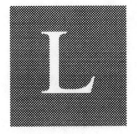

When I began my medical education almost 20 years ago, I had no idea what a medical article was. In those days I was a textbook man - a rather plodding fellow who liked his information organized, summarized, and neatly packaged between the covers of a book. The first time I actually saw an article I was sitting in pathology lab looking at a slide of my own blood. In between glances at neutrophils and lymphocytes, my lab partner handed me a copy of an article from a pediatric journal. "What's this?" I asked, glad for the chance to talk to a multicellular organism. "It's an article on CBCs," he said. "Did you know there's a shift to the right with viral infections?" "No," I said rather sheepishly. The only shifting I knew about was shifting dullness, and I had only learned about that the week before. Nevertheless, since ignorance is something medical students learn to live with, I leaned forward with my best "I'm really interested in this" face. "What else does it say?" I queried. "A lot," he said. "I'll copy it for you after class." At which point we went back to looking at doughnut -shaped RBCs, platelets, and the like.

I still remember how excited I was after class. Wow! I thought. So this is what the medical literature is all about. Copying articles and reading stuff that's so new it hasn't made it into the textbooks yet. When we got to the library, I actually felt taller, as though I had traversed some major evolutionary step in an instant. Little did I know, however, that one day I would look back on this afternoon with a somewhat different perspective.

The problem, I learned, is that it is impossible to keep up with the medical literature. This is not the fault of the medical literature itself, but rather of those individuals who keep adding to it as though it were an endangered species. Unfortunately, while most of us cannot keep up with our reading, we all know people who say they can. But is this really true? Are there people out there who do not need to eat or sleep? People who never need to change diapers, attend ballet recitals, or plant azaleas? People who take their journals with them wherever they go?

To settle this issue, I spent the last few years examining the reading habits of all the physicians I know. What I found out is that few physicians actually go to bed with their journals at night (this was a comforting observation). I also discovered that physicians go through stages in their reading just like other areas of development. And, as we all know, the important thing about developmental stages is finding out whether you are reaching your milestones. Therefore, I have compiled the information I collected into a Table for your review. If your reading habits are in sync with the listed categories, you can relax and should no longer feel guilty when you pick up a beer instead of a medical journal. (Remember, older golfers don't hit in the 70s anymore, so why should you?) On the other hand, if you don't "fit" anywhere on the Table, perhaps now is the time to take a sabbatical and open up that restaurant you've been talking about all these years.

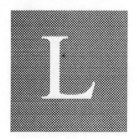

Howard J. Bennett's Classification for Reading Medical Articles

- Medical Student: Reads entire article but does not understand what any of it means.
- Intern: Uses journal as a pillow during nights on call.
- Resident: Would like to read entire article but eats dinner instead.
- Chief resident: Skips article entirely and reads the classifieds.
- Junior attending: Reads and analyzes entire article in order to pimp medical students.
- Senior attending: Reads abstracts and quotes the literature liberally.
- Research attending: Reads entire article, reanalyzes statistics, and looks up all references, usually in lieu of sex.
- Chief of service: Reads references to see if he was cited anywhere.
- Private attending: Doesn't buy journals in the first place but keeps an eye open for medical articles that make it into *TIME* or *Newsweek*.
- Emeritus attending: Reads entire article but doesn't understand what any of it means.

American Library Association
Public Library Association (c/o)
50 E. Huron Street, Chicago, IL 60611
312/944-6780

Medical Library Association
6 N. Michigan Ave, Ste. 300, Chicago, IL 60602
312/419-9094

Special Libraries Association
1700 18th St., NW, Washington, D.C. 20009
202/234-4700

Licensure
Licensing: What Doctors Should Know

Douglas N. Cerf

An increasing public awareness and demand for protection, coupled with the growth in the number and sophistication of fraudulent practitioners over the past 10 years, has resulted in stronger and more complex state licensing boards and licensing statutes throughout the country. As might be expected, the rate of change differs widely among the states' licensing boards, depending on each state's resources and Medical Practice Acts as well as on legislative, media, and public expectations. All states, however, have improved dramatically over the decade and will continue to improve, although at different rates.

Within this context, a physician seeking licensure for the first time or in another state should anticipate the possibility or necessary delays for investigation of credentials and past practice, as well as the need to comply with increasingly stringent licensing standards. To assist a physician in the quest for licensure, a rough set of ground rules is provided below. These suggestions, obviously will not apply in all cases but generally will help most physicians applying for licensure, as well as benefit the licensing board of the state in which the physician wishes to practice. The ground rules are as follows:

1. When contacting a licensing board for the first time, ask how long it takes to process applications and for a copy of its current licensing requirements. This will provide the physician with a solid idea of when to close an existing practice and/or plan a move, as well as with information about the potential problem areas to be addressed in completing an application.

2. At the initial contact in writing, the physician should provide the licensing board with a resume or curriculum vitae. This will allow a licensing board to evaluate potential problem areas early in the process. In short, the initial contact should be used to develop a set of reasonable expectations about the duration and complexity of the licensing process in a state. A physician who fails to develop appropriate expectations will likely end up frustrated with the licensing process. More important; unreasonable expectations can result in financial jeopardy due to the premature closing of a practice or failure to meet a starting date with an employer in the new state.

3. A physician should never try to hide derogatory information from a licensing board. It is much better to come forward with the information, assist the board in obtaining records and other necessary data, and present the reasons why the situation should not result in the denial of the license. Full and frank disclosure of all information requested is by far the best approach to being successfully licensed. A physician should remember that in most states, making a false statement on a license application is grounds for denial or future restriction.

4. A physician who is actively involved in the licensing process often can shorten the length of time it takes to get licensed. Personally contacting the medical schools, training programs, and appropriate hospitals and then following up will motivate these institutions to more expeditiously verify credentials. Following up with the licensing boards in other states where the physician holds or has held a license also may assist in shortening the time for licensure. It is important to note that there is a difference between follow up and overutilization of phone contact, which often delays the processing of requested verification materials, since the physician's application or request may need to be pulled from the "stack" to answer an inquiry. A short note to the organization processing the request for information thirty days after the initial letter or form was mailed may be a better course to follow than frequent phone contact.

5. A physician should not confuse reciprocity with endorsement. In medical licensing, reciprocity has largely become a thing of the past, as most states' legislatures wish to establish their own eligibility criteria and require licensure from a credentialing process based upon original documents or direct contact with educational training or licensing boards. Endorsement of the licensing examination scores of another state is really the only form of reciprocity left in medical licensing, and even it has mutated to the point that it can hardly be called endorsement. A physician should be prepared to engage in the gathering and submission of original documents.

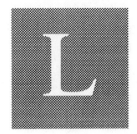

6. A wise physician will exercise patience and courtesy in the licensing process. State licensing boards, in most cases, do the best job possible with the resources provided them. The staffs of licensing boards are there to do the best possible job of protecting the public. This requires taking the time necessary to fairly evaluate each application for licensure.

Since this article was originally written for the 1988 Edition of U.S. Medical Licensure Statistics and Current Licensure Requirements, many innovative changes have occurred to increase cooperation among national and state agencies to expedite the processing of licensure applications. The first effort worth recognizing is the AMA's National Physician Credentials Verification Service, or AMA/NCVS, which will contain source-verified credential on a physician's medical school, graduation, postgraduate training, and other data necessary for licensure and hospital credentialing. Benefits to the physician who is an AMA/NCVS subscriber include time savings (no starting from scratch on each application) and convenience (assurance that an accurate record of his/her credentials is available whenever needed).

Some states will use this service as the primary source for licensure, while others will use it as a check-off procedure to assist that all organizations are contacted for information. Either way, the net result will be a swing toward one-step credentials verification not only for licensure but for hospital privileges and obtainment of malpractice insurance.

Organizations such as the Federation of State Medical Boards of the United States, the American Medical Association, the National Board of Medical Examiners, the Educational Commission for Foreign Medical Graduates, and the state medical boards are taking steps toward technological advances with data transmission in order to expedite the sharing of data. Ultimately, this will further reduce delays in processing credentials.

Each of these organizations will allow the quick and necessary exchange of information necessary to determine whether physicians meet licensing standards for licensure in participating states.

Both physicians and state licensing boards will soon be able to benefit from a less restrictive flow of data that, in the past, relied on completing similar forms each time a new license or a change in hospital privileges was pursued.

Finally, physicians willing to inform themselves and work cooperatively with a licensing board need not find licensing an unpleasant experience. Members of the medical profession should never forget that the business of licensing boards is to protect the public from unprofessional and incompetent physicians. However licensing boards also strive to ensure a process that protects the legal rights and privileges of physicians. While maintaining this balance often appears bureaucratic and cumbersome, the end result is improved health care for the people of our country.(LIC)

Federation of State Medical Boards
of the United States, Inc.
6000 Western Place/Suite 707
Ft. Worth, TX 76107
817/735-8445

National Board of Medical Examiners
3930 Chestnut St., Philadelphia, PA 19104
215/590-9500

National Clearinghouse on Licensure,
Enforcement and Regulation
Council of State Governments
Ironworks Pike, PO Box 11910
Lexington, KY 40578
606/231-1939

US Medical Licensure Statistics and Current Licensure Requirements Chicago, American Medical Association, 1993. ISBN 0-89970-544-8 OP399091

Licensure, State

Alabama: Mr. Larry D. Dixon, Exec. Dir.
Alabama State Board of Medical Examiners
PO Box 946, Montgomery, AL 36102-0946
205/242-4116

Alaska: Pam Ventgen, CMA Exec. Secy.
Alaska State Medical Board,
3601 C. Street, #722, Anchorage, AK 99503
907/561-2878

Arizona: Mr. Douglas N. Cerf, Exec. Dir.
Arizona Board of Medical Examiners
2001 W. Camelback Rd., Suite 300
Phoenix, AZ 85015
602/255-3751

Arkansas: Joe Verser, MD, Secy. Treasurer
Arkansas State Medical Board
PO Box 102, Harrisburg, AR 72432-0102
501/578-2448

California: Mr. Kenneth Wagstaff, Exec. Dir.
Medical Board of California
1430 Howe Ave., Sacramento, CA 95825
916/920-6411

Canal Zone:
Previous holders of a Canal Zone license may obtain information concerning their license from:
Office of Health and Safety,
Panama Canal Commission
APO Miami, FL 34011

Colorado: Mr. Thomas J. Beckett, Program Administrator
Board of Medical Examiners,
1525 Sherman St., Rm. 132
Denver, CO 80203-1750
303/866-2468

Connecticut: Joseph Gillen, Section Chief
Connecticut Division of Medical Quality Assurance
150 Washington St, Hartford, CT 06106
203/566-7398

Delaware: Ms. Rosemarie S. Vanderhoogt, Admin. Officer
Delaware Board of Medical Practice, O'Neil Bldg.,
PO Box 1401, Dover, DE 19903
302/736-4522

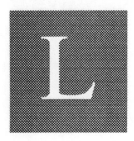

District of Columbia: Mr. John P. Hopkins, Exec. Dir.
District of Columbia Board of Medicine
605 G. Street, S.W., Room 202-Lower Level, Washington, DC 20001
202/727-9794

Florida: Mrs. Dorothy Faircloth, Exec. Dir.
Florida Board of Medical Examiners
1940 N. Monroe St., Suite 110
Tallahassee, FL 32399-0450
904/488-0595

Georgia: Andrew Watry, Exec. Dir.
Composite State Board of Medical Examiners
166 Pryor St., SW, Atlanta, GA 30303
404/656-3913

Guam: Ms. Tina T. Blas, RN, Administrator
Guam Board of Medical Examiners
Department of Public Health and Social Services
PO Box 2816, Agana, Guam 96910
671/734-2951

Hawaii: Mr. John Tamashiro,
Board of Medical Examiners
PO Box 3469, Honolulu, HI 96801
808/548-4392

Idaho: Mr. Donald L. Deleski, Exec. Dir.,
State Board of Medicine
280 N. 8th St, Suite 202, Boise, ID 83720
208/334-2822

Illinois: Nikki Sollar, Dir.
Department of Professional Regulation
320 W. Washington, 3rd Floor
Springfield, IL 62786
217/785-0820

Indiana: Mr. Patrick J. Turner, Exec. Dir.
Indiana Health Professions Services Bureau
One American Square, Suite 1020, Box 82067
Indianapolis, IN 46282
317/232-2960

Iowa: Mr. William S. Vanderpool, Exec. Dir.
Board of Medical Examiners
State Capitol Complex, Executive Hills West,
1209 E. Court Avenue
Des Moines, IA 50319-0075
515/281-5171

Kansas: Ms. Susan Lambrecht
Licensing Supervisor
Board of Healing Arts
900 SW Jackson, Suite 553
Topeka, KS 66612-1256
913/296-7413

Kentucky: Mr. C. Wm. Schmidt, Exec. Dir.
Kentucky Board of Medical Licensure
310 Whittington Parkway, Suite 1B
Louisville, KY 40222
502/429-8046

Louisiana: Ms. Paula M. Mensen
Ad. Services Asst.
Louisiana State Board of Medical Examiners
830 Union St., Suite 100
New Orleans, LA 70112-1499
504/524-6763

Maine: Mr. David R. Hedrick, Exec. Dir.
Maine Board of Registration and Medicine
State House Station #137, Augusta, ME 04333
207/289-3601

Maryland: Mr. J. Michael Compton, Exec. Dir.
Maryland Board of Physician Quality Assurance
4201 Patterson Ave., 3rd Floor
Baltimore, MD 21215
301/764-4777

Massachusetts: Ms. Barbara Neuman, Exec. Dir.
Massachusetts Board of Registration and
Discipline in Medicine
10 West Street, Boston, MA 02111
617/727-3086; 617/727-3087

Michigan: Ms. Marcia Malouin,
Licensing Supervisor
Michigan Board of Medicine,
Bureau of Health Services
611 W. Ottawa St., PO Box 30018
Lansing, MI 48909
517/373-0680

Minnesota: Mr. H. Leonard Boche, Exec. Dir.
Board of Medical Examiners
2700 University Avenue West, #106
St. Paul, MN 55114-1080
612/642-0538

Mississippi: Frank Jay Morgan, Jr., MD
Exec. Officer
Mississippi State Board of Medical Licensure
2688-D Insurance Center Dr., Jackson, MS 39216
601/354-6645

Missouri: Mr. Gary R. Clark, Exec. Secy.
Missouri State Board of Registration
of the Healing Arts
PO Box 4, Jefferson City, MO 65102
314/751-0171

Montana: Carol Berger Norling, Admin. Asst.
Montana State Board of Medical Examiners
1424 9th Ave., Helena, MT 59620-0407
406/444-4284

Nebraska: Ms Katherine A. Brown, Assoc. Dir.
Nebraska State Board of Medical Examiners
301 Centennial Mall S., PO Box 95007
Lincoln, NE 68509-5007
402/471-2115

Nevada: Mr. David K. Boston, Exec. Dir.
Nevada State Board of Medical Examiners
1105 Terminal Way, Suite 301, Reno, NV 89510
702/688-2559

New Hampshire: William T. Wallace, MD
Exec. Secy.
Board of Registration in Medicine
Health and Welfare Bldg., 6 Hazen Dr.
Concord, NH 03301
603/271-4503

New Jersey: Charles A. Janousek, Exec. Secy.
New Jersey Board of Medical Examiners
28 W. State St., Rm. 602, Trenton, NJ 08608
609/292-4843

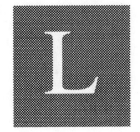

New Mexico: Mr. Bill Schmidt, Exec. Secy.
New Mexico State Board of Medical Examiners
491 Old Santa Fe Trail, Room 129
Santa Fe, NM 87504
505/827-7317

New York: Thomas Monahan, Assoc. Exec. Secy.
State Board for Medicine
State Education Dept., Cultural Education Center,
Room 3023,
Empire State Plaza, Albany, NY 12230
518/474-3841

North Carolina: Bryant D. Paris, Jr., Exec. Secy.
North Carolina Board of Medical Examiners
PO Box 26808, Raleigh, NC 27611
919/828-1212

North Dakota: Mr. Rolf P. Sletten
Exec. Secy. Treas.
Board of Medical Examiners
418 E. Broadway Ave., Suite C-10
Bismarck, ND 58501
701/223-9485

Ohio: Mr. Raymond Q. Bumgarner
Ohio State Medical Board
77 S. High St., 17th Floor
Columbus, OH 43266-0315
614/466-3934

Oklahoma: Carole A. Smith, Admin.
Oklahoma State Board of Medical Examiners
PO Box 18256, Oklahoma City, OK 73118
405/848-6841

Oregon: John J. Ulwelling, Exec. Secy.
Board of Medical Examiners
1500 1st Ave., Suite 620
Portland, OR 97201-5826
503/229-5770

Pennsylvania: Loretta M. Frank, Admin. Asst.
Pennsylvania State Board of Medicine
Bureau of Professional and Occupational Affairs
PO Box 2649, Harrisburg, PA 17105
717/787-2381

Puerto Rico: Sr. Pablo Valentin Torres, J.D.
Executive Director Puerto Rico Board
of Medical Examiners
Call Box 13969, Santurce, PR 00908
809/723-1617

Rhode Island: Milton Hamolsky, MD, Chief
Administrative Officer
Rhode Island Board of Licensure and Discipline
Department of Health
75 Davis Street, Room 205, Providence, RI 02908
401/277-3855

South Carolina: Mr. Stephen S. Seeling, JD
Exec. Dir.
South Carolina State Board of Medical Examiners
PO Box 12245, Columbia, SC 29211
803/734-8901

South Dakota: Mr. Robert D. Johnson, Exec. Sec.
South Dakota State Board of Medical and
Osteopathic Examiners
1323 S. Minnesota Ave., Sioux Falls, SD 57105
605/336-1965

Tennessee: Ms. Louise Blair
Regulatory Board Admin.
Tennessee Board of Medical Examiners
283 Plus Park Blvd., Nashville, TN 37219-5407
615/367-6231

Texas: G. Valter Brindley, Jr., MD, Exec. Dir.
Texas State Board of Medical Examiners
PO Box 149134, Austin, TX 78714-9134
512/834-7728

Utah: David E. Robinson, Dir.
Utah Division of Occupational and
Professional Licensing
160 E. 300 S., PO Box 45802
Salt Lake City, UT 84110
801/530-6628

Vermont: Ms. Vera A. Jones
Vermont State Board of Medical Practice
26 Terrace St., Montpelier, VT 05602
802/828-2674

Virginia: Hilary H. Connor, MD, Exec. Dir.
Virginia State Board of Medicine
1601 Rolling Hills Dr., Richmond, VA 23229-5005
804/662-9960

Virgin Islands: Jane Aubain, Admin. Asst.
Virgin Islands Board of Medical Examiners
48 Sugar Estate, Saint Thomas, VI 00802
809/776-8311

Washington: Ms. Gail Zimmerman, Exec. Secy.
Washington Board of Medical Examiners
1300 South Quince St, Olympia, WA 98504
206/753-3129

West Virginia: Mr. Ronald D. Walton
Executive Dir.
West Virginia Board of Medicine
101 Dee Dr., Suite 104, Charleston, WV 25311
304/348-2921

Wisconsin: Mrs. Deanna Zychowski, Exec. Secy.
Wisconsin Medical Examining Board
PO Box 8935, Madison, WI 53708
608/266-2811

Wyoming: Ms. Beverly Hacker, Exec. Secy.
Wyoming State Board of Medical Examiners
2301 Central Ave., Room 343, Barrett Building,
Cheyenne, WY 82002
307/777-6463

Life Insurance

American Council on Life Insurance
Strategic Research Department
1001 Pennsylvania Ave., NW
Washington, D.C. 20004-2599
202/624-2000

Association of Life Insurance
Medical Directors of America
Travelers Insurance Co., One Tower Square
Hartford, CT 06183-1030
203/277-4193

Lipid Diseases

National Lipid Diseases Foundation
1201 Corbin Street, Elizabeth, NJ 07201
201/527-8000

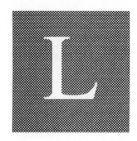

Lipo-Suction

American Society of Lipo-Suction Surgery
(affiliated with Newman Cosmetic Surgery Center)
1455 City Line Ave., Philadelphia, PA 19151
215/896-6677

American Society of Plastic
and Reconstructive Surgeons
444 E. Algonquin Rd., Arlington Heights, IL 60005
708/228-9900
Referral Line 800/635-0635

Literacy

Literacy Volunteers of America
5795 Widewaters Parkway, Syracuse, NY 13214
315/445-8000

Barbara Bush Foundation for Family Literacy
1002 Wisconsin Ave., NW
Washington, DC 20007
No phone number

Liver Diseases

American Association for the
Study of Liver Disease
6900 Grove Rd., Thorofare, NJ 08086
609/848-1000

American Liver Foundation
1425 Pompton Ave., Cedar Grove, NJ 07009
800/223-0179
201/256-2550 (in NJ)

Liver transplant status
Refer to National Institutes of Health
9000 Rockville Pike, Bethesda, MD 20892
301/496-5787

Living Will

AMA Policy: Living Wills, Durable Powers of Attorney and Durable Powers of Attorney for Health Care: The AMA believes that (1) state medical associations should encourage the 40 legislatures that have not enacted a durable power of attorney for health care statute to enact the model state bill adopted by the AMA in 1986; and (2) physicians should encourage their patients to document their wishes regarding the use of life-prolonging medical treatments.

Choice in Dying
250 W. 57th St. Rm. 831, New York, NY 10107
212/246-0493 800/248-2122

Guidelines for the appropriate use of do-not-resuscitate orders. Council on Ethical and Judicial Affairs, American Medical Association. JAMA. 1991 Apr 10; 265(14): 1868-71
Cardiopulmonary resuscitation (CPR) is routinely performed on hospitalized patients who suffer cardiac or respiratory arrest. Consent to administer CPR is presumed since the patient is incapable at the moment of arrest of communicating his or her treatment preference, and failure to act immediately is certain to result in the patient's death. Two exceptions to the presumption favoring CPR have been recognized, however. First, a patient may express in advance his or her

preference that CPR be withheld. If the patient is incapable of expressing a preference, the decision to forgo resuscitation may be made by the patient's family or other surrogate decision maker. Second, CPR may be withheld if, in the judgment of the treating physician, an attempt to resuscitate the patient would be futile. In December 1987, the American Medical Association's Council on Ethical and Judicial Affairs issued a series of guidelines to assist hospital medical staffs in formulating appropriate resuscitation policies. The Council's position on the appropriate use of CPR and do-not-resuscitate orders is updated in this report.

Medical Directive forms:
($5 for 2 forms with
a self-addressed, stamped envelope)
Medical Directive
c/o Harvard Medical School Health Letter
164 Longwood Ave
Boston, MA 02115

JAMA Article of Note: The Medical Directive.
Emanuel, L.L., Emanuel, E.J. JAMA. 1989 Jun 9;
261(22): 3288-93

JAMA Article of Note: Advanced Medical Directive.
David Orentlicher, D. JAMA. 1990 May 2; 263(17):
2365-67

JAMA Article of Note: Persistent vegetative state and the decision to withdraw or withhold life support. Council on Scientific Affairs and Council on Ethical and Judicial Affairs. JAMA. 1990 Jan 19; 263(3): 426-30
Persons with overwhelming damage to the cerebral hemispheres commonly pass into a chronic state of unconsciousness (ie, loss of self-awareness) called the vegetative state. When such cognitive loss lasts for more than a few weeks, the condition has been termed a persistent vegetative state, because the body retains the functions necessary to sustain vegetative functions. Recovery from the vegetative state does occur, but many persons in persistent vegetative states live for months or years if provided with nutritional and other supportive measures. The withdrawal of life support from these persons with loss of higher brain function is a controversial issue, as highlighted by public debates and judicial decisions. This article provides criteria for the diagnosis of permanent unconsciousness and reviews the available data that support the reliability of these criteria. Significant legal decisions have been made with regard to withdrawal of life support to patients in persistent vegetative states, and the trends in this area are discussed.

Loans

National Association of Residents and Interns
292 Madison Ave., New York, NY 10017
212/949-5900 800/221-2168

The Loan Application Process

A loan officer will request the type of information outlined in the Loan Application Checklist. In addition, some banks may require the applicant to complete the bank's loan application. Once the physician or group has submitted all requested documents, the loan officer will verify the information and evaluate the application. The approval process generally is completed within one to four weeks after all requested documents are provided.

Loan Application Checklist

The following checklist indicates the type of information that should be included in the physician's loan application package.

Market and Service Analysis:

New and existing practices include:
- Type of services to be provided
- Market area to be served

New practices, programs, or market include:
- Estimated demand in market area for services to be provided
- Estimated fees for service
- Estimated collection rate
- List of competitors and estimated volume of business provided
- Identification of where patients will come from and how they will be attracted to the practice

Existing practices include:
- Historical volumes and net revenues

Financial Information:

New and existing practices include:
- Projected income statement for practice (for one to five years; in some cases, month-by-month projections are suggested for the first year)
- Projected cash flow statement (for one to five years)
- Projected capital expenditures
- Estimated repayment term

Existing practices include:
- Three years of audited historical financial statements or corporate and personal tax returns

General Information:

New and existing practices may include:
- Physicians' credentials, including places of education and training
- Credentials of business management, including education and experience
- Personal statement of net worth
- Personal tax returns
- Long-term plans for the business
- Personal and professional references
- Guantor, or third party support in some cases
- Terms of purchase agreement (if buying an existing practice or buying into a practice)
- Nature of partnership agreement (if applicable)

Conclusion

The requirements to obtain a loan vary from institution to institution. A well-developed business plan will provide a significant portion of the information required by lenders and also will assist the physician or group in realistically evaluating the potential of the practice. In addition, the applicant stands a better chance of getting the loan by appearing fully prepared, since loan application reviews include a subjective component.(FIN)

Physicians beginning practice
American Professional Practice Association
292 Madison Ave., New York, NY 10017
212/949-5900

Locations for Practice
Checklist for Deciding Where to Practice

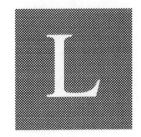

Geographic Factors
- Which areas need physicians? Check with the AMA's Physicians Placement Service, and the placement service of your specialty society.
- How many other doctors practice in the area? What are their specialties? How old are they? Check the local telephone classified directory, and the AMA's Physician Characteristics and Distribution in the U.S.
- Will the town support a physician in your specialty? Where do people go now for the type of medical service you provide? If they go outside the community, will they break existing medical ties to come to you?
- Is the town without a doctor? Why? How long has it been without one and why did the last physician leave?
- What is the trade area? Does the town have a bank, stores, or facilities that will draw people to it? Are there new or recent retail and commercial enterprises?
- Is the area gaining or losing population? Is the area prosperous or depressed? Compare per capita income with other areas in the state of similar size.
- What is the tax delinquency rate? Check with the local or county taxing body.
- What are the vacancy rates for apartments and commercial property? Check with the local real estate board.
- Has major industry moved into the area recently, or is it expected?
- Is the local construction industry vigorous, or in a decline?
- Are bank deposits going up or down, and how do they compare with areas of similar population? Your local bank can furnish you with data from the Federal Reserve system.
- Is the local economy subject to seasonal fluctuations or the fortunes of a single company or industry?

Professional factors
- Can you practice your kind of medicine in this community?
- Can you obtain adequate, well-located, reasonably-priced office space with ample parking and transportation facilities?
- If you are associating with another physician or a group, are office facilities well-located and well-equipped?
- Is there a good hospital? How far from your prospective office?
- Will you be able to obtain hospital privileges?
- Are special diagnostic and therapeutic facilities available in the area?
- Is there a good pharmacy? A good laboratory?
- Are other doctors in the community receptive to your coming? Are qualified practitioners in other specialties and subspecialties available for consultation? If you're going into solo practice, are there doctors with whom you can share coverage?
- Will allied health personnel be available when you need them?
- Will there be opportunities for continuing medical education and professional growth? How do physicians in the area get along together? Will you be able to develop the

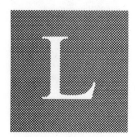

referral sources you need among other physicians?

- Is there hostility between local hospitals that involves the medical staffs?
- Is the country medical society active, and what level of participation will be expected of you?
- Are nursing home or other extended care facilities available?

Economic factors

- Can you make a good living in the area? Will living expenses be drastically different from those to which you've been accustomed? How do doctors' incomes compare with those of MDs in other similarly populated parts of the state?
- Do doctors' fees seem in line with charges for other services? Have they kept pace or lagged behind?
- Can you rent or buy office space and equip it at a reasonable price?
- Is there good housing, fairly priced? How about state and local taxes? Are they in line with income and living costs?
- Will banks or other institutions provide the financial backing you need to set up practice?
- What is the prevailing salary level for medical office personnel?

Personal factors

- Can you and your spouse live the kind of life you want in the community?Will the rest of your family like living there?
- Will you fit into the community? Religion, ethnic background, and personal lifestyle might be considerations.
- Is good housing available? Are there good schools? Churches? Are there community organizations that interest you?
- Are there shopping facilities within reasonable distance that offer a range of high quality goods and services?
- Are there congenial people in the area with ages and interests that are similar to those of you and your marriage partner? Will the recreational and cultural outlets meet the needs of yourself and your family? (BUS)

Locum Tenens
More and More Medical Practices Are Using Locum Tenens

"Locum tenens," the Latin term for someone holding a place, has a specific connotation in the medical field. The term has been adapted to physicians who hold temporary positions for other physicians when they must be absent from their practices.

Locum tenens physicians take temporary assignments to fill vacancies in solo practices, on hospital staffs, in group practices, and in managed care organizations. Temporary assignments are both short- and long-term, ranging from one-week to one-year commitments. Today, there is a growing demand for locum tenens physicians.

Locum tenens help practices balance workloads and test new services in the marketplace. During times of peak patient loads, such as flu season, locum tenens enable practices to balance staffing shortages without burdening the permanent medical staff. As marketplace demand for additional services occurs, locum tenens can be employed to test new services, thus ascertaining consumer acceptance before hiring permanent staff. When new medical centers open, locus tenens can be used to free up the time of the medical directors to concentrate on administrative activities, and to test the market before hiring staff for the demonstrated patient volume.

Checklist for Locum Tenens Recruitment

- If possible, begin the process of recruitment three to four months in advance.
- Select the prospective candidates you wish to interview.
- Interview candidates over the telephone. Request that candidates submit the necessary documentation and recommendations.
- Verify all credentials.
- Verify that the locum tenens and the medical practice have adequate malpractice coverage. Check references.
- Make locum tenens offer and negotiate contract terms.
- Obtain state licensure and malpractice insurance, as needed.
- Arrange for travel and housing, as needed.
- Prepare the practice, hospital, and pharmaceutical staff for the arrival of the locum tenens. Welcome the locum tenens and provide adequate orientation to the practice, hospital, pharmacy, and community.
- Monitor the work of the locum tenens.(LOC)

Lung Diseases
Disorders of the Lung

The lungs are continuously exposed to airborne particles, such as bacteria, viruses, and allergens, all of which can cause lung disorders. Most of these disorders do not interfere with oxygen supply; those that do are a major threat to health.

Infection. Infective disorders are common, especially tracheitis (inflammation of the lining of the windpipe) and croup (a virus infection of young children). Bronchitis (inflammation of the bronchi), bronchiectasis (swelling of the bronchi), and bronchiolitis (inflammation of the bronchioles) commonly follow colds or influenza. Pneumonia (inflammation of the lung) is usually caused by infection by viruses or bacteria. Fungal infections of the lungs, such as aspergillosis, actinomycosis, histoplasmosis, and candidiasis, are relatively uncommon.

Allergies. Bronchial asthma, in which the muscles of the bronchi contract and obstruct the free passage of air, often occurs in sensitized people exposed to pollens, house mites, fungal spores, animal dander, and many other agents. Allergic alveolitis (inflammation of the alveoli) may be caused by many organic dusts, such as moldy hay.

Tumors. Lung cancer is one of the most common of all malignant tumors; in most cases it is associated with cigarette smoking. Secondary malignant tumors, which have spread from other parts of the body to the lungs, are common. However, benign tumors affecting the lung are uncommon.

Injury. Lung injury usually results from penetration of the chest wall. Pneumothorax (air in the pleural cavity) and hemothorax (blood in the pleural cavity) are usually caused by a penetrating injury;

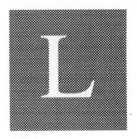

either may cause collapse of the lung. Injury can also occur from the inhalation of poisonous dusts, gases, or toxic substances. Silicosis and asbestosis are caused by inhalation of silica and asbestos, respectively; they may lead to progressive fibrosis of the lung.

Impaired Blood And Oxygen Supply. The most serious disorder is pulmonary embolism, in which a blood clot formed in one of the major veins breaks free and is carried to the lungs. The clot may block the pulmonary arteries and cause death. Heart failure may cause pulmonary edema, in which the lungs become filled with fluid. Respiratory distress syndrome, which may affect newborn babies or adults, has many causes. In this condition, leakage of fluid into the alveoli seriously interferes with oxygen supply. Emphysema, in which the walls of the alveoli break down so that the area for oxygen exchange is reduced, is frequently seen in people suffering from chronic bronchitis and asthma.

Investigation. Lung disorders are investigated by chest X ray, bronchoscopy, pulmonary function tests, sputum analysis, blood tests, and physical examination. Sometimes a biopsy of lung tissue is taken for analysis.(ENC)

American Lung Association
1740 Broadway, New York, NY 10019
212/315-8700

LUNGLINE
National Jewish Hospital Asthma Center
800/222-LUNG (800/222-5864)
8:30 AM-5:00 PM MST

Lung Associations, Statewide

American Lung Association of Alabama
PO Box 55209, Birmingham, AL 35255
205/933-8821

American Lung Association of Alaska
605 Barrow St, Suite 2
Anchorage, AK 99501-3688
907/276-5864

American Lung Association of Arizona
102 W McDowell Road, Phoenix, AZ 85003
602/258-7505

American Lung Association of Arkansas
211 Natural Resources Drive
Little Rock, AR 72205
501/224-5864

American Lung Association of California
424 Pendleton Way, Oakland, CA 94621-2189
415/638-5864

American Lung Association of Colorado
1600 Race St, Denver, CO 80206-1198
303/388-4327

American Lung Association of Connecticut
45 Ash St, East Hartford, CT 06108
203/289-5401

American Lung Association of Delaware
1021 Gilpin Ave, Suite 202, Wilmington, DE 19806
302/655-7258

American Lung Association of the
District of Columbia

475 H St NW, Washington, DC 20001
202/682-5864

American Lung Association of Florida
PO Box 8127, Jacksonville, FL 32239-8127
904/743-2933

American Lung Association of Georgia
2452 Spring Road, Smyrna, GA 30080
404/434-5864

American Lung Association of Hawaii
245 N Kukui St, Honolulu, HI 96817
808/537-5966

American Lung Association of Idaho
1111 S Orchard, Suite 245, Boise, ID 83705-1966
208/344-6567

American Lung Association of Illinois
PO Box 19239, Springfield, IL 62794-9239
217/528-3441

American Lung Association of Indiana
9410 Priority Way W Drive
Indianapolis, IN 46240-1470
317/573-3900

American Lung Association of Iowa
1025 Ashworth Road, West Des Moines, IA 50265
515/224-0800

American Lung Association of Kansas
PO Box 4426, Topeka, KS 66604-2419
913/272-9290

American Lung Association of Kentucky
PO Box 969, Louisville, KY 40201-0969
502/363-2652

American Lung Association of Louisiana
333 St. Charles Ave, Suite 500
New Orleans, LA 70130-3180
504/523-5864

American Lung Association of Maine
128 Sewall St, Augusta, ME 04330
207/622-6394

American Lung Association of Maryland
1840 York Road, Suite K-M
Timonium, MD 21093-5156
301/560-2120

American Lung Association of Massachusetts
803 Summer St, 3rd Floor
South Boston, MA 02127-1609
617/269-9720

American Lung Association of Michigan
403 Seymour Ave, Lansing, MI 48933-1179
517/484-4541

American Lung Association of Minnesota
490 Concordia Ave, Saint Paul, MN 55103-2441
612/227-8014

Mississippi Lung Association
PO Box 9865, Jackson, MS 39206-9865
601/362-5453

American Lung Association of Eastern Missouri
1118 Hampton Ave, Saint Louis, MO 63139-3196
314/645-5505

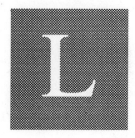

American Lung Association of Western Missouri
2007 Broadway, Kansas City, MO 64108
816/842-5242

American Lung Association of Montana
Christmas Seal Bldg, 825 Helena Ave.
Helena, MT 59601
406/442-6556

American Lung Association of Nebraska
8901 Indian Hills Drive, Suite 107
Omaha, NE 68114-4057
402/393-2222

American Lung Association of Nevada
PO Box 7056, Reno, NV 89510-7056
702/825-5864

American Lung Association of New Hampshire
PO Box 1014, Manchester, NH 03105
603/669-2411

American Lung Association of New Jersey
1600 Route 22 E, Union, NJ 07083
201/687-9340

American Lung Association of New Mexico
216 Truman Ave NE, Albuquerque, NM 87108
505/265-0732

American Lung Association of New York State
8 Mountain View Ave, Albany, NY 12205-2899
518/459-4197

American Lung Association of North Carolina
PO Box 27985, Raleigh, NC 27611-7985
919/832-8326

American Lung Association of North Dakota
PO Box 5004, Bismarck, ND 58502-5004
701/223-5613

American Lung Association of Ohio
PO Box 16677, Columbus, OH 43216-6677
614/279-1700

American Lung Association of Oklahoma
PO Box 53303, Oklahoma City, OK 73152-3303
405/524-8471

American Lung Association of Oregon
PO Box 115, Portland, OR 97207
503/224-5145

American Lung Association of Pennsylvania
Olde Liberty Square
4807 Jonestown Road, Suite 251
Harrisburg, PA 17109
717/540-8506

Asociacion Puertorriquena del Pulmon
GPO Box 3468, San Juan, PR 00936
809/756-5664

Rhode Island Lung Association
10 Abbott Park Place, Providence, RI 02903-3703
401/421-6487

American Lung Association of South Carolina
1817 Gadsden St, Columbia, SC 29201
803/765-9066

South Dakota Lung Association
208 E 13th St, Sioux Falls, SD 57102-1099
605/336-7222

American Lung Association of Tennessee
PO Box 399, Nashville, TN 37202-0399
615/329-1151

American Lung Association of Texas
PO Box 26460, Austin, TX 78755-0460
512/343-0502

American Lung Association of Utah
1930 S 1100 E, Salt Lake City, UT 84106-2317
801/484-4456

Vermont Lung Association
30 Farrell St, South Burlington, VT 05403
802/863-6817

American Lung Association of the Virgin Islands
PO Box 974, St. Thomas, VI 00801-4624
809/774-2077

American Lung Association of Virginia
PO Box 7065, Richmond, VA 23221-7065
804/355-3295

American Lung Association of Washington
2625 3rd Ave, Seattle, WA 98121-1213
206/441-5100

American Lung Association of West Virginia
PO Box 3980, Charleston, WV 25339
304/342-6600

American Lung Association of Wisconsin
1330 N 113th St, Suite 190
Milwaukee, WI 53226-3212
414/258-9100

American Lung Association of Wyoming
PO Box 1128, Cheyenne, WY 82003-1128
307/638-6342

Lupus

Lupus Foundation of America, Inc.
4 Research Place, Suite 180, Rockville, MD 20850
301/670-9292 800/558-0121

Lyme Disease

The Lyme Borreliosis Foundation
PO Box 462, Tolland, CT 06084
203/871-2900

Rush Lyme Disease Center
1653 W. Congress Parkway, Chicago, IL 60612
312/942-5963 (312/942-LYME)

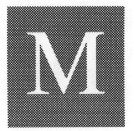

Macular Diseases
Association for Macular Diseases
210 E. 64th St., New York, NY 10021
212/605-3719

Magnetic Resonance Imaging
Society for Magnetic Resonance Imaging
213 West Institute Place, Chicago, IL 60610
312/751-2590

Mammography
JAMA Article of Note: Early Detection of Breast
Cancer. Council on Scientific Affairs. JAMA. 1984
Dec 7; 252(21): 3008-11

Recommendations
American College of Radiology
1891 Preston White Dr., Reston, VA 22091
703/648-8900

Management
American Management Association
135 W. 50th St., New York, NY 10020
212/586-8100

Marijuana
JAMA Article of Note: Marijuana. Its health
hazards and therapeutic potentials. Council on
Scientific Affairs. JAMA. 1981 Oct 16; 246(16):
1823-7

Potsmokers Anonymous
316 E. Third St., New York, NY 10009
212/254-1777

Marketing
How to Develop a Marketing Program

Basic Questions:

What are the choices?
Evaluate the current situation: identify
opportunities and challenges (i.e., market
research).

What is the next step?
Formulation of realistic objectives

How is that accomplished?
Development of market strategies

What will it cost?
Allocation of resources

What progress has been made?
Monitoring of results

Marketing Enhancement Checklist
- Is practice marketing a recognized priority? Do
  all office personnel recognize its importance?
- Is there a practice marketing plan? Are all
  personnel involved?
- Has the practice identified the target markets to
  be served?
- Is there systematic follow-up with patients?
- Is there systematic contact with referral sources?
- Does the physician participate in outreach or
  satellite programs?
- Is the practice using the hospital's marketing
  resources to the physicians' advantage?

Marketing to Other Physicians
The reader might find it strange that physicians
need to market to other physicians, but, in fact,
this can be one of the most useful aspects of a
marketing plan. This is especially true of
secondary-care and specialty physicians who
derive many of their patients from referrals. In
addition, there are circumstances in which
physicians can be of significant assistance to one
another in mutual marketing efforts. The following
options should be considered in a marketing
program to other physicians:
- Affiliation with a multispecialty clinic so that
  appropriate linkages can be made with other
  medical specialists
- Affiliations with practitioners who are able to
  provide backup services and coverage for solo
  practitioners
- Participation in medical-society and other
  physician-group meetings, especially meetings
  involving physicians in the immediate service
  area
- Participation in meetings of the medical staff of
  the main hospital with which the practitioner is
  affiliated.

American Marketing Association
250 S. Wacker Dr., Suite 200, Chicago, IL 60606
312/648-0536

American Society for Healthcare Marketing
& Public Relations
c/o American Hospital Association
840 North Lake Shore Drive, Chicago, IL 60611
312/280-6359

Marketing Research Information:
FIND/SVP
625 Avenue of the Americas, New York, NY 10011
212/645-4500

Marriage Counselling
American Association of Marriage
and Family Therapy
1717 K St. NW, Suite 407
Washington, DC 20006
202/429-1825

Massage Therapy
American Massage Therapy Association
1130 W. North Shore Ave.
Chicago, IL 60626-4670
312/761-2682 (312/761-AMTA)

Matching Program

National Resident Matching Program
2450 N Street, NW, Suite 201
Washington, DC 20037
202/828-0676

- *Residents who were not matched:*
  Neurology/Psychiatry
  American Psychiatric Association
  202/682-6000
- Obstetrics and Gynecology
  American College of Obstetricians and
  Gynecologists
  202/638-5577
- Otolaryngology
  American Academy of Otolaryngology--Head
  and Neck Surgery
  202/289-4607
- Plastic Surgery
  University of Louisville
  502/588-6880

All others, contact appropriate specialty society.

Maternal and Child Care

National Center for Education
in Maternal and Child Health
38th and R. Sts., NW, Washington, DC 20057
202/625-8400

Maxillofacial Surgery

Oral and Maxillofacial Surgeon alternate titles:
oral surgeon. Performs surgery on mouth, jaws,
and related head and neck structure: Executes
difficult and multiple extraction of teeth. Removes
tumors and other abnormal growths. Performs
preprosthetic surgery to prepare mouth for
insertion of dental prosthesis. Corrects abnormal
jaw relations by mandibular or maxillary revision.
Treats fractures of jaws. Administers general and
local anesthetics. May treat patients in
hospital.(DOT)

American Society of Maxillofacial Surgeons
129 Oakbrook Center Mall, Oak Brook, IL 60521
708/571-3470

Mayo Clinic

Mayo Clinic
200 First St., SW, Rochester, MN 55905
507/282-2511

Mayo, Charles Horace 1865-1939

JAMA. 1939 Jun 3; 112(22): 2342

Charles Horace Mayo noted as a surgical genius,
a great medical administrator and a genial
physician, died in Chicago of pneumonia, May 26.
The younger of the two world-famed Mayo
brothers was born in Rochester, Minn., July 19,
1865, the son of William Worrall Mayo and Louise
Wright Mayo. After an education in the Rochester
High School and at the Niles Academy he
attended Chicago Medical College, later known as
Northwestern University, and received his degree
in medicine in 1888. As a young boy he began,
almost from childhood, to live in a medical

atmosphere and to become inspired toward
medicine as a career. After his graduation in
medicine he returned to Rochester, where his
urge toward research and his surgical genius led
to innumerable investigations in medicine and in
surgery. His first published statement entitled
"Report of Clinic in St. Mary's Hospital, Rochester,
Minnesota, January 19, 1891," which was
published in the Northwest Lancet in November of
that year. From that time on hardly a year passed
without a contribution by either Dr. Charles H.
Mayo alone or with his brother, or with some of
the younger men who soon became attracted to
them. These contributions cover every phase of
medicine and surgery and in later years embrace
as well the fields of philosophy, economics and
statesmanship.

In the field of scientific medical organizations Dr.
Charles H. Mayo was president of the Western
Surgical Association in 1904, the Minnesota State
Medical Association in 1905, the Society of
Clinical Surgery in 1911, the Clinical Congress of
Surgeons of North America in 1914, the American
Medical Association in 1916, the American
College of Surgeons in 1924, the American
Surgical Association in 1931 and the Minnesota
Public Health Association form 1932 to 1936.

Dr. William J. Mayo, Dr. Charles Horace Mayo and
their distinguished father made a small village
become one of the most notable medical centers
of the world. Throughout their careers these
distinguished leaders devoted themselves to the
advancement of organized medicine. The medical
society of the county in which they practiced was
founded by Dr. William Worrall Mayo. Dr Charles
H. Mayo was widely known not only as a surgical
genius, as a great surgical teacher, as an inspired
organizer, as a leader in medical advancement
and as a citizen of his city, county, state and of the
nation, but also as a warm hearted, genial, faithful,
true humanitarian, easily approachable,
unostentatious, ready to trade wits and banter,
always in the most kindly and sympathetic
manner. Such men come but infrequently in any
civilization and their places are not easily filled as
the world moves on.

Many of the greatest universities in the world
conferred honorary degrees on him. Thus the
master of arts degree was conferred by the
Northwestern University in 1904, fellowship in the
Royal College of Surgeons in England in 1920 and
in the Royal Society of Medicine in 1926, and
master in surgery by Trinity College of Dublin in
1925. He was made doctor of public health by the
Detroit College of Medicine and Surgery in 1927
and doctor of science by Princeton University in
1917, the University of Pennsylvania in 1925 and
the University of Leeds in England in 1909. He
also received the honorary degree of LL.D. from
the University of Maryland in 1909, Kenyon
College in 1916, Northwestern University in 1921,
the University of Edinburg in Scotland in 1925,
Queen's University in Belfast, Ireland in 1925,
University of Manchester in England in 1929,
Hamline University in 1930 and Carleton College
in 1932.

A number of great nations also honored him with
citations for distinguished service, the record
including officier de l'Ordre national de la legion
d'honneur, France, 1925; officier de l'Instruction
publique et des beaux-art, France, 1925, and

Cross of Knight Commander of the Royal Order of the Crown of Italy, 1932, as well as citations from many other countries.

During the World War he and his brother, Dr. William J. Mayo, alternated between Rochester where they maintained graduate study for physicians entering the service, and the personnel department in Washington. They served also as consultants in surgery. Dr. Charles H. Mayo was commissioned Major on April 19, 1917, Colonel June 15, 1918, and Brigadier General Nov. 22, 1921. He received the distinguished service by the National Organization of the American Legion and was presented with a commemorative plaque, the special ceremony being conducted by President Franklin D. Roosevelt in person in 1934.

The list of his membership in distinguished civic and medical organizations, both American and foreign, is far too long to list. To many of these he gave personally of himself and of his advice, in others he held honorary membership only. He gave also freely of himself and of his work to many scientific and general publications. He served as health officer of the city of Rochester since May 1, 1912, and as a member of the school board of that city from 1915 to 1923.

In 1915 Drs. William J. and Charles H. Mayo established the Mayo Foundation for Medical Education and Research in Rochester, affiliating this organization with the University of Minnesota. Their first contribution was $1,500,000, which has now been increased to more than $2,650,000. In order to perpetuate this institution, the Mayo Properties Association was established in 1919 to hold all the property, endowments and funds of the Mayo Clinic and to insure the permanence of the institution for public understanding that the moneys and property can never inure to the benefit of any individual.

Mayo, William James 1861-1939

JAMA. 1939 Aug 5; 113 (6): 524

Dr. William J. Mayo, former President of the American Medical Association, recognized throughout the world as a brilliant surgeon, a great organizer, as esteemed leader in the field of medicine, died at his home in Rochester, Minn., July 28, aged 78; an operation for perforating ulcer of the stomach had been performed April 22. But a few months have passed since the death of the younger of the two brothers, Dr. Charles H. Mayo. Their careers were inseparable. Their passing this life so closely together was no doubt as they themselves might have wished it.

The career of Dr. William J. Mayo will be fully recorded in many biographies in which space will be available for proper consideration of its many facets. Since the sixteenth century, the Mayo family has been one closely associated with science. The father of the two boys, Dr. William Worrall Mayo, was born in Manchester, England, May 31, 1819; after training as a physicist and chemist he came to the United States in 1845. In 1847 he removed to Lafayette, Ind., where he studied medicine with Dr. Eleazar Deming. He then completed his medical studies in the University of Missouri and graduated in 1854. After practicing briefly in Laporte, Ind., Dr. William Worrall Mayo removed to Minnesota, settling

eventually in Rochester in 1863, where he was in charge of the draft board during the Civil War. The father of these boys was himself a competent surgeon, one of the first physicians in the West to use the microscope, founder of the Minnesota State Medical Association and its president in 1873. Dr. William Worrall Mayo died in Rochester in 1911. He and Mrs. William Worrall Mayo had three daughters and two sons.

The elder son, William James Mayo, was born in LeSueur, Minn., June 29, 1861. The family removed to Rochester when he was slightly over 1 1/2 years old. The boy attended the public school in Rochester and the high school and thereafter spent one year in a private school for languages and science and two years in Niles Academy. During their youth, both William and Charles accompanied their father on his rounds and had an opportunity to observe both surgical operations and postmortem examinations. For a time, both clerked in the drug store. With their father they learned to use the microscope. In 1880, William J. Mayo went to the University of Michigan, Ann Arbor, and completed a three year course which had just been established to replace the former two year medical course. In his medical education Dr. William J. Mayo had an opportunity to be associated with the anatomist Ford and with Victor C. Vaughan, and his training in surgery was under Donald McLean, then professor of surgery. When he was 22, Dr. William J. Mayo completed his medical studies in the university and received his degree.

In November 1884, one year later, Dr. Will married Miss Hattie M. Damon of Rochester. Through many years the close association of Mrs. Mayo with Dr. William J. Mayo in extending hospitality, in the organization of many aspects of the clinic and in carrying a great share of the responsibility for his success and happiness has been widely recognized.

In 1884, Dr. William J. Mayo spent two months in New York City taking the first course given in the New York Post-Graduate School. In 1885 he took a course in the New York Polyclinic. For many years he and Dr. Charles alternated in spending week-ends in Chicago with Christian Fenger. Frequently they traveled abroad to observe surgery as practiced in every nation in the world.

In 1885, Dr. William J. Mayo read his first paper before the Southern Minnesota Medical Association, and his literary contributions to every phase of medical science and art and practice have been innumerable.

From 1889 until 1905, the Drs. Mayo carried on their work in St. Mary's Hospital in Rochester, an institution which they, with their father, had aided in establishing and one which is now known throughout the world largely because of their work. The record of surgical procedures performed indicate an early tendency toward selection of abdominal surgery by Dr. Will, leaving many of the other fields to Dr. Charles. As Dr. Will himself said, "Charlie soon had me driven to cover by being a better surgeon, and I began to specialize in abdominal work and in operations on the ureters and kidneys." As the repute of their work spread, they soon began to associate with themselves younger men who had shown special predilection for surgical work, the first to be selected being Dr.

E. Starr Judd, who had charge of the third operating room in 1905. From that time on, the surgical developments in Rochester were so rapid that additional wings continued to be added to the hospital, an annex was opened and additional hospitals were built. As it became apparent that internal medicine and diagnosis, with the work of the laboratory, would be of prime importance, these developments were particularly encouraged. Throughout the record of the growth and development of this monumental institution to the proud position which it now occupies signs of the leadership of Dr. William J. Mayo appear again and again. Early in his career Dr. Will conceived the idea of a permanent endowed institution in Rochester to be connected with a university. He elaborated the concept of the Mayo Foundation and he gave freely of himself, of his funds and of his life for its perpetuation.

The honors and recognitions given to him indicate how widely recognized were his achievements for the good of mankind, including a citation for distinguished service given by the American Legion with a commemorative plaque, which was presented by the President of the United States in person in 1934.

Dr. William J. Mayo became associated early with medical organizations. He served as president of his county and state medical associations. He was chairman of the Section on Surgery and Anatomy of the American Medical Association, 1898-1899, and President of the American Medical Association, 1906-1907. He was also president of the American Surgical Association, of the American College of Surgeons, of the Congress of American Physicians and Surgeons, and of the Inter-State Postgraduate Medical Association of North America.

During the World War he was commissioned Major in the Medical Reserve Corps on April 9, 1917, and Colonel of the Medical Corps of the National Army on June 15, 1918. He served as chief consultant for all surgical services during the period of the war and was stationed in the office of the Surgeon-General in Washington. He was commissioned Brigadier-General in the Reserve Corps in 1921 and since then has served at various times as consultant in surgery to the War Department.

His memberships in medical organizations, in military organizations and in civic bodies were far too numerous even for listing. Most of the important foreign medical societies of the world had elected him an honorary member.

His contributions to medical literature, previously mentioned, were well beyond 300 in number, beginning with a report of an operation for ovarian tumor and covering many phases of medical and surgical science, a wide variety of commencement and honorary addresses, a number of descriptive letters of travel and philosophic contributions to the problems of our day.

In 1915, Drs. William J. and Charles H. Mayo donated $1,500,000 to establish the Mayo Foundation for Medical Education and Research in Rochester in affiliation with the University of Minnesota. In 1919 the brothers formed the Mayo Properties Association to hold all the properties, endowments and fund of the Mayo Clinic to insure the permanence of the institution for public service. Again in 1934 the Mayo Properties Association presented a gift of $500,000 to the University of Minnesota, making a total of $2,800,000 that the brothers had given to the Mayo Foundation. In sending this contribution, Dr. William J Mayo wrote, in part:

"Our father recognized certain definite social obligation. He believed that any man who had better opportunity than others; greater strength of mind, body, or character, owed something to those who had not been so provided; that is, that the important thing in life was not to accomplish for oneself alone, but for each to carry his share of collective responsibility....The fund which we had built up and which had grown far beyond our expectations had come from the sick, and we believed that it ought to return to the sick in the form of advanced medical education, which would develop better-trained physicians, and to research to reduce the amount of sickness....The people's money, of which we have been the custodians, is being irrevocably returned to the people from whom it came....The practice of medicine in Rochester is carried on in the same manner as by other members of the regular medical profession throughout the state and nation. All classes of patients, without regard to race or creed, social or financial standing, receive necessary care without discrimination...."

These words reflect the great character, the human kindliness, the profound human sympathy that were the part of Dr. William James Mayo. It has been said that opportunity and great occasions make great men. Exception to this rule is present in the lives of Drs. William J. and Charles H. Mayo. They made a small village into one of the most notable medical centers of the world wholly through a genius for surgery and for medical leadership. Throughout their careers they devoted themselves to the advancement of scientific medicine and of the medical profession which they served so nobly and which gloried so greatly in their achievements.

In 1906, when Dr. William J. Mayo read his presidential address to the American Medical Association, he forecast and considered some of the great problems that concern medical practice today. He attacked abuses of medical care by public service corporations and the abuses of medical charity by those able to pay. He condemned all attempts by those not trained in the science and art of medicine to dominate its functions. To the very end he contended for this point of view. And in a note written just a few days before his death, he urged continued work for the advancement and stabilization of medical science and the traditions of medical practice.

All the world pauses in the midst of its turmoil and stress to give him honor and to pay him in his death the tribute that is so justly his due - a great physician, a superb surgeon, a magnificent leader, a beloved man!

Medicaid

The Medicaid Program, through grants to States, provides medical services to the needy and the medically needy. The Administration is responsible for working with the States to develop approaches toward meeting the adequate medical care.

The Medicare/Medicaid Programs include a quality assurance focal point to carry out the quality assurance provisions of the Medicare and Medicaid Programs; the development and implementation of health and safety standards for providers of care in Federal health programs; and the implementation of the End Stage Renal Disease Program and the Professional Review provisions.(USG)

Contact State (or local) Department of Public Aid for information regarding Medicaid

Medical Assistant

History: Since its founding in 1956, the American Association of Medical Assistants (AAMA) has been the only professional association devoted exclusively to the profession of medical assisting. The AMA, an early supporter if AAMA, still provides assistance, in recognition of the fact that AAMA serves an important role in improving the educational preparation and continuing education opportunities for the medical assistant.

The first certification examination was administered in 1963, preceding the establishment of the accreditation program. In 1966, AAMA began work on formal curriculum standards in collaboration with the AMA. A task force of physicians and medical assistants surveyed existing medical assistant programs a nd drew up tentative standards, which were adopted in 1969. About three years were spent in laying a solid groundwork for a two-year associate degree program. In 1971, after two years of actual accreditation activity, the initial standards were revised to allow for the accreditation of one-year educational programs.

Occupational Description: Medical assisting is a multiskilled allied health profession: practitioners work primarily in ambulatory settings such as medical offices and clinics. Medical assistants function as members of the healthcare delivery team and perform administrative and clinical procedures.

Job Description: Medical assistants are allied health professionals who assist physicians in their offices or other medical settings. In accordance with respective state laws, they perform a broad range of administrative and clinical duties, as indicated by the 1990 Developing a Curriculum (DACUM) occupational analysis.

Administrative duties include scheduling and receiving patients, preparing and maintaining medical records, performing basic secretarial skills and medical transcription, handling telephone calls between the physician and other individuals, and managing practice finances.

Clinical duties include asepsis and infection control, taking patient histories and vital signs, performing first aid and CPR, preparing patients for procedures, assisting the physician with examinations and treatments, collecting and processing specimens, performing selected diagnostic tests, and preparing and administering medications as directed by the physician.

Both administrative and clinical duties involve maintenance of equipment and supplies for the practice. A medical assistant who is sufficiently qualified by education and/or experience may be responsible for supervising personnel, developing and conducting public outreach programs to market the physician's professional services, and participating in the negotiation of leases and of equipment and supply contracts.

Employment Characteristics: More medical assistants are employed by practicing physicians than any other type of allied health personnel. Medical assistants are usually employed in physicians' offices, where they perform a variety of administrative and clinical tasks to facilitate the work of the physician. The responsibilities of medical assistants vary, depending on whether they work in a clinic, hospital, large group practice, or small private office. With a demand from more than 200,000 physicians, there are and will probably continue to be almost unlimited opportunities for formally educated medical assistants.

According to the 1991 CAHEA Annual Supplemental Survey, entry level salaries average $14,555.(ALL)

AMA Division of Allied Health
312/464-4628

Locating a medical assistant

There are many ways to find and hire a competent medical office assistant. It's important to select the right assistant, particularly if a physician is just starting a practice. An inexperienced or inefficient assistant could prove an expensive investment at a time when the physician can least afford financial mistakes. It is suggested that physicians do the following:

- Check with the local medical society for possible job candidates; many run formal or informal placement services for such employees.
- Contact the local chapter of the American Association of Medical Assistants for suggestions. AAMA has chapters in nearly all states today.
- Get in touch with schools in the area with accredited training programs for medical assistants and medical secretaries, whose graduates may be seeking positions. Some run rotating externship programs in physicians' offices.
- If schools offering specialized training programs aren't operating locally, call community college placement offices, other secretarial schools or high schools to inquire about possible good applicants.
- Talk with other physicians; they may know of suitable applicants.
- Call the local hospital(s) personnel department for leads.
- Get assistance in locating good job candidates when using a professional management consultant to help launch a practice.

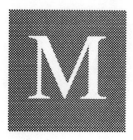

- Ask detail people and medical supply sales people if they know of assistants coming onto the job market.
- Utilize the services of personnel agencies.
- Advertise in local newspapers and professional journals.

Thinking Through Employment Needs

Before screening potential employees, the physician should analyze office needs and formulate a detailed job description which lists the duties each employee will perform.

Schools training medical assistants approved by AAMA-AMA expect their graduates to be able to perform a wide range of front office and clinical duties. The duties an assistant performs will vary, depending upon the type of practice. For example, a specialty may require an individual have additional professional training, and perhaps hold a license from the state, they handle certain tasks, operate specific equipment, or perform specialized procedures. If so, professional schools or hospitals training the kind of individuals needed or other placement agencies will have to be consulted to find suitable candidates.

Before interviewing job candidates the physician should write a job description. Each job description should include a brief job summary, a list of qualifications, and specific requirements.

Once the kind of assistant has been defined, a list of specific duties to be performed should be drawn up, It should include the minimum qualifications the ideal applicant will have in terms of experience, education, and skills, thus increasing the chances of finding the right person for the position. The physician may have personal preferences about educational background, special training, age and personality qualities.

Educational qualifications and skills certainly are important since there is no room for incompetence in a medical setting. Personality is also extremely important because the medical assistant deals with patients. Any assistant chosen should be sincerely interested in people, friendly, cheerful, sympathetic and courteous. Sometimes a job candidate may be highly efficient but the personality may be unsuited to a medical office where the service philosophy must be paramount.

Techniques to help find the right employee
To prepare an advertisement that will attract suitable job applicants the physician should consider some assistance from the newspaper advertising staff.

One point, however, must not be overlooked. The physician cannot discriminate on the base of age, sex, race, religion, marital status, physical defects that would not interfere with reasonable demands of the job, or national origin or ancestry. In recent years such discrimination has been specifically prohibited by the federal government, imposes restrictions on questions that can be asked of job applicants and mandates certain payment schedules and other provisions through the Equal Employment Opportunity Commission and the Wage and Hour Division of the Department of Labor. Fair Employment Practice laws in the states also prohibit any discrimination in hiring and are strictly enforced, with fines imposed for violations. The purpose of these rules and

regulations are to prevent discrimination in the hiring of minorities, women, older persons, the handicapped and others at an employment disadvantage. If unaware of these proscriptions on hiring, one could inadvertently break the law and face legal proceedings, with the possible outlay of thousands of dollars in a settlement to a disappointed and/or disgruntled minority applicant.

Briefly, an ad should be worded screen applicants. Advertising for an "assistant," may get clerical applicants as well as clinical applicants. Advertising only for a "secretary" may attract business secretaries without the special interest and training in the desired medical field.

Unless a physician wants to spend many hours personally talking with many applicants, only a few of them really suited to your needs, it's a good idea to say in an ad: "Reply by letter only, enclosing a resume." The physician might even say that replies should be hand written since legible writing is particularly important in a medical office. Generally, it's advisable to use a box number for replies. As the responses come in, they should be examined for their quality - how well they are completed often indicates how well the applicant will perform on the job. (BUS - Adaptation)

American Association of Medical Assistants
20 N. Wacker Dr., Chicago, IL 60606
312/899-1500

Medical Associations

American Medical Association
515 N. State St., Chicago, IL 60610
312/464-5000

American Medical Women's Association
801 N. Fairfax St., Ste 400, Alexandria, VA 22314
703/838-0500

Australian Medical Association
42 Macquarie Street
Barton, ACT (Australian Capital Territory) 2600
(06) 270-5400 / FAX (06) 270-5499

British Medical Association
BMA House, Tavistock Square
London WCIH 9JP, England
(01) 387-4499

Canadian Medical Association
1867 Alta Vista Dr., Box 8650
Ottawa, Ontario K1G 0G8
613/731-9331

Christian Medical and Dental Society
1616 Gateway Blvd. PO Box 830689
Richardson, TX 75083
214/783-8384

Mexican Medical Association
No longer exists--has disbanded (8/90)

National Medical Association
1012 10th St. NW, Washington, DC 20001
202/347-1895

Pan American Medical Association
222 Kent Terrace, West Palm Beach, FL 33407
407/832-0296

Royal College of Physicians
11 St. Andrew's Place
London NW1 4LE, ENGLAND
Telephone: 01-935-1174

Royal College of Surgeons
35-43 Lincoln's Inn Fields
London WC2A 3PN, ENGLAND
Telephone: 01-405-3474

Southern Medical Association
35 Lake Shore Dr., PO Box 190088
Birmingham, AL 35219-0088
205/945-1840

World Medical Association
(Association Medicale Mondiale-AMM)
28, Avenue des Alpes,
F-01210 Ferney-Voltaire, France
Telephone 50 40 7575
FAX 50 40 5937

Medical Illustration

JAMA Cover Essay.John Curtis Creed, MD
1986 Sept 26; 256(12): 1541

By the mid-1400s, the independent republic of
Florence became the preeminent cultural and
artistic center of Italy. At the epicenter of the
Italian Renaissance was the court of Lorenzo de'
Medici, whose patronage, and that of the Medici
family, had attracted to Florence an
unprecedented concentration of genius in every
branch of the arts. Among the painters, sculptors,
architects, poets, musicians, and philosophers
associated with the Medici during this illustrious
period was Leonardo da Vinci (1452-1519), who
was born in the nearby village of Vinci.

At the Medici court, philosophers had evolved
complex aesthetic ideas based on the writings of
the ancient Greeks and Romans, and it is most
likely from these thinkers that Leonardo was
introduced to the writings of the Roman architect
Vitruvius. Written in the first century BC, Vitruvius'
books on architecture described principles of
numeric proportions and geometric rhythm that
would set the classical style for Italian architecture
in the Renaissance. In addition to Leonardo, the
architects Alberti, Brunelleschi, and Bramante
were also greatly influenced by Vitruvius. So
prevalent was interest in Vitruvius that in 1542 a
Vitruvian Academy of Learning was founded in
Rome. Leonardo's drawing Vitruvian Man
illustrates a passage from Vitruvius' book on
temples, which Leonardo quotes in the text that
borders the drawing.

Among Vitruvius' writings, two passages in
particular had a special influence on Renaissance
builders. In the introduction to the book on the
design to temples, he describes the inherent
harmony of the measured proportions of the
human body, and then goes on to state that the
plan of church buildings should reflect the same
underlying mathematical harmonies. Next, as
proof of man's symmetry and harmony, he
describes how, with hands and feet extended, a

man exactly subtends the most divine, perfect
geometric figures of a circle and a square. It is
these important paragraphs that Leonardo
illustrates and quotes in his drawing Vitruvian
Man, also known as Man in Circle and Square.

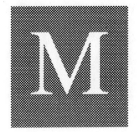

The image of a man in a circle and square was
regarded in the Renaissance as an icon
symbolizing the creation of man in the image of
God. Art historian Kenneth Clark has written that
"it is impossible to exaggerate what this simple
looking proposition meant to the men of the
Renaissance...it was the foundation of the whole
philosophy." Leonardo's friend, the mathematician
Luca Pacioli, summarized the metaphysical
interest in this concept in his book Divina
Proportione.

After having considered the right arrangement of
the human body the ancients proportioned all their
works, particularly the temples, in accordance with
it. For in the human body they find the two main
figures without which it is impossible to achieve
anything, namely the perfect circle ... and the
square.

Leonardo left Florence sometime between 1481
and 1483 to serve the powerful and militaristic
Duke of Milan, Lodovico Sforza. In a letter to
Lodovico, boasting of his many talents, Leonardo
cited first his skill as an architect and military
engineer, adding only later, "and I can do in
painting whatever may be done as well as any
other, be he whom he may." When Lodovico
commissioned Leonardo to design a church in
Pavia, in 1490, Leonardo naturally turned to
Vitruvius' classic work on temples for guidance,
Leonardo probably drew Vitruvian Man that same
year.

During his years in Milan, Leonardo is thought to
have been associated with the celebrated
architect Bramante, also at the court of Lodovico
Sforza. Both of them designed church buildings in
the style characteristic of the Italian Renaissance,
that is, following a central plan based on the
Vitruvian perfect circle. During the period when
Leonardo drew Vitruvian Man, he filled his
notebooks with sketches for church buildings
based on overlying patterns of circles and
squares. In fact, one of these sketches
corresponds very closely to Bramante's first
scheme for St. Peter's in Rome.

In the text accompanying Vitruvian Man, Leonardo
writes (in mirror-image print, from right to left),
"Vitruvius the architect says in his work on
architecture that the measurements of the human
body are determined by nature as follows: that
four fingers make one palm and four palms make
one foot, six palms make one cubit." Having
calibrated the scale below the figure in units of
"thumbs" and "palms," he then goes on to note
several other Vitruvian measurements, including
"the length of a man's outspread arms is equal to
his height."

Leonardo draws here with sharp, clear lines and
bold, horizontal cross-hatching, as he did when
drawing for demonstration and clarity. Instead of
straining the figure in order to center both the
circle and the square on the umbilicus, as other
artists had done, Leonardo lowers the square to
the symphysis pubis and widens the stance,
forming the third geometric figure, the equilateral

triangle, along the lower extremities. This alteration creates a pleasing sense of balance and stability. Some authors have postulated that the divine circle, centered on the umbilicus, might be taken as a generative, maternal symbol, while the square, centered on the pubis, could be thought of as a product of the man, "foursquare," representing the earth and masculinity. However, Leonardo makes it clear that he depicts not an abstraction but a physical, human subject: the feet rest naturally on the surfaces and the arms stretch easily to the boundaries.

In this single drawing, one can begin to sense the breadth of Leonardo's legacy. In it, the historian can identify the links between ancient Rome and the high Renaissance courts of Lorenzo de' Medici and Lodovico Sforza. The mathematician might find the Vitruvian mathematical and geometric formulas intriguing. The student of architecture can see in the drawing the conceptual basis for the Renaissance centrally planned church. The physician can recognize Leonardo's proficiency in the study of human anatomy. And, finally, the philosopher can interpret in the in the drawing Leonardo's vision of man - harmoniously created in the image of God, reaching to touch perfection.

note: *Vitruvian Man*, 1490, DaVinci, Leonardo. Italian. Pen and ink on paper. 34.3 x 22.3 cm.

Medical Illustrator
History: Formal educational programs for the medical illustrator date back to the early 1900s with Max Broedel's school at Johns Hopkins. The Association of Medical Illustrators (AMI) was established in 1945. Under the auspices of the AMI, standards were developed by which the organization has accredited medical illustration programs in this country since 1967.

In 1986, the AMI expressed a desire to have educational programs for the medical illustrator accredited by the Committee on Allied Health Education and Accreditation (CAHEA) of the American Medical Association (AMA). This desire stemmed from the recognition that professional medical illustrators programs were more closely related to allied health than to the visual arts.

An Ad Hoc Committee on Outside Accreditation of the AMI worked with staff of the AMA Division of Allied Health Education and Accreditation to modify the existing standards to comply with the format recommended by CAHEA. The resulting Essential and Guidelines of an Accredited Educational Program for the Medical Illustrator were adopted by the AMI and the AMA Council on Medical Education in 1987.

Occupational Description: The term medical illustrator applies to persons of professional competence in the discipline of medical illustration. Medical illustrators create visual material designed to facilitate the recording and dissemination of medical, biological, and related knowledge through communication media. The medical illustration profession embraces not only production of such material but also consultant, advisory, and administrative functions. Medical illustration employs a variety of artistic techniques, ranging from drawing, painting, sculpting, layout, design, and typography to computer graphics and electronic imaging.

With a strong foundation in biological sciences, physiology, pathology, and general medical knowledge, combined with a high degree of proficiency in the artistic skills, medical illustrators are able to depict subjects with extreme accuracy and realism or to interpret and reduce a complex idea to a simple explanatory diagram or schematic concept.

Job Description: Through the medical graphics they create, medical artists are communicators and teachers. Although some medical illustrators specialize in a single art medium or confine their interest to one of the medical specialties, the majority handle an ever-changing variety of assignments. They work with many different media to produce the highly accurate and authentic illustrations used in the publication of medical books, journals, films, video tapes, exhibits, posters, wall charts, and computer programs. Materials prepared by medical illustrators may also be used for projection in the classroom or for professional group presentations.

A medical artist may also work as a member of a research team to provide illustrations or to participate directly in the research problem. Some specialize in preparing prosthetics or in preparing models for instructional purposes.

In addition to the production of graphics and three-dimensional works, medical illustrators may serve as producers/directors or designers in the development of instructional programs. They may also organize and administer biomedical communication centers or illustration services at major teaching hospitals, health science centers, or elsewhere.

Employment Characteristics: The majority of medical illustrators are employed by medical schools and large medical centers that conduct teaching and research programs; others are in private, state, and federal hospitals; clinic; and dental and veterinary schools. Many work independently on a free-lance basis for medical publishers, for pharmaceutical houses and advertising agencies, in commercial settings, or for lawyers. Medical illustrators with appropriate background and professional experience are qualified to direct an illustration service unit or a biomedical communication center.

AMA Allied Health Department
312/464-4622

Association of Medical Illustrators
1819 Peachtree St, NE, Suite 560
Atlanta, GA 30309
404/350-7900

Medical Laboratory Technician
History: The American Society of Clinical Pathologists (ASCP) began program accreditation review as one of the functions of its Board of Registry of Medical Technologists in 1933, working with the AMA Council on Medical education. The first set of Essentials of an Acceptable School for Clinical Laboratory Technicians was prepared by the ASCP Board of Registry and subsequently adopted by the AMA House of Delegates in 1937. The first list of 211 accredited programs was issued by the ASCP Board of Registry in 1933. The program title was

changed to medical technology in 1947 with that year's revised Essentials/

The American Society for Medical Technology (ASMT) was organized in 1932. ASMT joined ASCP in periodic revisions of the Essentials and was represented on the ASCP Board of Registry and the ASCP Board of Schools (established in 1949). The ASMT was recognized by the Council on Medical Education as one of the organizations collaborating with the AMA in accrediting educational programs.

In 1972, representatives of ASMT and ASCP began talks that culminated in the Incorporation of the National Accrediting Agency for Clinical Laboratory Sciences (NAACLS) in October 1973 as an organization that is independent of the professional organizations and to which the authority to approve Essentials was delegated. NAACLS is the first agency of its kind to conduct the process of detailed program review and recommendations upon which CAHEA accredits programs.

Units within NAACLS include the review board, three program review committees, and the executive office staff. The board is the governing unit. The bylaws provide for sponsoring and participating organization representation on the board. ASCP and ASMT are sponsoring organizations. Current participating organizations are the American Society for Microbiology and the National Society for Histotechnology. In addition to the representatives from these professional organizations, the membership of the board includes two college educators, one public member, a technologist laboratory administrator, and one technician practitioner.

The program review committees include technologist and pathologist program officials, and educator/practitioners.

In addition to the work associated with conducting program reviews, NAACLS provides workshops and publishes a periodic newsletter, as well as information for students and occasional monographs dealing with issues in accreditation.

Histologic Technician/Technologist

Occupational Description: Physicians (usually pathologists) and other scientists specializing in biological sciences or related clinical areas, such as chemistry, work in partnership with medical laboratory workers to analyze blood, tissues, and fluids from humans (and sometimes animals), using a variety of precision instruments. The results of these tests are used to detect and diagnose disease and other abnormalities.

The main responsibility of the histologic technician/technologist in the clinical laboratory is preparing sections of body tissue for examination by a pathologist. This includes the preparation of tissue specimens of human and animal origin for diagnostic, research, or teaching purposes. Tissue sections prepared by the histologic technician/technologist for a variety of disease entities enable the pathologist to diagnose body dysfunction and malignancy.

Job Description: Histotechnicians process sections of body tissue by fixation, dehydration, embedding, sectioning, decalcification, microincineration, mounting, and routine and special staining. Histotechnologists perform all the functions of the histotechnician as well as the more complex procedures for processing tissues. They identify tissue structures, cell components, and their staining characteristics, and relate them to physiological functions; implement and test new techniques and procedures; make judgments concerning the results of quality control measures; and institute proper procedures to maintain accuracy and precision. Histotechnologists apply the principles of management and supervision when they function as section supervisors and of educational methodology when they teach students.

Employment Characteristics: Most histologic technologists work in hospital laboratories, averaging a 40-hour week. Salaries vary depending on the employer and geographic location.

Occupational Description: Laboratory tests play an important role in the detection, diagnosis, and treatment of many diseases. Medical laboratory workers perform these tests under the supervision or direction of pathologists (physicians who diagnose the causes and nature of disease) and other physicians, or scientists who specialize in clinical chemistry, microbiology, or the other biological sciences. Medical laboratory workers develop data on the blood, tissues, and fluids in the human body by using a variety of precision instruments.

Job Description: Medical laboratory technicians (associate degree) perform all of the routine tests in an up-to-date medical laboratory and can demonstrate discrimination between closely similar items and correction of errors by use of pre-set strategies. The technician has knowledge of specific techniques and instruments and is able to recognize factors which directly affect procedures and results. Form confirmation of results, the technician conducts more than one test for each specialty area. The technician also monitors quality control programs within predetermined parameters.

Employment Characteristics: Most medical laboratory personnel work in hospital laboratories, averaging a 40-hour week. Salaries vary depending on the employer and geographic location.

According to a 1990 CAHEA Annual Supplementary Survey, entry level salaries average $18,460 (ALL).

AMA Department of Allied Health
312/464-4625

Medical Practice Acts

Code of Alabama 1975
Title 34; Chapter 24 "Physicians and other
Practitioners of the Healing Arts"
sections 34-24-1 through 34-24-406

Alaska Statutes 1987
Title 8: Chapter 64 "Medicine"
sections 08.64.010 through 08.64.380

Arizona Revised Statutes Annotated 1992
Title 32; Chapter 13 "Medicine and Surgery"
sections 32-1401 through 32-1491

Arkansas Code of 1987 Annotated:
Official Edition 1992
Title 17; Chapter 93 "Physicians and Surgeons"
sections 17-93-101 through 17-93-505

West's Annotated California Codes 1990
Division 2; Chapter 5 "Medicine"
sections 2.5.2000 through 2.5.2505

Colorado Revised Statutes 1985
Title 12; Article 36 "Medical Practice"
sections 12-36-101 through 12-36-136

General Statutes of Connecticut 1987
Title 20; Chapter 370 "Medicine and Surgery"
sections 20-8 through 20-14g

Delaware Code Annotated 1974
Title 24; Chapter 17 "Medical Practices Act"
sections 1701 through 1795

District of Columbia Code 1989
Title 2; Chapter 33 "Health Occupations"
sections 2-3301.0 through 2-3312.1

West's Florida Statutes Annotated 1991
Title 32; Chapter 458 "Medical Practice"
sections 458.001 through 458.349

Code of Georgia Annotated 1985
Chapter 84-9 "Medical Practitioners"
sections 84-901 through 84-936

Hawaii Revised Statutes 1985
Title 25; Chapter 453 "Medicine and Surgery"
sections 453-1 through 453-33

Idaho Code 1979
Title 54; Chapter 18 "Physicians and Surgeons"
sections 54-1801 through 54-1841

Smith-Hurd Illinois Annotated Statutes
Chapter 111 "Physicians";
sections 4401 through 4479

Burns Indiana Statutes Annotated:
Code Edition 1991
Title 25; Article 22.5 "Medicine, Physicians
Surgeons and Osteopaths"
sections 25-22-2-2 through 25-22-59-14.5

Iowa Code Annotated 1989
Title 8; Chapter 148 "Practice of Medicine
and Surgery"
sections 148.1 through 148.13

Kansas Statutes Official 1985
Chapter 65; Article 28 "Healing Arts"
sections 65-2801 through 65-28,122

Kentucky Revised Statutes Official Edition 1990
Title 26; Chapter 311 "Physicians,
Osteopaths and Podiatrists"
sections 311.010 through 311.992

Louisiana Statutes Annotated 1988
Title 37; Chapter 15 "Physicians, Surgeons,
Osteopaths, and Midwives"
sections 37:1261 through 37:1360.27

Maine Revised Statutes Annotated 1964
Title 32; Chapter 48 "Board of Registration
in Medicine"
sections 3263 through 3300

Annotated Code of Maryland 1991
Title 14 "Physicians"
sections 14-101 through 14-702

Annotated Laws of Massachusetts 1991
Title XVI; Chapter 112 "Registration of Physicians
and Surgeons"
sections 112:2 through 112:12CC

Michigan Statutes Annotated 1988
Title 14; Part 170 "Medicine"
sections 14.15(17001) through 14.15(17088)

Minnesota Statutes Annotated 1988
Chapter 147 "Physicians and
Surgeons, Osteopaths"
sections 147.01 through 147.33

Mississippi Code 1972 Annotated
Title 73, Chapter 25 "Physicians"
sections 73-25-1 through 73-25-95

Vernon's Annotated Missouri Statutes 1988
Title XXII; Chapter 334 "Physicians and Surgeons,
Physical Therapists and Athletic Trainers"
sections 334.010 through 334.748

Montana Code Annotated 1991
Title 37; Chapter 3 "Medicine"
sections 37-3-101 through 37-3-405

Revised Statutes of Nebraska 1943
Chapter 71 "Practice of Medicine and Surgery"
sections 71-1,102 through 71-1,107.30

Nevada Revised Statutes 1985
Title 54; Chapter 630 "Physicians and Assistants"
sections 630-003 through 630-411

New Hampshire Revised Statutes Annotated 1984
Title XXX; Chapter 329 "Physicians and Surgeons"
sections 329:1 through 329:31

New Jersey Statutes Annotated 1991
Title 45; Chapter 9 "Medicine and Surgery"
sections 45:9-1 through 45:9-58

New Mexico Statutes of 1978 Annotated
Chapter 61; Article 6 "Medicine and Surgery"
sections 61-6-1 through 61-6-35

McKinney's Consolidated Laws of New York Annotated 1985
Title 8; Article 131 "Medicine"
sections 6520 through 6529

General Statutes of North Carollina 1985
Chapter 90; Article 1 "Practice of Medicine"
sections 90-1 through 90-21.21

North Dakota Century Code Annotated
Title 43; Chapter 47-17 "Physicians and Surgeons"
sections 43-17-01 through 43-17-42

Page's Ohio Revised Code Annotated
Title 47; Chapter 4731 "Physicians ..."
sections 4731.01 through 4731.99

Oklahoma Statutes Annotated 1989
Title 59; Chapter 11 "Medicine"
sections 481 through 536.11

Oregon Revised Statutes 1985
Title 52A; Chapter 677 "Regulation of Medicine, Podiatry and Related Medical Services"
sections 677.010 through 677.810

Purdon's Pennsylvania Statutes Annotated
Title 63; Chapter 12 "Physicians and Surgeons"
sections 422.1 through 422.45

General Laws of Rhode Island
Chapter 37 "Board of Medical Licensure and Discipline"
sections 5-37-1 through 5-37-32

Code of Laws of South Carolina 1976
Title 40; Chapter 47 "Physicians, Surgeons and Osteopaths"
sections 40-47-660 through

South Dakota Codified Laws
Title 36; Chapter 36-4 "Physicians and Surgeons"
sections 36-4-1 through 36-4-40

Tennessee Code Annotated
Title 63; Chapter 6 "Medicine and Surgery"
sections 63-6-101 through 63-6-503

Vernon's Texas Annotated Civil Statutes
Chapter 6 "Medicine"
articles 4495b through 4512m

Utah Code Annotated 1953
Title 58; Chapter 12 "Practice of Medicine and Surgery and the Treatment of Human Ailments"
part 5 "Medical Malpractice Act"
sections 58-12-26 through 58-12-43

Vermont Statutes Annotated 1989
Title 26; Chapter 23 "Medicine and Surgery"
sections 1311 through 1449

Code of Virginia 1950, Annotated
Title 54.1; Chapter 29 "Medicine and Other Healing Arts"
sections 54.1-2900 through 54.1-2993

West's Revised Code of Washington Annotated
Title 18; Chapter 18.71 "Physicians"
sections 18.71.01. through 18.71.941

West Virginia Code
Chapter 30; article 3 "West Virginia Medical Practice Act"
sections 30-3-1 through 30-3-17

West's Wisconsin Statutes Annotated
Chapter 448, Chapter 448 "Medical Practices"
sections 448.01 through 448.40

Wyoming Statutes Annotated
Title 33; Chapter 26 "Physicians and Surgeons"
sections 33-26-101 through 33-26-511

Medical Records
Record Retention
Whether retiring or selling the practice, a physician should start making arrangements for handling the office's medical records at least three months before closing. What are the rules for record retention after closing an office?

How Long Should Medical Records Be Kept?
There are no hard and fast rules. When there is no legal requirement, which is the case in most states, records should be kept for the period of the statute of limitations for professional liability (the length of time in which a suit can be filed).

The time period varies from state to state, but is usually under ten years. The local state or county medical society should be contacted in order to find out what the local laws are.

It should be noted, too, that the statute of limitations does not begin running for children until they reach the age of majority-usually eighteen. In many states, the statute of limitations is two years from the date of discovery. If the practice specialty is pediatrics or obstetrics or otherwise involves treatment of children, some records should be retained possibly a minimum of thirty years.

It may be advantageous to retain some records for a "reasonable amount of time" beyond the statute. Records should be available in the event that patients want them. Of course, only four or five patients in a couple of thousand may actually contact their physician for the record. But it may make a dramatic difference to that person if the record is available. For instance, women whose mothers took DES during their pregnancy have been grateful to physicians who retained records containing the information.

How to Decide Which Records to Keep? Unless unlimited storage space is available, it will be necessary to set some guidelines for which records to keep and which to purge. As a rule, the physician can discard records of patients seen only once for a routine checkup or procedure and of patients with uncomplicated problems who haven't been seen in a number of years.

Deceased patients' records can be destroyed a few years after their death. Once the estate is closed, and any statute of limitations for wrongful death actions has run, no suits for professional liability can be brought.

The physician should retain records of active patients. How is active defined? Where is the cutoff in terms of the date of the last visit or the complexity of the case? Once again, the judgment call is the physician's to make.

Even if a physician is a part of a group practice or partnership that will retain the patient's records after the physician leaves, purging inactive records before terminating the business relationship is a good idea. Inactive files should not take up valuable space from colleagues.

In What Form Should a Medical Record be Transferred? The physician owns the original hard copy of the record and therefore should keep it. If a patient requests the forwarding of a file to a new doctor, the original physician has two options. He or she can either photocopy the entire contents, letting the new physician decide what to retain, or a summary of the record can be made. The summary is preferable if there are notes in short hand or if the physician's handwriting is illegible.

What if Patient Owes on Account? Is the Physician Obliged to Transfer the Patient's Record If Requested? The physician can't refuse to forward a record because a patient owes money. Nor should such information be in the medical record. If it is, it may be a violation of state or federal laws.

Should a Copy of the Record be Given to the Patient? A number of states have passed laws granting patients the access to their medical records. Note, however, that you should provide a copy, not the original.

What Are the Options for Storing Medical Records? When closing a practice, the physician faces the decision of where to store medical records. There are several options:
- The local medical society must be contacted. Some have storage centers or know of others in the community.
- Is there room in the physician's basement, attic, or garage? Does the physician intend to stay in that location? Are these places dry and safe?
- The physician should check out storage companies in the area and what they charge for retrieving a record.

What About Microfilm? Microfilming records may or may not be the answer to the physician's storage problems. The initial cost can be high, depending on the size and number of charts. The major cost is for labor to prepare the record for filming. The physician may want to select only certain material for filming, which will require review of each record. Then there is the removing of staples and paper clips and putting the papers in the proper sequence.

What Can Be Done with X-ray Film? If the physician retains the report in the x-ray, the information is probably sufficient, If, for any reason, the x-ray might be needed later, it should be kept. X-rays may be turned in for their silver value. The physician should call the local medical society to find out who in the area might be interested in the films for their silver content.

How Are Records Destroyed? The physician should find a way in which the records will not fall into the hands of someone outside who might use them. If a refuse service picks up the records, the physician should make sure they will be burned. The records should be cut or torn in half before being disposed. (CLO - Adaptation)

American Association for Medical Transcription
PO Box 576187, Modesto, CA 95357
800/982-2182; 209/576-0883

American Health Information Management Association (Formerly American Medical Records Association)
919 N. Michigan Ave., Ste 1400
Chicago, IL 60611
312/787-2672 800/621-6828

Medical Information Bureau
PO Box 105, Essex Station, Boston, MA 02112
617/426-3660

"Medical Records: Getting Yours"
Available for $5.00:
Health Research Group, Publications Manager
2000 P St, NW, Suite 700, Washington, DC 20036

"Your Health Information Belongs to You"
American Health Information Management Association
919 N. Michigan Ave., Ste 1400
Chicago, IL 60611
312/787-2672, 800/621-6828

Principles of Medical Record Documentation

The following principles of medical documentation have been developed jointly by representatives of the American Health Information Management Association, the American Hospital Association, the American Managed Care and Review Association, the American Medical Association, the American Medical Peer Review Association, the Blue Cross and Blue Shield Association, and the Health Insurance Association of America. Although their joint development is not intended to imply either endorsement of or opposition to specific documentation requirements, all seven groups share the belief that the fundamental reason for maintaining an adequate medical record should be its contribution to the high quality of medical care.

- *Principles of Documentation*:
  The medical record should be complete and legible.
- The documentation of each patient encounter should include: the date; the reason for the encounter; appropriate history and physical exam; review of lab, x-ray data, and other ancillary services, where appropriate; assessment; and plan care (including discharge plan, if appropriate).
- Past and present diagnoses should be accessible to the treating and/or consulting physician.
- The reasons for and results of x-rays, lab tests, and other ancillary services should be documented or included in the medical record.
- Relevant health risk factors should be identified.

- The patient's progress, including response to treatment, change in treatment, change in diagnosis, and patient non-compliance, should be documented.
- The written plan for care should include, when appropriate: treatments and medications, specifying frequency and dosage; any referrals and consultations; patient/family education; and specific instructions for follow-up.
- The documentation should support the intensity of the patient evaluation and/or the treatment, including thought processes and the complexity of medical decision-making.
- All entries to the medical record should be dated and authenticated.
- The CPT/ICD-9 codes reported on the health insurance claim form or billing statement should reflect the documentation in the medical record.

Medical Record Administrator

History: Standards for educational programs for medical record administrators (formerly librarians) were established in 1935 by the American Medical Record Association (AMRA) through its committee on training. The first four programs for medical record administrators were accredited in that year, three of which were hospital-based and one of which was a college-based program. In 1942, AMRA invited the American Medical Association (AMA) to serve as the official accrediting agency for educational programs for medical record administrators. This responsibility was accepted by the House of Delegates of the AMA. Essentials for educational programs for medical record administrators were initially developed and adopted in 1943 and were subsequently revised in 1952, 1960, 1967, 1974, 1981, and 1988.

In 1953, the Essentials for educational programs for medical record technicians were established and approved by both the American Medical Record Association and the American Medical Association. The first educational programs for medical record technicians were hospital-based. Over the years there has been a gradual transition from hospital-based educational programs for medical record administrators and medical record technicians to college- and university-based programs. In 1965, 1976, 1983, and 1988, the American Medical Record Association in collaboration with the AMA Council on Medical Education revised and adopted the Essentials for educational programs for medical record technicians. In 1988, one set of Essentials was adopted addressing both the medical record technician and administration programs.

Occupational Description: Medical records administrators manage health information systems consistent with the medical, administrative, ethical and legal requirements of the health care delivery system. Although medical record administrators are not often directly involved in patient contact, their work with the medical and hospital administrative staff is of critical importance to patient care. Because medical record administrators deal with patient records and information, they should not be confused with medical librarians who work chiefly with books, periodicals, and other medical publications.

Job description: The medical record administrator is the professional responsible for the management of health information systems consistent with professional standards and the medical administrative, ethical, and legal requirements of the health care delivery system. The medical record administrator possesses the administrative knowledge and skills necessary to plan and develop health information systems which meet standards of accrediting and regulating agencies; design health information systems appropriate for various sizes and types of health care facilities; manage the human, financial, and physical resources of a health information service; participate in medical staff and institutional activities including utilization management, risk management, and quality assessment; collect and analyze patient and facility data for reimbursement, facility planning, marketing, risk management, quality assessment and research; serve as an advocate for privacy and confidentiality of health information; plan and offer inservice educational programs for health care personnel.

Employment Characteristics: The demand for medical record administrators is greatest in hospitals. Other growing areas of employment are ambulatory and long-term health care facilities, state health departments, peer review organizations, government agencies, and private industry. Medical record administrators interested in teaching may accept faculty appointments in academic programs for medical record administrators and medical record technicians.

According to the 1990 CAHEA Annual Supplemental Survey, entry level salaries average $22,918. (ALL)

Medical Record Technician

Occupational Description: the medical record is a permanent document prepared for each person treated in a health care facility. It contains the "who, what, why, where, when, and how" details of patient care during diagnosis and treatment, as well as information of medical, scientific, and legal value. Medical record technicians (MRT) are important members of the health care team. Traditionally, medical record technicians have been employed in the medical record department of hospitals. With the increasing expansion of health care needs, opportunities for employment are also available in ambulatory health care facilities, industrial clinics, state and federal health agencies, long-term care facilities, and in a number of other areas.

Job Description: The medical record technician is the professional responsible for maintaining components of health information systems consistent with the medical, administrative, ethical, legal accreditation, and regulatory requirements of the health care delivery system. In all types of facilities, and in various locations within a facility, the medical record technician possesses the technical knowledge and skills necessary to process, maintain, compile, and report health information data reimbursement, utilization management, quality assessment and research; abstract and code clinical data using appropriate classification systems; and analyze health records according to standards. The medical record technician may be responsible for functional supervision of the various components of the health information system.

Employment Characteristics: Although the demand for medical record technicians is greatest in hospitals, other growing areas of employment may include nursing homes, out-patient clinics, rehabilitation centers, state and local health departments, and large group medical practices.

According to the 1990 CAHEA Annual Supplemental Survey, entry level salaries average $18,170.

AMA Allied Health Department
312/464-4622

Medical Schools, U.S.
Association of American Medical Colleges
2450 N Street, N.W., Washington, DC 20037
202/828-0400

Alabama
University of Alabama School of Medicine
UAB Station, Birmingham, AL 35294
205/934-1111

University of South Alabama College of Medicine
307 University Boulevard, Mobile, AL 36688
205/460-7174

Arizona
University of Arizona College of Medicine
Arizona Health Sciences Center
1501 North Campbell Ave., Tucson, AZ 85724
602/626-6214

Arkansas
University of Arkansas College of Medicine
4301 W. Markham St., Little Rock, AR 72205
501/686-5000

California
Loma Linda University School of Medicine
Loma Linda, CA 92350
714/824-4462

Stanford University School of Medicine
300 Pasteur Dr., Stanford, CA 94305
415/723-6951

University of California
Davis School of Medicine, Davis, CA 95616
916/752-0331

University of California
Irvine College of Medicine, Irvine, CA 92717
714/856-5925

University of California, Los Angeles
UCLA School of Medicine
10833 La Conte Ave.
Los Angles, CA 90024
213/825-9111

University of California, San Diego
School of Medicine, La Jolla, CA 92093
619/534-3713

University of California, San Francisco
School of Medicine
San Francisco, CA 94143-0410
415/476-2342

University of Southern California
School of Medicine
1975 Zonal Ave., Los Angeles, CA 90033
213/224-7001

Colorado
University of Colorado School of Medicine
4200 E. Ninth Ave., Denver, CO 80262
303/399-1211

Connecticut
University of Connecticut School of Medicine
263 Farmington Ave., Farmington, CT 06032
203/679-2000

Yale University School of Medicine
333 Cedar St., PO Box 3333
New Haven, CT 06510
203/423-4771

District of Columbia
George Washington University
School of Medicine and Health Sciences
2300 Eye St., N.W., Washington, DC 20037
202/994-3266

Georgetown University School of Medicine
3900 Reservoir Rd., N.W., Washington, DC 20007
202/687-1164

Howard University College of Medicine
520 W. St., N.W., Washington, DC 20059
202/806-6270

Florida
University of Florida College of Medicine
Box J-215, J. Hillis Miller Health Center
Gainesville, FL 32610
904/392-3701

University of Miami School of Medicine
1600 N.W. 10th Ave., PO Box 016960 (R59)
Miami, FL 33101
305/547-6545

University of South Florida College of Medicine
12901 Bruce B. Downs Blvd.
Tampa, FL 33612-4799
813/974-4950

Georgia
Emory University School of Medicine
Woodruff Health Sciences Center
Administration Building
1440 Clifton Rd., N.E., Atlanta, GA 30322
404/727-5650

Medical College of Georgia School of Medicine
1120 Fifteenth St., Augusta, GA 30912
404/721-0211

Mercer University School of Medicine
1550 College St., Macon, GA 31207
912/744-2600

Morehouse School of Medicine
720 Westview Dr., S.W., Atlanta, GA 30310-1495
404/752-1500

Hawaii
University of Hawaii
John A. Burns School of Medicine
1960 East-West Rd., Honolulu, HI 96822
808/948-8287

Illinois
Loyola University of Chicago
Stritch School of Medicine
2160 S. First Ave., Maywood, IL 60153
708-216-9192

Northwestern University Medical School
303 E. Chicago, Ave., Chicago, IL 60611
312/908-8649

Rush Medical College of Rush University
600 S. Paulina St., Chicago, IL 60612
312/942-6913

Southern Illinois University School of Medicine
801 N. Rutledge, PO Box 19230
Springfield, IL 62794
217/782-3318

University of Chicago
Pritzker School of Medicine
5841 S. Maryland Ave., Chicago, IL 60637
312/702-1000

University of Health Sciences/
Chicago Medical School
3333 Green Bay Rd., North Chicago, IL 60064
312/578-3000

University of Illinois College of Medicine (UIC)
PO Box 6998 (M/C 784), Chicago, IL 60680
312/996-3500

UIC - College of Medicine at Peoria
One Illini Dr., PO Box 1649, Peoria, IL 61656
309/671-3000

UIC - College of Medicine Rockford
1601 Park Ave., Rockford, IL 61107
815/395-5600

Indiana
Indiana University School of Medicine
Indiana University Medical Center
1120 S. Drive, Indianapolis, IN 46202-5114
317/274-8157

Iowa
University of Iowa College of Medicine
200 Human Biology Research Facility
Iowa City, IA 52242
319/335-8050

Kansas
University of Kansas Medical Center School of
Medicine
39th and Rainbow Blvd., Kansas City, KS 66103
913/588-5283

Kentucky
University of Kentucky College of Medicine
A.B. Chandler Medical Center
800 Rose St., Lexington, KY 40536-0084
606/233-5000

University of Louisville School of Medicine
Health Sciences Center, Louisville, KY 40292
502/588-5184

Louisiana
Louisiana State University,
School of Medicine New Orleans
1542 Tulane Ave., New Orleans, LA 70112-2822
504/568-4006

Louisiana State University,
School of Medicine in Shreveport
PO Box 33932, Shreveport, LA 71130-3932
318/647-5000

Tulane University School of Medicine
1430 Tulane Ave., New Orleans, LA 70112
504/588-5263

Maryland
Johns Hopkins University School of Medicine
720 Rutland Ave., Baltimore, MD 21205
301/955-5000

JAMA Theme Issue: Johns Hopkins
JAMA. 1989 Jun 2; 261(21)
A theme issue of JAMA which commemorates the
centennial of this medical institution. Subjects
range from DNA markers in Huntington's disease,
the attitudes and practices of medical students
and house staff regarding alcoholism, to a essay
about Johns Hopkins' first century. The cover
features a 1906 portrait of the four founders of the
institution by American painter John Singer
Sargent.

Uniformed Services University
of the Health Sciences
F. Edward Hebert School of Medicine
4301 Jones Bridge Rd.
Bethesda, MD 20814-4799
301/295-3013

University of Maryland School of Medicine
655 W. Baltimore St., Baltimore, MD 21201
301/328-7410

Massachusetts
Boston University School of Medicine
80 E. Concord St., Boston, MA 02118
617/638-8000

Harvard Medical School
25 Shattuck St., Boston, MA 02115
617/732-1000

Tufts University School of Medicine
136 Harrison Ave., Boston, MA 02111
617/956-6565

University of Massachusetts Medical School
55 Lake Ave, North, Worcester, MA 01655
508/856-0011

Michigan
Michigan State University
College of Human Medicine
East Lansing, MI 48824
517/353-1730

University of Michigan Medical School
1301 Catherine Rd., Medical Sciences Building I
Ann Arbor, MI 48109-0624
313/763-9600

Wayne State University School of Medicine
540 E. Canfield, Detroit, MI 48201
313/577-1460

Minnesota
Mayo Medical School
200 First St., S.W., Rochester, MN 55905
507/384-3671

University of Minnesota, Duluth
School of Medicine
10 University Drive, Duluth, MN 55812
218/726-7571

University of Minnesota Medical
School-Minneapolis
UMHC Box 293, 420 Delaware St., S.E.,
Minneapolis, MN 55455
612/624-1188

Mississippi
University of Mississippi School of Medicine
2500 N. State St., Jackson, MS 39216
601/984-1000

Missouri
Saint Louis University School of Medicine
1402 South Grand Blvd, Saint Louis, MO 63104
314/577-8000

University of Missouri
Columbia School of Medicine
One Hospital Drive, Columbia, MO 65212
314/884-1566

University of Missouri
Kansas City School of Medicine
2411 Holmes Street, Kansas City, MO 64108
816/276-1800

Washington University School of Medicine
660 South Euclid Avenue, Saint Louis, MO 63110
314/362-5000

Nebraska
Creighton University School of Medicine
California at 24th Street, Omaha, NE 68178
402/280-2900

University of Nebraska College of Medicine
42nd Street and Dewey Ave., Omaha, NE 68105
402/559-4000

Nevada
University of Nevada School of Medicine
Reno, NV 89577-0046
702/784-6001

New Hampshire
Dartmouth Medical School
Hanover, NH 03756
603/646-7505

New Jersey
University of Medicine and Dentistry of New Jersey
New Jersey Medical School
185 South Orange Ave, Newark, NJ 07103-2757
201/456-4300

University of Medicine and Dentistry of New Jersey
Robert Wood Johnson Medical School
675 Hoes Lane, Piscataway, NJ 08854-5635
201/463-1966

New Mexico
University of New Mexico School of Medicine
Albuquerque, NM 87131
505/277-2413

New York
Albany Medical College
47 New Scotland Ave., Albany, NY 12208
518/445-5582

Albert Einstein College of Medicine of Yeshiva
University
1300 Morris Park Ave., Bronx, NY 10461
212/430-2000

Columbia University College of Physicians and
Surgeons
630 West 168th St., New York, NY 10032
212/305-3592

Cornell University Medical College
1300 York Ave., New York, NY 10021
212/746-5454

Mount Sinai School of Medicine of the City
University of NY
One Gustave L. Levy Place, New York NY 10029
212/241-6500

New York Medical College
Sunshine Cottage, Valhalla, NY 10595
914/993-4000

New York University School of Medicine
550 First Ave., New York, NY 10016
212/340-7300

State University of New York
Health Science Center at Brooklyn,
College of Medicine
450 Clarkson Ave., Brooklyn, NY 11203
718/270-1000

State University of New York at Buffalo
School of Medicine and Biomedical Sciences
3435 Main St., Buffalo, NY 14214
716/831-2775

State University of New York at Stony Brook
Health Sciences Center
School of Medicine, Stony Brook, NY 11794
516/444-2080

State University of New York
Health Science Center of Syracuse,
College of Medicine
750 East Adams St., Syracuse, NY 13210
315/473-5540

University of Rochester School
of Medicine and Dentistry
601 Elmwood Ave., Rochester, NY 14642
716/275-3407

North Carolina
Bowman Gray School of Medicine
of Wake Forest University
300 South Hawthorne Road
Winston-Salem, NC 27103
919/748-2011

Duke University School of Medicine
PO Box 3005, Durham, NC 27710
919/684-8111

East Carolina University School of Medicine
Greenville, NC 27858-4354
919/551-2201

University of North Carolina at Chapel Hill
School of Medicine, Chapel Hill, NC 27599
919/966-4161

North Dakota
University of North Dakota School of Medicine
501 North Columbia Road
Grand Forks, ND 58201
701/777-2514

Ohio
Case Western Reserve University
School of Medicine
2119 Abington Road, Cleveland, OH 44106
216/368-2000

Medical College of Ohio
Caller Service No. 10008, Toledo, OH 43699
419/381-4172

Northeastern Ohio Universities
College of Medicine
4209 State Route 44, PO Box 95
Rootstown, OH 44272
216/325-2511

Ohio State University College of Medicine
370 West Ninth Ave., Columbus, OH 43210
614/292-5674

University of Cincinnati College of Medicine
231 Bethesda Ave., Cincinnati, OH 45267
513/558-7391

Wright State University School of Medicine
PO Box 927, Dayton, OH 45401-0927
513/873-3010

Oklahoma
University of Oklahoma College of Medicine
PO Box 26901, Oklahoma City, OK 73190
405/271-2265

Oregon
Oregon Health Sciences University
School of Medicine
3181 S.W. Sam Jackson Park Road
Portland, OR 97201
503/279-8311

Pennsylvania
Hahnemann University School of Medicine
Broad and Vine Streets, Philadelphia, PA 19102
215/448-7604

Jefferson Medical College
of Thomas Jefferson University
1025 Walnut Street, Philadelphia, PA 19107
215/928-6000

Medical College of Pennsylvania
330 Henry Ave., Philadelphia, PA 19129
215/842-6000

Pennsylvania State University College of Medicine
500 University Drive, PO Box 850
Hershey, PA 17033
717/531-8521

Temple University School of Medicine
3400 North Broad Street, Philadelphia, PA 19140
215/221-3655

University of Pennsylvania School of Medicine
36th and Hamilton Walk, Philadelphia, PA 19104
215/898-8034

University of Pittsburgh School of Medicine
Alan Magee Scaife Hall of the Health Professions
Pittsburgh, PA 15261
412/648-9891

Puerto Rico
Ponce School of Medicine
PO Box 7004, Ponce, PR 00732
809/840-2551

Universidad Central del Caribe School of Medicine
Call Box 60-327, Bayamon, PR 00621-6032
809/798-3001

University of Puerto Rico School of Medicine
Medical Sciences Campus, G.PO Box 5067
San Juan, PR 00936
809/758-2525

Rhode Island
Brown University Program in Medicine
97 Waterman Street, Providence, RI 02912
401/863-3313

South Carolina
Medical University of South Carolina
College of Medicine
171 Ashley Ave., Charleston, SC 29425
803/792-2300

University of South Carolina School of Medicine
Columbia, SC 29208
803/733-3210

South Dakota
University of South Dakota School of Medicine
2501 West 22nd Street, Sioux Falls, SD 57105
605/339-6648

Tennessee
East Tennessee State University
James H. Quillen College of Medicine
PO Box 23320A, Johnson City, TN 37614
615/929-6315

Meharry Medical College School of Medicine
1005 D.B. Todd Jr. Boulevard
Nashville, TN 37208
615/327-6337

University of Tennessee, Memphis
College of Medicine
800 Madison Ave., Memphis, TN 38163
901/528-5539

Vanderbilt University School of Medicine
21st Avenue South at Garland Ave.
Nashville, TN 37232
615/322-2145

Texas
Baylor College of Medicine
One Baylor Plaza, Houston, TX 77030
713/798-4951

Texas A&M University College of Medicine
147 Medical Science Building
College Station, TX 77843
409/845-7743

Texas Tech University
Health Sciences Center, School of Medicine
3601 4th Street, Lubbock, TX 79430
806/743-3000

University of Texas
Southwestern Medical School
5323 Harry Hines Boulevard, Dallas, TX 75235
214/688-3611

University of Texas Medical School at Galveston
301 University Boulevard, Galveston, TX 77550
409/761-1011

University of Texas Medical School at Houston
PO Box 20708, Houston, TX 77225
713/792-2121

University of Texas Medical School at San Antonio
7703 Floyd Curl Drive, San Antonio, TX 78284
512/567-4420

Utah
University of Utah School of Medicine
50 North Medical Drive, Salt Lake City, UT 84132
801/581-7201

Vermont
University of Vermont College of Medicine
School of Medicine, Burlington, VT 05405
802/656-2150

Virginia
Eastern Virginia Medical School
Medical College of Hampton Roads
PO Box 1980, Norfolk, VA 23501
804/446-5600

Virginia Commonwealth University
Medical College of Virginia, School of Medicine
1101 East Marshall Street, Richmond, VA 23298
804/786-9793

University of Virginia School of Medicine
Medical Center Box 395, Charlottesville, VA 22908
804/924-0211

Washington
University of Washington
School of Medicine, Seattle, WA 98195
206/543-1060

West Virginia
Marshall University School of Medicine
Huntington, WV 25755
304/696-7000

West Virginia University School of Medicine
Morgantown, WV 26506
304/293-4511

Wisconsin
Medical College of Wisconsin
8701 Watertown Plank Road
Milwaukee, WI 53226
414/257-8296

University of Wisconsin Medical School
1300 University Ave., Madison, WI 53706
608/263-4900

Medical Science Knowledge Program
Medical School Entrance Exam(MSKP)

Registration:
Association of American Medical Colleges
202/828-0400

Test centers:
National Board of Medical Examiners
215/349-6400

Medical Students
American Medical Students Association
1890 Preston White Dr., Reston, VA 22091
703/620-6600

Medical Technology (Technologists)

Med Tech Explains the Differential
The normal individual has a large marrow reserve...which can be released in response to sudden need.

Bartley, J. "Medicine and Poetry" JAMA. 1992 Sept 2; 268(9): 1061

Introduction to Hematology
After work,
exhausted,
"eye muscles
strained to buttons
behind my lids,
I dream them: cells
forming and falling
in eggshell white
protein skies:

lymphocytes
with china-blue rims,
their centers dark
as if a heavy-handed child
has colored them in,

neutrophils,
imperfect spheres
with azurophilic
flecks of dust,
their nuclei
a series of fists
joined by inky filaments.

The fragile, ashen monocytes
with ragged vacuolated edges,
tissue paper flowers,
wandering ghosts;
sometimes
an exotic Turk,
dark angry prowler
in an indigo mask,
or plasma cells,
sensuous half-mooned
harbingers of pain,
Cassandras of the marrow's
passion turned obsession.

Then come the blasts,
those overblown balloons
with pale uncertain
centers,
released
before the end
of the parade.

I wake with vertigo
as if I too
were floating
in the microscope's
white glare,
falling
from a source
I cannot name.

Medical Technology
Occupational Description: Laboratory tests play an important role in the detection, diagnosis, and treatment of many diseases. Medical technologists perform these tests in conjunction with pathologists (physician who diagnose the causes and nature of disease) and other physicians, or scientists who specialize in clinical chemistry, microbiology, or the other biological sciences. Medical technologists develop data on the blood, tissues, and fluids in the human body by using a variety of precision instruments.

Job Description: In addition to the skills possessed by medical laboratory technicians, medical technologists perform complex medical analyses, fine line discrimination and correction of errors. They are able to recognize interdependency of tests and have knowledge of physiological conditions affecting test results in order to confirm these results and to develop data which may be used by a physician in determining the presence, extent, and, as far as possible, the cause of disease.

Medical technologists assume responsibility for, and are held accountable for, accurate results. They establish and monitor quality control programs and design or modify procedures as necessary. Tests and procedures performed or supervised by medical technologists in the clinical laboratory center on major areas of hematology, microbiology, immunohematology, immunology, clinical chemistry, and urinalysis.

Employment Characteristics: Most medical technologists are employed in hospital laboratories. The remainder are chiefly employed in physicians' private laboratories and clinics, by the armed forces, by city, state, and federal health agencies, in industrial medical laboratories, in pharmaceutical houses, in numerous public and private research programs dedicated to the study of specific diseases, and as faculty of accredited programs preparing medical laboratory personnel. Salaries vary depending on the employer and geographic location.

According to the 1990 CAHEA Annual Supplemental Survey, entry level salaries average $24,252.(ALL)

AMA Department of Allied Health
312/464-4625

American Society for Medical Technology
2021 L Street, NW, Ste 400
Washington, DC 20036
202/785-3311

Medical Waste
JAMA Article of Note: Infectious medical wastes. Council on Scientific Affairs. JAMA. 1989 Sept 22-29; 262(12): 1669-71
A number of recent incidents involving improper handling and disposal of hospital waste have prompted the demand for more stringent legislation to cover the management of infectious hospital waste. Resolution 53 (December 1987 Interim Meeting) called for the American Medical Association to promote the passage of federal legislation for the proper disposal of infectious hospital waste. This resolution has prompted a Council on Scientific Affairs report on the current status of infectious hospital waste management and of state

and federal regulations to control such waste. The Council has concluded that existing federal and state regulations for the management of hazardous waste--in conjunction with the accreditation program of the Joint Commission on Accreditation of Healthcare Organizations and the guidelines of the Environmental Protection Agency and the Centers for Disease Control, if adhered to and properly enforced--should be adequate to ensure that the public and environment are not endangered. Therefore, the Council does not favor additional federal legislation at this time and recommends that this report be accepted in lieu of Resolution 53.

Medicare

Medicare Glossary:
"Reform 1: a change in form; removing faults and abuses 2: a new way to get paid

Howard Larkin AMNews 7/6-13/92 p.17+

Medicare hasn't just changed the way it pays. It's also changed the language. Here's a glossary of terms in current use by government and private payers.

Actual Charge – Physician's billed charge. The amount Medicare many other payers pay if lower than the Medicare payment schedule amount or insurer charge screen.

Adjusted Average Per Capita Cost (AAPCC) – A measure of the average cost of treating Medicare patients in a locality. Health maintenance organizations with Medicare risk contracts are paid a capitated rate of 95% of the AAPCC.

Adjusted Historical Payment Basis (AHPB) – Similar to, but differing in important ways, the old prevailing charge, the AHPB is a crucial factor in calculating Medicare payments during the transition to the full resource-based relative value scale payment schedule in 1996. The way AHPB is calculated largely explains greater-than-expected 1992 payment cuts. Like the old prevailing charge, the AHPB for each service is based on the average charge for that service in each of the approximately 230 Medicare localities. Unlike the prevailing charge, the AHPB includes all charges for a given service in a locality regardless of provider status, combining figures for physicians of all specialties and, in some cases, non-physician providers as well. The result not only eliminates specialty differentials, it also lowers the average for some services below the prevailing charge for fully licensed physicians. For 1992, the AHPB was also updated for inflation (+1.9%) and adjusted to compensate for the so-called transition asymmetry (-5.5%). In 1992, Medicare payments may not move more than 15% of the full RBRVS payment schedule rate above or below the AHPB for each service. But since the AHPB is in many cases lower than individual physician' 1991 profiles, payment cuts for 1992 are often more than 15% from 1991 rates. Meanwhile, payment hikes for some services that are up the entire 15% from the

AHPB are up less than 15% from the actual 1991 rates.

Adverse Selection – The tendency of people with poorer health or expectations of health problems to apply for or continue health care coverage to a greater degree than people in better health or with expectations of better health. Adverse selection is blamed for spiraling health costs in small group plans; as premiums rise healthy people drop out which, in turn, causes premiums to rise more for those left in the risk group. Some groups have also claimed that adverse selection is largely responsible for indemnity insurance costs being higher than HMO costs, a claim the HMO industry disputes.

Approved Amount – Physician payment for a service that includes the Medicare payment amount plus the patient's 20% co-payment.

Assignment – Practice of accepting as payment in full the amount approved by Medicare or other payer. For Medicare, physicians accepting assignment receive 80% of the approved amount from Medicare and bill patients for the remaining amount, once the patient's deductible is met.

Balance Billing – Practice of billing patients for payments exceeding the Medicare or other payer-approved amount. Physicians not participating in Medicare may balance-bill Medicare patients, but no more than 120% of the approved amount for non-participating physicians.

Baseline Adjustment – A 6.5% reduction in the conversion factor used by Medicare to translate the adjusted RBRVS into dollar payments. The baseline adjustment was substituted in the final payment reform regulations after a storm of objections to reductions in the proposed rule of about 10%, including a "behavioral offset" to compensate for projected volume increases by physicians hoping to replace income lost to payment cuts.

Behavioral Offset – A proposed reduction in the conversion factor used by Medicare to translate the adjusted RBRVS into dollar payments. The reduction was to compensate for volume increases that HCFA projected would result from physicians trying to maintain income in the face of lower payments. The proposal ignited a storm of protest by the AMA and other medical groups, who argued HCFA had no basis for assuming volume increases. The behavioral offset was dropped from the final payment reform regulations, replaced by the baseline adjustment.

Budget Neutrality – A requirement in the legislation mandating Medicare physician payment reform that total expenditures be no more than would have been spent if the old customary, prevailing and reasonable charge system were maintained. The budget neutrality requirement prompted a number of adjustments to the conversion factor used to translate the RBRVS into dollar payments, including the highly controversial behavioral offset.

Capitation – A method of payment, frequently employment by HMOs, in which doctors or hospitals are paid a flat fee for each person to whom service is provided, regardless of how many services any individual consumes. The object is to shift risk for controlling resource utilization to the service provider.

Carrier – Regarding Medicare, private companies that administer Medicare Part B (physician insurance) services under contract with HCFA. There are 54 carriers around the nation; most are Blue Cross/Blue Shield plans or commercial health insurance companies.

Coinsurance – Requirement that insured individuals pay a fixed percentage of medical costs. For Medicare Part B, beneficiaries pay 20%. Private insurers typically require 20% coinsurance as well, though the trend has been to lower or eliminate coinsurance for HMO or preferred provider organization coverage while raising it for traditional indemnity plans.

Conversion Factor (CF) – A multiplier Medicare uses to translate geographically adjusted values from the RBRVS into dollar payment amount for specific services. The 1992 conversion factor is $31,001, so a service with an adjusted relative value of 1.00 would be paid at $31, a service with a relative value of 2.00 at $62, etc. The conversion factor will be updated annually.

Current Procedural Terminology (CPT) – A coding system describing physician services developed by the AMA and updated annually. Medicare and most other health insurers require physicians to use CPT codes in filing claims.

Customary Charge – A physician's median charge for a given service during a specified period. Medicare used physicians' customary charge as part of a formula to set payments under the old customary, prevailing and reasonable charge system.

Customary, Prevailing and Reasonable (CPR) Method – Medicare's method for setting payments before Jan. 1, 1992, when implementation of payment reform began. Under CPR, for a given service doctors were paid the lowest of their actual billed charge, their own customary charge (the individual doctor's median charge for the service) or the prevailing charge (the median charge of all physicians or specialists in the Medicare locality providing the service). CPR essentially locked into place wide variations in pay for similar services provided in different locations.

Deductible – A set amount of medical expenses a patient must pay to become eligible for insurance benefits. For Medicare Part B the annual deductible in 1992 is $100. Physicians and outpatient services deductibles for private insurance typically run $100 or more. Many companies have raised deductibles to $250 or $500 to cut their own benefit costs and to encourage workers to join managed care plans.

Department of Health and Human Services – Department of the federal government responsible for administering health and social welfare programs, including Medicare and the federal portion of Medicaid.

Electronic Media Claim (EMC) – Claims submitted electronically. All Medicare carriers and many commercial insurers are equipped to receive claims via modem, computer tape or computer disc.

Evaluation and Management Services (E/M) – Sometimes characterized as cognitive services, these are patient evaluation and management functions performed during patient office visits, outpatient visits, and hospital visits or consultations. They consist largely of taking patient history, patient examination and medical decision-making. These three factors form the primary basis for assigning new E/M codes developed by the CPT editorial panel for 1992 and adopted by Medicare as part of payment reform. Under payment reform, Medicare will generally pay more for E/M services relative to procedural services than under the old CPR system.

Explanation of Medicare Benefits (EOMB) – A statement detailing what billed services are or are not covered by Medicare and the amount due from Medicare and the patient.

Final Rule – Regulations published in the Nov. 25, 1991, Federal Register implementing payment reform. The final rule includes values assigned individual services under the RBRVS, list of geographic cost indices for modifying the values and details of how payment reform will be implemented.

Gaming – The practice of tailoring documentation and billing practices to take maximum advantage of peculiarities of reimbursement systems and policies. This term can refer to legitimate strategies for maximizing receipts, such as billing for visits performed outside a global service package. More frequently it refers to questionable or even fraudulent activities such as itemizing and billing separately components of a service or altering coding patterns to avoid audits.

Geographic Practice Cost Index (GPCI) – Pronounced "gypsies," these indices are used to modify Medicare payments to reflect differences in physician costs in different areas. GPCI values have been developed for the cost of living, practice costs in each Medicare locality relative to the national average. If costs in a given area are below the national average, GPCI values are less than 1.00; if costs are higher, GPCI values are more than 1.00. For each service, relative values for physician work, practice expense and professional liability insurance costs are multiplied by the corresponding GPCI value. The products are added together and multiplied by the conversion factor to arrive at a payment amount. Physician groups have criticized the accuracy of the GPCIs, which will be reviewed and updated.

Global Charge – The sum of the profession and technical components of a service both are provided and billed by the same physician.

Global Surgical Package (or Global Service) – A standard Medicare surgery payment policy that provides a single payment for a group of services including preoperative care for one day before surgery, all intraoperative care and follow-up care for 90 days after surgery. Initial consultations for surgery are not included in the package. The standardized package replaces various global packages defined by individual Medicare carriers before payment reform. Many private insurers also have global surgical payment policies.

Health Care Financing Administration (HCFA) – Agency within the Dept. of Health and Human Services that administers the Medicare program. HCFA is responsible for developing Medicare payment regulations to implement Medicare law and for overseeing Medicare carrier operations.

Health Care Financing Administration's Common Procedural Coding System (HCPCS) – Codes HCFA requires when billing services and supplies. HCPCS includes CPT codes to describe physician services as well as codes to describe non-physician services and supplies.

Health Professional Shortage Area (HPSA) – Areas identified by the Public Health Service as medically underserved. Physicians in dedicated HPSAs are paid a bonus of 10% above Medicare payment schedule amount and are exempt from certain Medicare payment rules, notably the rules that mandate lower payments for physicians in their first years of private practice.

Limiting Charge – Limit set by law on how much non-participating physicians may bill Medicare patients. It mostly replaced the maximum actual allowable charge (MAAC) on Jan. 1, 1991. The limiting charge for 1992 is the lower of the MAAC or 120% of the approved charge for non-participating physicians.

Locality – Geographic areas defined by Medicare for determining payment amounts. There are now about 230 Medicare localities, some covering entire states, others counties, groups of counties or metropolitan areas. Payment reform reduces wide variations in payments among localities, sometimes within a few miles of each other, experienced under the old CPR system.

Maximum Actual Allowable Charge (MAAC) – Limit on amount non-participating physicians could bill Medicare patients under the old CPR system. Will be phased out by the limiting charge in 1993.

Medicare Economic Index (MEI) – Used to update Medicare payments, the MEI is a measure of general and medical inflation. Under the new system the MEI will update the conversion factor used to transform relative value units into dollar payment amounts. The increases will be subject to limits imposed by the Medicare volume performance standards, which require payment cuts if service volume grows beyond a certain point.

Medical Payment Schedule – A new basis for setting physician Medicare payments, the payment schedule replaced the old CPR system on Jan. 1, 1992, and is the cornerstone of payment reform. It is based on the RBRVS developed at the Harvard University School of Public Health. The Harvard RBRVS takes into account the resource cost of physician work, practice overhead and professional liability insurance. RBRVS values are adjusted for geographic differences in practice costs and multiplied by a conversion factor to arrive at a dollar payment figure. Payment schedule amounts includes both the 80% paid by Medicare and the 20% patient co-payment. In 1992, about 30% of Medicare services are paid at the schedule amount, and the others are paid based on a blend of the payment schedule and historical charges. Transition to the full Medicare payment schedule will be complete in 1996.

Medicare Volume Performance Standard (MVPS) – A national spending goal for Medicare Part B services, the MVPS will be used to control spending growth by cutting physician payments if volume grows any faster than projected. Essentially, if the MVPS is exceeded in one year, physician payment updates are cut the next year. The cuts are made by reducing the Medicare Economic Index to compensate for the amount actual Part B expenditures exceeded the MVPS target. That, in turn, reduces the conversion factor by which Medicare multiplies relative values for each service to arrive at a dollar payment amount. The MVPS is established annually by Congress either according to recommendations by HHS, the Physician Payment Review Commission and groups such as the AMA, or by a statutory formula. model fee schedule - A preliminary payment schedule HCFA developed in 1990. The model fee schedule included relative values for 1,400 services studied in Phase I of the Harvard RBRVS study and preliminary geographic practice cost indices. Payments or certain "overvalued" procedures were also cut based on the model fee schedule.

Non-participating Physician (non-par) – A physician who has elected not to sign a Medicare participation agreement. Non-participating physician must collect from patients for services, but are free to bill Medicare patients for more than the Medicare approved amount for a service. However, bills may not exceed the lower of the MAAC or limiting charge, which this year is 120% of the approved amount for non-par physicians and will be reduced to 115% next year. Approved amounts for non-participating physicians are set at 95% of approved amounts for participating physicians in the same locality. Non-participating physicians may accept assignment on a case-by-case basis.

Notice of Proposed Rulemaking (NPRM) – HCFA's proposed rules to implement physician payment reform published June 5, 1991. HCFA received a record 95,000 comment letters on the

proposal, which was modified considerably before final rules were issued Nov. 25, 1991.

OBRA 89 (Omnibus Budget Reconciliation Act of 1989) – Legislation mandating Medicare physician payment. OBRA 89 specifies that the new system be based on as RBRVS and that its implementation be budget neutral - that is, costing no more than would have been spent under the old CPR system. The legislation also contains a number of more specific directions, notably a ban on payment for reading electrocardiograms when done in conjunction with providing another service.

Outlier – A point in a statistical distribution that is outside a certain range, usually defined as two or three standard deviations from the mean. Often refers to a case or hospital stay that is unusually long or expensive for its type, or to a physician practice that uses an abnormally high or low volume of resources.

Participating Physician (par) – A physician who has signed a Medicare participation agreement, which binds the physician to accept assignment on all Medicare claims within the calendar year. Participating physicians are paid 80% of approved charges directly from Medicare and must bill patients for the 20% co-payment, but may not bill for more. Some private insurers, notably Blue Cross and Blue Shield plans, have similar participation programs.

Physician Payment Review Commission (PPRC) – An advisory committee created by Congress to review and evaluate Medicare physician proposals.

Physician Work – One of three factors used to determine the relative value of physician services, the other two being practice expense and professional liability insurance costs. The physician work component reflects the time, technical skill, training, and physical and mental effort required to provide a service.

Practice Expense – One of three factors used to determine the relative value of physician services, the other two being physician work and professional liability insurance costs. The practice expense component reflects practice overhead involved in providing a service, including rent, staff salary and benefits and medical equipment and supplies.

Prevailing Charge – One factor Medicare used to set physician payments under the CPR system used before payment reform. The prevailing charge was set at the customary, or median, charge of the 75th percentile of physicians delivering a particular service in a particular Medicare locality. Increases in the prevailing charge were capped by the Medicare Economic Index.

Professional Component – Portion of payment for a service covering physician work, practice costs and professional liability insurance as opposed to the technical component, which covers the use of equipment and supplies and technician salaries.

Professional Liability Insurance (PLI) Component – One of three factors used to determine the relative value of physician services, the other two being physician work and practice expenses. The PLI component reflects the cost of insurance indemnifying physicians against professional liability claims for a particular service.

Relative Value Scale (RVS) – An index of physician services that assigns values to individual services relative to other services. Such scales are generally based on historical charges (charge-based) or on resources consumed to provide services (resource-based). Various relative value scales have been used by insurers as the basis of payment schedules. Typically, relative values are multiplied by a conversion factor to arrive at a dollar payment amount.

Relative Value Unit (RVU) – Basic element of measure for the Medicare RBRVS. Each service is assigned relative value units for physician work, practice expenses and professional liability insurance. The three added together are the relative value of the service. Without geographic modifiers, the middle of the five codes that cover office visits for established patients under the new CPT coding system (99213) is equal to 1.00 RVU while quadruple coronary bypass surgery (33513) is equal to 76.37 RVUs. RVUs are modified by geographic practice cost index values to compensate for regional variations in practice costs.

Resource-based Relative Value Scale (RBRVS) – A relative value scale developed by a Harvard research team that assigns values to physician services based on the resource cost of providing those services. As the basis of Medicare's new payment schedule, it is the cornerstone of physician payment reform. The RBVRS payment schedule is intended to even out regional payment differences that existed under the old CPR system as well as establish a rational basis for setting payments for office visits and other "cognitive" services relative to surgery and other "procedural" services. The scale was developed in three phases. Medicare's new payment schedule is based on Phase III values. RBRVS assigns relative value units to each physician service for physician work, practice expenses and professional liability insurance costs required to perform that service. Values for each of these three components are modified to reflect local cost variations, by multiplying them by geographic practice cost index values established for each Medicare locality. The RBRVS will undergo constant revision to keep up with changes in technology and medical practice.

Specialty Differential – Under Medicare's old CPR system some carriers paid physicians from different specialties different amounts for providing the same service. Legislation mandating payment reform required that specialty differentials be eliminated.

Technical Component – Portion of payment for physician services covering equipment, supplies and technician salary, as opposed to the professional component, which covers physician work, practice overhead and professional liability costs.

Transition Asymmetry – Phenomenon of payments for services that will increase, rising faster than payments that will decrease during transition to Medicare's RBRVS payment schedule between 1992 and 1996. The transition asymmetry threatened to push overall Medicare spending higher than it would have been under old CPR system, a violation of the budget-neutrality requirement in the legislation mandating physician payment reform. To compensate, HCFA reduced the adjusted historical price basis used to blend historical and RBRVS charges during the transition by 5.5%.

Transition Offset – A 5.5% cut in the adjusted historical price basis to offset transition asymmetry.

Unbundle – The practice of billing separately, for higher reimbursement, components of an integral service. Also known as code fragmentation.

Upcode – The practice of coding services at a higher level than justified by their content.

The **Medicare** Program is a Federal health insurance program for persons over 65 years of age and certain disabled persons. It is funded through social security contributions, premiums, and general revenue. The Administration develops and implements policies related to program recipients, the providers of services such as hospitals, nursing homes, physicians, and the contractors who process claims. It also coordinates with the States to develop departmental programs, activities, and organizations that are closely related to the Medicare Program.(USG)

Complaints regarding fraud, waste, abuse, etc.
Department of Health and Human Services
(Inspector General's Hotline)
800/368-5779, 301/597-0724 (in MD)

Contact local Medicare office
Contact state department of public aid

JAMA Theme Issue: Relative Value Studies
JAMA. 1988 Oct 28; 260(16)
With the RBRVS being officially applied in 1991, this issue's presentation of the thoughts involved in the development of a payment scale for physicians is noteworthy. Discussions of values for specific procedures, measurement of intraservice work, and the potential effects of a relative value scale, plus supportive editorials, are included.

Federal Register
RBRVS Information--November 25, 1991
Government Printing Office
North Capitol and H Streets, NW
Washington, DC 20401
Publication orders and inquiries
202/783-3238
Information
202/275-3648

Medicare Physician Payment Reform: The Physicians' Guide. Chicago; American Medical Association. 1992. Two volumes.
ISBN 0-89970-419-0. OP059691

Physicians' Medicare Guide (Loose leaf manual for Medicare Part B--includes full descriptions of the CPT codes from the AMA's CPT book including RBRVS) updated monthly. Available from:
Commerce Clearing House
4025 W. Peterson Ave, Chicago, IL 60646
312/583-8500

Physician Payment Review Commission
2120 L St., NW, Suite 510, Washington, DC 20037
202/653-7220

Unique Physician Identification Number (UPIN)
Physicians: Contact Medicare Carrier

Insurance Carriers:
Contact the Privacy Act Office
301/966-3000

Medicare Carriers
Certain staff members at state or local medical societies may be of assistance with questions about medical necessity review process. Many state and some local medical societies have well established liaisons between the Medicare insurance carrier and the medical society. Because of this, medical society staff may have inside or firsthand information about how to approach problems a physician may be experiencing.
However, at times a physician may find it useful to communicate directly with the Medicare insurance carrier when a medical policy question regarding a particular claim needs addressing, or to obtain materials on specific carrier medical policy. The following list identifies the appropriate carrier to be contacted in these incidences. Remember, that it is advantageous to communicate with the carrier in writing in order to establish a written record of the information requested and received.

Alabama
Blue Cross & Blue Shield of Alabama
Provider Affairs Dept.
PO Box 995, Birmingham, AL 35283
205-985-0191

Alaska
Medicare Aetna Life & Casualty
Policy and Procedures
200 S.W. Market, PO Box 1997
Portland, OR 97207
800-547-6333

Arizona
Medicare Aetna Life & Casualty
Cost Containment Section
PO Box 37200, Phoenix, AZ 85069
602-870-0041

Arkansas
Medicare Arkansas Blue Cross & Blue Shield
Medicare Services Unit, PO Box 1418
Little Rock, AR 72203
501-378-2320

California
Medicare Transamerica Occidental
Life Insurance Company
Box 54905, Los Angeles, CA 90054
Participating:800-423-2508
Non-participating:213-742-3934
for Los Angeles, Orange, San Diego, Ventura,
Imperial, San Luis Obispo, and Santa Barbara
counties.

Medicare Claims Dept., Blue Shield of California
Medical Review, Chico, CA 95976
Northern CA:916-743-1587
Southern CA:714-824-0176
for the remainder of the state

Colorado
Colorado Blue Cross and Blue Shield
Medicare Communications
PO Box 173500, Denver, CO 80127
Denver only 303-831-1221; all others
800-824-9500

Connecticut
Medicare The Travelers Insurance Co.
Medical Review Unit
PO Box 9000, Meriden, CT 06454-9000
participating:800-824-0369
non-participating 203-639-3000

Delaware and District of Columbia
Medicare Pennsylvania Blue Shield Medical Affairs
PO Box 65, Camp Hill, PA 17089-0202
717-731-2333

Florida
Medicare Blue Cross & Blue Shield of Florida, Inc.
Provider Education Dept., Medicare Part B
PO Box 2078, Jacksonville, FL 32231-0048
participating 904-634-4994,
non-participating:904-634-4988

Georgia
Medicare Aetna Georgia
PO Box 3018, Savannah, GA 31402-3018
non-participating:800-927-0934

Hawaii
Medicare Aetna Life & Casualty
Honolulu, HI
participating PO Box 2700, 96803
808-524-1240
non-participating PO Box 3947, 96812
808-524-1240

Idaho
Medicare Equicor Inc., Medical Review Section
PO Box 8048, Boise, ID 83707
208-342-7763

Illinois
Medicare Claims Health Care Service Corp.
PO Box 4433, Marion, IL 62959
participating 618-997-2349 non-participating
618-997-3190

Indiana
Medicare Part B Associated Insurance
Companies, Inc.
PO Box 240, Indianapolis, IN 46206
participating:800-237-9754
non-participating:800-851-0877
Indianapolis area
participating:317-842-2542
non-participating:317-845-2992

Iowa
Medicare Iowa-South Dakota
Health Services Corp
Des Moines, IA 50309
participating Box 9146, 515-244-0445
non-participating Box 10491, 515-245-4881

Kansas
Medicare Blue Cross and Blue Shield
of Kansas City
PO Box 419840 Kansas City, MO

Kentucky
Medicare Blue Cross and Blue Shield of Kentucky
Customer Support Department
100 East Vine Str., Lexington, KY 40507
606-233-1465

Louisiana
Medicare Blue Cross & Blue Shield of Louisiana
Medicare Services
PO Box 95024, Baton Rouge, LA 70895-9024
800-624-3364, 504-237-5102,5201

Maine
Medicare Blue Cross & Blue Shield of
Massachusetts/Tri-State
Medicare B, PO Box 1010, Biddeford, ME 04005
207-284-1002

Maryland
Medicare Blue Cross & Blue Shield of Maryland
1946 Greenspring Dr., Timonium, MD 21093
301-561-4063

Massachusetts
Medicare B Blue Shield of Massachusetts, Inc.,
Provider Communications
1022 Hingham Str., Rockland, MA, 02371
617-956-2150

Michigan
Medicare Part B, Blue Cross & Blue Shield of
Michigan
Government Provider Inquiry
PO Box 2201, Detroit, MI 48231
Detroit:313-255-8222 or 800-483-8760

Minnesota
Medicare The Travelers Insurance Co., Medical
Providers Service
8120 Penn Ave., South, Bloomington, MN 55431

Mississippi
Medicare The Travelers Insurance Co., Medical
Providers Service
795 Woodlands Parkway, Ridgeland, MS 39157
601-977-0208

Missouri
Medicare Blue Shield of Kansas City
PO Box 419840, Kansas City, MO 64141-6840
local 816-756-1601 or 800-654-9629

Montana
Medicare Blue Cross & Blue Shield of Montana,
Utilization Review/Medicare
PO Box 4310, Helena, MT 59604
406-444-8224

Nebraska
Blue Cross Blue Shield of Kansas (Nebraska)
Edit and Profit Unit
PO Box 3512, Topeka, KS 66601-3512
800-633-1003

Nevada
Medicare B, Aetna Life & Casualty
PO Box 37230, Phoenix, AR 85069
602-870-0041

New Hampshire
Medicare Blue Cross Blue Shield of
Massachusetts/Tri-State
2 1/2 Beacon Str., Concord, NH 03301
603-225-2883

New Jersey
Medicare B Pennsylvania Blue Shield
PO Box 400011, Camp Hill, PA 17140-0011

New Mexico
Medicare B Aetna Life and Casualty
Oklahoma City, OK
participating: PO Box 24600, 73124; 405-843-9379
Non-participating: PO Box 25500, 73125;
505-843-7711 (Albuquerque) 800-423-2925

New York
Medicare Empire Blue Cross and Blue Shield ,
622 Third Ave., 39th Flr., New York, NY 10017
212-490-5151

Medicare B Blue Shield of Western New York
Binghamton, NY:
Participating: PO Box 5207, 13902-5207;
800-331-2933, Unassigned PO Box 600,
13902-0600 800-442-0148

Medicare B Group Health Incorporated. 88 West
End Ave.,
PO Box 1608 Ansonia Station
New York, NY 10023
Participating: 212-721-1214.
Non-participating: 212-721-1218

North Carolina
Medicare B Equicor of North Carolina
Medicare Administration
1 Triad Center, Ste 240, 7736 McCloud Rd
Greensboro, NC 27409
919-655-0341

North Dakota/South Dakota/Wyoming
Medicare B Blue Cross Blue Shield of
North Dakota
Provider Services Unit
4510-13th Ave., SW, Fargo, ND 58121-0001
701-282-1090 (Fargo), 800-828-5740

Ohio/West Virginia
Medicare B, Nationwide Mutual Insurance
Company (Ohio)
Medicare, Provider Relations,
PO Box 16788 Columbus, OH 43216
614-464-9924; 800-255-1844(Ohio): 800-245-4435

Oklahoma
Medicare B Aetna Life & Casualty
Participating: PO Box 24700
Oklahoma City, OK 73124
405-843-0379.
Non-participating: 701 NW 63rd St., Ste. 100,
73116-7693, 405-848-7711, 800-522-9079

Oregon
Medicare B Aetna Life & Casualty
Policy and Procedures
200 SW Market St., PO Box 1997
Portland, OR 97207
503-222-3118, 800-325-9308

Pennsylvania
Medicare B Pennsylvania Blue Shield,
Camp Hill, PA
Participating: PO Box 890318, 17089-0318,
717-763-5700
Non-participating: PO Box 890301, 17089-0301,
717-763-5700

Rhode Island
Medicare B Professional Relations Dept.,
Blue Cross & Blue Shield of Rhode Island
444 Westminster St, Providence, RH 02901.
Participating: 401-274-4889.
Non-participating: 401-274-9527

South Carolina
Medicare B Blue Cross & Blue Shield
of South Carolina
300 Arbor, Ste. 1300 Columbia, SC 29223.
Participating: 803-735-1205.
Non-participating: 803-735-0624

South Dakota see North Dakota.

Tennessee
Medicare B, Equicor, Inc.,
PO Box 1465, Nashville, TN 37202
615-244-5680

Texas
Medicare Blue Cross & Blue Shield of Texas, Inc.
PO Box 650301, Dallas, TX 75265-030111
214-669-7395

Utah
Medicare B Blue Cross BS of Utah
Beneficiary and Provider Services
PO Box 30270, Salt Lake City, UT 84130-0269
801-481-6169(Salt Lake City); 800-426-3477

Vermont
Medicare B Blue Shield of Massachusetts/Tri State
1 Burlington Square, Burlington, VT 05401
802-863-9711

Virginia
Medicare B The Travelers Insurance Co.,
Richmond, VA, 23261-6463
Participating: PO Box C32086, 804-330-6228.
Non-Participating: PO Box 26463.

Washington
Medicare B King County Medical Blue Shield
Medical Professional Affairs
PO Box 21248, Seattle, WA 98111
206-464-3772

West Virginia: see Ohio

Wisconsin
Medicare B, Physician Services
PO Box 1787, Madison, WI
Participating: 608-221-4121
Non-participating: 608-221-3218

Wyoming: see North Dakota

American Samoa and Guam:
see Hawaii

Puerto Rico and Virgin Islands
Medicare B, Seguros De Servicio De Salud De
Puerto Rico, Inc.
Office Medical Coordinator, Call Box 71391
San Juan, Puerto Rico 00936
809-749-4900

Medicare Carrier Review. 2nd ed. American
Medical Association, Chicago. 1988. 64pp.
ISBN 0-89970-410-7. OP059890

Meetings, Medical
"World Meetings Series" by World Meetings
Publications, Macmillan Publishing Company, 866
Third Ave., New York, NY 10022
Fax: 212/319-1216

"World Meetings: Medicine" ISSN 0161-2875
two year listing of upcoming medical meetings
updated quarterly.

"World Meetings: United States and Canada"
ISSN 0043-8693
two year listing of upcoming scientific, technical
and medical meetings.

"World Meetings: Outside United States
and Canada"
ISSN 0043-8693/
two year listing of upcoming scientific, technical
and medical meetings.

"Scientific Meetings" Scientific Meetings
Publications, PO Box 81662
San Diego, CA 92138
ISSN# 0487-8965
619-270-2910
Quarterly listing of future meetings of technical
scientific, medical and management organizations
and universities.

"Medical Meetings"
ISSN 0093-1314 The Laux Company, 63 Great
Rd., Maynard, MA 01754.
Bi-monthly publication to aid in the planning of
medical meetings.

Mental Health
The Surprise Party

Harold I. Eist, MD "A Piece of My Mind" JAMA.
1983 Jun 24; 249(24): 2632

In understanding the experience of mentally ill
individuals, we should recognize the courage they
often exhibit even while engaging in superficial
ordinary human interactions. Unless we
appreciate this, their responses of isolation and
withdrawal because of interpersonal terror will
seem inexplicable. Two clinical examples help to
clarify this point.

An alcoholic woman began talking about her son,
who had been psychotic since childhood, and I
wondered if there would ever be any end to her
grief. Alcohol had destroyed her liver, but it had
not washed away the grief. She mentioned with a
slight smile that finally she was beginning to
accept the many losses her son's illness
represented.

"We had him home from the hospital Sunday, and
Mary, the friend I told you about who also has a
schizophrenic son, brought him over. The two
boys have known each other since they were kids
and there they were, both of them on the couch,
acting like the other one didn't exist."

Her remark took me back 17 years to a medication
group I had run for chronically schizophrenically ill
patients at a Veterans Administration hospital.
During my weekly sessions with the group, as
each of the ten assiduously avoided eye contact
with the other, I often thought, "You guys don't
need a psychiatrist -you need an air traffic control
operator."

Six weeks prior to my leaving this group, I
announced I was moving on to another service.
Each patient responded by firmly fixing his eyes
on a distant point. I wondered if there was any
concern on the part of the group members at my
leaving, but I couldn't tell for sure.

As the group assembled at the last meeting, one
of the members, who was uncharacteristically well
groomed, emptied a bag of doughnuts in the
center of the group-room table. Each member of
the group filed to the table and took a doughnut.

"The last one's for you, Doc." one of them said.
"It's a surprise party." Suddenly it hit me that these
terribly isolated men had gotten together in spite
of their fearfulness and had planned a party for

me. Furthermore, in the face of crippling illness, they had carried it off.

We ate our doughnuts silently, no one looking at anyone else, and then we discussed medications. I shook hands with each of them, and someone said, "Hope you enjoy your new job."

"Me too," I answered, full of sadness, gratitude, and new-found understanding.

National Alliance for the Mentally Ill
2101 Wilson Blvd, Ste 302, Arlington, VA 22201
703/524-7600

National Depressive and
Manic Depressive Association
222 S. Riverside Plaza, Suite 2812
Chicago, IL 60606
312/993-0066

National Institute of Mental Health
Office of Scientific Information
Public Inquiries Section
5600 Fishers Lane, Room 15C-17
Rockville, MD 20857
301/443-4513

National Mental Health Association
1021 Prince Street, Alexandria, VA 22314
703/684-7722
800/969-NMHA (800/969-6642)

Mental Retardation
American Association on Mental Retardation
1719 Kalorama Rd. NW, Washington, DC 20009
202/387-1968

Midwives
American College of Nurse-Midwives
1522 K St. NW, Suite 1000
Washington, DC 20005
202/289-0171

Informed Homebirth/Informed Birth and Parenting
PO Box 3675, Ann Arbor, MI 48106
313/662-6857

Planned Parenthood Federation of America
810 Seventh Ave., New York, NY 10019
212/541-7800

Position on Midwifery:
American College of Obstetricians
and Gynecologists
409 12th St., SW, Washington, DC 20024
202/638-5577

Military Medicine
Association of Military Surgeons
of the United States
9320 Old Georgetown Road, Bethesda, MD 20814
301/897-8800

The Society of Medical Consultants
to the Armed Forces
4301 Jones Bridge Road
Bethesda, MD, 20814-4799
301/295-3106

Minority Health
JAMA Theme Issue: African American Health
JAMA. 1989 Jan 13: 261(2)
A portrait of Martin Luther King, Jr. graces the cover of this issue of JAMA, which focuses on the health of black Americans. Federal agencies, the CDC, HCFA, PHS, NIH and HRSA all contributed essays from their point of view on the issues affecting the health of African Americans. Also included are medical perspectives discussing the state of medical education for African Americans, and reviews of books discussing fuller treatment of several facets of the points raised herein.

JAMA Article: Black-white disparities in health care. Council on Ethical and Judicial Affairs. JAMA. 1990 May 2; 263(17): 2344-6
Persistent, and sometimes substantial, differences continue to exist in the quality of health among Americans. Blacks have higher infant mortality rates and shorter life expectancies than whites. Underlying the disparities in the quality of health among Americans are differences in both need and access. Moreover, recent studies have suggested that even when blacks gain access to the health care system, they are less likely than whites to receive certain surgical or other therapies. These studies have examined treatments in several areas, including cardiology and cardiac surgery, kidney transplantation, general internal medicine, and obstetrics. Whether the disparities in treatment decisions are caused by differences in income and education, sociocultural factors, or failures by the medical profession, they are unjustifiable and must be eliminated. In this report, the Council on Ethical and Judicial Affairs of the American Medical Association emphasizes the need for (1) greater access to necessary health care for black Americans, (2) greater awareness among physicians of existing and potential disparities in treatment, and (3) the continued development of practice parameters, including criteria that would preclude or diminish racial disparities in health care decisions.

JAMA Article: Hispanic health in the United States. Council on Scientific Affairs. JAMA. 1991 Jan 9; 265(2): 248-52
Hispanics are the fastest growing minority in the United States. Typically, they are divided into five subgroups: Mexican American, Puerto Rican, Cuban American, Central or South American, and "other" Hispanics. Risk factors for morbidity and mortality vary among these subgroups. Use of health care services is affected by perceived health care needs, insurance status, income, culture, and language. Compared with whites, Hispanics are more likely to live in poverty, be unemployed or underemployed, and have little education and no private insurance. Hispanics are at an increased risk for certain medical conditions, including diabetes, hypertension, tuberculosis, human immunodeficiency virus infection, alcoholism, cirrhosis, specific cancers, and violent deaths. Proportionate to their representation in the population, there are few Hispanic health providers, emphasizing the need for all medical personnel to be knowledgeable about Hispanic health care needs.

Missing Children

Childfind Hotline
800/426-5678

Missing Child Hotline
National Center for Missing and Exploited Children
800/843-5678 9 a.m.-Midnight

MEDWATCH
800/I-AM-LOST (800/426-5678)
(Sponsored by Wyeth Laboratories)

Multiple Births

Center for Study of Multiple Birth
333 East Superior St., Suite 476
Chicago, IL 60611
312/266-9093

National Organization of Mothers of Twins Club
12404 Princess Jeanne, N.E.
Albuquerque, NM 87112
505/275-0955

Twinline
2131 University Ave., Suite 234
Berkeley, CA 94704
415/644-0861

Muscle Disorders

The most common muscle disorder is injury, followed by symptoms caused by a lack of blood supply to a muscle (including the heart). In addition, there are a number of other rarer disorders of muscle.

Genetic Disorders: The muscular dystrophies cause progressive weakness and disability. Some types appear at birth, some in infancy, and some develop as late as the fifth or sixth decade. One type of cardiomyopathy, a general term for disease of the heart muscle, is inherited.

Infection: The most important infection of muscle is gangrene, which may complicate deep wounds (especially those contaminated by soil). Tetanus is acquired in a similar way, causing widespread muscle spasm through the release of a powerful toxin.

Viruses: (especially influenza B) may also infect muscles (causing myalgia), as may the organism causing toxoplasmosis. Trichinosis is an infestation of muscle with the worm Trichinella Spirilis, which is acquired be eating undercooked meat (usually pork).

Injury: Muscle injuries, such as tears and sprains, are very common; they cause bleeding into the muscle tissue. Healing leads to formation of a scar in the muscle, which shortens its natural length. Blunt muscle injury may result in hematoma formation from bleeding into the muscle. Rarely, bone may form in the hematoma causing myositis ossificans.

Tumors: Primary muscle tumors may or may not be cancerous. Noncancerous tumors are called myomas, those affecting smooth muscle are leiomyomas, and those affecting skeletal muscle are rhabdomyomas. Myomas of the uterus are among the most common of all tumors. Cancerous tumors are called myosarcomas and are very rare; cancers of the skeletal muscle are known as rhabdomyosarcomas.
Secondary tumors, which spread from a primary site of cancer elsewhere in the body, very rarely involve muscle.

Hormonal and Metabolic Disorders: Muscle contraction depends on the maintenance or proper levels of sodium, potassium, and calcium in and around muscle cells. Any alteration in the concentration of these substances affects muscle function. For example, a severe drop in the level of potassium (hypokalemia) causes profound muscle weakness and may stop the heart. A drop in blood calcium (hypocalcemia) causes increased excitability of muscles and, occasionally, spasms.

Thyroid disease is often associated with muscle disorders, the most common being a swelling of the small muscles that move the eyes, causing a bulging eyeball.

Adrenal failure causes general muscle weakness.

Impaired Blood Supply: Muscles depend on a good blood supply for normal function. Cramp is usually caused by a lack of blood flow, sometimes associated with severe exertion. Peripheral vascular disease, which restricts the blood supply, causes claudication (muscle pain on exercise). Angina pectoris (chest pain caused by lack of blood supply to heart muscle) occurs in coronary heart disease. The compartment syndrome is pain in muscles as a result of swelling that limits the blood supply. It is brought on by injury or exercise, occurring often in athletes with well-developed muscles.

Poisons and Drugs: Several toxic substances can damage muscle. They include alcohol, which can cause damage following a prolonged drinking bout. Other substances that may cause muscle damage include aminocaproic acid, chloroquine, clofibrate, emetine, and vincristine.

Autoimmune Disorders: Myasthenia gravis is a disorder of transmission of nerve impulses to muscles; it usually begins by causing droopin of the eyelids and double vision. Other diseases with an autoimmune basis that may affect muscles are lupus erythematous, rheumatoid arthritis, scleroderma, sarcoidosis, and dermatomyositis.

Investigation: Muscle disorders are investigated by EMG (electromyography), which measures the response of muscles to electrical impulses, and by muscle biopsy.(ENC)

Muscular Dystrophy Association
3561 E. Sunrise Dr, Tucson, AZ 85718
602/529-2000 800/223-6666

Myasthenia Gravis Foundation
53 W. Jackson, #1352, Chicago, IL 60604
800/541-5454

National Multiple Sclerosis Society
205 E. 42nd St., New York, NY 10017
212/986-3240 800/624-8236

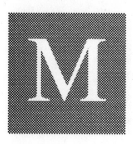

Museums, Medical

Historical Museum of Medicine and Dentistry
230 Scarborough Street
Hartford, CT 06105
203-236-5613
Weekday Hours 10:00 AM to 4:00 PM

International College of Surgeons
1516 N. Lake Shore Dr., Chicago, IL 60610
312/787-6274
Tuesday through Saturday 10:00 AM to 4:00 PM
Sunday 11:00 AM to 5:00 PM

Museum of Ophthalmology
655 Beach Street
San Francisco, CA 94133
415-561-8500
Weekday Hours 8:00 AM to 5:00 PM

National Museum of Health and Medicine
(Walter Reed Army Medical Center)
Dahlia and 14th Streets, NW
Washington, DC 20306
202-576-2348
Weekday hours 9:30 AM to 4:30 PM
Weekend Hours 11:30 AM to 4:30 PM.

Narcolepsy

American Narcolepsy Association
335 Quarry Road, Belmont, CA 94002
415/591-7979

Narcolepsy and Cataplexy Foundation of America
1410 New York Avenue, Suite 2D MB22
New York, NY 10021
212/628-6315

Narcotics

Narcotics Anonymous
PO Box 9999, Van Nuys, CA 91409
818/780-3951

Narcotic Educational Foundation of America
5055 Sunset Blvd., Los Angeles, CA 90027
213/663-5171

National Health Care

National Health Care Anti-Fraud Association
1255 23rd St., N.W./Suite 800
Washington, DC 20037
202/659-5955

Physicians for a National Health Program
Cambridge Hospital
1493 Cambridge St, Cambridge, MA 02139
617/498-1000

National Institutes of Health

The National Institutes of Health (NIH) is the principal biomedical research agency of the Federal Government. By conducting, supporting, and promoting biomedical research, NIH seeks to improve the health of all American people through increasing the understanding of processes underlying human health, disability, and disease; advancing knowledge concerning the health effects of interactions between humans and the environment; developing methods of preventing, detecting, diagnosing, and treating disease; and disseminating research results for critical review and ultimately for medical application. In the pursuit of this mission, NIH supports biomedical and behavioral research domestically and abroad, conducts research in its own laboratories and clinics, trains promising young researchers, and promotes acquiring and distributing medical knowledge. Focal points have been established to assist in developing NIH-wide goals for health research and research training programs related to women and minorities, coordinating program direction, and ensuring that research pertaining to women's and minority health is identified and addressed through research activities conducted and supported by the NIH. Research activities conducted by NIH will determine much of the quality of health care for the future and reinforce the quality of health care currently available.(USG)

National Institutes of Health
9000 Rockville Pike, Bethesda, MD 20892
301/496-5787

Major Components:
National Cancer Institute. Research on cancer is a high priority program as a result of the National Cancer Act, which made the conquest of cancer a national goal. The Institute developed a National Cancer Program to expand existing scientific knowledge on cancer cause and prevention as well as on the diagnosis, treatment, and rehabilitation of cancer patients.

Research activities conducted in the Institute's laboratories or supported through grants or contracts include many investigative approaches to cancer, including chemistry, biochemistry, biology, molecular biology, immunology, radiation physics, experimental chemotherapy, epidemiology, biometry, radiotherapy, and pharmacology. Cancer research facilities are constructed with Institute support, and training is provided under university-based programs. The Institute, through its cancer control element, applies research findings as rapidly as possible in preventing and controlling human cancer.

National Cancer Institute
For further information, call 301-496-5737.
Public inquiries 301/496-5583

National Heart, Lung, and Blood Institute
The Institute provides leadership for a national program in diseases of the heart, blood vessel, blood, and lungs, and in the use of blood and the management of blood resources.

It conducts studies and research into the clinical use of blood and all aspects of the management of blood resources, and supports training of manpower in fundamental science and clinical disciplines for participation in basic and clinical research programs relating to heart, blood vessel, blood, and lung diseases.

It coordinates with other research institutes and with all Federal agency programs relating to the above diseases, including programs in hypertension, stroke, respiratory distress, and sickle cell anemia.

The Institute plans, conducts, fosters, and supports an integrated and coordinated program of research, investigations, clinical trials and demonstrations relating to the causes, prevention, methods of diagnosis and treatment (including emergency medical treatment) of heart, blood vessel, lung, and blood diseases through research performed in its own laboratories and through contracts and research grants to scientific institutions and to individual scientists.

The Institute also conducts educational activities, including the dissemination of educational materials about these diseases, with emphasis in the prevention thereof, for health professionals and the lay public, and maintains continuing relationships with institutions and professional associations and with international, national, and State and local officials, and voluntary agencies and organizations working in these areas.

National Heart, Lung and Blood Institute
For further information, call 301-496-2411
Public Inquiries 301/496-4236.(USG)

National Office of Alternative Medicine
301/402-2466

National Institute of Arthritis and Musculoskeletal and Skin Diseases
301/468-3235

National Eye Institute
301/496-5248

National Institute of Alcohol Abuse and Alcoholism
National Clearinghouse for Alcohol Information
301/443-3860

National Institute of Allergy and Infectious Diseases
Public Response 301/496-5717

National Institute of Child Health and Human Development
Public Information 301/496-5133

National Institute of Dental Research
Information 301/496-4261

National Institute of Diabetes
Digestive and Kidney Disease 301/496-3583

National Institute of General Medical Sciences
301/496-7301

National Institute of Neurological Disorders and Stroke
Health Reports 301/496-5751

National Institute on Aging
301/496-1752

National Institute on Drug Abuse
National Clearinghouse for Drug Abuse
301/443-6500

National Institute of Mental Health
Public Communication 301/443-4515

Natural Childbirth
American Society for Psychoprophylaxis in Obstetrics (ASPO/Lamaze)
1840 Wilson Blvd./Suite 204, Arlington, VA 22201
703/524-7802

International Childbirth Education Association (ICEA)
PO Box 20048, Minneapolis, MN 55420
612/854-8660

Naturopathy
The term "naturopathy" was coined in 1895 by John Scheel, a practitioner in New York City, to describe his methods of health care. In 1902, he sold rights to the term to Benedict Lust, who had come to the United States in 1892 to promote hydrotherapy. Lust was largely responsible for naturopathy's growth in this country.

Before 1961 the doctor of naturopathy (ND) degree could be obtained at a few chiropractic schools; now it is available only from two full-time schools of naturopathy and a few correspondence schools. In 1987 the U.S. Secretary of Education approved the Council on Naturopathic Medical Education as an accrediting agency for the full-time schools. The leading naturopathic institution, Bastyr College in Seattle, has also received full accreditation from the Northwest Association of Schools.

Naturopaths are licensed as independent practitioners in seven states and the District of Columbia, and may legally practice in a few others as well. The American Association of Naturopathic Physicians has about 400 members. The total number of practitioners is unknown but includes chiropractors and acupuncturists who practice naturopathy. Bastyr College offers degrees in naturopathy, acupuncture, nutrition and Oriental medicine. During the past two years, it has also teamed with the National Nutritional Foods Association to produce educational programs for health food retailers.(ALT)

Doctor, Naturopathic: Diagnoses, treats, and cares for patients, using system of practice that base treatment of physiological functions and abnormal conditions on natural law governing human body: Utilizes physiological, psychological, and mechanical methods, such as air, water, light, heat, earth, phytotherapy, food and herb therapy, psychotherapy, electrotherapy, physiotherapy, minor and orificial surgery, mechanotherapy, naturopathic corrections and manipulation, and natural methods or modalities, together with natural medicines, natural processed foods, and herbs and nature's remedies. Excludes major surgery, therapeutic use of x rays and radium, and use of drugs, except those assimilable substances containing elements or compounds of body tissues and are physiologically compatible to body processes for maintenance of life. (DOT)

American Association of Naturopathic Physicians
PO Box 20386, Seattle, WA 98102
206/323-7610

Nephrology
American Society of Nephrology
1101 Connecticut Ave, N.W.
Washington, DC 20036
202/857-1190

Board Certification
American Board of Internal Medicine
3624 Market St., Philadelphia, PA 19104
215/243-1500
800/441-ABIM (800/441-2246)

Neurofibromatosis
National Neurofibromatosis Foundation
141 Fifth Avenue, Suite 7-S, New York, NY 10010
800/323-7938

Neurological Surgery
(for use of the profession only)
American Academy of Neurological Surgery,
Dept. of Neurosurgery, University of Tennessee
956 Court Ave., Memphis, TN 38163
901/528-6374

American Association of Neurological Surgeons
22 S. Washington, Park Ridge, IL 60068
708/692-9500

American Board of Neurological Surgery
Smith Tower, Suite 2139, 6550 Fannin St.
Houston, TX 77030-2701
713/790-6015

Congress of Neurological Surgeons
Mayfield Neurological Institute
506 Oak St., Cincinnati, OH 45219
513/872-2656

Neurology

Neurologist: alternate titles: nerve specialist:
Diagnoses and treats organic diseases and
disorders or nervous systems: Orders and studies
results of chemical, microscopic, biological, and
bacteriological analyses of patient's blood and
cerebro-spinal fluid to determine nature and
extent of disease or disorder. Identifies presence
of pathological blood conditions or parasites and
prescribes and administers medications and
drugs. Orders and studies results of
electroencephalograms or x-rays to detect
abnormalities in brain wave patterns, or
indications of abnormalities in brain structure.
Advises patient to contact other medical
specialist, as indicated. (DOT)

American Academy of Neurology
2221 University Ave. SE, Suite 335
Minneapolis, MN 55414
612/623-8115

American Board of Psychiatry and Neurology
500 Lake Cook Rd, Suite 335, Deerfield, IL 60015
708/945-7900

New England Journal of Medicine

New England Journal of Medicine
ISSN 0028-4793
Massachusetts Medical Society
1440 Main St., Waltham, MA 02254
800/843-6356

Nuclear Energy

JAMA Article of Note: Medical Perspective on
Nuclear Power. Council on Scientific Affairs.
JAMA. 1989 Nov 17; 262(19): 2724-9

Nuclear Medicine

American Board of Nuclear Medicine
900 Veteran Ave., Rm. 12-200
Los Angeles, CA 90024
213/825-6787

American College of Nuclear Medicine
145 W. 58th St., New York, NY 10019
212/582-3919

American College of Nuclear Physicians
1101 Connecticut Ave., NW, Ste 700,
Washington, DC 20036
202/857-1135

The Society of Nuclear Medicine
136 Madison Ave., New York, NY 10016-6760
212/889-0717

Nuclear Medicine Technologist

History: The Joint Review Committee on
Educational Programs in Nuclear Medicine
Technology was formed by the Society of Nuclear
Medicine, Society of Nuclear Medical
Technologists, American College of Radiology,
American Society of Clinical Pathologists,
American Society for Medical Technology, and
American Society of Radiologic Technologists.
The first meeting of the Joint Review Committee
was held in January 1970.

The Society of Nuclear Medical Technologists,
one of the original sponsors, terminated its
corporate status as a professional organization in
1975 and relinquished its sponsorship of the Joint
Review Committee. Current representation of
collaborating sponsors on the review committee
includes two members appointed by each of the
following organizations: American College of
Radiology, American Society for Medical
Technology, American Society of Clinical
Pathologists, American Society of Radiologic
Technologists, Society of Nuclear Medicine,
Society of Nuclear Medicine, and Society of
Nuclear Medicine-Technologist Section. The
current sponsorship maintains a balance between
physicians and technologists.

The responsibilities of the Joint Review Committee
include coordinating the preparation and revision
of educational standards for adoption by
collaborating organizations and conducting
program reviews. The committee meets twice
annually to review educational programs and
prepare recommendations on accreditation status
for final action by the Committee on Allied Health
Education and accreditation.

The first Essentials of an Accredited Educational
Program for the Nuclear Medicine Technologist
were adopted by the collaborating organizations in
1969. The Essentials were substantially revised in
1976 and 1984.

Occupational Description: Nuclear medicine is the
medical specialty that utilizes the nuclear
properties of radioactive and stable nuclides to
make diagnostic evaluations of the anatomic or
physiologic conditions of the body and to provide
therapy with unsealed radioactive sources. The
skills of the nuclear medicine technologists
complement those of the nuclear medicine
physician and of other professionals in the field.

Job Description: Nuclear medicine technologists
perform a number of tasks in the areas of patient
care, technical skills, and administration. When
caring for patients, they acquire adequate
knowledge of the patients' medical history to
understand and relate to their illness and pending
diagnostic procedures for therapy; instruct the
patient prior to and during procedures; evaluate
the satisfactory preparation of the patient prior to
commencing a procedure; and recognize
emergency patient conditions and initiate
lifesaving first aid when appropriate.

Nuclear medicine technologists apply their
knowledge of radiation physics and safety
regulations to limit radiation exposure; prepare
and administer radiopharmaceuticals; use
radiation detection devices and other kinds of
laboratory equipment that measure the quantity
and distribution of radionuclides deposited in the

patient or in a patient specimen; perform in-vivo and in-vitro diagnostic procedures; utilize quality control techniques as part of a quality assurance program covering all procedures and products in the laboratory; and participate in research activities.

Administrative functions may include supervising other nuclear medicine technologists, students, laboratory assistants, and other personnel; participating in procuring supplies and equipment; documenting laboratory operations; participating in departmental inspections conducted by various licensing, regulatory, and accrediting agencies; and participating in scheduling patient examinations.

Employment Characteristics: The employment outlook in nuclear medicine technology is excellent. Opportunities may be found in major medical centers and in small hospitals. Opportunities are also available for obtaining positions in clinical research, education, and administration. Salaries vary depending on the employer and geographic location.

According to the 1990 CAHEA Annual Supplemental Survey, entry level salaries average $26,118.(ALL)

AMA Allied Health Department
312/464-4634

Nuclear War

JAMA Theme Issue: Weapons of Destruction
JAMA. 1989 Aug 4; 262(5)
Yearly JAMA commemorates the August 6, 1945 bombing of Hiroshima by printing details from the *Hiroshima Murals* of Iri and Toshi Maruki on the cover. Occasionally, the issue refects concerns of the use of these weapons, and the technology that supports them, on society. Discussions here are specific to chemical and biological warfare, radiation safety, and radioactive wastes. Previous issues (August 1, 1986; August 2, 1985) concentrate on nuclear war, in general, and the Chernobyl accident.

Nurse Attorneys

American Association of Nurse Attorneys
113 W. Franklin St., Baltimore, MD 21201
301/752-3318

Nurse Midwives

Provides medical care and treatment to obstetrical patients under supervision of Obstetrician. Delivers babies, and instructs patients in prenatal and postnatal health practices: Participates in initial examination of obstetrical patient, and is assigned responsibility for care, treatment, and delivery of patient. Examines patient during pregnancy, utilizing physical findings, laboratory test results, and patient's statements to evaluate condition and ensure that patient's progress is normal. Discusses case with Obstetrician to assure observation of specified practices. Instructs patient in diet and prenatal health practices. Stays with patient during labor to reassure patient and to administer medication. Delivers infant and performs postpartum examinations and treatments to ensure that patient and infant are responding normally. When deviations from standard are encountered during pregnancy or delivery, administers stipulated emergency measures, and arranges for immediate contact of Obstetrician. Visits patient during postpartum period in hospital and at home to instruct patient in care of self and infant and examine patient. Maintains records of cases for inclusion in establishment file. Conducts classes for groups of patients and families to provide information concerning pregnancy, childbirth, and family orientation. May direct activities of other workers. May instruct in midwifery in establishment providing such training. (DOT)

American College of Nurse-Midwives
1522 K St. NW, Suite 1000
Washington, DC 20005
202/289-0171

Nursing

Nurse, General Duty: alternative titles: nurse, staff: Provides general nursing care to patients in hospital, nursing home, inffffirmary, or similar health care facility: Administers prescribed medications and treatments in accordance with approved nursing techniques. Prepares equipment and aids physician during treatments and examinations of patients. Observes patient, records significant conditions and reactions, and notifies superior or physician of patient's condition and reaction to drugs, treatments, and significant incidents. Takes temperature, pulse, blood pressure, and other vital signs to detect deviations from normal and assess condition of patient. May rotate among various clinical services of insititution, such as obstetrics, surgery, orthopedics, outpatient and admitting, pediatrics, and psychiatry. May prepare rooms, sterile instruments, equipment and supplies, and hand items to surgeon, obstetrician, or other medical practitioner. May make beds, bathe, and feed patients. May serve as leader for group of personnel rendering nursing care to number of patients.(DOT)

Nurse Practitioner alternate titles: primary care nurse practitioner. Provides general medical care and treatment to patient in medical facility, such as clinic, health center, or public health agency, under direction of physician: Performs physical examinations and preventive health measures within prescribed guidelines and instructions of physician. Orders, interprets, and evaluates diagnostic tests to identify and assess patient's clinical problems and health care needs. Records physical findings, and formulates plan and prognosis, based on patient's condition. Discusses case with physician and other health professionals to prepare comprehensive patient care plan. Submits health care plan and goals of individual patients for periodic review and evaluation by physician. Prescribes or recommends drugs or other forms of treatment such as physical therapy, inhalation therapy, or related therapeutics procedures. May refer patients to physician for consultation or to specialized health resources for treatment. May be designated according to field of specialization as Pediatric Nurse Practitioner. Where state law permits, may engage in independent practice.(DOT)

Nurse, Licensed Practical: Provides prescribed medical treatment and personal care services to ill, injured, convalescent, and handicapped persons in such settings as hospitals, clinics, private homes, schools, sanitariums, and similar institution: Takes and records patients' vital signs. Dresses wound, gives enemas, douches, alcohol rubs, and massages. Applies compresses, ice bags, and hot water bottles. Observes patients and reports adverse reactions to medication or treatment to medical personnel in charge. Administers specified medication, orally or by subcutaneous or intermuscular injection, and notes time and amount on patients' charts. Assembles and uses such equipment as catheters, tracheotomy tubes, and oxygen suppliers. Collects samples, such as urine, blood, and sputum, from patients for testing and performs routine laboratory tests on samples. Sterilizes equipment and supplies, using germicides, sterilizer, or autoclave. Prepares or examines food trays for prescribed diet and feeds patients. Records food and fluid intake and output. Bathes, dresses, and assists patients in walking and turning. Cleans rooms, makes beds, and answers patients' calls. Washes and dresses bodies of deceased persons. Must pass state board examination and be licensed. May assist in delivery,care, and feeding of infants. May inventory and requisition supplies. May provide medical treatment and personal care to patients in private home settings and be designated Home Health Nurse, Licensed Practical. (DOT)

Nurse Anesthetist: Administers local, inhalation, intravenous, and other anesthetics prescribed by Anesthesiologist to induce total or partial loss of sensation or consciousness in patients during surgery, deliveries, or other medical and dental procedures: Fits mask to patient's face, turns dials and sets gauges of equipment to regulate flow oxygen and gases to administer anesthetic by inhalation method, according to prescribed medical standards. Prepares prescribed solutions and administers local, intravenous, spinal, or other anesthetic, following specified methods and procedures. Notes patient's skin color and dilation of pupils and observes video screen and digital display of computerized equipment to monitor patient's vital signs during anesthesia. Initiates remedial measures to prevent surgical shock or other adverse conditions. Informs physician of patient's condition during anesthesia.(DOT)

American Academy of Nurse Practitioners
45 Foster St, Suite A, Lowell, MA 01851
512/442-4262

American Association of Colleges of Nursing
One Dupont Circle, NW, Suite 530
Washington, DC 20036
202/463-6930

American Nurses Association
600 Maryland Ave, SW, Suite 100W
Washington, DC 20024
202/554-4444

National League of Nursing
10 Columbus Circle, New York, NY 10019
212/582-1022

Prescriptive privileges for controlled substances by nurses; State breakdown,

Discussion and Summary
Katherine H. Chavigny. 1993.

Alaska**
Legal Authority: Statutory authority for independent prescription privileges for qualified nurse practitioners (NPs).
Restrictions: No restrictions NPs prescribe controlled substances, Schedule II-V

Arizona**
Legal Authority: Full prescriptive authority under the nurse practice and pharmacy acts for NPs upon application to the Board of Nursing.
Restrictions: Schedule II and III drugs limited to 48 hour supply

Connecticut**
Legal Authority: Nurse practice acts requires certification in advanced practice. The only title regulated is Advanced Practice Registered Nurse (APRN). Definitions vary but usually applies to Nurse Midwives, NPs, Nurse Anesthetists, and, often, Clinical Nurse Specialists.

Restrictions: APRN must apply for extra license to prescribe which includes controlled substances.

Washington D.C.
*Legal Authority***:** NP authorized in health occupation act under the jurisdiction of the board of nursing.

Restrictions: Must work with MD or DOs and prescribe Schedule II-V drugs by exiting federal laws.

Maryland
Legal Authority: NPs certified to practice by the board of nursing and with written agreements with responsible MDs.

Restrictions: Prescription of controlled substances with written agreement of physician.

Montana**
Legal Authority: The board of nursing recognizes nurse specialists and requires certification. Regulations for prescribing drafted by a joint board.

Restrictions: Nurse specialist can prescribe all medications under their own DEA numbers.

New Hampshire
Legal Authority: NPs are registered under the board of nursing and required certification.
Restrictions: May prescribe Schedule II-V from an official formulary from a board with one MD.

New York
Legal Authority: New York education act authorizing title and scope of practice of nurse practitioner.

Restrictions: Includes prescribing all drugs/devices when in a collaborative relationship with physicians. Nurses have applied for DEA numbers without success.

North Dakota
Legal Authority: Licenses APRN -- RNs in advanced practice, such as NPs, Nurse Midwives, and Nurse Anesthetists.

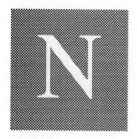

Restrictions: Statements required form a physician clarifying RN prescriptive practices

Wisconsin
Legal Authority: Authority from the nurse practice act with broad definition of nursing. There is NO use of the word "prescribe". Instead, RNs prescribe as a "delegated medical act" under a specific chapter in the administrative code.

Restrictions: Registered nurses may prescribe as a "delegated medical act" all drugs as long as the regulations of administrative code are met.

Discussion:
Plenary prescriptive privileges: Four states, Alaska, Arizona, Connecticut, and Montana have now authorized plenary prescriptive privileges i.e., prescription of all drugs including controlled substances without any protocols identified with physicians. The first three states use the title "nurse practitioner" in the statutes. The title includes adult nurse practitioners, pediatric nurse practitioners, family nurse practitioners, geriatric nurse practitioners, and school nurse practitioners, and perhaps women nurse practitioners.

In Connecticut, the statutes authorize nurses in "advanced practice" to prescribe controlled substances. The title "Advanced Practice RN" expands the categories of nurses with prescriptive privileges to include not only nurse practitioners but also nurse anesthetists, nurse midwives, and perhaps clinical nurse specialists who work in hospitals. Advanced practice definitions are still being sought by organized nursing.

Five other states have authorized the prescription of controlled substances; Washington DC, Maryland, New Hampshire, New York, and North Dakota. In these states, nurse prescription is a defined collaborative arrangement with physicians and/or, as in New Hampshire, an official formulary is required.

Special note is made of Wisconsin, where registered nurses may prescribe as a delegated medical act. The title use here is "registered nurse" and therefore applies to all registered nurses as soon as they are licensed. The administrative code calls for strict supervision by physicians; however, it does include prescribing controlled substances; therefore it is included in the list of state where nurses prescribe Schedule II-V drugs.

Summary. There are ten states where nurses can prescribe controlled substances. In four states, Alaska, Arizona, Connecticut, and Montana, nurse prescription is "plenary" and nurses may prescribe controlled substances, Schedule II-V without physician intermediaries and without physician protocols. In one state, Wisconsin, prescribing controlled substances by RNs is a "delegated medical act".

**Independent of physician collaboration either in practice and/or using physician protocols.

Nursing Assocations, Statewide
Alabama State Nurses' Association
360 N. Hull St, Montgomery, AL 36104-3658
205/262-8321

Alaska Nurses' Association
237 E 3rd Ave, Suite 3, Anchorage, AK 99501
907/274-0827

Arizona Nurses' Association
1850 E Southern Ave, Suite 1
Tempe, AZ 85282-5832
602/831-0404

Arkansas Nurses' Association
117 S Cedar St, Little Rock, AR 72205
501/664-5853

California Nurses' Association
1855 Folsom St, Suite 670
San Francisco, CA 94103
415/864-4141

Colorado Nurses' Association
5453 E Evans Place, Denver, CO 80222
303/757-7483

Connecticut Nurses' Association
377 Research Parkway, Suite 2D
Meriden, CT 06450
203/238-1207

Delaware Nurses' Association
2634 Capitol Trail, Suite A, Newark, DE 19711
302/368-2333

District of Columbia Nurses' Association
5100 Wisconsin Ave, NW, Suite 306
Washington, DC 20016
202/244-2705

Florida Nurses' Association
PO Box 536985, Orlando, FL 32853-6985
407/896-3261

Georgia Nurses' Association
1362 W Peachtree St, NW, Atlanta, GA 30309
404/876-4624

Guam Nurses' Association
Box 3134, Agana, GU 96910

Hawaii Nurses' Association
677 Ala Moana Blvd, No. 301, Honolulu, HI 96813
808/531-1628

Idaho Nurses' Association
200 N 4th St, Suite 20, Boise, ID 83702-6001
208/345-0500

Illinois Nurses' Association
20 N Wacker Drive, Suite 2520, Chicago, IL 60606
312/236-9708

Indiana State Nurses' Association
2915 N High School Road
Indianapolis, IN 46224-2969
317/299-4575

Iowa Nurses' Association
100 Court Ave, Suite 9LL, Des Moines, IA 50309
515/282-9169

Kansas State Nurses' Association
700 SW Jackson, Suite 601

Topeka, KS 66603-3731
913/233-8638

Kentucky Nurses' Association
PO Box 2616, Louisville, KY 40201
502/637-2546

Louisiana State Nurses' Association
712 Transcontinental Drive, Metairie, LA 70001
504/889-1030

Maine State Nurses' Association
283 Water St, PO Box 2240
Augusta, ME 04338-2240
207/622-1057

Maryland Nurses' Association
5820 Southwestern Blvd.
Baltimore, MD 21227-4404
301/242-7300

Massachusetts Nurses' Association
340 Turnpike St, Canton, MA 02021
617/821-4625

Michigan Nurses' Association
2310 Jolly Oak Road, Okemos, MI 48864
517/349-5640

Minnesota Nurses' Association
1295 Bandana Blvd, N, Suite 140
St. Paul, MN 55108
612/646-4807

Mississippi Nurses' Association
135 Bounds St, Jackson, MS 39206
601/982-9182

Missouri Nurses' Association
206 E Dunklin St, PO Box 325
Jefferson City, MO 65102-0325
314/636-4623

Montana Nurses' Association
PO Box 5718, Helena, MT 59604
406/442-6710

Nebraska Nurses' Association
941 O Street, Suite 711, Lincoln, NE 68508
402/475-3859

Nevada Nurses' Association
3660 Baker Lane, Suite 104, Reno, NV 89509
702/825-3555

New Hampshire Nurses' Association
48 West St, Concord, NH 03301
603/225-3783

New Jersey State Nurses' Association
320 W State St, Trenton, NJ 08618
609/392-4884

New Mexico Nurses' Association
909 Virginia NE, Suite 101
Albuquerque, NM 87108
505/268-7744

New York State Nurses' Association
2113 Western Ave, Guilderland, NY 12084
518/456-5371

North Carolina Nurses' Association
Box 12025, Raleigh, NC 27605-2025
919/821-4250

North Dakota Nurses' Association
212 N 4th St, Bismarck, ND 58501
701/223-1385

Ohio Nurses' Association
4000 E Main St, Columbus, OH 43213-2950
614/237-5414

Oklahoma Nurses' Association
6414 N Santa Fe, Suite A
Oklahoma City, OK 73116
405/840-3476

Oregon Nurses' Association
9600 SW Oak St, Suite 550, Portland, OR 97223
503/293-0011

Pennsylvania Nurses' Association
2578 Interstate Drive, PO Box 8525
Harrisburg, PA 17105
717/657-1222

Colegio de Professionales de la Enfermeria de
Puerto Rico
PO Box 363647, San Juan, PR 00936-3647
809/753-7197

Rhode Island State Nurses' Association
345 Blackstone Blvd, Providence, RI 02906
401/421-9703

South Carolina Nurses' Association
1821 Gadsden St, Columbia, SC 29201
803/252-4781

South Dakota Nurses' Association
1505 S Minnesota, Suite 6, Sioux Falls, SD 57105
605/338-1401

Tennessee Nurses' Association
545 Mainstream Drive, Suite 405
Nashville, TN 37228-1207
615/254-0350

Texas Nurses' Association
300 Highland Mall Blvd, Suite 300
Austin, TX 78752-3718
512/452-0645

Utah Nurses' Association
1058 E 900th S, Salt Lake City, UT 84105
801/322-3439

Vermont State Nurses' Association
500 Dorset St, South Burlington, VT 05403
802/864-9390

Virgin Islands Nurses' Association
PO Box 2866, Veterans Dr. Sta.
St. Thomas, VI 00803
809/776-7397

Virginia Nurses' Association
1311 High Point Ave, Richmond, VA 23230
804/353-7311

Washington State Nurses' Association
2505 2nd Ave, Suite 500, Seattle, WA 98121
206/443-9762

West Virginia Nurses' Association
PO Box 1946, Charleston, WV 25327
304/342-1169

Wisconsin Nurses' Association
6117 Monona Drive, Madison, WI 53716
608/221-0383

Wyoming Nurses' Association
1603 Capitol Ave, Room 305
Cheyenne, WY 82001
307/635-3955

Nursing Homes

Referrals are made by a personal physician

Accreditation:
Joint Commission on Accreditation
of Healthcare Organizations
One Renaissance Blvd.
Oakbrook Terrace, IL 60181
708/916-5600

American Health Care Association
1201 L St., NW, Washington, DC 20005
202/833-2050

American Association of Homes for the Aging
1129 20th St., NW, Suite 400
Washington, DC 20036
202/296-5960

Complaints: Contact state or local Department of Public Health.

Nutrition
American College of Nutrition
722 Robert E. Lee Drive
Wilmington, NC 28412-0927
919/452-1222

American Society for Parenteral
and Enteral Nutrition
8603 Fenton St., Suite 412
Silver Spring, MD 20910
301/587-6315

Food and Nutrition Information Center
National Agricultural Library Bldg., Rm 304
Beltsville, MD 20705
301/504-5414

Food Safety
U.S. Department of Agriculture Meat
and Poultry Hotline
800/535-4555

Four Basic Food Groups:
Human Nutrition Information Service
U.S. Department of Agriculture
6505 Bellcrest R., Hyattsville, MD 20782
301/436-8617

Nutrition Programs in Medical Schools
American Society for Clinical Nutrition
9650 Rockville Pike, Bethesda, MD 20814
301/530-7110

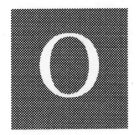

Obesity

American Society of Bariatric Physicians
5600 S. Quebec, Suite 1600
Englewood, CO 80111
303/779-4833

Gastroplasty Support Group
c/o Lumbomyr Kuzmak, MD,
657 Irvington Avenue, Newark, NJ 07106
201/374-1717

National Association to Aid Fat Americans
PO Box 188620, Sacramento, CA 95818
916/443-0303

Obsessive Compulsive Disorder

The Obsessive Compulsive Disorder
(OCD) Foundation
PO Box 9573, New Haven, CT 06535
203/772-0565

Obstetrics and Gynecology

Obstetrician: Treats women during prenatal, natal, and postnatal periods: Examines patient to ascertain condition, utilizing physical findings, laboratory results, and patient's statements as diagnostic aids. Determines need for modified diet and physical activities, and recommends plan. Periodically examines patient, prescribing medication or surgery, if indicated. Delivers infant, and cares for mother for prescribed period of time following childbirth. Performs cesarean section or other surgical procedure as needed to preserve patient's health and deliver infant safely. May treat patients for diseases of generative organs (DOT).

American Board of Obstetrics and Gynecology
4225 Roosevelt Way, NE, Suite 305,
Seattle, WA 98105
206/547-4884

American College of Obstetricians
and Gynecologists
409 12th St., SW, Washington, DC 20024-2188
202/638-5577

American Association of
Gynecologic Laparoscopists
13021 E. Florence Ave.
Santa Fe Springs, CA 90670
213/946-8774

Occupational Health Services
Guidelines for Physicians Contracting Occupational Health Services

Physicians providing occupational health care, either as an employee or as a contractor, must negotiate certain basic rules with the management at the onset of the relationship. As in most contractual relationships, the physician's requests and preferences are more likely to be heard and respected prior to the signing of a contract. Parkinson[1] has outlined several areas for discussion between the physician and employer:

- **Physician Visibility and Accessibility** Physicians who agree to provide medical consultation in the workplace must inspect the workplace at regular intervals. Workers must have access directly to the physician, either individually or through a joint health and safety committee of workers and management, if the industry is large enough to have such a committee.
- **Industrial Hygiene** If a full-time industrial hygienist is not available, the physician must alert management to the need for periodic industrial hygiene consultation, in order to correct deficient work practices and maintain effective hygiene at the worksite.
- **Workers' Compensation Education and Prevention** The physician has an obligation to inform a worker if a disease possibly is related to the worker's occupation. If necessary, the physician must assist the worker or representative in filing the documentation necessary for establishment of a claim.
- **Education and Prevention** The physician should participate actively in illness prevention at the workplace and should have access to the workplace for programs of education and health promotion.

Also, the physician must maintain skills in occupational medicine and have the support of the company for continuing his or her education. In addition to NIOSH educational resource centers the American Occupational Medical Association offers a "basic curriculum" in occupational medicine. The program involves a three-part course offered in two-day segments on a yearly rotating basis.

- **Communication** The physician should establish the right to communicate directly with individual workers and with labor representative on matters affecting health and safety. Health and safety should not become matters that are resolved by confrontations of labor and management.
- **Record-Keeping** Thorough and confidential records should be kept, preferably in a standardized format that is amenable to easy extraction of data by hand or computer. The data should be available for use in epidemiologic studies. An annual or periodic report should be prepared using information gathered from employee medical examinations, that are either preventive or illness-related. When combined with industrial hygiene data, such reports may uncover relationships between workplace exposures and illnesses or injuries.
- **Preplacement Examinations** The employer must furnish a description of the physical and mental requirements of the job under consideration. The physician will furnish the prospective employer with a statement of the patient's suitability for placement based on these requirements. No other information should be supplied. Only the patient, not the potential employer, should be notified of medical conditions that require follow-up. The employers should receive no information about medical diagnoses or laboratory evaluations. Of course, the decision to hire rests with the employer.

- **Periodic Government Mandated Examinations** Employers as well as employees should be notified of evidence indicating adverse effects of occupational exposures. Recommendations concerning maintenance of health through elimination of exposure should be made to both. Only the employee should be given information regarding medical follow-up that may be necessary.
- **Chief Executive Officer Support** As part of any employment contract, physicians offering occupational health services should have an agreement with the company's chief executive officer about the about guidelines (preferably this agreement should be in writing). In addition, all physical-worker-management interactions should be guided by the American Occupational Medical Association's Code of Ethical Conduct for Physicians.

Conclusions

Several aspects of family medicine coincide with providing occupational health care. The continuity of care provided by family physicians increases the likelihood of detecting delayed or chronic health effects due to occupational exposures. Training in behavioral skills allows for better recognition of disturbed biorhythms due to shiftwork, substance abuse, or job stress. The care of other family members due to agents brought home by an employee. Worker-related effects involving children or spouse may be detected more readily when the entire family is seen by the same physician. The traditional advocacy role of the family physician may encourage greater confidence among workers if the same physician is seen at the workplace.

An awareness of community resources, such as visiting nurses, public welfare agencies, industrial health coalitions, local health departments, other medical practitioners and voluntary health agencies is necessary for optimal patient care by both the occupational and the family physician. Cooperative health ventures between industries and physicians may be important resources in communities where industries do not have large corporate medical departments but do have an active interest in the well-being of working people.(FAM)

Reference:

1. Parkinson DHK: Occupational health in family medicine education. Address presented at National Conference on Occupational and Environmental Health Education in Family Medicine, Kansas City, MO, Sept 13, 1983.

Guiding Principles for Occupational Medical Exam.

The physician and the medical staff, and the employee-patient should appreciate the unique role of the occupational medical staff. They are there to serve the patient as well as the company for which the patient works. Thus the staff must take extra care to protect the confidentiality of the physician-patient relationship. And the patient must understand that, although his or her medical information is confidential, the physician's opinion regarding the patient's health status and his or her ability to perform tasks are frequently used in employment determinations by the patient's employer.

The examination should be supervised by, or personally conducted by, the physician. A nurse or other adequately trained member of the health service team can obtain basic data from the examinee, such as the history (including occupational history); vision and audiometric testing; height and weight, blood pressure, pulse and temperature; and, depending upon training, physical assessment to differentiate normal from abnormal. In addition, the assistant can perform urinalysis, pulmonary function tests, ECGs, and other appropriate laboratory procedures. A female attendant should be present when women are being examined.

It is the duty of the physician to interpret medical findings and to make decisions regarding their work significance. Health counseling requires special training and should be performed by the physician or by designated professional personnel.

It is fundamental that the physician must have the first hand knowledge from personal observation of the various jobs within the industry being served. Information showing physical demands, working conditions, and accident and health hazards of each job classification facilitates appropriate placement.

Scope of the Examination

The nature of the industry, its inherent hazards, the variation in jobs, and physical demands and health exposures are determinants of the nature and scope of the medical examination. It is essential that each examination be thorough and suitable for its purpose. What may be adequate in one case may be quite insufficient in another. For example, the physical demands on an ironworker engaged in construction of a skyscraper are quite different from those of the sedentary typist. The value of different examination procedures and their cost in time and dollars must be assayed. After carefully studying the problems involved, the physician should advise management concerning the scope of the examination.

It might be economically unsound for an essentially nonhazardous industry to include extensive laboratory and x-rays tests of all employees. On the other hand, a brief and superficial examination can be false economy and be misleading to employer and employee alike. Some large companies extend their capability for employee health appraisals by use of multiphasic health testing, performed by allied health personnel but reviewed by the physician.

The best type of examination program is one that emphasizes flexibility according to need, rather than one that has a set and invariable routine. A flexible plan provides for a basic minimum examination but recognizes the difference among individuals, age groups, and jobs. This permits the examining physician to devote less time time and fewer procedures to the evidently young individual in a nonhazardous job. Another worker in a potentially more hazardous job should receive more searching attention. Frequency of examination should vary with age, sex, occupation, and individual findings.

Opinions vary considerably as to what constitutes a minimum examination. The following is suggested:

1. **History**

a. Personal

b. Family

c. Social

d. Occupational

2. **General Health**

a. Blood pressure

b. Resting pulse

c. Height

d. Weight

e. General appearance

3. **Physical examination**

a. Skin, eyes, ears, nose, teeth and mouth

b. Chest - lungs and heart

c. Palpable lymph nodes

d. Peripheral blood nodes

e. Abdomen - especially for hernias

f. Genitalia and anus

g. Spine and extremities

h. Brief neurologic examination

i. Brief mental status examination

4. **Laboratory**

a. Visual and hearing acuity

b. Urinalysis

Types of Examinations

The various kinds of examinations may be classified as: (1) initial or preplacement; (2) periodic; and (3) special.

Pre-placement Examinations: Previously called "pre-employment examinations, pre-placement examinations are made for the express purpose of determining and recording the physical condition of the prospective worker and assigning the worker to a suitable job in which impairments, if any, will not affect personal health and safety, or the health and safety of others. The prospective worker or his or her personal physician must be advised of conditions needing attention.

Periodic Examination: Periodic examinations of employees may be voluntary or mandatory for continued employment.

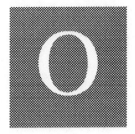

If voluntary, it is usually customary to make the examination on or near the birthday of each individual. This usually results in a reasonable spread of examination over the calendar year and eliminates peak loads. If the operations involved are relatively non-hazardous, intervals between examinations can be as long as two or three years.

Periodic examinations are usually required for workers who are exposed to processes or materials that are definite or suspected health hazards, or whose work involves responsibility for the safety of others. Noise, heavy metals, certain chemicals, radiation, temperature and barometric extremes, and mineral and vegetable fibers and dusts, for example, are capable of causing occupational disease or injury. Usually, process controls keep workers reasonably safe. However, caution dictates the advisability of periodic medical examination to be certain that the engineering controls are effective. This also enables early detection of the hypersusceptible individual and the worker whose unsafe personal practices defeat the control measures. Regulations and standards developed under occupational safety and health legislation often require mandatory medical or biological monitoring of workers exposed to specific hazards in certain industries.

The frequency of examination will vary in accordance with legislation, the quality of the engineering control, the severity of the exposure and the individual findings on each examination. Thus, some exposures might justify examinations or laboratory tests of the workers on a monthly or quarterly basis, while in other cases annual or biennial examinations may be adequate. In some instances, laboratory tests at regular intervals will suffice as the primary focus of a periodic examination program, accompanied by complete examinations at less frequent intervals.

Examinations of executives may be regarded as a special type of periodic examination. While not new, they are becoming more popular and are justified by their advocates on the premise that business executives carry heavy responsibilities, including the welfare of large numbers of employees.

While some companies require their executives to participate in these programs, considerable advantage accrues when the programs are voluntary promoted by a thorough campaign, inasmuch as individuals seeking examination are more cooperative and appreciative of the service. Practices vary regarding use of in-plant medical departments. If the in-plant health facility is adequately staffed and equipped, it is preferable to do these examinations within the department since counseling for health maintenance is often more effective in this setting. Otherwise, executives should be sent to outside facilities well-qualified to perform the required services. Emphasis should be on health evaluation and counseling.

Special Examination: Special examinations may indicated at the time of a transfer from one job to

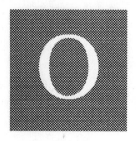

another. The control of communicable disease by examination of food handlers is an example of a special purpose examination; in many jurisdictions, this is required by law.

Many organizations find it worthwhile to make "return to work" examinations of employees who have been absent more than a specified number of days due to illness or injury. This is done to control communicable disease as well as to determine suitability for return to work. Upon return to work following such absence, a new evaluation of physical capacities may be necessary. Rehabilitation procedures may be necessary to reduce disability and improve the range of employability.

Another special examination is the health evaluation of a problem employee, that is, an individual who is having performance or attendance problems on the job, which may be the result of some health problem. Problem employees are usually referred to the physician by the supervisor, although they may be referred by family, friend, union or self. Not infrequently, chronic illness, alcoholism or a social problem is discovered and an appropriate referral for treatment and rehabilitation can be made by the occupational health physician.(OEM)

Occupational Medicine
American College of Occupational Medicine (formerly American Occupational Medical Assn.) 55 W. Seegers, Arlington Heights, IL 60005 708/228-6850

Board Certification
American Board of Preventive Medicine Department of Community Medicine Wright State University, P.O. Box 927 Dayton, OH 45401 513/278-6915

Occupational Physician alternate titles: company doctor; physician, industrial. Diagnoses and treats work-related illnesses and injuries of employees, and conducts fitness-for-duty physical examinations: Attends patients in plant or hospital, and reexamines disability cases periodically to verify progress. Oversees maintenance of case histories, health examination reports, and other medical records. Formulates and administer health programs. Inspects plant and makes recommendations regarding sanitation and elimination of health hazards. (DOT)

Nurse, Staff, Occupational Health Nursing alternate titles: nurse, staff, industrial. Provides nursing service and first aid to employees or persons who become ill or injured on premises of department store, industrial plant, or other establishment: Takes patient's vital signs, treats wounds, evaluates physical condition of patient, and contacts physician and hospital to arrange for further medical treatment, when needed. Maintains record of persons treated, and prepares accident reports and insurance forms. Develops employee programs, such as health educations, accident prevention, alcohol abuse counseling, curtailment of smoking, and weight control regimes. May assist physician in physical examination of new employees. (DOT)

Occupational Health and Safety
How to deal with requirements of OSHA safety rules

Mike Mitka AMNews 5/18/92 p. 23+

The effective dates for the Occupational Safety and Health Administration's bloodborne-pathogen standards are coming fast and furious.

Earlier this month physicians, in their role as employers, had to have written exposure-control plans in place. By June 4, employees must receive education on bloodborne-disease transmission and must be trained in universal precautions. Employers must begin maintaining employee records, including information on training, occupational injuries and vaccinations.

On July 6, 1992, engineering - meaning the physical isolation of potentially infectious materials - and work practice controls must be in place and protective equipment must be in place and protective equipment must be in use. Free hepatitis B vaccinations and postexposure treatment must be available. All hazardous material labels should be in place.

The standards are meant to protect all workers who could be "reasonably anticipated" to face contact with blood and other potentially infectious materials.

Physicians appear willing to meet the standard, but confusion still remains. Michael Zarski, an American Medical Association legislative counsel, has complied the following list of key points that physicians should be aware of.

Physicians must have completed by May 5 the Exposure Control Plan, which is designed to document what risks are present in the workplace and what protective measures are being utilized.

The plan must contain a exposure determination list, a schedule and methods for implementing the OSHA regulations and protocols for evaluation of exposure incidents.

Exposure Determination List. The list cites the job classifications in which all employees risk exposure, that is, unprotected contact with blood or other potentially infectious material. It also lists job classifications in a facility in which some employees risk exposure and procedures performed on site in which occurred without use of personal protective equipment.

Schedule and methods for implementation. These must include brief descriptions of how a facility complies with regulations on workplace and engineering controls, personal protective equipment, housekeeping, hepatitis B vaccination, postexposure evaluation and follow-up, labels, signs and recordkeeping.

For workplace and engineering controls, the standard emphasizes hand washing and procedures for minimizing needlesticks and the splashing and spraying of blood. It also requires appropriate packaging and labeling of specimens, regulated wastes and contaminated equipment.

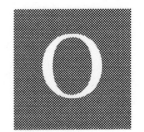

Personal protective equipment - such as gloves, gowns, masks, mouthpieces and resuscitation bags - must be provided at no cost to employees, and its appropriate use required.

A written housekeeping schedule must be maintained noting that employees are responsible for ensuring that equipment and surfaces are cleaned with an appropriate disinfectant and decontaminated immediately after a spill or leakage occurs and at the end if a work shift.

A hepatitis B vaccination must be made available at no costs to all employees within 10 working days of an assignment involving potential occupational exposure to blood. The OSHA-approved waiver form must be signed by any employee declining the vaccine.

Post-exposure evaluation and follow-up requires that specific procedures will be made available at no cost to all employees who have had an exposure incident. The follow-up must include a confidential medical evaluation.

Labels and signs must be used on all hazardous items.

Recordkeeping requires that confidential medical records will be kept for all employees with occupational exposure for at least 30 years after the person leaves employment. Training records of workers at risk to occupational exposure must also be kept for at least three years following the date of the training sessions.

Protocols for evaluation of exposure incidents. A written procedure must be maintained that includes four key elements. They are:
• The name of the contact person for exposure accidents.
• The name of the person who will evaluate the exposure incident to determine if any procedures should be changed.
• A requirement for written documentation of the incident that includes the name of the exposed individual, the source of exposure, a description of what happened and the date and time.
• A requirement for written evaluation of the exposure incident including any suggestions for procedure changes and a record of how these changes were implemented.
Physicians-employers seeking more detailed information about the standards should contact their OSHA are office.

Periodic updating needed

The Exposure Control Plan is the most important document to be maintained by physicians regarding the Occupational Safety and Health Administration bloodborne pathogens standard.

In the unlikely event of an OSHA inspection, the Exposure Control Plan will be used by the inspector as a key to how well a physician is complying.

The plan is not a passive document. It will need periodic updating:
• At least annually.
• When new tasks and procedures that affect occupational exposure are added.

• When tasks and procedures affecting occupational exposure are changed or modified.
• When new employee positions with occupational exposure risk are added or when employee positions are changed to include the exposure.

Clearinghouse for Occupational
Safety and Health Information
4676 Columbia Parkway, Cincinnati, OH 45226
800/356-4674
513/533-4674 (in Ohio)

Occupational Safety and Health Administration
Department of Labor
200 Constitution Ave., NW
Washington, DC 20210
202/523-8151

OSHA Regional Offices

Region I: CT, MA, ME, NH, RI, VT
133 Portland St, 1st Floor, Boston, MA 02114
617/565-7164

Region II: NJ, NY, PR, VI
201 Varick St, Room 670, New York, NY 10014
212/337-2378

Region III :DC, DE, MD, PA, VA, WV
Gateway Building, Suite 2100,
3535 Market St, Philadelphia, PA 19104
215/596-1201

Region IV: AL, FL, GA, KY, MS, NC, SC, TN
1375 Peachtree St, NE, Suite 587
Atlanta, GA 30367
404/347-3573

Region V: IL, IN, MI, MN, OH, WI
230 S. Dearborn St, Room 3244
Chicago, IL 60604
312/353-2220

Region VI: AR, LA, NM, OK, TX
525 Griffin St, Room 602, Dallas, TX 75202
214/767-4731

Region VII: IA, KS, MO, NE
911 Walnut St, Room 406, Kansas City, MO 64106
816/426-5861

Region VIII: CO, MT, ND, SD, UT, WY
Federal Bldg, Room 1576, 1961 Stout St.
Denver, CO 80294
303/844-3061

Region IX: American Samoa, AZ, CA,
Guam, HI, NV
71 Stevenson St, Room 415
San Francisco, CA 94105
415/744-6670

Region X: AK, ID, OR, WA
1111 Third Ave, Suite 715, Seattle, WA 98101
206/553-5930

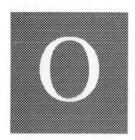

Occupational Therapy

History: In 1933, the American Occupational Therapy Association (AOTA) requested that the Council on Physical Therapy AMA undertake review and evaluation of occupational therapy programs. The AMA Board of Trustees referred the request to the Council on Physical Therapy and the Council on Medical Education and Hospitals.

The Council on Physical Therapy had been created in 1925 "to investigate and report on the value and merits of all non-medicinal apparatus and contrivances offered for sale to physicians and hospitals, and to publish in the Journal from time to time results of its investigations." The Council on Medical Education and Hospitals was selected as the proper body to undertake the reviews because of its experience in all phases of medical education, including the investigation of medical schools, teaching hospitals, and programs for the education of technicians in specialties that are closely allied to medical service. The review of occupational therapy programs, which began in 1933, was carried out in conjunction with other activities of the Council.

In 1934 and 1935, joint meetings were held with representatives of the American Occupational Therapy Association, the AMA Council on Physical Therapy, and the Council on Medical Education and Hospitals to establish Essentials for educational programs. The Essentials were adopted by the AMA House of Delegates in 1935.The Essentials were revised in 1938, 1943, 1949, 1965, 1973, and 1983.

During the 1950s, educational programs for assistant level personnel in occupational therapy were developed. In 1958, AOTA formalized the implementation of a plan for the Certified Occupational Therapy Assistant, approved educational standards, and assumed responsibility for review and approval of the educational programs. There were originally two sets of educational standards for the occupational therapy assistant. One set was for the certificate programs, generally hospital based, that were a year or less in length. The second was for the associate degree programs at community and junior colleges. In 1975, the Essentials and Guidelines of an Approved Educational Program for the Occupational Therapy Assistant (modeled after the Essentials established for the professional level programs) were established and adopted, and hospital based programs were discontinued. Educational standards were revised in 1983 and again in 1990. During 1990, at the request of the AOTA, CAHEA and the OTA programs into the CAHEA accreditation system.

The American Occupational Therapy Association has placed its emphasis on objectivity and consistency in reviewing, revising, and coordinating its accreditation process and evaluation documents. In addition, attention has been directed toward decreasing time and costs for both the institution and the AOTA Accreditation Committee in preparing documentation required for the accreditation process.

The role of collaborating organizations in accreditation is vitally important. The American Occupational Therapy Association is involved in the accreditation process through adoption of Essentials and review of programs. The Association participates in drafting and revising Essentials and its governing body formally adopts Essentials. The Association provides experts to survey programs to ascertain whether the educational programs meet the Essentials, and to provide representatives for the AOTA Accreditation Committee to meet as a review committee to evaluate programs for accreditation. A representative from the American Occupational Therapy Association also serves on the CAHEA Panel of Consultants.

Occupational Therapy Assistant

Occupational Description: Under the direction of an occupational therapist, the occupational therapy assistant directs an individual's participation in selected tasks to restore, reinforce, and enhance performance; facilitate learning of those skills and functions essential for adaptation and productivity; diminish or correct pathology; and promote and maintain health. The occupational orientation of the assistant is that of guiding the individual's goal-directed use of time, energy, interest, and attention. A fundamental concern is the development and maintenance of the capacity throughout the life span, to perform with satisfaction to self and others those tasks and roles essential to productive living and to the mastery of self and the environment.

Under the therapist's direction, the assistant participates in the development of adaptive skills and performance capacity, and is concerned with factors which promote, influence or enhance performance as well as those that serve as barriers or impediments to the individual's ability to function. The occupational therapy assistant provides service to those individuals whose abilities to cope with tasks of living are threatened or impaired by development deficits, the aging process, poverty and cultural differences, physical injury or illness, or psychological and social disability.

Job Description: Entry-level occupational therapy assistant technical education prepared the individual to:
- Collaborate in providing occupational therapy services with appropriate supervision to prevent deficits and to maintain or improve functions in the activities of daily living, work, and play/leisure and in the underlying components, e.g., sensorimotor, cognitive, and psychosocial.
- Participate in managing occupational therapy service.
- Direct activity programs.
- Incorporate values and attitudes congruent with the profession's standards and ethics.

Employment Characteristics: OTAs assist in the planning and implementation of treatment of a diverse population in a variety of settings such as nursing homes, hospitals and clinics, rehabilitation facilities, long-term care facilities, extended care facilities, sheltered workshops, schools and camps, private homes, and community agencies. Recent AOTA studies indicate that the mean average salary is $17,841.

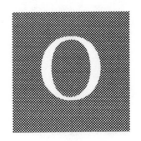

Occupational Therapist

Occupational Description: Occupational therapy is the application of purposeful, goal-oriented activity in the evaluation, diagnosis, and/or treatment of persons whose abilities to cope with the tasks of living are impaired by physical injury, illness, or emotional disorder, congenital or development disability, or the aging process, in order to achieve optimum functioning, to prevent disability, or to maintain health. Individuals are helped to attain the highest possible functional independence in self care, work, and leisure.

Job Description: Specific occupational therapy services include, but are not limited to, education and training in activities of daily living (ADL); the design, fabrication, and application of orthoses (splints); guidance in the selection and use of adaptive equipment; therapeutic activities to enhance functional performance; prevocational evaluation and training; and consultation concerning the adaptation of physical environments for the handicapped. These services are provided to individuals or groups, and to both in-patients and out-patients.

Employment Characteristics: The wide population served by occupational therapists is located in a variety of settings such as hospitals, clinics, rehabilitation facilities, long-term care facilities, extended care facilities, schools, camps and the patient's own homes. Occupational therapists both receive referrals from and make referrals to the appropriate health, educational or medical specialists.

According to the 1990 CAHEA Annual Supplemental Survey, entry level salaries average $28,238.

AMA Allied Health Department 312/464-4628

American Occupational Therapy Association
1383 Piccard Drive, Suite 300
P.O. Box 1725, Rockville, MD 20850-4375
301/948-9626

Office Laboratories

Commission on Office Laboratory
Assessment(COLA)
8701 Georgia Avenue, Suite 610
Silver Spring, MD 20910
301/588-5882

Oncology

American Society of Clinical Oncology
435 N. Michigan Ave., Suite 1717
Chicago, IL 60611
312/644-0828

American Society for Therapeutic
Radiology and Oncology
1891 Preston White Drive, Reston, VA 22091
703/648-8903

Board Certification:
Medical Oncology
American Board of Internal Medicine
3624 Market St., Philadelphia, PA 19104
215/243-1500, 800/441-ABIM (800/441-2246)

Society for Oral Oncology
c/o Carol S. Beckert, D.D.S.
Affiliated Pediatric Dental Specialists
3901 Beaubien Blvd., Detroit, MI 48201

Gynecologic Oncology, Maternal
and Fetal Oncology
American Board of Obstetrics and Gynecology
4225 Roosevelt Way, NE, Ste. 305
Seattle, WA 98105
206/547-4884

Radiation Oncology
American Board of Radiology
2301 W. Big Beaver Road, Suite 625
Troy, MI 48084
313/643-0300

Ophthalmic Medical Technician

History: Established in 1969, the Joint Commission on Allied Health Personnel in Ophthalmology (JCAHPO) represents all segments of ophthalmology, including representatives of the American Academy of Ophthalmology, the Association of University Professors of Ophthalmology, the Contact Lens Association of Ophthalmologists, the Society of Military Ophthalmologists, the Canadian Ophthalmological Society, the American Ophthalmological Society, the American Association of Certified Allied Health Personnel in Ophthalmology (AACAHPO), the American Orthoptic Council, the American Society of Ophthalmic Nurses, and the American Association of Certified Orthoptists. JCAHPO and AACAHPO are the agencies jointly designated to collaborate with the American Medical Association in the accrediting of educational programs.

In February 1974, the AMA Council on Health Manpower approved the concept of the Ophthalmic Medical Assistant and agreed that a need for a single category of ophthalmic assistant had been demonstrated. To develop educational Essentials, the Council on Medical Education worked with representatives of the American Association of Certified Allied Health Personnel in Ophthalmology (AACAHPO), the American Association of Medical Assistants (AAMA), the American Association of Ophthalmology (AAO), the American Academy of Ophthalmology and Otolaryngology (AAOO), the Association of University Professors in Ophthalmology (AUPO), the Contact Lens Association of Ophthalmologists (CLAO), the Joint Commission on Allied Health Personnel in Ophthalmologists (JCAHPO), and the Society of Military Ophthalmologists (SMO).

It was agreed that in the establishment of Essentials and the accreditation of educational programs for the ophthalmic medical assistant, the interests of ophthalmological medicine would be represented by JCAHPO and the interests of the allied health occupations by AACAHPO and AAMA. These three organizations developed and adopted the Essentials of an Accredited Educational Program for the Ophthalmic Medical Assistant, which was then adopted by the AMA House of Delegates at its June 1975 meeting. The review committee changed its name to the "Joint Review Committee for Ophthalmic Medical Personnel" in 1988. AACAHPO changed its name to "Association of Technical Personnel

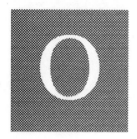

Ophthalmology." Under the Essentials approved in 1988, "ophthalmic medical assistant" was omitted and no longer accredited by CAHEA. The Essentials now include two levels of programs, "ophthalmic medical technician" and "ophthalmic medical technologist" which are accredited by CAHEA.

Occupational Description: Ophthalmic medical technicians and technologists are skilled persons qualified by academic and clinical training to carry out diagnostic and therapeutic procedures under the direction and responsibility of the physician.

Job Description: Ophthalmic medical technicians and technologists by performing tasks delegated to them, such as collecting data, and administering treatment ordered by ophthalmologists. They are qualified to take a medical history, administer diagnostic tests, make anatomical and functional ocular measurements, test ocular functions (including visual acuity, visual fields and sensorimotor functions), administer topical ophthalmic medications, and instruct the patient (as in home care and in use of contact lenses). Duties include assisting in ophthalmic surgery in the office or hospital; making optical measurements; assisting in the fitting of contact lenses; adjusting and making minor repairs on spectacles. Ophthalmic medical technicians and technologists may also maintain ophthalmic and surgical instruments, as well as office equipment.

Ophthalmic medical technologists perform all duties performed by technicians but are expected to do so at a higher level of expertise and to exercise considerable clinical technical judgement. Additionally, technologists may be expected to perform ophthalmic clinical photography and fluorescence angiography, ocular motility and binocular function tests, electrophysiological and microgiological procedures as well as provide instruction and supervision of the ophthalmic personnel and patients. (Ophthalmic medical technologist programs are designated with an asterisk in the program listing.)

Employment Characteristics: Ophthalmic medical technicians and technologists render supportive services to the ophthalmologist. They are employed primarily by ophthalmologists, but may be employed by medical institutions, clinics or physician groups and assigned to an ophthalmologist who is responsible for their direction. They may be involved with patients of an ophthalmologist is responsible. Salaries vary depending on employers and geographic location.

According to the 1990 CAHEA Annual Supplemental Survey, entry level salaries average $26,500.

AMA Department of Allied Health
312/464-4634

American Association of Certified Allied Health Personnel in Ophthalmology
1702 Deepwood Drive, Jeffersonville, IN 47130
812/948-8897

Ophthalmology

Ophthalmologist alternate titles: eye specialist: oculists. Diagnoses and treats diseases and injuries of eye: Examines patients for symptoms indicative of organic or congenital ocular disorders, and determines nature and extent of injury or disorder. Performs various tests to determine vision loss. Prescribes and administers medications, and performs surgery, if indicated. Directs remedial activities to aid in regaining vision, or to utilize sight remaining, by writing prescriptions for corrective glasses, and instructing patient in eye exercises. (DOT)

American Academy of Ophthalmology
P.O. Box 7424, 655 Beach
San Francisco, CA 94120
415/561-8500

American Board of Ophthalmology
111 Presidential Blvd., Suite 241
Bala Cynwyd, PA 19004
215/664-1175

Optometric Associations, Statewide

Alabama Optometric Association
400 S Union St, Suite 435, Montgomery, AL 36104
205/834-1057

Alaska Optometric Association
700 Katlian, Suite C, Sitka, AK 99835
907/747-6644

Arizona Optometric Association
3625 N 16th St, Suite 119, Phoenix, AZ 85016
602/279-0055

Arkansas Optometric Association
University Tower Bldg, Suite 819
Little Rock, AR 72204
501/661-7675

California Optometric Association
PO Box 2591, Sacramento, CA 95812-2591
916/441-3990

Colorado Optometric Association
410 17th St, Suite 2060, Denver, CO 80202-4433
303/892-8898

Connecticut Optometric Association
638 Prospect Ave, Hartford, CT 06105
203/233-0022

Delaware Optometric Association
PO Box 446, Elkton, MD 21921
301/392-4157

Optometric Society of the District of Columbia
4948 St Elmo Ave, Suite 302
Bethesda, MD 20814
301/656-8650

Florida Optometric Association
PO Box 13429, Tallahassee, FL 32317
904/877-4697

Georgia Optometric Association
PO Box 301, Avondale Estates, GA 30002
404/296-3130

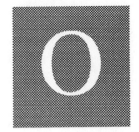

Hawaii Optometric Association
3221 Waialae Ave, No. 390, Honolulu, HI 96816
808/732-1004

Idaho Optometric Association
1016 E Locust St, Emmett, ID 83617
208/365-2471

Illinois Optometric Association
1301 W 22nd St, Suite 302, Oak Brook, IL 60521
708/573-8012

Indiana Optometric Association
201 N Illinois St, Suite 1920
Indianapolis, IN 46204
317/237-3560

Iowa Optometric Association
5721 Merle Hay Road, Suite 14A
Johnston, IA 50131
515/278-1697

Kansas Optometric Association
1266 SW Topeka Blvd, Topeka, KS 66612
913/232-0225

Kentucky Optometric Association
PO Box 572, Frankfort KY 40602
502/875-3516

Louisiana State Association of Optometrists
2576 Toulon Drive, Suite 1
Baton Rouge, LA 70816
504/292-9995

Maine Optometric Association
RFD 1, Box 1610, Litchfield, ME 04350-9730
207/268-4631

Maryland Optometric Association
113 W Franklin St, Baltimore, MD 21201
301/727-7800

Massachusetts Society of Optometrists
101 Tremont St, Room 608, Boston, MA 02108
617/542-9200

Michigan Optometric Association
530 W Ionia St, Suite A, Lansing, MI 48933
517/482-0616

Minnesota Optometric Association
1821 University Ave, Suite 269S
St. Paul, MN 55104
612/646-2883

Mississippi Optometric Association
PO Box 16441, Jackson, MS 39236-0441
601/956-7412

Missouri Optometric Association
417 E High St, Jefferson City, MO 65101-3274
314/635-6151

Montana Optometric Association
PO Box 908, Helena, MT 59624
406/442-1432

Nebraska Optometric Association
216 N 8th St, Suite 219, Lincoln, NE 68501
402/474-7716

Nevada Optometric Association
PO Box 709, Verdi, NV 89439
702/345-6153

New Hampshire Optometric Association
8 N State St, Concord, NH 03301
603/225-6311

New Jersey Optometric Association
88 Lakedale Drive, Trenton, NJ 08648
609/695-3456

New Mexico Optometric Association
PO Box 11585, Albuquerque, NM 87112
505/299-5617

New York State Optometric Association
90 S Swan St, Albany, NY 12210
518/449-7300

North Carolina State Optometric Association
114 N Pine St, PO Box 1206
Wilson, NC 27894-1206
919/237-6197

North Dakota Optometric Association
418 E Broadway, Bismarck, ND 58501
701/258-6766

Ohio Optometric Association
169 E Livingston Ave, Columbus, OH 43215
614/224-2600

Oklahoma Optometric Association
Lincoln Plaza Office Center
4545 N Lincoln Blvd, Suite 105
Oklahoma City, OK 73105
405/524-1075

Oregon Optometric Association
17898 SW McEwan Road, Portland, OR 97224
503/639-5036

Pennsylvania Optometric Association
PO Box 3312, Harrisburg, PA 17105
717/233-6455

Rhode Island Optometric Association
PO Box 8845, Warwick, RI 02888-8845
401/461-7550

South Carolina Optometric Association
2730 Devine St, Columbia, SC 29205
803/799-6721

South Dakota Optometric Association
116 N Euclid, PO Box 1173, Pierre, SD 57501
605/224-8199

Tennessee Optometric Association
992 Davidson Drive, Suite F, Nashville, TN 37205
615/353-0246

Texas Optometric Association
1016 La Posada, Suite 174, Austin, TX 78752
512/451-8476

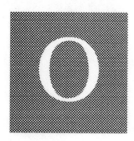

Utah Optometric Association
230 West 200 South, Suite 2110
Salt Lake City, UT 84101
801/364-9103

Vermont Optometric Association
26 State St, PO Box 1531, Montpelier, VT 05601
802/233-1197

Virginia Optometric Association
Old City Hall, 1001 E Broad St, Suite 110,
Richmond, VA 23219
804/643-0309

Washington Optometric Association
555 116th NE, Suite 166
Bellevue, WA 98004-5274
206/455-0874

West Virginia Optometric Association
Morrison Bldg, 815 Quarrier St, Suite 415,
Charleston, WV 25301
304/345-4710

Wisconsin Optometric Association
5721 Odana Road, Madison, WI 53719
608/274-4322

Wyoming Optometric Association
PO Box 3050, Cheyenne, WY 82003
307/632-8819

Optometry

Optometrist. Examines eye to determine nature and degree of vision problem or eye disease and prescribes corrective lenses or procedures: Examines eyes and performs various tests to determine visual acuity and perception and to diagnose diseases and other abnormalities, such as glaucoma and color blindness. Prescribes eyeglasses, contact lenses, and other vision aids or therapeutic procedures to correct or conserve vision. Consults with and refers patients to opthalmologist other health care practitioner if additional medical treatment is determined necessary. May prescribe medications to treat eye diseases if state laws permit. May specialize in type of services provided, such as contact lenses, low vision aids or vision therapy, or in treatment of specific groups, such as children or elderly patients. May conduct research, instruct in college or university, act as consultant, or work in public health field. (DOT)

American Optometric Association
243 N. Lindbergh Blvd., St. Louis, MO 63141
314/991-4100

Optometric Assistant. Performs any combination of following tasks to assist optometrist: Obtains and records patient's preliminary case history. Maintains records, schedules appointments, performs bookkeeping, correspondence, and filing. Prepares patient for vision examination; assists in testing for near and far acuity, depth perception, macula integrity, color perception, and visual field, utilizing ocular testing apparatus. Instructs patient in care and use of glasses or contact lenses. Works with patient in v ision therapy. Assists patient in frame selection. Adjusts and repairs glasses. Modifies contact lenses. Maintains inventory of materials and cleans instruments. Assists in fabrication of eye glasses or contact lenses. (DOT)

Organ Donations
Custodian

Victor T. Wilson, MD "A Piece of My Mind" JAMA. 1987 Oct 9: 258(14): 1898

This patient, this beautiful 4-year old boy, was brought in by helicopter from the scene of a head-on auto collision. The nurse recounts the familiar story: an unrestrained back-seat passenger, found under the front dash in the crushed plastic and steel mess. He was extracted with pneumatic jaws and immobilized on a board. Ringer's lactate brought the blood pressure up. Oxygen through an endotracheal tube pinkened his lips. He did not move then and does not now. His pupils do not shrink from light. His skull is in pieces and his brain on CT scan is distorted, cut by white jags of hemorrhage. The flurry of deep-line placements, roentgenograms, burr holes, and blood tests have settled into routine intensive care. Pressor drips infuse. His vital signs are stable now.

Bandaged and crying, his parents are led to him. Their shock, guilt, and grief are the same as they are every time, with every child like him, but still I must turn away from it. I think of my own sweet son and feel dread.

The neurological examination remained barren throughout the night: no reflexes, no tone, and no brain-stem signs. I remove his ventilator briefly and wait for him to breathe. Ho does not. This morning the unassailable judgment of a cerebral perfusion scan is accomplished. The boy is dead.

This is where my job usually ends. Tubing would be disconnected, machines turned off. The coroner would come. But now we ask gently and urgently of his parents that they give a great gift. Would they donate his organs? At first they are repulsed. Then their anger melts and they see in it a hope and a comfort. They whisper, and embrace, and agree.

I check on the other patients in the unit. The teenager with asthma is better. I kid him about his tattoo and he grins. The baby recovering from repair of a heart defect is not ventilating well. After some adjustments she breathes easier and grabs my finger.

A curious feeling takes me: as physician to these other children, I continue to work, hoping they will get better, that we will best the disease. But for the dead boy there is no hope and no struggle. For him I am now merely custodian of organs.

The transplant surgeons arrive. Is the heart still good? A last diagnostic flourish of echocardiogram, Swan-Ganz catheter, and isoenzymes suggests it is. The ward clerk wonders how to bill the child's supplies, now that he is no longer a patient. His blood pressure falls slowly. A little fluid, a little more pressor drip, and he is nudged back to a tenuous homeostasis. I stand at the bedside and touch his warm toes. "He is gone, isn't he?" his mother asks. I tell her yes.

Potential recipients rush to the hospital. Heart, kidneys, eye, and pancreas will be harvested. His parents have said their good-byes and have gone. I sit in his room and watch him, looking for the difference, but he still looks like a live little boy. In midafternoon he is wheeled past me to the operating room, the beautiful dead boy I cared for today. His vital signs are stable.

American Council on Transplantation
700 N. Fairfax, suite 505, Alexandria, VA 22314
703/836-4301
800-622-9010 for free donor cards only

Association of Organ Procurement Organizations
(Contact if donating party is mistakenly billed)
1250 24th St, NW, Suite 280
Washington, DC 20037
202/466-4353

Entire Body
Anatomical Gift Association
2240 W. Fillmore, Chicago, IL 60612
312/733-5283

Lions Club International, (Eye Donor Registry)
300 22nd St., Oak Brook, IL 60570
708/986-1700

Living Bank
P.O. Box 6725, Houston, TX 77265
800/528-2971
800/527-2971 (Donor Registration)

Medic Alert Organ Donor Program Foundation
P.O. Box 1009, Turlock, CA 95381
209/668-3333 (only for ID bracelets)

National Kidney Foundation
30 E. 33rd St., 11th Fl, New York, NY 10016
212/889-2210

Organ Transplant Fund
5120 S. Main, Downers Grove, IL 60515
708/963-1220

National Society to Prevent Blindness
500 E. Schaumburg, IL 60173
708/843-2020

Uniform Donor Cards
United Network for Organ Sharing
P.O. Box 13770, 1100 Boulder Parkway
Suite 5000
Richmond, VA 23225
800/24-DONOR (800/243-6667)

Heart Donor

Reetika Varirani "Poetry and Medicine"
JAMA. 1992 Apr 15; 267(15): 2015

You gave your son his first Erector set.
Ever since, the house always lacked a hinge-
his loosened closet door on which you leaned
your narcotic frame. Neighbors crowded like crows
on the drive after the medics slipped in -
no siren-: or, downstairs we couldn't hear.
But your son would see you smoothly led
down hospital corridors on a chrome-wheeled cot
driving a spirit with no heart: your heart
for science, that we not wonder why a piece
survives a whole; so that someone should use it
as a man would take a tool for the day's work;
as your son used his to unmake latches
and all the other world came into view.

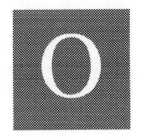

Orphan Drugs

In 1982, the Office of Orphan Products Development was established within the Food and Drug Administration, an agency of the Department of Health and Human Services (HHS). The Orphan Drug Act (Public Law 97-414) to encourage the development of drugs to treat rare diseases became law in January 1983 and was amended in 1984, 1985, and 1988. The Act defines an orphan drug as one used for the diagnosis, treatment, or prevention of a disease or condition affecting less than 200,000 people in the United States. If more than 200,000 people are affected, a drug has orphan status when the cost of developing and making it available would not be expected to be covered by sales in the United States. Application for an orphan designation must be made prior to filing a New Drug Application (NDA) or Product License Application (PLA). More than 400 products have been given orphan designations. (DE)

National Information Center for Orphan Drugs and Rare Diseases
P.O. Box 1133, Washington DC 20013
800/336-4797

National Organization for Rare Disorders
P.O. Box 8923, New Fairfield, CT 06812
203/746-6518

Office of Orphan Drugs
Food and Drug Administration
5600 Fishers Lane, Rockville, MD 20857
301/443-3170

Pharmaceutical Manufacturers Association
Commission on Drug for Rare Disorders
1100 15th St., Suite 900, NW
Washington, DC 20005
202/835-3561

Orthomolecular Medicine

Orthomolecular Medical Society
Huxley Institute for Biosocial Research
900 N. Federal Highway, Boca Raton, FL 33432
800/847-3802

Orthopaedics

American Academy of Orthopaedic Surgeons
6300 N. River Rd., Rosemont, IL 60018
708/823-7186

American Board of Orthopaedic Surgery
737 N. Michigan Ave., Suite 1150
Chicago, IL 60611
312/664-9444

American Orthopaedic Association
6300 N. River Rd., Rosemont, IL 60018
708/318-7330

American Orthopaedic Society for Sports Medicine
2250 E Devon, Suite 115, Des Plaines, IL 60018
708/803-8700

Orthotics

Orthotist. Provides care to patients with disabling conditions of limbs and spine by fitting and preparing orthopedic braces, under direction of and in consultation with physician: Assists in formulation of specifications for braces. Examines and evaluates patient's needs in relation to disease and functional loss. Formulates design of orthopedic brace. Selects materials, making cast measurements, model modifications, and layouts. Performs fitting, including static and dynamic alignments. Evaluates brace on patient and makes adjustments to assure fit, function, and quality of work. Instructs patient in use of orthopedic brace. Maintains patient records. May supervise Orthotics Assistants and other support personnel. May supervise laboratory activities relating to development of orthopedic braces. May lecture and demonstrate to colleagues and other professionals concerned with orthotics. May participate in research. May perform functions of Prosthetist and be designated Orthotist-Prosthetist (DOT).

Orthotics Assistant. Assists Orthotist in providing care and fabricating and fitting orthopedic braces to patients with disabling conditions of limbs and spine: Under guidance of and in consultation with Orthotist, makes assigned casts, measurements, model modifications, and layouts. Performs fitting, including static and dynamic alignments. Evaluates orthopedic braces on patient to ensure fit, function, and workmanship. Repairs and maintains orthopedics braces. May be responsible for performance of other personnel. May also perform functions of Prosthetics Assistant and be designated Orthotics-Prosthetics Assistant(DOT).

American Academy of Orthotists and Prosthetists
717 Pendleton St, Alexandria, VA 22314
703/836-7118

American Board for Certification in
Orthotics and Prosthetics
717 Pendleton St, Alexandria, VA 22314
703/836-7114

Ostoepathic Medicine

Osteopathic physician alternate titles: doctor, osteopathic; osteopath. Diagnoses and treats diseases and injuries of human body, relying upon accepted medical and surgical modalities: Examines patient to determine symptoms attributable to impairments in musculoskeletal system. Corrects disorders and afflictions of bones, muscles, nerves, and other body systems by medicinal and surgical procedures, and, when deemed beneficial, manipulative therapy. Employs diagnostic images, drugs, and other aids to diagnose and treat bodily impairments. May practice medical or surgical specialty. (DOT)

American Osteopathic Association
142 E. Ontario, Chicago, IL 60611
312/280-5800

Osteopathic Schools
California
College of Osteopathic Medicine of the Pacific
College Plaza, Pomona, CA 91766-1889
714/623-6116

Florida
Southeastern University of Health Sciences
College of Osteopathic Medicine
1750 NE 168th St., North Miami Beach, FL 33162
305/949-4000

Illinois
Chicago College of Osteopathic Medicine
555 31st St., Downers Grove, IL 60515
708/971-6080

Iowa
University of Osteopathic Medicine
and Health Sciences
College of Osteopathic Medicine and Surgery
3200 Grand Ave., Des Moines, IA 50312
515/271-1400

Maine
University of New England College of
Osteopathic Medicine
Hills Beach Road, Biddeford, ME 04005
207/283-0171

Michigan
Michigan State University
College of Osteopathic Medicine
Fee Halls, East Lansing, MI 48824
517/355-9611

Missouri
University of Health Sciences
College of Osteopathic Medicine
2105 Independence Blvd, Kansas City, MO 64124
816/283-2000

Kirksville College of Osteopathic Medicine
800 West Jefferson St, Kirksville, MO 63501
816/626-2121

New Jersey
University of Medicine and Dentistry of New Jersey
School of Osteopathic Medicine
40 East Laurel Road, Stratford, NJ 08084
609/346-6990

New York
New York College of Osteopathic Medicine
New York Institute of Technology
Old Westbury, Long Island, NY 11568
516/626-6947

Ohio
Ohio University College of Osteopathic Medicine
Grosvenor Hall
Athens, Ohio 45701-2979
614/593-2500

Oklahoma
College of Osteopathic Medicine of Oklahoma
State University
1111 West 17th St, Tulsa, OK 74107
918/582-1972

Pennsylvania
Philadelphia College of Osteopathic Medicine
4150 City Ave, Philadelphia, PA 19131
215/871-1000

Texas
Texas College of Osteopathic Medicine
3500 Camp Bowie, Fort Worth, TX 76107
817/735-2000

West Virginia
West Virginia School of Osteopathic Medicine
400 North Lee St, Lewisburg, WV 24901
304/645-6270

Osteoporosis
American Brittle Bone Society
1256 Merrill Dr., West Chester, PA 19382
215/692-6248

National Institute of Arthritis and
Musculoskeletal and Skin
Diseases, 9000 Rockville Pike
Bethesda, MD 20892
301/496-4000

National Osteoporosis Foundation
2100 M Street, NW, Suite 602
Washington, DC 20037
202/223-2226

Ostomy
United Ostomy Association
36 Executive Park, Suite 120, Irvine, Ca 92714
714/660-8624

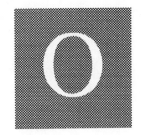

Otolaryngology
Otolaryngologist alternate titles:
otorhinolaryngologist. Diagnoses and treats
diseases of ear, nose, and throat: Examines
affected organs, using equipment such as
audiometers, prisms, nasocopes, microscopes,
x-ray machines, and fluoroscopes. Determines
nature and extent of disorder, and prescribes and
administers medications, or performs surgery.
Performs tests to determine extent of loss of
hearing due to aural or other injury, and speech
loss as a result of diseases or injuries to larynx.
May specialize in treating throat, ear, or nose and
be designated Laryngologist; Otologist;
Rhinologist.(DOT)

American Academy of Otolaryngology-
Head and Neck Surgery
1 Prince St, Alexandria, VA 22314
703/836-4444

American Board of Otolaryngology
5615 Kirby Dr., Suite 936, Houston, TX 77005
713/528-6200

American Academy of Otolaryngic Allergy
8455 Colesville Rd., Suite 745
Silver Spring, MD 20910
301/588-1800

Otology
American Otological Society
4500 San Pablo Rd., Jacksonville, FL 32224-9369
904/223-2146

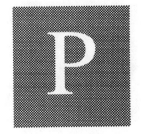

Paget's Disease

Paget's Disease Foundation
165 Cadman Plaza East, Brooklyn, NY 11201
718/596-1043

Pain

American Academy of Pain Medicine
5700 Old Orchard Rd., Skokie, IL 60077
708/966-9510

American Pain Society
PO Box 186, Skokie, IL 60076
708/475-7300

Board Certification
American Board of Anesthesiology
100 Constitution Plaza, Hartford, CT 06103
203/522-9857

Pain Management Guidelines
Agency for Healthcare Policy Research
PO Box 8547, Silver Spring, MD 20907
800/358-9295

Pancreas

American Pancreatic Association
University of Missouri
Department of Surgery, Room M580
Columbia, MO 65212
314/882-7942

Panic Attack

Panic Attack Sufferers' Support Group
1042 East 105th St., Brooklyn, NY 11236
718/763-0190

Paralysis

American Paralysis Association
PO Box 187, Short Hills, NJ 07078
800/225-0292
201/379-2690 (in NJ)

Parkinson's Disease

National Parkinson Foundation
1501 N.W. Ninth Ave., Miami, FL 33136
305/547-6666
800/327-4545, 800/433-7022 (FL only)

American Parkinson Disease Association
116 John Street, New York, NY 10038
800/223-2732
(In New York: 800/732-9550)

Paternity Testing

JAMA Article of Note: Guidelines for Reporting
Estimates of Probability of Paternity. Council on
Scientific Affairs. JAMA.1985 Jun 14;
253(22): 3298.

Pathology

Pathologist alternate titles: medical pathologist:
Studies nature, cause, and development of
diseases, and structural and functional changes
caused by them: Diagnoses, from body tissue,
fluids, secretions, and other specimens, presence
and stage of disease, utilizing laboratory
procedures. Acts as consultant to other medical
practitioners. Perform autopsies to determine
nature and extent of disease, cause of death, and
effects of treatment. May direct activities of
pathology department in medical school, hospital,
clinic, medical examiner's office, or research
institute. May be designated according to specialty
as Clinical Pathologist; Forensic Pathologist;
Neuropathologist; Surgical Pathologist.(DOT)

JFK's death - the plain truth from the MDs who did the autopsy.

JAMA.1992 May 27;267(20):2794-2803

There are two and only two physicians who know
exactly what happened - and didn't happen -
during their autopsy of President John F. Kennedy
on the night of November 22, 1963, at the Naval
Medical Center at Bethesda, Md. The two, former
US Navy pathologists James Joseph Humes, MD,
and "J" Thornton Boswell, MD, convened last
month in a Florida hotel for two days of
extraordinary interviews with JAMA editor George
D. Lundberg, MD, himself a former military
pathologist, and this reporter about the events of
that fateful night. It is the only time that Humes
and Boswell have publicly discussed their famous
case, and it was the result of seven years of
efforts by Lundberg to persuade them to do so.

Bullets came from above and behind
The scientific evidence they documented during
their autopsy provides irrefutable proof that
President Kennedy was struck by only two bullets
that came from above and behind from a
high-velocity weapon that caused the fatal
wounds. This autopsy proof, combined with the
bullet and rifle evidence found at the scene of the
crime, and the subsequent detailed
documentation of a six-month investigation
involving the enormous resources of the local,
state, and federal law enforcement agencies,
proves the 1964 Warren Commission conclusion
that Kennedy was killed by a lone assassin, Lee
Harvey Oswald.

Humes, who was in charge, calls it "probably the
least secret autopsy in the history of the world." It
was Humes and Boswell who opened the casket
when the President's body was brought by
ambulance from Andrews Air Force Base after the
flight from Dallas. It was Humes and Boswell who
lifted the former President from his casket and
placed him on the examining table to begin a
four-hour autopsy. (They were joined later at the
autopsy table Army Lt. Col. Pierre Finck, MC, who
participated as an expert consultant; Finck, who
now lives in Switzerland, declined to come to
Florida for the joint interview.) Humes says he is
breaking his 29-year silence "because I am tired
of being beaten upon by people who are
supremely ignorant of the scientific facts of the
President's death."

Coincidentally, on the second day of the
interviews, Boswell told the group that a Fort
Worth physician, Charles Crenshaw, MD, had
appeared on TV that very morning to argue the
claim in his recent book, *JFK: Conspiracy of
Silence*, that when allegedly observed the dead
President at Dallas' Parkland Hospital, he was
positive that the bullets struck Kennedy from the
front, not the back, "as the public has been led to
believe." Crenshaw, who was a surgical resident
in 1963, is not mentioned in the **Warren**

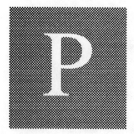

Commission's 888-page summary report and his 203-page, generously spaced paperback was written with the aid of two assassination-conspiracy buffs. Crenshaw's book is only the latest in a long parade of conspiracy theories purporting to tell how Kennedy was really killed, including the 1991 release of Oliver Stone's film, *JFK*. Humes and Boswell had agreed to the JAMA interview without the slightest idea that Crenshaw's book had been published.

Now, his face incredulous with disbelief, Humes exploded with his summation. Pointing toward the window, the exasperated pathologist said, "If a bullet or a BB were fired through that window, it would leave a small hole where it entered and a beveled crater where it exited. That is what 'J' and I found when we examined the President's skull. There was a small elliptical entrance wound on the outside of the back of the skull, where the bullet entered, and a beveled larger wound on the inside of the back of the skull where the bullet tore through and exploded out the right side of the head. When we recovered the missing bone fragments and reconstructed this gaping wound where the bullet exited, we found this same pattern - a small wound where the bullet struck the inside of the skull and beveled larger wound where it exited. This is always the pattern of through-and through wound of the cranium - the beveling or crater effect appears on the inside of the skull at the entrance wound and on the outside of the skull at the exist wound. The crater effect is produced when the bony tissue of the skull turns inside out where the bullet leaves."

'A foolproof finding'

He concludes, "in 1963, we proved at the autopsy table that President Kennedy was struck from above and behind by the fatal shot. The pattern of the entrance and exit wounds in the skull proves it, and if we stayed here until hell freezes over, nothing will change this proof. It happens 100 times out of 100, and I will defend it until I die. This is the essence of our autopsy, and it is supreme ignorance to argue any other scenario. This is a law of physics and it is foolproof - absolutely, unequivocally, and without question. The conspiracy buffs have totally ignored this central scientific fact, and everything else is hogwash. There was no interference with our autopsy, and there was no conspiracy to suppress the findings."

Though the evidence is less well defined, Humes emphasizes that his autopsy found that the other bullet that struck Kennedy, the so-called "magic bullet" that was the first to hit Kennedy and that also hit Texas Gov. John Connally, was also fired from above and behind. He says, "There was an 'abrasion collar' where this bullet entered at the base of the President's neck, and this scorching and splitting of the skin from the heat and scraping generated by the entering bullet is proof that it entered from behind. Unfortunately, at the time of the autopsy, the tracheostomy performed on the President at Dallas in an attempt to save his life obliterated the exit wound through the front of his neck near the Adam's apple. Soft-tissue wounds are much more iffy than bone wounds, but there is no doubt from whence cometh those bullets - from rear to front from a high-velocity rifle."

Still, the other scenarios continue to be painted. "Recently," Humes notes, "there were about 300 people at a convention in Dallas, each hawking a different conspiracy theory about how the President was killed. I think this kind of general idiocy is a tragedy - it almost defies belief - but I guess it is the price we pay for living in a free country. I can only question the motives of those who propound these ridiculous theories for a price and who have turned the President's death into a profit-making industry."

Humes and Boswell had a long, long day 29 years ago, and, in many ways, it has never ended. The 6-foot, 4-inch, physician energetic Humes is a commanding presence, and he says. "I was in charge of the autopsy - period. Nobody tried to interfere - make that perfectly clear." The 5-foot, 9-inch, pipe-puffing Boswell is precise and methodical, and he says, "We documented our findings in spades. It's all there in the records. And Jim is not the kind of guy anybody pushes around." Their comments on the record are essential because polls show, in the wake of the film JFK and the glut of conspiracy-theorist authors, that many, if not most Americans disbelieve the Warren Commission finding that Oswald, "acting alone and without assistance," killed Kennedy. To set the record straight, they agreed to relive for JAMA their actions of Friday, November 22, 1963.

American Association of Pathologists
9650 Rockville Pike, Bethesda, MD 20814
301/530-7130

American Board of Pathology
5401 W. Kennedy Blvd., PO Box 25915
Tampa, FL 33622
813/286-2444

American Society of Clinical Pathologists
2100 W. Harrison St. Chicago, IL 60612
312/738-1336

College of American Pathologists
325 Waukegan Rd., Northfield, IL 60093
708/446-8800

National Association of Medical Examiners
1402 S. Grand Blvd., St. Louis, MO 63104
314/577-8298

United States and Canadian
Academy of Pathology
3643 Walton Way, Augusta, GA 30909
404/733-7550

Patient Rights

AMA's Patient Bill of Rights

The AMA is concerned about patients as well as physicians. The AMA feels a great responsibility to the people it serves. The AMA Principles of Medical Ethics for physicians is an example of this commitment. The AMA Patient Bill of Rights is another. Both help ensure the rights of the patient. Physicians who belong to the AMA support these six rights:

I. The patient has the right to receive information from physicians and to discuss the benefits, risks and costs of appropriate treatment alternatives.

II. The patient had the right to make decisions regarding the health care that is recommended by his or her physician.

III. The patient has the right to courtesy, respect, dignity, responsiveness and timely attention to his or her needs.

IV. The patient has the right to confidentiality.

V. The patient has the right to continuity of health care.

VI. The patient has a basic right to have available adequate health care. (CHO)

American Hospital Association
840 N. Lake Shore Dr., Chicago, IL 60611
312/280-6000

Patient Education

National Council on Patient
Information and Education
666 Eleventh Street, NW, Suite 810
Washington, DC 20001
202/347-6711

National Health Information Center
PO Box 1133, Washington, DC 20013-1133
800/336-4797

Pediatrics

Pediatrician: Plans and carries out medical care program for children from birth through adolescence to aid in mental and physical growth and development: Examines patients to determine presence of disease and to establish preventive health practices. Determines nature and extent of disease or injury, prescribes and administers medications and immunizations, and performs variety of medical duties. (DOT)

Ambulatory Pediatric Association
6728 Old McLean Village Dr., McLean, VA 22101
703/556-9222

American Academy of Pediatrics
141 Northwest Point Blvd.
Elk Grove Village, IL 60007
800/433-9016 (outside IL)
708/228-5005 (in IL)

American Board of Pediatrics
111 Silver Cedar Court, Chapel Hill, NC 27514
919/929-0461

American Pediatric Surgical Association
Children's Hospital National Medical Center
111 Michigan Avenue, NW
Washington, DC 20010
202/745-2153

Children in Hospitals
31 Wilshire Park, Needham, MA 02192
617/444-3877

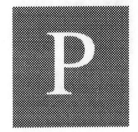

Peer Review

What Every Doctor Needs to Know: Peer Review Organizations

Peer Review Organizations (PROs) were established by Congress in 1982 to determine if the health care services provided to Medicare patients receiving hospital inpatient, HMO or ambulatory surgical care were medically necessary, appropriate and of a quality that meets professionally recognized standards. PROs review a sample of health care services provided to Medicare patients throughout the United States and its territories according to the requirements of the PRO Scope of Work.

When will the new PRO Scope of Work begin?

The PRO Scope of Work outlines the medical review requirements that PROs must meet to carry out their contract with the Health Care Financing Administration (HCFA), which is the federal agency responsible for implementing the PRO program. Most PROs will implement the new Fourth Scope of Work during 1993, some as early as April 1. As it has done in the past, HCFA will phase-in the new scope of work in four contract "cycles," each covering a staggering three-year period. Approximately 13 PROs are included in each cycle.

What changes will occur now?

Under this new scope of work, the PRO program will move from dealing with individual clinical errors toward helping physicians and hospitals improve medical care by analyzing patterns of care and their outcomes. When pattern analyses are completed, PROs will share their findings with hospital medical and administrative staffs to identify means to improve outcomes and quality of care. PROs also plan to focus review on the management of Medicare patients who have acute myocardial infarction, coronary angioplasty, or coronary artery bypass grafts. HCFA will also:

- Minimize case review and emphasize treatment pattern analyses,
- Replace the existing Quality Intervention Plan "point" system with a more "educational" Quality Review Process,
- Require physician reviewers to be licensed in the state where the services are performed and to care routinely for Medicare patients at least 20 hours per week,
- Request and consider comments from state medical associations and others in formulating new review criteria, and will distribute the

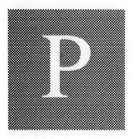

revised criteria to the medical community before implementation,

• For the first time, require PROs to provide additional due process protections for physicians by allowing them to obtain a second level reconsideration following a PRO's initial quality determination,

• Require PROs to evaluate the potential impact on the physician reviewers if their names are released to those under review, and

• Require PROs each quarter to provide individual hospitals, state medical and hospital associations, and relevant specialty societies with reports on the types and patterns of quality, utilization, and documentation concerns identified by their state's PRO.

Summary:

Persons Covered by Immunity: The individuals exempt from liability for good faith actions taken within their statutorily authorized duties usually include members of peer review committees, consultants to, or employees of peer review committees, and persons providing information to such committees.

Types of Committee Covered: The state statutes generally pertain to peer review committees formed by medical societies, as well as to those bodies created by a hospital or medical staff.

Responsibilities of Committee: The various statutory duties of peer review committees, the functions they perform under state law, and the degree to which these activities are subject to the immunities provided are addressed in the statutory provisions. The language varies from state to state.

Non-discoverability and Confidentiality: The proceedings and records of peer review committee typically are confidential and non-discoverable. In the statutes of twenty-two states, an important clarification states that information, documents or records otherwise available from original sources are not to be construed as immune from discovery or use in any civil action against a health care provider arising out of the matters which are the subject of evaluation and review by the committee merely because they were presented during proceedings of the peer review committee. In addition, any person who testifies before such a committee, or who is a member of such committee, may not be prevented form testifying as to matters within his knowledge, but such witness cannot be asked about his testimony before the committee or about opinions formed by him as a result of such proceedings. The following state laws contain this provision: Alaska, Arkansas, Florida, Georgia, Indiana, Kentucky, Massachusetts, Minnesota, Mississippi, Missouri, Montana, Nebraska, New Mexico, North Carolina, North Dakota, Pennsylvania, Rhode Island, South Carolina, Tennessee, Vermont, West Virginia and Wisconsin.

An exception that is present in the peer review non-discoverability provisions of a number of state laws permits a physician to obtain access to peer review materials when challenging the curtailment, suspension, termination or denial of staff privileges. Examples of state statutes which contain this exception are: Alaska, Arizona,

California, Colorado, Connecticut, Hawaii, Illinois, Kansas, Kentucky, Louisiana, Mississippi, Missouri, New Hampshire, Oregon, Rhode Island, South Dakota and Washington.(SPR)

Health Care Quality Improvement Act of 1986 Public Law #99-660 Title IV; enacted on November 14, 1986

Subsequent amendments to PL-99-660: section 402 in PL#100-77 enacted December 1, 1987

amended section 402 in section 6103(e(6)) in PL# 101-239, enacted 12-19-89

American College of Medical Quality (formerly American College of Utilization Review Physicians) 1531 S. Tamiami Trail, Suite 703 Venice, FL 34292 813/497-3340

American Medical Peer Review Association 810 First St, NE, Ste. 410, Washington, DC 20002 202/371-5610

Perfusionist

History: The field of cardiovascular perfusion emerged in the mid-1950s, with its practitioners trained on the job until the mid-1970s. Over that period members of the occupation were identified by various titles: perfusion technologist/technician, pump technician, extracorporeal technologists, extracorporeal perfusionist, cardiovascular perfusionist and others. The preferred title now in wide use is perfusionist. Often trainees come from other disciplines: nursing, respiratory therapy, biomedical engineering, operating room technicians, monitoring technicians, and the laboratory.

In 1968, the American Society of Extra-Corporeal Technologists (AmSECT) began a program of certification for perfusionists. In 1975, this program was turned over to a new agency established to conduct certifications as an independent activity: the American Board of Cardiovascular Perfusion (ABCP). The ABCP also adopted also adopted minimum standards for training programs as developed by AmSECT and began evaluation and accreditation activities. AmSECT, with the cosponsorship of the American Association of Thoracic Surgeons (AATS) and the Society of Thoracic Surgeons (STS), petitioned the AMA for recognition of the occupations and, in December 1976, the Committee on Emerging Health Manpower recommended approval; the CME granted recognition in that same month.

In 1977, four collaborating organizations sponsored the formation of the Joint Review Committee for Perfusion Education (JRC-PE); they were the AATS, ABCP, AmSECT, and STS. Over the period 1978-1979, the JRC-PE and others developed the Essentials and Guidelines for an Accredited Educational Program for the Perfusionist. The Essentials were adopted in 1980 and accreditation of programs was begun in 1981. The Essentials were revised in 1984 and in 1989. In 1985, the Perfusion Program Directors Council became an additional sponsor, as did the Society of Cardiovascular Anesthesiologist in 1989.

Occupational Description: A perfusionist is a skilled person, qualified by academic and clinical education, who operates extracorporeal circulation equipment during any medical situation where it is necessary to support the patient's circulatory or respiratory function. The perfusionist is knowledgeable concerning the variety of equipment available to perform extracorporeal circulation functions and is responsible, in consultation with the physician, for selecting the appropriate equipment and techniques to be used.

Job Description: Perfusionists conduct extracorporeal circulation and ensure the safe management of physiologic functions by monitoring the necessary variables. Perfusion (extracorporeal circulation) procedures involve specialized instrumentation and/or advanced life support techniques, and may include a variety of related functions. The perfusionist provides consultation to the physician in the selection of the appropriate equipment and techniques to be used during extracorporeal circulation.

During cardiopulmonary bypass, the perfusionist may administer blood products, anesthetic agents, or drugs through the extracorporeal circuit on prescription. The perfusionist is responsible for the induction of hypothermia and other duties, when prescribed. Perfusionists may be administratively responsible for purchasing supplies and equipment as well as for personnel and departmental management. Final medical responsibility for extracorporeal perfusion rests with the surgeon-in-charge.

Employment Characteristics: Perfusion is still a relatively new occupation, and the demand for perfusionists often exceeds the supply. Perfusionists may be employed in hospitals, by surgeons, and as part of a medical service group. They may work weekend and night duty, including emergency calls. They may also work on an on-call system, depending on the number of perfusionists employed by the institution.(ALL)

AMA Allied Health Department
312/464-4628

American Society of Extra-Corporeal Technology
1980 Isaac Newton Square, Reston, VA 22090
703/435-8556

Pesticides
National Coalition Against the Misuse of Pesticides
530 Seventh St. SE, Washington, DC 20003
202/543-5450

National Pesticide Telecommunication Network
Texas Tech. University Health Sciences Center
School of Medicine, Rm. S-129, Thompson Hall
Texas Tech University, Lubbock, TX 79409
800/858-7378

Rachel Carson Council, Inc.
8940 Jones Mill Rd., Chevy Chase, MD 20815
301/652-1877

Pharmacology
American Society for Pharmacology and Experimental Therapeutics
9650 Rockville Pike, Bethesda, MD 20814
301/530-7060

American Society for Clinical Pharmacology and Therapeutics
1718 Gallagher Road, Norristown, PA 19401-2800
215/825-3838

Pharmacy
Pharmacist alternate titles: druggist. Compounds and dispenses prescribed medications, drugs, and other pharmaceuticals for patient care, according to professional standards and state and federal legal requirements: Reviews prescriptions issued by physician, or other authorized prescriber to assure accuracy and determine formulas and ingredients needed. Compounds medications, using standard formulas and processes, such as weighing, measuring, and mixing ingredients. Directs pharmacy workers engaged in mixing, packaging, and labeling pharmaceuticals. Answers questions and provides information to pharmacy customers on drug interactions, side effects, dosage and storage of pharmaceuticals. Maintains established procedures concerning quality assurance, security of controlled substances, and disposal of hazardous waste drugs. Enters data, such as patient name, prescribed medication and cost, to maintain pharmacy files, charge system, and inventory. May assay medications to determine identity, purity, and strength. May instruct interns and other medical personnel on matters pertaining to pharmacy, or teach in college of pharmacy. May work in hospital pharmacy and be designated Pharmacists, Hospital (DOT).

Pharmacist Assistant: Mixes and dispenses prescribed medicines and pharmaceutical preparations in absence of or under supervision of Pharmacist : Compounds preparations according to prescriptions issued by medical, dental, or veterinary officers. Pours, weighs, or measures dosages and grinds, heats, filters, or dissolves and mixes liquid or soluble drugs and chemicals. Procures, stores, and issues pharmaceutical materials and supplies. Maintains files and records and submits required pharmacy reports. (DOT)

Pharmacy Technician: alternate titles: pharmacy clerk. Performs any combination of following duties to assist Pharmacist in hospital pharmacy or retail establishment: Mixes pharmaceutical preparations, fills bottles with prescribed tablets and capsules, and types labels for bottles. Assists Pharmacist to prepare and dispense medication. Receives and stores incoming supplies. Counts stock and enters data in computer to maintain inventory records. Processes records of medication and equipment dispensed to hospital patient, computes charges, and enters data in computer. Prepares intravenous (IV) packs, using sterile technique, under supervision of hospital pharmacist. Cleans equipment and sterilizes glassware according to prescribed methods. (DOT)

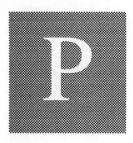

American Pharmaceutical Association
2215 Constitution Ave. NW
Washington, DC 20037
202/628-4410

Pharmaceutical Manufacturers Association
1100 15th St., NW, Washington, D.C. 20005
202/835-3400

Phobias

A persistent, irrational fear of, and desire to avoid, a particular object or situation. Many people have minor phobias, experiencing some anxiety when unable to avoid contact with spiders, for example. However, these phobias do not impair the ability to cope with day-to-day life. It is only when a fear causes significant distress and interferes with normal social functioning that it is considered a psychiatric disorder.

Types: Simple phobias, also known as specific phobias, are the most common. They may involve fear of particular animals (most often dogs, snakes, spiders, or mice) or of particular situations, such as enclosed spaces (claustrophobia), heights, or air travel. Animal phobias usually start in childhood, but other forms may develop at any time. Treatment is not usually required, unless the feared object is so common that it is not easily avoided (e.g., fear of elevators in a person who lives in a large city).

Agoraphobia (fear of open spaces or entering public places) is a more serious type of phobia, often causing severe impairment and disruption of family life. It is the most common phobia for which treatment is sought. The disorder usually starts in the late teens or early 20s.

Social phobia, which is relatively rare, is fear of being exposed to the scrutiny of others. Examples include fear of eating, speaking, or performing in public, using public toilets, or writing in the presence of others. The disorder usually begins in late childhood or early adolescence.(ENC)
Phobia Society of America

6000 Executive Blvd, Ste 200
Rockville, MD 20852
301/231-9350

Photobiology

American Society for Photobiology
8000 Westpark Drive, Suite 400
Mc Lean, VA 22102
703/790-1745

Photographs, Medical

Historical:
National Library of Medicine
Prints and Photographs Collection
Bethesda, MD 20209
301/496-5961

Bettman Archive, Inc.
902 Broadway, 5th Fl, New York, NY 10010
212/777-6200

Smithsonian Institution
National Museum of History and Technology
14th St. & Constitution Ave. NW
Washington, DC 20560
202/357-1960

World Health Organization
525 23rd St, NW, Washington, DC 20037
202/861-3200

Physical Examination

JAMA Article of Note: Physical Examination Guidelines or Medical Evaluation of Healthy Persons. Council on Scientific Affairs. *JAMA*.1983 Mar 25;249(12):1626-33

For Pilots:
JAMA Article of Note: A Review of the Medical Standards for Civilian Airmen. JAMA.1986 Mar 28;255(12):1589-99

Physical Medicine

Physiatrist: alternate titles: physical medicine specialist. Specializes in clinical and diagnostic use of physical agents and exercises to provide physiotherapy for physical, mental, and occupational rehabilitation of patients: Examines patient, utilizing electrodiagnosis and other diagnostic procedures to determine need for and extent of therapy. Prescribes and administers treatment, using therapeutic methods and procedures, such as light therapy, diathermy, hydrotherapy, iontophoresis, and cryotherapy. Instructs Physical Therapist and other personnel in nature and duration or dosage of treatment, and determines that treatments are administered as specified. Prescribes exercises designed to develop functions of specific anatomical parts or specific muscle groups. Recommends occupational therapy activities for patients with extended convalescent periods and for those whose disability requires change of occupation.(DOT)

American Academy of Physical
Medicine and Rehabilitation
122 S. Michigan Ave., Suite 1300
Chicago, IL 60603-6107
312/922-9366

American Board of Physical
Medicine and Rehabilitation
Northwest Center, 21 First St. SW, Suite 674,
Rochester, MN 55902
507/282-1776

Association of Academic Physiatrists
290 Norristown Rd, PO Box 977
Blue Bell, PA 19422
215/825-5000

Physical Therapy

Physical Therapist alternate titles: physiotherapist. Plans and administers medically prescribed physical therapy treatment for patients suffering from injuries, or muscle, nerve, joint and bone diseases, to restore function, relieve pain, and prevent disability: Reviews physician's referral (prescription) and patient's condition and medical records to determine physical therapy treatment required. Tests and measures patient's strength, motor development sensory perception, functional capacity, and respiratory and circulatory efficiency, and records findings to develop or revise treatment programs. Plans and prepares written treatment program based on evaluation of patient data. Administers manual exercises to improve and maintain function. Instructs, motivates, and assists patient to perform various physical activities, such as nonmanual exercises, ambulatory functional activities, daily-living activities, and in use of assistant and supportive devices, such as crutches, canes, and prostheses. Administers treatments involving application of physical agents, using equipment, such as hydrotherapy tanks and whirlpool baths, moist packs, ultraviolet and infrared lamps, and ultrasound machines. Evaluates effects of treatment at various stages and adjusts treatments to achieve maximum benefit. Administers massage, applying knowledge of massage techniques and body physiology. Administers traction to relieve pain, using traction equipment. Records treatment, response, and progress in patient's chart or enters information into computer. Instructs patient and family in treatment procedures to be continued at home. Evaluates, fits, and adjusts prosthetic and orthotic devices and recommends modification to Orthotist. Confers with physician and other practitioners to obtain additional patient information, suggest revisions in treatment program, and integrates physical therapy treatment with other aspects of patient's health care. Orients, instructs and directs work activities of assistants, aides, and students. May plan and conduct lectures and training programs on physical therapy and related topics for medical staff, students, and community groups. May plan and develop physical therapy research programs and participate in conducting research. May write technical articles and reports for publications. May teach physical therapy techniques and procedures in educational institutions. May limit treatment to specific patient group or disability or specialize in conducting physical therapy research. In facilities where assistants are also employed, may primarily administer complex treatment, such as certain types of manual exercises and functional training, and monitor administration of other treatments. May plan, direct, and coordinate physical therapy program and be designated Director, Physical Therapy. Must comply with state requirement for licensure. (DOT)

Physical Therapist Assistant: alternate titles: physical therapy assistant; physical therapy technician. Administers physical therapy treatments to patients, working under direction of and as assistant to Physical Therapist: Administers active and passive manual therapeutic exercises, therapeutic massage, and heat, light, sound, water, and electrical modality treatments, such as ultrasound, electrical stimulation, ultraviolet, infrared, and hot and cold packs. Administers traction to relieve neck and back pain, using intermittent and static traction equipment. Instructs, motivates, and assists patients to learn and improve function activities, such as preambulation, transfer, ambulation, and daily-living activities. Observes patients during treatments and compiles and evaluates data on patients' responses to treatments and progress and report orally or in writing to the physical therapist. Fits patient and supportive devices, such as crutches, canes, walkers, and

wheelchairs. Confers with members of physical therapy staff and other health team members, individually and in conference, to exchange, discuss, and evaluate patient information for planning, modifying, and coordinating treatment programs. Gives orientation to new Physical Therapist Assistants and directs and gives instructions to Physical Therapy Aides. Performs clerical duties, such as taking inventory, ordering supplies, answering telephone, taking messages, and filling out forms. May measure patient's range-of-joint motion, length and girth of body parts, and vital signs to determine effects of specific treatments or to assist Physical Therapist to compile data for patient evaluations. May monitor treatments administered by Physical Therapy Aides.(DOT)

American Physical Therapy Association
1111 N. Fairfax St., Alexandria, VA 22314
703/684-2782

Physicians
American College of Physicians
Independence Mall West, Sixth St. at Race,
Philadelphia, PA 19106
215/351-2400

Association of American Physicians
Stuart Kornfeld, MD
Department of Hematology,
Washington University Medical School
660 S. Euclid Ave, St. Louis, MO 63110
314/362-8803

Doctors Ought to Care (DOC)
3243 E. Murdock, Ste 303, Wichita, KS 67208
316/688-3976

Physician's Assistants
Physician's assistants: Rx for stress. PAs can help lift burden on busy physician

Howard Larkin AMNews 3/25/91 p.13+

Odon, Ind. - At this time last year Bob Webb, MD, saw about 40 patients a day at his solo practice in this town of 1,500. After early hospital rounds he'd open his office around 10 a.m. and work until 7:30 or 8 p.m.

"I was swamped," the board-certified family practice specialist says. The hours weren't doing much for his home life - or his patients' tempers.

That's all changed. Dr. Webb now opens at 9 a.m., and although his caseload has grown to about 65 patients per day he usually makes it home by 5:30 or 6 p.m.

Dr. Webb didn't add a partner. He hired John Smith, a physician's assistant, to help out.

As other physicians in specialties ranging from internal medicine to cardiac surgery have found, physician's assistants can help build patient volume without increasing practice costs as much as adding new associates.

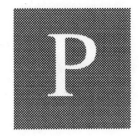

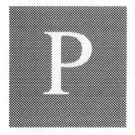

In rural areas, that can mean the difference between a financial viable practice and one that isn't. In urban areas, physician's assistants can help lower costs to better compete for managed care business.

But the biggest payoff may be relieving stress, says Gary Matthews, vice president and director of consulting for Atlanta-based Paragon Health Management. "The most crisis-driven recruitment needs are by stress, not economic opportunity."

If stress is the problem, hiring a physician's assistant, who can take over tasks such as taking histories, preparing charts, treating minor problems, and assisting in surgery, can make more sense than adding an associate, Matthews says.

"You hire a doctor to relieve stress and six or 12 months down the road you realize you paid an arm and a leg. Then you have buyer's remorse and that raises problems. The biggest reason partnership and associate relationships fall apart is stress."

But controversy remains over how broad a role the nation's 22,000 physicians should play. Much of it revolves around whether PAs should be allowed to prescribing narcotics.

The AMA, which is involved in accrediting 52 PA training programs around the country, opposes PAs prescribing or dispensing drugs. However, 26 states allow PAs limited prescribing or dispensing privileges. Most ban PAs prescribing narcotics.

In all states PAs must work under the supervision of a licensed physician, though requirements vary on how closely they must be supervised.

The AMA supports state legislation removing barriers to practice for physician's assistants as well as regulation requiring their supervision by licensed physicians. The AMA opposes direct payment to PAs by Medicare or other payers.

"Physician assistants are still very much a dependent profession," says Wayne Bottom, associate professor and director of the physician's assistant program at the University of Florida in Gainesville. "They can't practice without a doctor."

PAs are steadily gaining acceptance - and demand is increasing. For every PA graduating in 1990 there were nine job offers, according to the American Academy of Physician Assistants in Alexandria, VA., which maintains job listings for PAs.

Early this year New Jersey became the last state to allow PAs when regulators approved a pilot licensing program. The measure passed over objections from the Medical Society of New Jersey, but local medical groups in other states have supported PAs, particularly in rural areas.

Access is one reason.

With Smith's help "we're offering a service that wouldn't otherwise be available," says Dr. Webb, who describes his practice as an "aggressive clinic." Located in an area designated as medically underserved, his office features a

trauma room, lab, x-ray and stress-testing equipment, and room to add another doctor.

The clinic is a hit with local residents, including a group of Amish dependent on horse-drawn wagons, who used to travel at least 22 miles to the nearest hospital for those services. Now, about 30 new patients a week come to Dr. Webb's practice, which has grown to serve about 5,500 residents from farms and nearby towns.

Recruiting physician's assistants to rural areas is often easier than attracting physicians, Bottom says. But it is getting more difficult as demand for PAs grows in surgical specialties and in teaching hospitals, which are now using them to relieve residents, whose hours are restricted by law.

Economics are another reason PAs are gaining ground. Revenues from 25 extra patient visits per day "more than amply pays for what a physician assistant makes," Dr. Webb says.

What they made in 1990 ran from about $30,000 to $35,000 at the low end for PAs in pediatrics to a high of $40,000 to $45,000 for those in surgery, say the American Academy of Physician Assistants. PAs in cardiac surgery make the most, with some topping $100,000 annually. PAs can do roughly 80% of all services for adults in ambulatory settings and 90% of services for children, says the University of Florida's Bottom. In surgery, they often serve as first assistants and perform many prep and follow-up services.

He estimates that PAs in ambulatory settings bring in about two-thirds to three-fourths the revenue of a physician while being paid one-fourth to one-third the salary.

Because Dr. Webb's clinic is in an area designated as underserved, even Medicare will pay for ambulatory visits to PAs. In other areas, Medicare payments are limited to PA services in hospitals or nursing homes. Most other insurers pay PA services, some at 100% of the rate paid for the same service performed by a physician.

Most insurers in Milwaukee pay less for work done by PAs than by physicians, says Leonard Kleinman, MD, who heads a four-partner cardiac surgery group that employs seven PAs. Still, the PAs more than pay for themselves and have helped the three-physician core of the group increase open heart surgeries from about 250 to 1,000 annually. "There's no way we could do that amount of work without the PAs."

Dr. Kleinman's group hired its first PA 18 years ago. "The amount of work they do has increased as time goes by," Dr, Kleinman says. Group PAs take histories, prepare discharge summaries, and make rounds.

They also do procedures once reserved for physicians, including harvesting veins, inserting aortic balloons, and even closing the chest.

That has drawn some criticism from general surgeons, who once did those jobs, but Dr. Kleinman says PAs have done it without any problem and at lower cost. "Our mortality and morbidity rates are better than average."

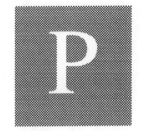

The lower cost of PAs helps the group keeps its costs down in an environment increasingly dominated by managed care. About 25% of the group's revenue come from HMO and PPO payers, Dr. Kleinman says.

But equality is an issue, says Joseph Riggs, MD, president of the Medical Society of New Jersey. The society opposes New Jersey's pilot licensing program because "it will not produce better care or lower cost. It will simply cause confusion for patients and will lessen the quality of care," he says.

PAs are a poorly trained substitute for physicians, Dr. Riggs says.

Dr. Webb, who was a physician's assistant before going to medical school, disagrees. "The point is they are not a substitute, they are an extender. A physician assistant can't practice without direct supervision."

Under Indiana law, Dr. Webb must sign off on any work his physician's assistant, John Smith, does within 24 hours. When Dr. Webb is out of town, Smith is supervised by another physician in a town 22 miles away.

Physician's assistants actually enhance quality of care by making it possible to spend more time with patients and allowing the physicians to concentrate on complicated cases that require more time, Dr. Webb says.

Supervising physicians are also liable for malpractice claims arising form their assistant's actions. That isn't a problem for Dr. Webb. In Indiana his liability insurance covers his PA as it covers other employees.

In other states, physicians pay an additional premium to cover physician assistants. In Dr. Kleinman's group the premiums for physician's assistants are lower than for doctors.
Still, Smith can take over many tasks that Dr. Webb once did, including providing first aid and seeing unscheduled patients with minor problems such as sore throats. "When I start the day my book is open," Smith says. "That gives him a lot of freedom."

American Academy of Physician's Assistants
940 N. Washington, Alexandria, VA 22314
703/836-2272

National Commission on Certification of
Physician's Assistants
2845 Henderson Mill Road NE, Atlanta, GA 30341
404/493-9100

Physician Assistant Practice
The concept of the physician's assistant arose in the mid-1960s and early 1970s when a number of institutions and creative members of their faculty and staff began exploring new territory in American medical education. Their goal was to assist physicians, in the care of their patients. In the process, they developed curricula that taught individuals a body of clinical knowledge and skills that previously had largely been limited to the professional preserve of the physician.

In its restricted meaning, "physician assistant" is the title used since the latter 1970s to identify the person prepared in the clinical knowledge and skills that are common to primary care medicine. Initially, this practice was identified as an assistant to the primary care physician.

In its general meaning, "physician assistant" is used to encompass the primary care physician assistant, as described above, but it has been applied also to personnel such as surgeon's assistants, radiologist's assistants and others. While several of these forms of assisting physicians are very small in number, three occupations with listings in this Directory have obtained recognition from the American Medical Association: anesthesiologist's assistant, physician assistant, and surgeon assistant.

Physician Assistant and Surgeon Assistant
History: The profession of the physician assistant originated in the mid-1960s with leadership form Duke University, the University of Colorado, the University of Washington, and Wake Forest University. The early 1970s brought a rapid growth in the number of such educational programs, which were supported initially with $6.1 million appropriated under the authority of the Health Manpower Act of 1972. This funding also supported some of the initial organization and administration of the national program for the accreditation of education programs, in this field, specifically those designed to prepare individuals as assistants to primary care practitioners.

Interest in the development of national accreditation standards for the education of assistants to primary care physicians was first expressed by the American Society of Internal Medicine. By 1971, standards had been developed collaboratively by a committee composed of representatives from the American Academy of Family Physicians, American Academy of Pediatrics, the American College of Physicians, the Association of American Medical Colleges, the American College of Obstetrics and Gynecology, the American Society of Internal Medicine, the nursing profession, and educators of the physician assistant. These standards were adopted in that year by the American Medical Association, the American Academy of Family Physicians, the American Academy of Pediatrics, the American College of Physicians, and the American Society of Internal Medicine (ASIM). (The ASIM withdrew its sponsorship of accreditation in September 1981.)

Early in 1972, the medical specialty organizations which had adopted the new educational standards established the Joint Review Committee on Educational Programs for the Assistant to the Primary Care Physician. A principal function of the committee was to assess the extent to which applicant programs were in compliance with the Essentials for the Assistant to the Primary Care Physician and to formulate recommendations for accreditation to the AMA Council on Medical Education. This committee was composed of three representative from each of the four sponsoring organizations. In April of 1973, the committee appointed three graduate physician's assistants to serve as members-at-large for one-year terms. By March 1974, the sponsors of the committee and the American Medical Association had recognized

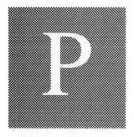

the American Academy of Physician Assistants as the fifth sponsor of the review committee.

Essentials for the surgeon assistant were adopted by the American College of Surgeons in 1973 and by the American Medical Association in 1974. These standards were revised in 1982 and again in 1990. Originally, the American College of Surgeons Committee on Allied Health Personnel reviewed applicant programs' compliance with these standards.

As a result of discussions initiated in 1975, the review committees for the assistant to the primary care physician and surgeon assistant were brought together in 1976 into a unified accreditation review committee. On petition from the Association of Physician Assistant Programs, the collaborating sponsoring organizations of the accreditation review it as the seventh sponsor of the committee in 1978. The committee was renamed the Accreditation Review Committee on Education for the Physician Assistant in 1988.

Following a two-year consultation with accredited educational programs, sponsors, of the accreditation service, and other interested parties, revised Essentials were adopted for the education of assistants to primary care physicians in 1978. Following a similar consultation, the revised Essentials were adopted in 1985 as standards for the education of physician assistants. Accreditation standards for physician and surgeon assistant education and training were consolidated in 1990 and supported by all of the collaborating sponsor organizations.

Accreditation was offered from 1970 through 1975 for orthopaedic and urologic physicians assistants. Unlike the Essentials for the education of the surgeon assistant and the physician assistant, the standards for education of the orthopaedic and urologic assistants did not require education and training to competence in eliciting a comprehensive health history and in performing a comprehensive physical examination. Accreditation for these programs was discontinued due to the withdrawal of support by the American Academy of Orthopaedic Surgeons and the American Urological Association.

Occupational Description: The physician assistant is prepared academically and through supervised clinical practice provides health care services with the direction and supervision of a qualified and licensed doctor of medicine or osteopathy. The functions of the physician assistant include performing diagnostic, therapeutic, preventive and health maintenance services in any setting in which the physician renders care, in order to allow more effective and focused application of the physician's particular knowledge and skills. Individuals choosing to prepare as surgeon assistants preform a number of functions and tasks formerly done only by surgeons in pre-, intra-, and postoperative care within a variety of appropriate settings such as a hospital surgical suite, a surgical clinic, an emergency room, and an office practice. Physician and surgeon assistants are accountable for their own actions, as well as being accountable to their supervising physician.

Job Description: The role of the physician assistant demands intelligence, sound judgement, intellectual honesty, the ability to relate effectively with people and the capacity to react to emergencies in a calm and reasoned manner. An attitude of respect for self and others, adherence to the concept of privilege and confidentiality in communicating with patients, and a commitment to the patient's welfare are essential attributes.

Service performed by physician assistants include, but are not limited to, the following:

- *Evaluation:* Initially approaching a patient of any age group, in any setting to elicit a detailed and accurate history, perform an appropriate physical examination, delineate problems, and record and present the data.
- *Monitoring:* Assisting the physician in conducting rounds in acute and long-term inpatient care settings, developing and implementing patient management plans, recording progress notes and assisting in the provision of continuity of care in office-based and other ambulatory care settings.
- *Diagnostics:* Performing and/or interpreting at least to the point of recognizing, deviations, from the norm, common laboratory. radiologic, cardiographic, and other routine diagnostic procedures used to identify pathophysiologic processes.
- *Therapeutics:* Performing routine procedures such as injections, immunizations, suturing and wound care, managing simple conditions produced by infection or trauma, assisting in the management of more complex illness and injury, which may include assisting the surgeons in the conduct of operations and taking initiative in performing evaluation and therapeutic procedures in response to life-threatening situations.
- *Counseling:* Instructing and counseling patients regarding compliance with prescribed therapeutic regimens, normal growth and development, family planning, emotional problems of daily living and health maintenances.
- *Referral:* Facilitating the referral of patients to the community's health and social service agencies when appropriate.

Employment Characteristics: A study published in 1990 indicated that just under half of physician graduates were working with family physicians and internists. Almost 36 worked in a private solo practice or private partnership practice. Similarly, 36 were working in one of a variety of hospital settings, including county, city, and private hospital, Veterans Adminstration hospitals, academic medical centers, and the like. The rest worked in such diverse settings as health maintenance organizations, industrial health clinics, military facilities, and prisons.

The normal work week for a majority of PA's exceeds 45 hours. Almost half devote more than 40 hours to direct patient contact, with one in five working over 50 hours a week. Similarly, about half report spending some additional hours of the week on call. It is anticipated that the demand for PA's will continue to increase in the coming decade.

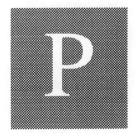

Salaries vary depending on the experience and education of the individual, the economy of a given region, and the nature of the practice and job responsibilities. According to a recent survey, entry level salaries average $33,337. Experienced PA's commonly earn in the $40,000-$60,000 range. It is anticipated that the demand for physician assistants will continue to exceed the supply during the immediate future. (ALL)

AMA Allied Health Department
312/464-4622

Physician Broadcasters
National Association of Physician Broadcasters
515 N. State St, Chicago, IL 60610
312/464-5484

Physician Credentials
For Professionals
Data Bank (Information prior to 1990)
Federation of State Medical Boards
of the United States
6000 Western Place/Suite 707
Fort Worth, TX 76107
817/735-8445

National Physician Credentials Verification Service
800/677-NCVS (800/677-6287)

National Practitioner Data Bank
(Established under the Health Care Quality
Improvement Act)
UNISYS Corporation
8301 Greensboro Dr., Suite 1100
McLean, VA 22102
800/767-6732

For Public
To receive a free biography of an MD
(Requests must be in writing.)
Send stamped self-addressed envelope to:
AMA Department of Physician Data Services
515 N. State, Chicago, IL 60610

Doctor Certification Line
American Board of Medical Specialties
800/776-2378 (information on board certification)

"Directory of Medical Specialists"
Marquis Who's Who, Macmillan Directory Division
3002 Glenview Road, Wilmette, IL 60091
708/441-2387
800/621-9669 (outside IL)

Physician Earnings
Physicians Earnings, 1981-1990
James W. Moser

The medical practice environment continues to evolve, with important consequences for the monetary rewards to physicians. While the new Medicare Fee Schedule did not go into effect until January 1, 1992, restraint on payment growth - if not outright reductions - affected many procedures under the old payment system still in effect through 1990. Physicians have become more involved with alternative, "managed care" delivery systems. Utilization review activities have continued to become more prevalent. With health

care access and cost problems continuing to escalate, many in the socio-political-medical arena are calling for health care system reform, so the future holds the prospect of further dramatic changes in the medical practice environment.

The impacts of these and other factors have important implications for physicians earnings. This report presents and discusses time trends and patterns across specialties and geographic regions in physician net income. The general period of study is from 1981 to 1990, with special emphasis given to the newly-reported figures for 1990. Physician net income, or earnings, is defined to be net income after expenses but before taxes. Income includes all earnings from medical practice, including contributions into deferred compensation plans. A physician is defined as a nonfederal M.D. involved at least 20 hours per week in patient care activities. Both office-based and hospital-based physicians are included; however, residents, clinical fellows, and physicians whose primary activities are research or administration are excluded.(SCM)

Physician Fees
Contact local medical society or state board of medicine
In Washington DC only:
Commission of Licensure to Practice
the Healing Arts
605 G St. NW, Rm. 202, Washington, DC 20001

Physician Patient Relations
The Knee

Constance J. Meyd "A Piece of My Mind"
JAMA.1982 Dec. 24-31;248(24):403.

We are on attending rounds with the usual groups: attending, senior resident, junior residents, and medical students. There are eight of us. Today we will learn how to examine the knee properly. The door is open. The room is ordinary institutional yellow, a stained curtain between the beds. We enter in proper order behind our attending physician. The knee is attached to a woman, perhaps 35 years old, dressed in her own robe and nightgown. The attending physician asks the usual questions as he places his hand on the knee: "This knee bothers You?" All eyes are on the knee; no one meets her eyes as she answers. The maneuvers begin - abduction, adduction, flexion, extension, rotation. She continues to tell her story, furtively, pushing her clothing between her legs. Her endeavors are hopeless, for the full range of knee motion must be demonstrated. The door is open. Her embarrassment and helplessness are demonstrated. More maneuvers and a discussion of knee pathology ensue. She asks a question. No one notices. More maneuvers. The door is open. Now the uninvolved knee is examined - abduction, adduction, flexion, extension, rotation. She gives up. The door is open. Now a discussion of surgical technique. Now review the knee examination. We file out through the open door. She pulls the sheet up around her waist. She is irrelevant.

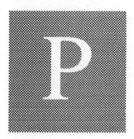

Communicate...or Litigate

Flora Johnson Skelly AMNews 6/29/92 p.29+

"Happy patients don't sue." That has long been a pet phrase among risk managers all over the country. What it means is this: If your patients like you, they are far less likely to sue you - even if you make a mistake in their care - than if they are neutral toward you. And if they're angry at you...watch out! You may not even have to make a medical mistake in order to find yourself on the receiving end of a lawsuit.

In *Medical-Legal Survival: A Risk Management Guide for Physicians* (University Hospital Consortium, 1991), a committee of authors writes: "The malpractice problem is essentially a human relations problem. The critical variable in the filing of a malpractice suit is not the clinical error nor the iatrogenic injury but rather his perceptions of the patient or his/her family."

Is this widely held belief accurate? If so, what can you do to make your patients happier (and therefore less litigious)?

Human motives are notoriously difficult to pin down, and so studies of why patients sue their physicians are rare. Conclusive evidence of a link between poor communication and litigation is lacking.

Says J. Gregory Carroll, PhD, manager of communications training for the Pharmaceutical Division of Miles Inc, in New Haven, Conn., "Unfortunately, there is no clear-cut prospective clinical trial or anything very close to it."

But that doesn't say the evidence isn't suggestive.

For example, there is abundant evidence that patients' decisions to sue correlate poorly with evidence of medical negligence. Says James Orlikoff, president of Orlikoff & Associates, a Chicago health-care consulting firm, and former director of the American Hospital Assn.'s Institute on Quality of Care and Patterns of Practice: "Many sue who have no reason to do so, legally. Many have legal reasons to sue but choose not to."

Faced with evidence such as this, observers have concluded that medical negligence alone, and even the desire for financial compensation, cannot in itself why most people sue. Many suggest that poor doctor-patient communication must be at least one important factor.

"What motivates a patient to become a plaintiff?" says Orlikoff. "All you're left with [if you rule out medical negligence] is patient interaction, how the patient feels about the provider and the hospital, if the patient is angry - those are the issues that really frame the whole issue of malpractice.

"The data is inferential, but it's there."

Correlation, if not cause
A number of studies, though inconclusive, do show strong correlations between patients' perceptions of their providers and their tendency to file claims. Says Dr. Carroll: "There is actually a fair degree of evidence that the two are linked."

The most recent of these studies was published in the March 11 Journal of the American Medical Association. Gerald B. Hickson, MD, and colleagues at Vanderbilt University in Nashville interviewed members of more than 100 families who had closed malpractice claims in Florida, asking them why they had chosen to sue.

The study found that patients who sue "are not a homogeneous group in that they offer an array of reasons for claiming." Frequently, people said they were moved to sue because someone outside the family - sometimes even a physician - suggested that they do so.

However, family members frequently cited poor communication by the physician as a reason for suing. "Most respondents complained about at least one aspect of physician-family communication," wrote with the authors, adding that their results "suggest that communication problems between physicians and their patients contribute to many decisions to file malpractice claims."

The study authors also noted that poor communication seems to present a liability risk even when the physician otherwise provides "technically adequate care."

In an interview, Dr. Hickson says that this study should not be "overinterpreted." After all, the family members interviewed had already sued their physician. "Individuals [who have sued] may need to feel some degree of hostility toward their physicians in order to justify what they've done. You don't go through the legal process without developing some anger."

On the other hand, he says, "we were surprised at the number of complaints that seemed to be related to communication."

He and his colleagues are currently engaged in research that will attempt to determine more precisely what moves people to sue. "Specifically, we hope to get at the issue of whether being liked by a patient makes a difference."

In the meantime, however, Dr. Hickson says, "The common wisdom [that patients don't sue physicians they like] makes sense."

Insurers offer discounts
Many medical liability insurers already assume that the common wisdom is true. Says Dr. Carroll: Risk managers find it's difficult to predict how people are going to react. But experience tells them that a lot of what affects that decision [whether to sue] is the relationship with the health care provider."

Several insurance companies now offer discounts on liability premiums to physicians who take a four-and-a-half-hour course on physician-patient communication. The course was developed by Miles, which is training health care professionals around the country to teach it.

The first company to offer the course was Northwest Physicians Mutual Insurance Co. in Salem, Ore., which grants physicians a 7.5% discount on their liability premiums if they take it.

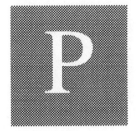

"There is some feeling in the industry that about 70% of malpractice suits have at least a relationship to communication by the physician or his staff, and therefore that improving those communication skills gets to the heart of the cause," say Robert E. Taylor, MD, the company's medical director.

Northwest Physicians Mutual cannot demonstrate that the Miles course, which has been taken by several hundred Oregon physicians since it was first offered in 1989, has had an impact on litigation. However, "there has been a tremendous interest in the subject," Dr. Taylor says.

The course also appears to have been well-received in other states.

In Colorado, Copic Insurance Co. of Englewood allows physicians to earn as much as a 15% discount on premiums by participating in a risk management program, one facet of which is the Miles course. "We have gotten feedback from participants stating that they have tried some of the techniques and felt very confident that those new skills did help avoid a patient-physician relationship deteriorating further," says Kathy Gardner, manager of the Dept. of Risk Management.

Uncommon courtesies
Asked about the communication problems most likely to provoke litigation, risk managers name an array of issues, both general and specific.

Almost all agree that treating patients discourteously or uncaring (or allowing staff to do so) is unwise. Says Barbara Brown, PhD, RN, head of the Risk Management Division of Virginia Professional Underwriters Inc.: Patients "will accept error, but they will not accept the feeling that they haven't been seen, haven't been heard and haven't been accepted.

"We've had cases," she adds where patients seem to have sued primarily because of "a feeling that no one cared about them."

In Virginia, Doctors Insurance Reciprocal, a risk retention group, and the subscriber-owned Virginia Insurance Reciprocal offer a variable discount to physicians who take risk management programs, one of which is the Miles course in communication.

Dr. Brown has been trained by Miles to teach this course. "In the seminars, physicians quickly agree that their decision process is 'find it, fix it'" she says, "and that procedures such as engaging the patient and empathizing with the patient are not taught in medical school. When they get into day-to-day practice, they have been made immune to the common courtesies that people expect."

In the physician-patient encounter, the physician may act just as he or she was trained to, Dr. Brown notes. But "there are humanistic issues that the patient expects will be dealt with." Brusqueness, failure to listen and failure to show an interest in the patient as a person all may contribute to the patient's sense that "the doctor doesn't care."

Not being listened to may be one of the most common patient complaints; 13% of patients in Dr. Hickson's study in Florida indicated that they had decided to sue because the doctor did not listen to them.

How does one listen well? In the Miles course, physicians are urged to ask "open-ended" questions, which allow the patient room to fully express concerns, and to resist the temptation to interrupt while the patient is talking.

Risk managers also stress that physicians must take time to answer patients' questions, explain procedures and make sure that patients feel they've been consulted about decisions in their care.

More than a signature
Risk managers not that communication problems also tend to crop up in certain situations. One is when the physician sets out to gain informed consent.

Many physicians seem to believe that having the patient sign the consent form is enough, these experts note. But, in the event of litigation, "that signature on the paper does no good," says Dr. Brown, adding that the physician must discuss "everything that could reasonably go wrong" with the patient - and do so in person.

Lee Johnson, JD, counsel for health care law for New York City's Medical Liability Mutual Insurance Co., agrees: "Doctors think informed consent is a form. They forget it's just evidence of a conversation. In most states, either by case law or statute, the patient is entitled to that conversation. The patient has to be able to ask questions; say, 'I didn't quite understand that'; have an opportunity to repeat back what the doctor has said in his or her own words. Only at the end of the full procedure does the patient sign the consent form."

Both Johnson and Dr. Brown further note that, in discussing the procedure with the patient, the physician should be careful not to make promises about outcomes. "Don't say, 'If I do this procedure, thus-and-so will happen,'" Dr. Brown says. "Say, 'Our experience indicates that (some proportion) of patients have (this result).'"

When the worst happens
One of the most difficult junctures in any physician-patient relationship occurs immediately following an adverse outcome.

The Florida study suggests that poor communication at this time may lead to many lawsuits. In the study, 70% of family members who sued said their physicians did not warn them about the possibility of long-term neurodevelopmental problems; 48% said the physician had attempted to mislead them; 32% complained that the physician "would not talk openly."

This doesn't mean the physicians actually did behave the way the family members said they did, the authors of the study note. The physicians may have attempted to communicate, but failed.

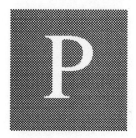

Dr. Hickson points out that patients who are in grief or in shock may not remember what a physician tells them. Sometimes the same message must be given more than once.

Patients also may want more information than physicians customarily impart, or information or a different type. "Several studies suggest that physicians and patients have differing ideas about the amount and type of information that can or should be transmitted" write the authors of the Florida study.

And finally, some families will find it difficult to accept that, sometimes, there's no way to know what happened or why. "It's important to let families know that there are certain aspects of medicine that we don't understand very well," says Dr. Hickson.

Invariably, physicians face "an enigma of how much to tell, how much to predict; they want families to understand that there may be problems, but not dash all hope," Dr. Hickson says. "Even the best communicators can come up short in the eyes of families struggling with grief."

Faced with such difficulties, some physicians may try to avoid communicating altogether. The Florida study found that some physicians "avoid families after bad outcomes, are not available, have brusque personalities, or, in fact, provide incorrect information."

This is because physicians "are human," Dr. Hickson says, "and have as much difficulty as anyone else in facing a bad outcome." But his study indicates it's unwise to give in to this temptation. Says Dr. Hickson: "Honesty is the best protection. Speaking as an individual, I think we're always better off disclosing everything."

Orlikoff agrees: "One of the best times to effectively communicate with patients or families is immediately after something bad has happened. Go in and get it out in the open; talk about what's going to be done."

On the other hand, speaking as a lawyer, Lee Johnson warns that physicians should not give patients information that might later be used against them or others in a court of law.

Physicians are legally required to disclose information needed for a patient's continued care, and certainly should not cover up any adverse event, she says. Nor is it wise to avoid a patient in the wake of such an event.

"We usually recommend that a physician see the patient more. If you were seeing the patient once a day before, see the patient twice a day now. Let the patient talk about his or her anger. Express your sympathy and concern. Ask, 'Is there anything I can do to help you?'"

But it's legally dangerous to try to explain why the adverse event occurred, assess blame or "confess" you own role in the affair. Unfortunately, Johnson says, anything you say really can be used against you.

Opening a complaint department

A third crucial juncture when good communication is needed is when the patient has a complaint.

Patients "often have complaints that they want to lodge against physicians, and currently the court system is the only effective way to do that," says Dr. Hickson. He believes that the medical profession as a whole should look for "alternative ways" for patients to voice their complaints. But in the meantime, being able to listen to a patient's complaint, without getting defensive, could stop a lawsuit.

Says Orlikoff: "Most hospital staff and physicians don't want to talk to a complaining patient. But the complaining patient is your friend. This patient is saying, 'We can work this out.' You would much rather hear the complaint from the patient than from the patient's attorney.

"If you close off the avenues of complaint, what you're saying is, 'If you're really upset, sue us.'"

When all is said and done, Orlikoff concludes, "Injuries don't file lawsuits. Lawyers don't file lawsuits. Patients do. And patients who like their doctors don't sue them."

How to get yourself sued for malpractice
Risk managers know that you don't have to make a medical mistake in order to get sued for malpractice. Sometimes just alienating your patients can be enough.

So, with tongue firmly planted in cheek, health care consultant James Orlikoff offers the following list of "ways to get sued for malpractice":

1. Don't greet patients warmly. Read the chart instead of saying hello.
2. Don't appear interested in patients. Avoid making eye contact.
3. Use body language that conveys superiority. If a patient is sitting down or lying on a bed, stand so you tower above him or her.
4. Don't listen. When patients are talking, interrupt frequently.
5. Don't encourage patients to talk. Ask only "closed questions," which require a limited response.
6. If you make a mistake, hide it or cover it up. If necessary, lie.
7. Don't explain anything to patients. In fact, use a tremendous amount of medical jargon.
8. Disregard patients' interest in specific information or specific treatments. If the patient asks a question, be hostile.
9. Don't treat patients with respect. Always use their first names without first asking how they want to be addressed. And be sure to make derogatory entries about patients in their medical records.
10. Don't treat patients as individuals. Treat them all the same. Better yet, treat every patient as a disease or body part.

Strategies to Please Patients:
The Patient Calls For An Appointment.

1. Handle Phone Calls Courteously and Professionally
- Always use good telephone etiquette.
- Do your best to ease patients' fears and communicate your concern over the phone.
- Never use the word "busy" when patients ask to speak to the physician.
- Uuse the "hold" button judiciously.

2. Send a welcome letter to the patient after she has made her appointment, thanking her and enclosing a patient information handbook and the time and date of the appointment.

The Patient Arrives For The Appointment

3. Acknowledge arriving patients upon their arrival.

4. Set high standards for your staff. Make sure each member of your staff reflects your own attitudes of courtesy and concern. The patient should be greeted by a staff that is uniformly cheerful, helpful, and courteous. An ability to communicate well with patients should be given a top priority in hiring new staff members.

5. Always address a patient by name as far as that is possible. Be very sensitive to patients' feelings in deciding whether to use formal or informal terms of address.

6. Appropriate professional dress and deportment should be displayed by each member of the staff.

7. Provide special personnel to handle patient needs (probably applicable only to larger practices):
- a) A receptionist and "official greeter" at the main door.
- b) An in-office escort service for elderly and infirm patients.
- c) A patient representative to handle patient requests and complaints.
- d) A transportation service to and from your office for elderly, patients, patients without cars, etc.

8. Explain all lengthy delays, and make sure that patients are given the opportunity to reschedule if they so desire.

9. Decorate your reception room to give it a warm and personal ambience. Some physicians use such things artwork, plants, flowers, aquariums, and professional interior decoration to enhance the attractiveness of their reception areas.

10. Provide interesting, up-to-date, and attractively-displayed reading material for your waiting patients. In some offices a television set (with the volume controlled) may be appropriate. Many patients might also appreciate a copy of the daily paper to read while they are (briefly) waiting. Parents often appreciate comic books or children's literature for their youngsters.

11. Provide refreshments. Make coffee, juice, or other refreshments available to your patients.

12. Provide educational materials to your patients.
- Such materials are not only an effective way to promote your practice; they are also greatly appreciated by patients and they usually result in patients who are more able and willing to assume responsibility in assisting you in the healing process. Many forms of educational material are available to you:
- Utilize free materials available from pharmaceutical and insurance firms, professional associations, and government agencies.

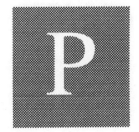

- Purchase commercial programs, many of which are quite attractive and explanatory.
- Write your own educational materials and personalize them to your patients.
- Establish a patient education center in your reception area in which you utilize printed materials and video- technology to inform and entertain your patients while they are (briefly) waiting to see you.
- Produce your own video or audio cassettes to explain preliminary or supplementary information to your patients.
- Conduct classes for small groups of your patients with common conditions in order to avoid repetitions and encourage experiences.
- Use good teaching aids -- diagrams, anatomical drawings, slides plastic models, etc. -- to help illustrate your explanations to patients.
- Establish an "office library" from which patients can borrow books, articles, cassettes, and other educational materials to review in the privacy of their homes.
- Inform patients about the local Tel-Med service and/or similar educational networks if such resources are available in your area.

13. Put up bulletin boards in your office on which to post pictures of your patients.
- This works especially well in pediatric and OB/GYN practices. In other offices, physicians train their staffs to be alert for news items about established patients, and all laudatory items -- promotion, awards, anniversaries, retirements, and the like -- are acknowledged on the practice bulletin board.

14. Provide play areas and/or special supervision for small children.

15. Provide separate waiting areas for "well patients" and "ill patients" where appropriate.

16. Provide washroom facilities for your patients that are sanitary and attractive.

17. Provide a telephone for your patients' use either in your reception area or in an adjoining hallway.

18. Provide conveniences for your patients, such as a changing table or suspension hooks in a pediatric office, or a set of jumper cables in your office in case a patient's automobile battery goes dead.

19. Prohibit smoking in your office, or at least make sure smoking areas are well-designated and well-ventilated.

20. Always use the patient's name. Glance at the patient's chart before entering the exam room if you need to refresh your memory.

21. Be a caring professional. Project at all times an air of professional competence and personal concern. Be affable, warm, and concerned, rather than cold, aloof, and indifferent.

22. Keep informed of the major interests and activities of each patient and his or her family.
- Bring up such interests in the conversations you have with each patient. Ask about the patient's family, how they're feeling and what they've been doing. Some physicians with less-than-perfect memories jot down personal notes about each patient and keep them in the patient's chart. A few physicians even ask their assistant to take a Polaroid photograph of each patient and attach it to the patient's chart to refresh the physician's memory.

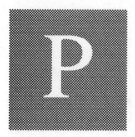

23. Spend adequate time with each patient. Surveys indicate that the degree of patient satisfaction is often directly correlated with the amount of time the physician spends with the patient. So spend an amount of time with each patient that a reasonable person would expect.

24. Answer patients' questions.
- The five questions that should always be answered by someone in your office are What is wrong with me? What caused it? What are you and I going to do about it? How long is it going to take? How much is it going to cost?
- Always allow enough time for the patient to ask about his or her legitimate concerns.
- Encourage patients to ask questions with a phrase like "Now is there anything else you'd like to ask about today?"
- Provide written forms and encourage patients to write down their questions before meeting with you.
- Don't be defensive or disinterested in answering patients' questions. Never give patients the impression that you're too busy to be bothered with their concerns.

25. Use layman's terms, as far as that is possible, in describing a patient's condition and how it will be managed.

26. Listen sincerely to what your patients have to say.

27. Maintain eye contact with your patients while you are speaking with them.

28. Pay attention to your body language. Facial expression, gestures, etc., convey important messages to your patients, and such messages are often remembered after what you said in an encounter has been forgotten. Make sure your non-verbal communication does not convey the wrong impressions. Frowns or scowls, for example, may be interpreted by patients in ways you never intended. Be careful not to let the fatigue or irritation of a long day enter into your communication with patients.

29. Dictate the medical record in the patient's presence. Many physicians do not recommend this, but other physicians see it as a valuable way to let patients know what the physician is doing for them. If you choose to dictate in this fashion, close by saying something like "Is there anything I missed that you think we ought to add to your record?"

30. Emphasize the advantages of compliance. Always phrase your advice or instructions to patients in terms of the advantages they will realize by following such advice or instructions.

31. Keep the patient's values and self-image in mind when countering his objection to your advice or instructions.

32. Never interrupt or contradict a patient's objections. It won't get you anywhere. Instead, listen, restate, paraphrase and explain.

33. Follow the golden rule in treating patients. Always treat each patient the way you would want to be treated if your were in his shoes.
- Examine patients thoroughly and gently. Where you sense that a patient wants and expects an examination, briefly examine her even if the examination in unnecessary.
- Explain to the patient the necessity of all treatments that are painful or embarrassing, and *prepare* the patient before initiating such treatment.
- Avoid unorthodox treatment, over-treatment, and/or experimentation with the patient.

34. Explain the necessity of all lab tests and X-ray examinations which you order, and the billing procedures for such examinations.

35. Involve the patient in his or her treatment where appropriate.

36. Inform patients about what happens after they leave. Let them know what you will be doing for them before their next visit, and the concern with which you will follow the progress of their cases.

37. Walk patients to the door, or in some other way bring your encounter with the patient to a cordial conclusion.

After the patient has gone

38. Call patients to see how they are doing a few days after their visit to your office. This won't be appropriate for every patient, of course, but most patients will greatly appreciate your concern. Try especially to phone or visit a surgery patient a few days after the operation.

39. Call close family members, where appropriate, to let them know the results of a serious operation.

40. Call with good lab results. Patients will appreciate knowing that all is well.

41. Send handwritten congratulatory notes to long-time patients to acknowledge their anniversaries, promotions, retirements, etc.

42. Send holiday cards., birthday cards, etc., to your patients where appropriate. Try to personalize such cards (e.g., one orthodontist sends holiday cards in which all of the reindeer wear braces, and his younger patients love it).

43. Send follow-up notices to patients to remind them of physicals, vaccinations, etc., which are due.

44. Send condolences and/or flowers to the family of a deceased patient, and offer words of comfort where appropriate. Also where appropriate, offer bereavement counseling to the deceased's family, reviewing the circumstances of the loved one's death with them and answering any questions they may have.

45. Send flowers to a new mother, or treat the new parents to a fine dinner.

46. Stamp "Thank You" on all patients' cancelled checks.

47. Put a suggestion box in your office. Suggestions or complaints found there can be followed up personally or in your practice newsletter.

48. Take periodic surveys or your patients to get their feedback on your practice.

49. Take periodic surveys of your employees to see what suggestions they can give you for improving your practice habits or enhancing your interpersonal skills.(COM)

Physics

American Association for Physicists in Medicine
335 E. 45th St., New York, NY 10017
212/661-9404

Health Physics Society
8000 Westpark Drive, Suite 400
Mc Lean, VA 22102
703/790-1745

Physiology

American Physiological Society
9650 Rockville Pike, Bethesda, MD 20814
301/530-7164

Plastic Surgery

American Academy of Facial Plastic &
Reconstructive Surgery
1101 Vermont Avenue, NW, Ste. 404,
Washington, DC 20005
202/842-4500
800/332-FACE (800/332-3223)

American Association for Accreditation of
Ambulatory Plastic Surgery Facilities,
1202 Allanson Rd, Mundelein, IL 60060
708/949-6058

American Association of Plastic Surgeons
c/o Melvin Spira, MD
Baylor College of Medicine
6560 Fannin St., Suite 800, Houston, TX 77030
713/798-6141

American Board of Plastic Surgery
7 Penn Center, Suite 400, 1635 Market St.,
Philadelphia, PA 19103
215/587-9322

American Society of Plastic
and Reconstructive Surgeons
444 E. Algonquin, Arlington Heights, IL 60005
708/228-9900
Referral Service 800/635-0635

Podiatrics and Podiatry

Podiatrist: Diagnoses and treats diseases and
deformities of human foot: Diagnoses food
ailments, such as tumors, ulcers, fractures, skin or
nail diseases, and congenital or acquired
deformities, utilizing diagnostic aids, such as
urinalysis, blood tests, and x-ray analysis. Treats
deformities, such as flat or weak feet and foot
imbalance, by mechanical and electrical methods,
such as whirlpool or paraffin baths and short wave
and low voltage currents. Treats conditions, such
as corns, calluses, ingrowing nails, tumors,
shortened tendons, bunions, cysts, and
abscesses by surgical methods, including
suturing, medication, and administration of local
anesthetics. Prescribes drugs. Does not perform
foot amputations. Correct deformities by means of
plaster casts and strappings. Makes and fits
prosthetic appliances. Prescribes corrective
footwear. Advises patient concerning continued
treatment of disorders and proper foot care to
prevent recurrence. Refers patients to physician
when symptoms observed in feet and legs
indicate systemic disorders, such as arthritis,
heart disease, diabetes, or kidney trouble. May
treat bone, muscle, and joint disorders and be
designated Podiatrist, Orthopedic; childrens' foot
diseases and be designated Popopediatrician, or
perform surgery and be designated Podiatric
Surgeon. (DOT)

Podiatric Assistant: assists Podiatrist in patient
care. Prepares patients for treatment, sterilizes
instruments, performs general office duties, and
assists Podiatrist in preparing dressings,
administering treatments, and developing x rays.
(DOT)

American Podiatric Medical Association
9312 Old Georgetown Rd., Bethesda, MD 20814
301/571-9200

Board Certification
American Board of Podiatric Orthopedics
108 Orange St, Suite #6, Redlands, CA 92373
714/798-8910

American Board of Podiatric Public Health
9 Hansen Court, Narberth, PA 19072
215/667-9183

American Board of Podiatric Surgery
1601 Dolores St, San Francisco, CA 94110
415/826-3200

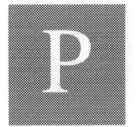

Poetry
In His Third Year of Dying

Joan I. Siegel "Poetry and Medicine" JAMA.1992
Dec 9: 268(22):3242

My father loses himself.
First it is his keys
then his words
then his children
wand when he finds them
they don't fit.

He raises his eyebrows to ask
"Where are my teeth?"
The words are wrong.
He waves them through the ceiling.

He cannot find himself
with his eyes open.

Maybe he looks in his sleep
for clues. Maybe he walks backward
through sleep looking for his mother.
Maybe he finds the boy he was
and hoists him on his shoulders

but the boy jumps down
and runs away.

American Physicians Poetry Association
Richard A. Lippin, MD, Exec. Dir.
230 Toll Drive, Southampton, PA 18966
215/364-2990

Poison Control Centers

American Association of Poison Control Centers
Arizona Poison and Drug Information Center
Health Sciences Center, Room 3204K
1501 N Campbell, Tucson, AZ 85725
602/626-1587

Poison Control Branch, Food and Drug
Administration
5600 Fishers Lane, Room 188-31
Rockville, MD 20857
301/443-6289

Polio

Polio Survivors Association
12720 La Reina Ave., Downey, CA 90242
213/923-0034

Post-Polio League for Information
5432 Connecticut Ave., N.W., Suite 204,
Washington, DC 20015
202/653-5010

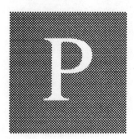

Political Associations

American Association of Physicians
for Human Rights
(Gay and Lesbian Physicians
and Medical Students)
2940 16th St., Suite 105
San Francisco, CA 94103
415/255-4547

Physician Committee for Responsible Medicine
PO Box 6322, Washington, DC 20015
202/686-2210

Physicians for Human Rights
100 Boylston Street, Suite 620, Boston, MA 02116
617/695-0041 FAX 617/695-0307

Physicians for a National Health Program
332 S. Michigan, Suite 500, Chicago, IL 60604
312/554-0382

Physicians for Social Responsibility
1000 16th St., NW, Ste 810
Washington, DC 20036
202/785-3777

People's Medical Society
(advocates citizen involvement in public
health issues)
462 Walnut St, Allentown, PA 18102
215/770-1670

Public Citizen Health Research Group (HRG)
2000 P St. NW, Washington D.C. 20036
202/872-0320

Publisher of "Public Citizen Health Resources
Group Health Letter" the HRG, monitors
government health agencies, analyzes proposed
legislation, testifies at hearings, and files lawsuits
when it believes that government agencies are too
lax in protecting consumers from dangerous
foods, drugs, or medical practices. Also
investigates and issues reports on the
effectiveness of state licensing boards and on
various other economic and quality-of-care
issues.(ALT)

Porphyria

American Porphyria Foundation
PO Box 11163, Montgomery, AL 36111
205/265-2200

Practice Development and Management

Making the Decision to Incorporate

Should a professional corporation for a medical
practice be formed? Unfortunately, there is no
simple answer to that question. First, the choice
depends on personal and professional
circumstances and interests - so much so that
incorporation might be ideal for one practitioner,
yet unwise for another. Second, the choice
involves some very complex questions, and it will
take careful analysis and planning to reach an
appropriate decision. Since the benefits and
drawbacks of that decision will be borne by the

physician, it is important to learn as much about
the subject as possible in order to make an
informed decision.

Many physicians avoid investigating the possibility
of forming a professional corporation because
they believe it will take too much time, or it will be
too complicated to figure out, or that it doesn't
matter one way or the other. As a result, some of
these practitioners may be paying more than they
should in taxes, or exposing themselves to
unnecessary legal and financial risks. A decision
against incorporation should never be made by
default.

A corporation is nothing more than a particular
form of legal organization for a business
enterprise - and it is only one form out of many.
Whatever current situation a practice is in, that
practice has a specific legal status, whether run by
a sole proprietor, a salaried employee, a
partnership, a shareholder in a professional
corporation, or some other status. Each kind of
legal status has a different impact on financial
operations, the taxes paid, and the potential legal
and business risks faced. Contrary to what some
people say, no one form of legal organization is
perfect for all physicians, or even for any particular
physician; each kind involves both benefits and
drawbacks. For example, some of the more
complex forms of legal organization may involve a
good deal more paperwork, administrative detail,
and start-up costs than the simpler forms. But the
trade-off might be a good one for many
physicians, in terms of tax savings, for example.
Carefully investigate both the good points and bad
points of incorporation as compared with other
forms or organization, to determine which is the
optimum choice. The following definitions should
provide a starting point.

A corporation is an artificial form of business
organization created by state laws, and
recognized by the federal government's tax and
other laws. A professional service corporation is a
specific kind of corporation, which has some
things in common with every other corporation, no
matter how large, but also has other aspects that
are specific to professional service corporations
and no other kind. Every state has laws governing
the formation and operation of corporations of all
kinds, and though the laws are generally similar,
any one state may have certain peculiarities in its
law that could affect a practice. By all means,
consult experts before making any final decisions.

The professional corporation is not a new concept.
The federal Revenue Act of 1918, enacted only
five years after the first income taxes were
authorized, contained a definition of a professional
service corporation as one that receives income
primarily from the rendering of professional
services, as opposed to the manufacturing of
goods or providing of nonprofessional services.
That definition is still a good starting point today.
However, until recently professional corporations
were quite rare, due primarily to the lack of state
professional service incorporation statutes and the
refusal of the Internal Revenue Service to
acquiesce to the idea that professional
corporations were entitled to the same federal tax
advantages that other kinds of corporations
enjoyed. However, the courts rejected the IRS
position in the late sixties, and the
professional-corporation approach has since been

widely adopted, particularly in the medical profession.

Perhaps the professional corporation's most important feature is that it separates a person from a practice, in a legal sense. The corporation has a separate existence, from the physician, even if that physician is the only stockholder, only officer, only director, and only employee. That can be an advantage compared with a sole proprietorship (the form a practice normally takes if a professional practices independently and takes no legal steps to form any other sort of organization). For example, if a sole proprietor owes a business debt, that debt can be collected from the sole proprietor's personal assets as well as his or her business assets. For federal tax purposes, all of the practice income and expenses are reported on the personal 1040 return.

Partners of partnerships fare the same in some states, where the practice is recognized as being separate from the personal affairs of the individual partners - but their tax status is generally no different from that of the solo practitioner. The partnership may have a legal status as a separate and distinct business, but the taxes that each partner pays are basically the same as if each partner were practicing independently, splitting all income and expense. Here it should be noted that while physicians may share office space or expenses, that does not necessarily mean those involved are or are not partners: partnership is a specific legal form that involves a sharing of income, costs, and business and legal risks within the scope of the partnership.

But if a practice incorporates, the corporation becomes an independent taxpaying completely separate from the physicians who are its shareholders. The way the group actually practices medicine won't change in any way, of course, but for accounting purposes the income and expenses of the corporation are kept absolutely and completely separate from the personal finances of the physician-shareholders. Once a corporation is created, it must obey a completely different set of state and federal laws with regard to legal rights and obligations, including tax obligations. These laws can be rather rigid; that is, the legal and financial advantages of some of these laws cannot be claimed unless all are obeyed quite strictly. A corporation may not simply be formed on paper and then forgotten about. For example, financial affairs must incorporate changes in procedure due to the incorporations. It cannot remain as it was prior. while conducting financial affairs prior to restructuring. Both the IRS and the courts may regard the corporation as nonexistent, and, therefore, it is possible to lose all the tax and legal advantages.

Professional corporation and professional service corporation, as used in this booklet, mean essentially the same thing. Each state has its own terminology to describe corporations that may be used by physicians and other professionals. In describing the applicable tax rules, the Internal Revenue Code generally uses the term professional service corporations, but the rules are applicable to all such entities regardless of the terminology used in the applicable state law. (PRO:Adaptation)

Forms Of Medical Practice

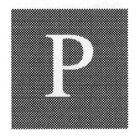

Sole Proprietorship: A sole proprietorship is an unincorporated business which is owned by a single individual. A sole proprietor may have a large number of employees, including other physicians, but so long as none of the employees is a part owner of the business it remains a sole proprietorship. Thus a sole proprietor is not the same thing as a solo practitioner.

For most purposes, the law makes no distinction between a sole proprietorship and its owner. The owner receives all the proceeds of the practice and is legally responsible for all its obligations. If the income from the practice is insufficient to pay its debts, the owner must pay them out of his or her personnel assets. The owner reports the practice income, and deducts the practice expenses on his personal income tax return, and pays taxes on the net income at rates applicable to personal earned income.

Another important aspect of a sole proprietor is that the owner, under the doctrine of respondeat superior, is legally responsible for acts committed by his or her employees within the scope of their employment. Thus, for example, if a patient files a professional liability suit involving a physician employed by a sole proprietor, he may sue the proprietor instead or in addition to the employee. If the suit is successful, a judgement will be rendered against the proprietor, even if the proprietor had no connection with the events giving rise to the lawsuit. And, as with general obligations of the business, the proprietor will be liable for such a judgement to the extent of all his or her assets, not just those assets connected with the practice. The only exceptions are assets in the proprietor's account in a qualified pension or other retirement plan, and, if the proprietor files for bankruptcy, assets which are exempt under the bankruptcy law.

Partnership: A partnership can be defined as association of two or more persons to carry on as co-owners a business for profit. Such an association includes a sharing of profits and, usually, losses from such business among the partners. The sharing of profits and losses is generally in accordance with a predetermined formula set forth in a partnership agreement, and is not necessarily equal.

Unlike a sole proprietorship, a partnership is, for some purposes, treated as a separate entity from the partners comprising it. Partnerships can generally own property, and in many states a partnership can sue or be sued in its own name. A partnership files an information return indicating the profits or losses attributable to each partner, but does not pay a separate federal income tax. The partners report such income or losses individually, in the same manner as sole proprietors.

An important aspect of partnership law is that each partner is an agent of the partnership for the purpose of its business and can legally bind the partnership by his or her acts unless the partner in fact has no authority to act in the particular matter and the person with whom he or she is dealing knows of such lack of authority. Thus, for example, a partner in a medical partnership could commit the partnership to purchase or lease office

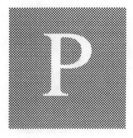

equipment even if the other partners are unaware of or opposed to such action.

Partners are also jointly and severally liable both for the debts of the partnership and the acts of the other partners within the scope of the partnership's business. Thus, for example, a patient who asserts a professional liability claim involving one partner may sue and, if successful, obtain a judgment against any of the partners. And such a judgment may be enforced against any partner to the extent of his or her entire assets, not just those used in the partnership's business. In addition, partners are jointly and severally liable for actions of employees of the partnership under the doctrine of respondeat superior in the same manner and to the same extent as sole proprietors are liable for the actions of their employees.(FOR)

Business Side of Medical Practice. Chicago; American Medical Associaiton ISBN 0-89970-343-7. OP385488

Financing a Medical Practice Start-Up, Acquisition, or Expansion. Chicago; American Medical Association. ISBN 0-89970-408-5. OP371990

Personnel policies:

Developing one's own employee policy manual.

The physician's own policies with regard to job descriptions, working hours, wages, and fringe benefits, which will need to be established before hiring the first assistant provide the basis for developing a policy manual - an important and useful guidebook for present and future employees. Here is a list of the policies a manual should set forth:

What Employees Need and Want to Know.

I. Introduction
- What's the purpose of this manual?
- How does it benefit me and my employer?
- Do I have any say if policies are revised?

II. The Work Week
- What are my working hours-daily, weekly?
- Explain my flex time arrangements or shifts
- Do I get a paid lunch and breaks? How long? Will we close the office for lunch or do we have to stagger our times?
- What are your OVERTIME policies?
- What type of time records does the office keep?
- When do I get my check? What happens when payday falls on a holiday? Can I get a salary advance if I need it?
- What about time paid for civic responsibilities, jury duty?
- Any exception to this because I'm a part-timer?

III. Sick Leave Policies
- How do I accumulate sick leave?
- When can I begin taking it?

- What if I don't use all the sick days I've earned?
- Can I carry over unused days until next year?
- What happens when I'm out for a long illness?
- If I'm a part-timer, do I get sick leave?
- Explain your "leave of absence" policies

IV. Personal Days
- What is a "personal day?" How many am I allowed?
- How much notice do you want if I'm going to use one?
- Can I use them in full or half day increments?

V. Holidays
- What Holidays are we paid for? New Years Day; Labor Day; Memorial Day; Thanksgiving Day; Independence Day; Christmas Day
- What happens when a holiday falls on a day when our office is normally closed?
- I'm a part-timer. Does the same apply to me?

VI. Vacations
- How is my vacation time computed?
- When can I take it? Can I take it a day at a time?
- When should I notify you of my vacation plans?
- Do we choose vacation preference based on seniority?
- Can I be paid in lieu of vacation not taken?
- Can I carry vacation time over to next year?
- What about part-timers?
- What if I'm sick during my vacation?
- What happens to earned vacation time if my employment is terminated?

VII. Benefits
- Do you offer any of the following: Medical Insurance; Dental Insurance; Life Insurance; Disability Insurance; Profit Sharing and/or Pension Plan; Credit Union; etc.
- When do I become eligible to receive benefits?
- What do I contribute? What do you contribute?
- What about uniform allowance?
- Do I receive educational reimbursement for such things as tuition and for what kinds of courses? For dues and meetings and for what kinds of Association? For attending workshops and Seminars?
- Do you offer free parking?
- Can I or my family receive free medical care in this office?
- Can I use office medical supplies?

VIII. Employment Responsibility
- How is my attitude important to the workings of this office?
- What are your ground rules for attendance and punctuality?
- Are personal phone calls allowed? What about long distance calls?
- Do you have dress code/appearance standards?
- What about smoking and eating on the job?
- How should I report work related injuries?

IX. Wage and Job Evaluation

- Is there a "probationary" period? What does this mean?
- How are salaries determined?
- When and how are they reviewed?
- Do you offer bonuses? Cost of living raises? Merit increases?
- How often is my job performance evaluated?
- Do I participate in this process?

X. Termination

- During the probationary period?
- How much notice should I give if I want to quit?
- If my work is unsatisfactory, do you have procedures for me to receive a second chance?
- Explain severance pay policies
- What are grounds for immediate dismissal?
- Are there grievance procedures?

XI. Confidentiality

- What is the physician-patient relationship?
- What about the release of medical information?
- Are financial and other records confidential as well?
- What are "medical ethics?"

(BUS Adaptation)

Value Enhancement Through Management

Practice Management: The Cornerstone of Value.

Although medical-practice marketing can be effective in creating value, the best marketing available will not solve problems if practice management is poor. Medical-practice management is the single most important element in creating value. Medical-practice management, refers to both clinical and office operations. It is essential that both of these be managed effectively and efficiently, not only to provide good patient care but also to give the practice the kind of economic value it strives toward.

All other things being equal, a well-managed medical practice will always have a higher value than one that is not well managed. This is because one of the key measurements of value is the ability to realize economic gains in amounts correlated with professional effort. If a physician is working hard treatment, the practice value inevitably suffers. Although many physicians rightly focus most of their efforts on treating patients, practice management is important from the standpoint of creating value as well as providing effective patient care. Medical practices that are well managed also tend to provide a higher caliber of patient care and take care of more patients.(ENH)

Physician's Guide to Professional Corporations, rev. ed. Chicago; American Medical Association ISBN 0-89970-353-4. OP378289

Planning Guide for Physicians' Medical Facilities Chicago; American Medical Association, 1986. ISBN 0-89970-261-9. OP385986

Retirement

Selecting a Corporate Retirement Plan Retirement plans that meet certain IRS requirements (i.e., qualified plans) offer significant tax advantages to physicians. Briefly, the major advantages are

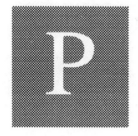

1. Amounts contributed by the professional corporation (or to the non-corporate entity in which the physician practices) to a qualified retirement plan are immediately deductible from the income of the corporation or other entity.

2. The physician does not have to pay current income tax on these contributions to the plan at the time they are made. Rather, the physician won't be taxed on those benefits until they're actually distributed to him or her.

3. Earnings and capital gains made by investments of the plan's funds are not subject to state or federal income taxes when received, but only after they're distributed to the physician. That means the yearly earnings of the plan compound tax-free, and therefore increase at a much greater rate than if they were subject to taxes.

4. Certain distributions from a qualified plan be taxed in advantageous ways:

- If the physician receives a lump-sum distribution of the benefits under the plan after age 59 1/2, the distribution can be subject to five-year averaging if it meets certain requirements. Under five-year averaging, the amount received is taxed in the year it is received, but it is taxed at rates that would have been applicable if it had been received over a five-year period.
- Individuals who are over 50 by January 1, 1986, may elect ten-year averaging under the rate schedule in effect in 1986, and in some cases may elect capital gains treatment for a portion of the distribution.
- In order to qualify for five-year averaging, ten-year averaging or capital gains treatment, however, the distribution must be received on account of certain specified events, and must meet several complex conditions.
- Certain distributions from qualified plans may be rolled over into an individual retirement account (IRA), and will not be taxed until they are withdrawn from the IRA. The rollover must occur no later than sixty days after the distribution is received, and this deadline cannot be extended for any reason.

A physician receiving a distribution from a plan should always seek the advice of a tax attorney or an accountant who is familiar with the physician's individual financial situation.

5. The amount of the participant's voluntary aftertax contributions to a plan generally is distribution tax-free, although there are limitations on the right of the participant to withdraw the voluntary contributions without being deemed to have also withdrawn a portion of the plan benefits that are subject to tax.

6. The first $5,000 of the death benefit from a deceased participant's accrued benefit from corporate contributions can pass to a beneficiary free of income tax.

There are basically two types of qualified plans: define-contribution plans and defined-benefit plans. Some plans, such as target-benefit plans, combine features of both type of plans.

Defined-Contributions Plans: Under this type of plan, contributions are made in an amount equal to a fixed percentage of each employee's salary or other compensation (hence the term defined-contribution). The employee's share of the contribution will be placed in his or her "account" in the plan, and that account will be adjusted from time to time by the employee's share of the plan's earnings, gains and losses. The plan doesn't say anything about how much the employee will receive in benefits when he or she retires. The employee will simply get a pension (or lump-sum distribution) equal in value to the amount held in his or her account at the time of retirement.

Defined-contribution plans come in two basic forms: profit-sharing and money-purchasing pension plans. The former is usually based on corporate profits, although it is now possible to make a contribution even in the absence of profits. The latter is usually a straight percentage of the employee's annual compensation. These two forms are very similar, but the distinctions can be important for financial and tax-planning purposes. Money-purchase pension plans require a fixed contribution every year, no matter what. On the other hand, a profit-sharing plan is much more flexible, since the corporation isn't required to make a contribution every year, and even when it does it can change from year to year. The primary advantage of a money-purchase plan is that the contribution can often go as high as 25 percent of a participant's compensation - but not more than $30,000 (1988 figure) per participant. However, the maximum contribution that can be made to a profit-sharing plan is generally 15 percent of compensation.

A professional corporation or a noncorporate entity should, in most cases, start out with a profit-sharing plan, since at first the practice's financial picture will be unclear, and this type is most flexible. Later, if retirement-plan contributions greater than 15 percent of employee compensation are desired, then a money-purchase pension plan can be adopted either instead of or in addition to the profit-sharing plan to make aggregate contributions of up to 25 percent of compensation. Many physicians practices will never need to contribute cannot be based on more than $200,000 (1988 figure) in compensation for any one employee. If the practice contributes 15 percent of $200,000 for its physician-owner, that amount is equal to $30,000 which is the maximum permissible contribution in any event.

Defined-Benefit Plans: A defined-benefit plan is one in which the amount of benefit that the employee will receive upon the retirement is guaranteed to be a certain amount - usually a specified percentage of the employee's compensation at the time of retirement. The contributions required to achieve that benefit level, however, can vary from year to year. In a defined-benefit plan, an actuary must figure, from the participant's age and other factors, how much must be contributed every year.

The most important feature of a defined-benefit plan is that the employer must contribute every year whatever sum is necessary to fund the plan adequately, which makes the plan very inflexible for financial-planning purposes. These plans are also complicated and often misunderstood by physicians and other corporate employees. However, for some physicians, defined-benefit plans may be an option worth exploring.

The primary advantage of a defined-benefit is that older physicians who have not previously maintained plans can often make larger contributions than are permissible in a defined-contribution plan. If an older physician has employees who are substantially younger than he or she is, that contribution can often be obtained at a substantially reduced cost for covering the staff than would be the case in a defined-contribution plan.

The primary advantage of a defined-benefit plan is that older physicians who have not previously maintained plans can often make larger contributions than are permissible in a defined-contribution plan. If an older physician has employees who are substantially younger than he or she, that contribution can often be obtained at a substantially reduced cost for covering the staff than would be the case in a defined-contribution plan.

Where several physicians are participating in the same plan, a defined-benefit plan will tend to favor the older participants, since the majority of contributions will be used to pay for benefits to the older physician participants. This may be an advantage if the group wishes to make substantially larger contributions on behalf of the older physicians than are made on behalf of the younger physicians. However, if younger physicians also wish to have substantial contributions made for them, a defined-benefit plan may, depending on their exact ages and certain other factors, actually reduce the maximum retirement-plan contributions that can be made on their behalf.

Target-Benefit Plans: A target-benefit plan has some features of a defined-benefit plan and some features of a defined-contributions plan. Its formula is structured as though it were a defined-benefit plan, and a contribution amount, based on that formula, is determined actuarially. Thus, older participants will generally receive larger contributions than younger ones. However, the formula used is only a "target" formula, and the targeted benefit is not guaranteed. Once the contribution amount is calculated, that amount is allocated to the participant's account as it would be in any other defined-contribution plan, and the participant's ultimate benefit from the plan is based on his or her account balance at the time of retirement. Target-benefit plans have become much more popular in recent years because of the increasing limitations on defined-benefit plans. (PRO)

Practice Parameters

The American Medical Association strongly supports the development of scientifically sound and clinically relevant practice parameters as a method to improve the quality of medical care. Practice parameters are strategies for patient

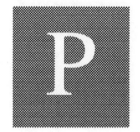

management developed to assist physicians in clinical decision making.(DIR)

What are Practice Parameters?

Practice parameters are strategies for patient management, developed to assist physicians in clinical decision-making. Based on thorough evaluation by relevant medical specialties of the best available scientific research and clinical experience, practice parameters describe the range of acceptable approaches to diagnosing, managing, or preventing specific diseases or conditions.

Reflecting the diversity of clinical medicine, practice parameters vary considerably in content, format, and degree of specificity. Over 45 physician organizations have developed approximately 1,500 practice parameters addressing a wide variety of clinical issues.

What is the Purpose of Practice Parameters?

Practice parameters enable physicians to stay abreast of the latest clinical research, assess the clinical significance of often conflicting research findings, and obtain the advise of recognized clinical experts. Practice parameters are *not* a cookbook, *nor* are they a substitute for individual clinical decision making; rather, practice parameters serve as educational tools, providing guidance to physicians when making complex decisions about patient care. After reviewing relevant practice parameters, physicians can determine which recommendations, either "as is" or modified, are most appropriate for the management or individual patients.(QAR)

Agency for Healthcare Policy Research
PO Box 8547, Silver Spring, MD 20907
800/358-9295

AMA joint Clinical Appropriateness Initiative with RAND Corporation
Parameters available through:
The RAND Corporation
1700 Main St, Box 2138, Santa Monica, CA 90407
310/393-0411

RAND/AMA set appropriateness guidelines for 7 procedures

Harris Meyer AMNews 4/6/92 p.3+,

In a major advance for practice guidelines, RAND, AMA and 12 top medical centers have rated the appropriateness and necessity of seven common procedures in thousands of clinical situations.

The ratings, which have been developed through extensive literature reviews and an expert consensus process, will provide the basis for organized medicine to draft better practice guidelines. It's hoped the ratings and subsequent guidelines will improve the quality and cost effectiveness of care, and pre-empt blunter solutions to uncontrolled U.S. medical costs, like rationing or spending caps.

Experts hope such guidelines can reduce large, unexplained variations in practice, such as those found in a separate RAND study published in the March 25 Journal of the American Medical Association. That report found differences of up to 50% in rates of hospitalization and prescription use between subspecialists and generalists, as well as between HMOs, large medical groups and small practices.

But the new ratings highlight broad disagreements on methods and goals among various players in the burgeoning guidelines movement and show that guidelines advocates have their work cut out for them.

The RAND-AMA effort used multispecialty physician panels and a highly structured consensus process to produce criteria for doing controversial procedures. In contrast, specialty societies have insisted that they alone can write standards for their practice areas and have used a grabbag of methods.

Meanwhile, the federal government, which began publishing guidelines last month, uses panels including non-physicians to make recommendations mostly for treatment of entire diseases rather than individual procedures.

The leader of the RAND effort called for guidelines developers to unite around the RAND approach and for funders to ante up for many more such studies.

"We need 100 to 150 of these ratings for the most costly and dangerous procedures right away to help make decisions about paying for care," said Robert Brook, MD, PHD, head of RAND's health science program.

"If physicians don't do it fast, they will lose control and all reform solutions will be economic."

This is the first time that all of organized medicine has worked with an outside scientific group to develop guidelines, which the AMA refers to as parameters. Experts say that medicine finally has acknowledged that it needs to come up with practice standards that are more credible and tougher.

But issues of who controls parameters, and how restrictive they should be, remain controversial among medical groups. There already are signs of unhappiness with the RAND ratings from doctors at some of the cooperating centers.

The AMA praised the new effort, which is part of its joint Clinical Appropriateness Initiative with RAND and the medical centers. The Association had made parameters a key ingredient of its proposals to improve quality, eliminate waste and expand insurance access.

"These ratings are an important and useful intermediate tool for developing practice parameters," said John Kelly, MD, head of the AMA's parameters effort. "but a considerable amount of work is needed by physician organizations before they are usable by practicing physicians."

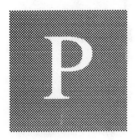

The ratings and literature reviews are contained in thick monographs available from RAND. The monographs cover coronary bypass surgery; coronary balloon angioplasty, coronary angiography; hysterectomy; cataract extraction, carotid endarterectomy; and abdominal aortic aneurysm surgery.

These procedures were chosen because of their high cost, high volume and wide variation of use. Monographs on the first two coronary procedures came out April 2. The others will follow shortly.

Each set of ratings, covering up to 1,000 indications, was done by a nine-member panel of recognized medical experts from a range of relevant specialties. Panelists were selected from specialty society nominations.

RAND, the Academic Medical Center Consortium, the Cardiac Advisory Committee of New York and the HMO Quality of Care Consortium headed individual studies. RAND directed the overall project.

RAND, a Santa Monica, Calif.-based research group that stands for research and development, had issued appropriateness ratings for some of the same procedures in the early 1980s, with little input from organized medicine. Its studies based on the ratings, which found up to a third of some of the procedures inappropriate, helped propel the push for better utilization controls.

But this is the first time RAND has had expert panels also rate the necessity of procedures - how "crucial" they are - for various indications. This new rating was added to measure underuse of services.

For RAND's panels, "appropriate" was defined to mean that the expected health benefit substantially exceeds the expected negative consequences, without reference to dollar cost. The RAND rating scale goes from 1 to 9; 1-3 is inappropriate, 4-6 uncertain and 7-9 appropriate.

"Necessary," which was also rated 1-9, was defined to mean that the procedure is appropriate, that it would be improper not to provide, that it offers a reasonable chance of benefiting the patient and that it delivers more than a small benefit. Physicians would be obliged to recommend the procedure for indications rated necessary, Dr. Brook said.

The necessity rating is important because most Americans soon will be in managed care and physicians need criteria to protect patients from managed care's bias to undertreat, he noted. Such a measure also could be used to help set a floor for basic health insurance, which many policymakers favor to lower costs.

No one expects the ratings in their current lengthy format to enter immediate wide use because they are not very handy for clinicians. But they are in the public domain, and there's nothing to stop payer and provider organizations from incorporating them into utilization review guidelines.

At least two companies now market computerized precertification systems based on detailed appropriateness criteria, derived partly from

RAND's prior work. One firm, Value Health Science, headed by a former RAND researcher, claims that its product saves client an average of 10% to 12% for the 27 procedures it covers.

An official at the other company, Aetna Health Plans, said appropriateness criteria are more effective in changing practice patterns in a managed care system than in a fee-for-service setting.

The AMA's Dr. Kelly, however, said the new ratings shouldn't be used for treatment and payment decisions until they are evaluated and translated into parameters by physician organizations. The AMA is working with a committee of relevant specialty societies to do just that for two of the procedures.

The AMA Committee is reconciling the ratings for carotid endarterectomy and abdominal aortic aneurysm surgery with parameters previously issued by specialty groups. There's "remarkable" overlap between the ratings and existing parameters, Dr. Kelly said.

When the parameters are complete, the AMA will take the lead in disseminating them.

How to effectively implement guidelines after dissemination, though, is one of the big unknowns in the field. To find out, more than 30 hospitals associated with the academic medical centers, the New York cardiac committee and the HMO consortium are comparing the ratings to their own utilization.

The academic centers, which include UCLA, Duke University and the Mayo Clinic, are scheduled to publish the comparative data for four procedures, without identifying the data by center. They also plan to use the ratings to modify their practice patterns if necessary.

But Jerome Grossman, MD, president of the New England Medical Center, an academic-center consortium member, sounded a note of dissatisfaction with the ratings. In using them, he said, too many procedures fell into the uncertain range, which he called "equivocal."

"That doesn't mean 'equivocal' about whether you should have done the procedure," he said. "It means equivocal about the consensus method's inability to reach agreement on whether particular indications are appropriate or not. This method doesn't give you the kind of clarity that's in patients' best interest."

The ratings' authors, though, defined uncertain to mean that the benefits and risks are nearly equal, the evidence is inconclusive or panel members split on the procedure's appropriateness.

The medical centers' physicians also had "concerns" about the ratings for certain indications, said David Witter, president of the Rochester, N.Y.-based consortium. They were skeptical because the criteria were crafted by multispecialty panels that included doctors like internists who don't do the procedures.

But the leader of the coronary bypass study said it's to be expected that some doctors would disagree with certain judgments.

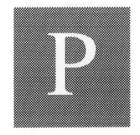

"The question is whether they are good general guidelines," said Lucian Leape, MD, who is also the overall project's co-principal-investigator. "They must be used with a mechanism to make exceptions for individual patients."

The consensus process that was developed by RAND and that produced these ratings has received wide praise for its rigor and its openness to retrospective scrutiny.

After reviewing the literature analysis, each expert rated the indications without contact with other panelists. The panel assembled and discussed the anonymously presented ratings.

Each panelist then confidentially rerated each indication. Agreement existed when no more than two individuals rate a particular indication outside one of the three-point regions (1-3, 4-6, 7-9).

After this, the experts rated the necessity of the procedure for indications the panel had found appropriate.

Critics say panelists are forced to rate combinations of indications so detailed that there's often no scientific evidence to guide them, thus reducing the rating's credibility. But supporters say there's no better alternative, short of thousands of expensive new clinical trials.

Funding for the studies was provided by the participating groups and by the Commonwealth Fund, Morgan Guaranty Trust, New York Community Trust, the John A. Hartford Foundation and the National Institute of Aging.

JE-Swartout, Ed. *Directory of Practice Parameters: Guidelines and Technology Assessments* 1992 ed. Chicago: American Medical Association. 1991. 158 pp. ISBN 0-89970-461-1. OP270292

Preadmission Criteria
"Reference Criteria for Short-Stay Hospital Review"
Order from NTIS (U.S. Dept. of Commerce): 5285 Port Royal Rd., Springfield, VA 22161 703/487-4650 (Order #PB81-179889)

Preferred Provider Organizations
A preferred provider organization (PPO) is an entity representing a group of physicians and/or hospitals that contracts with employers, insurance carriers, or third party administrators to provide comprehensive medical services on a fee-for-service basis to subscribers. The PPO contracts with physicians and hospitals to provide services at an established fee, generally at a discount from their usual charges.

How PPOs Evolved: Although relatively new on the health care scene, PPOs have had a dramatic impact on health care delivery in this country. While use of the term "PPO" is recent, the concept of the PPO arrangement can be traced to the Foundation for Medical Care (FMCs) of the 1950s, which placed their emphasis on providing medical services within the traditional fee-for-service framework. PPOs in the early 1980s were loosely affiliated groups of providers who agreed to discount their services in exchanged for assurances of new patients.

Discounted fees and utilization review were inherent in many PPOs at this time.

Initially, there was little regulation or control of PPOs by federal and/or state governments. The first state PPO legislation can be traced to California, which in 1982 enacted statutes designated to eliminate existing regulatory obstacles inhibiting PPO development. According to the American Medical Care Review Association (AMCRA), states had promulgated laws that could be interpreted as barring the channeling and selective contracting activities necessary to the effective operation of PPOs. These included the antidiscrimination and freedom-of-choice statutes often found in insurance codes; the antidiscrimination, freedom-of-choice, and "any willing provider" statutes found in legislation regulating health service corporations; and the various health maintenance organization acts. Because interpretation of these laws differed from state to state, the statutes tended to impose barriers to PPO development in about half the states and District of Columbia.

AMCRA also notes that states are attempting to encourage the development of PPOs through legislation and regulations. As of December 1986, 22 states had enabling provisions while only three states expressly prohibited the selective contracting and channeling activities essential to PPOs. Provisions in the new enabling measures, as well as preexisting regulations, protect consumers in PPOs, although it is still too early to assess their adequacy.

Because PPO arrangements are subject to the regulations that apply to the benefit plans they serve or to their sponsoring entities, they may be regulated in a variety of ways. This variations may create an imbalance that are less regulated and those that are subject to greater regulations. For example, a June 8, 1983 Federal Trade Commission advisory opinion (Health Care Management Associates: File No. 8330005) concluded that "the PPO program would likely improve competition in the health care sector and would not violate the Federal Trade Commission Act or any other antitrust statute." This opinion offered two important points - providers and payors must be free to participate in other programs, and competing providers and payors should not be involved in any agreement on PPO operations. In addition, according to the Justice Department, three key elements must be present to ensure that antitrust laws are not being violated. These are:

- - no anti-competition purposes;
- - the market share of the venture must not be so large that it forecloses effective competition; and
- - provider agreements must be secondary to the cooperative activity that promotes competition.

Characteristics of PPOs: As contractual units, PPOs differ widely. In fact, there is no "typical" PPO. Yet, for their differences, most PPO designs share many of the following characteristics:

- - A designated panel of health care professionals and/or institutions that serve as the contracted providers;
- - an established fee schedule that generally results in a discount of as much as 15 to 20 percent from usual, customary, and reasonable

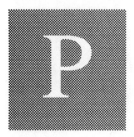

reimbursements for the employers or insurance carriers who are the purchasers of care;

- - medical services provided on a traditional fee-for-service basis;
- - a strong emphasis on utilization review and control;
- - usually no "lock-in" of the patient to specific health care providers; however, economic incentives such as the waiving or reducing of copayments or deductibles often are applied to encouraged used of contracted providers;
- - no formal risk-sharing arrangement by the physicians in a PPO as in the IPA model HMO; and
- - a strong effort to pay providers within a designated time period.

In most cases, PPO enrollees are not required to receive care from contract physicians or hospitals but their out-of-pocket expenses are increased if they do not. A few PPOs may not provide any benefits if patients do not utilize PPO panel physicians and hospitals. These arrangements are called "exclusive provider organization" (EPOs). According to AMCRA, as of January 31, 1988, 32 PPOs required a lock-in arrangement and could be classified as EPOs. AMCRA also reports that the majority (70.6 percent) of the 660 PPOs operate on a for-profit basis.

Most PPOs perform the functions of establishing a provider base of physicians and hospitals and marketing these providers to the payors. Utilization of review and claims processing usually are contracted out to third-party administrators, insurance companies, or professional review organizations. Some payors, however, process their own claims. Employers reimburse PPOs according to any one of several methods: an administrative fee, a monthly service fee, capitation, a percentage of claims, a per-claim fee, or a percentage of savings.

American Association of Preferred Providers
111 E. Wacker Drive, Chicago, IL 60604
312/644-6610

American Medical Care and Review Association
1227 25th St, NW, Suite 610
Washington, DC 20037
202/728-0506

Pregnancy
American College of Obstetricians
and Gynecologists
409 12th Street, SW, Washington, DC 20024-2188
202/638-5577

JAMA Article of Note: Legal Interventions During Pregnancy: court-ordered medical treatments and their legal penalties for potentially harmful behavior by pregnant women.
JAMA.1990 Nov 28;264(20):2663-70.

Premenstrual Syndrome
Premenstrual Syndrome Action
PO Box 16292, Irvine, CA 92716
714/854-4407

PMS Access Hotline
800/222-4767

Preventive Medicine
AMA Policy: Healthy People 2000 - Challenges in Preventive Medicine: It is the policy of the AMA that (1) physicians should become familiar with and increase their utilization of clinical preventive services protocols; (2) individual physicians as well as organized medicine at all levels should increase communication and cooperation with and support of public health agencies. Physician leadership in advocating for a strong public health infrastructure is particularly important; (3) physicians should promote and offer to serve on local and state advisory boards; (4) physicians and medical societies should advocate for the adoption of local/state health objectives for the year 2000; and (5) in concert with other groups, physicians should study local community needs, define appropriate health objectives, and work toward achieving health goals for the community.

Preventive medicine: The branch of medicine that deals with the prevention of disease by public health measures, such as the provision of pure water supplies; by health education aimed at discouraging smoking and the overuse of alcohol, promoting exercise, and giving advice about a prudent diet; by specific preventive treatments, such as immunization against infectious diseases; and by screening programs to detect diseases such as glaucoma, tuberculosis, and cancer of the cervix before they cause symptoms.

Most of the increase in the world's population during the 19th century was due to improvements in public health, particularly improvements in the overall standard of nutrition, and the provision of pure water supplies and proper sanitation. Today, these measures remain the priorities of preventive medicine in developing countries, and, along with a program of immunization in childhood, have been targeted as major objectives by the World Health Organization.

However, in developed countries, the primary objective is to persuade the adult population to adopt a healthier life-style. In the US, most premature death in adults (that is, deaths before the age of 65) are preventable, being due to accidents and/or linked to such factors as an unhealthy diet, smoking, and excessive drinking. Adoption of a healthier life-style, the wider use of screening for cancers, and measures to reduce accidents could lead to substantial improvements in the nation's health. (ENC)

American Board of Preventive Medicine
Department of Community Medicine
Wright State University
PO Box 927, Dayton, OH 45401
513/278-6915

American College of Preventive Medicine
1015 15th St. NW, Washington, DC 20005
202/789-0003

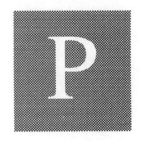

Primary Care

National Clearinghouse for
Primary Care Information
8201 Greensboro Dr., Suite 600
McLean, VA 22102
703/821-8955

Product Safety

Consumer Product Safety Commission
Household Product Safety Hotline
800/638-2772

Professional Liability

What Happens When a Suit Is Filed?

The steps in the legal process involving a malpractice claim will vary from state to state, and from jurisdiction to jurisdiction, as well as with the insurance company by which the physician is covered. This is important to remember, since your experience will probably differ from the steps listed here.

Keep in mind, too, that the first few steps will happen almost simultaneously - the complaint will be filed, the insurance company contacted, an attorney appointed, meetings with the attorney, etc. But while these activities may happen very quickly - in matter of two weeks to one month - the next series of activities may stretch on into years.

These are some of the step that you may encounter:

- *The patient consults a lawyer who will review the case*. Most lawyers work on a contingency fee, which means there is no cost to the plaintiff unless the case is won. If the case is won, the lawyer collects an average of 30% to 50% of the award. So in the first step, the plaintiff's attorney will evaluate the case to see if it is worth the time and money to get involved. The lawyer may choose not to take the case if it appears it cannot be won or settled for a reasonable gain.
- *The plaintiff's attorney will draft a complaint and file it with the court*. The physician will be served with a copy of the complaint and a summons to appear to answer the plaintiff's allegations. This is a critical time, because how the physician responds can influence the chances of a successful resolution. Many physicians react the wrong way. They get the notice of the complaint; comment to a colleague, "Can you believe this?"; and throw the document away. There is a time frame in which the physician's attorney must file the physician's response to the allegations. That time frame in many jurisdictions is 20 to 30 days.
- *The physician should contact his or her insurance company*, so an attorney can be assigned and the complaint can be answered, or a motion to dismiss can be filed. This is not the time to wait or hesitate. The plaintiff's lawyer has been working on the case for some time and has had access to the needed records to file the complaint. So in almost any situation, the physician's attorney will be catching up in terms of the time spent on case research and preparation.
- *The physician's attorney will review the case* to see how substantial it is, and how defensible it is. The strategy for defending against the claim begins here.

- *The physician should begin to research* by pulling the records on the case and putting them in a special file where they can't be misplaced or tampered with. A file in the physician's desk drawer is often the best place for the attorney calls. The physician's attorney will obtain any records that may be needed from a hospital. It is vital that the records not be altered in any way.
- *The physician may want* to search the literature for material pertinent to the case, such as an article that shows that the procedures use were acceptable or state-of-the-art for the patient's case. Material that will be helpful to the defense should be marked for future reference.
- *The physician will also want* to think about the case so that honest, candid answers can be given to his or her attorney.
- *The physician will be working with the attorney during this time*. Once again, it's vital that he or she be completely honest and candid about the case. He or she should ask for a thorough briefing about the case and the legal proceedings that will take place, as well as the physician's role in the proceedings. The physician will want to share with the attorney information gained from the research. He or she may help the lawyer formulate questions for the plaintiff's expert. Keep in mind a point made earlier - the lawyer knows the law; the physician knows medicine. Attorneys need physicians' help to win cases.
- *The physician will answer interrogatories,* a written process designed to streamline court proceedings by getting the facts on the table - facts such as agreeing that the person is a physician who is licensed to practice, the sequence of events, and other things that will help clarify the case.
- *The physicians will attend a deposition*. The deposition is similar to being in court. It usually occurs in a lawyer's office, where the parties come together, witnesses are sworn, and a court transcriber records the testimony. Since the transcript of the deposition may be used in the court proceedings, attorney will attempt to get witnesses to commit to as much as possible. If testimony is changed in court, the conflicting statements will weaken the case.
- *The physician will want*, and will be advised to answer questions calmly and succinctly, and not to volunteer information. In addition, the physician's attorney may not say much in terms of objecting to questions. And he or she may counsel the physician that if objections are made, they carry an important message for the physician. Careful preparation for the deposition is vital. The physician may spend hours on this, reading records and background material. The attorney will be the coach, and will tell the physician who will be at the deposition, when to speak, what questions probably will be asked, and how to respond. This can be a very stressful time - one in which the spouse will want to be especially supportive and understanding, since it will take the physician away from the family.
- The physician may want to take notes during the deposition that will be helpful to the attorney during the trial.

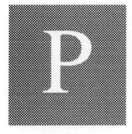

At this point, the attorney may meet with the spouse to explain the proceedings and how she or he can be involved.

- *A decision will have to be made on whether or not to settle.* This decision can be made at any point in the process. Again, if there has been an injury caused by negligence, most attorneys will advise that the case be settled as quickly as possible for the sake of the patient and the physician. The causation factor is a key. Unless the physician is clearly understood to have caused an injury, settlement may not be recommended.
- The decision to settle, if the case is defensible, is a difficult one for physician. Many feel that they should "fight" and should have their day in court. Some have insisted on going to trial, even when the plaintiff was willing to settle for a very small amount of money. On the other hand, some physicians prefer to settle and put the whole matter behind them. This is a decision that can only be made by the physician and attorney.

Remember that most claims are settled out of court.
- *There may be a pre-trial screening panel,* consisting often of a physician, attorney, and judge. Generally, these panels review the case, and listen to medical experts and presentations from the attorneys on both sides. The decision of the panel is not binding in most cases, but can be read into evidence at the trial. In some states, the panels become more significant, because those states have decided they should be used to weed out cases that are without legal merit.
- *If the decision is made to go to trial, the physician must be prepared to testify*, and must review all of the research compiled for the deposition - the medical literature, patient charts and records, the testimony given at the deposition. Close contact will be kept with the defense counsel who will advise on court procedures, strategies, and how to handle the cross-examination by the plaintiff's attorney. This cross-examination can be brutal, since the basis of a trial is to tear apart the opposing arguments.

The physician's presence at the trial will be extremely important, as will dress, demeanor, etc. Attorney and physician will work together, with the physician advising the attorney about possible errors on the part of the plaintiff's expert witness; and the attorney alerting the physician to tactics by the plaintiff's counsel. When testifying, he or she will be advised to answer questions succinctly, and not to volunteer information. The physician will have the opportunity to tell his or her story when the defense counsel asks for it.
- The case will be resolved.(SPP)

What Can Be Done About the Professional Liability Problem?

Patients want to be compensated for actual injuries caused by negligence, and no one argues that they should not be. But with the number of suits filed that are without legal merit, and the toll those suits are taking on physicians and on the delivery of health care in general, a solution must be found to the professional liability problem. And it must come from doctors, lawyers, insurance companies, and the public. No one can afford the cost - either monetary or emotional.

While no one will claim to have the final solution to the professional liability problem, suggestions for improving the situation include:

- reforms in the personal injury (tort) laws to control contingency fees, encourage periodic payments, reduce awards by amounts received from collateral sources, capping non-economic loss in the award, establish a reasonable statute of limitations, set up pretrial screening panels, limit dollar amounts of awards, etc.

- better peer review and discipline procedures in the medical profession
- educating physicians and the public about the liability problem and its costs and its effects on the delivery of medical care
- teaching physicians methods of practice that can minimize liability exposure

Beyond these general statements, observers and those involved have taken definite steps to try to alleviate the problem. Here are some of the ways the situation can be improved.

Physicians: According to many, there are steps individual physicians can take to decrease the risk of being sued for malpractice. These are some of the suggestions:

- Improve communication with patients so they understand the full implications of diagnosis and treatment.
- Foster realistic expectations about what medical care can do.
- Develop solid physician-patient relationships.
- Encourage patients to more actively participate in managing their own health care.
- Strive for continued scientific excellence by practicing both the art and the science of medicine.
- Practice only what they believe is within their own professional competence.
- Keep up with current literature.
- Go to medical meetings.
- Provide patient information in the office.
- Document office and hospital and hospital records as completely as possible; keep accurate, truthful, careful records.
- Keeps appointment on schedule so patients don't have to wait.
- Train staff carefully so they are courteous and helpful to patients.(SPP)

Coming Home

Adam O. Goldstein, MD "A Piece of My Mind"
JAMA. 1991 March 6; 265(9): 1099

Coming home after vacation is sometimes slightly sad. It's not that your trip was boring or too short. Rather, it's more like a bittersweet dream, when, having suddenly awakened, you are less upset to be awake than sorry you cannot return to your dream.

"Please take notice that..."

The first day back is always the worst. Restarting routines - unpacking, sorting mail, answering phone messages, washing clothes - these serve a purpose: to center yourself today for tomorrow's work, forgotten while vacationing. The first night back, a few phone calls to family and friends finish the grounding process. Tomorrow to work, to the hospital.

"...the undersigned will bring the above petition on the hearing before this court..."

The morning after holds such promise. Invigorated, a refreshed mind can attack daily challenges. Creativity runs high. Many tasks can be solved in a few short hours. The office desk is cleared, and the rooms are ready for patients. At times like this, patients, nurses, and physicians work together in mutual understanding, respect, and therapeutic alliance.

"...The petitioner's wife died after being admitted to the hospital..."

When the sheriff's deputy delivers the deposition, it is not even noon. A medical malpractice lawsuit. A surprise that is not so surprising. You take it in much the same manner as news of a friend of a friend's cancer death, with definite remorse but with a sense of fatality. During medical school and residency, you observed the increasing numbers of public medical malpractice cases. This greenhouse effect proceeds predictably. Again and again, you are told to CYA. As in championship chess, often the best defense is to seek a stalemate and not "lose." As in all sports, practice makes perfect, and you try practicing defensive medicine in clinics, offices, and hospitals.

"...She dies with the following as her diagnoses..."

You know much about the following medical malpractice; which types of patients are likely to sue, which types of patient communication skills lessen the risk, how important it is to document everything. Surgeons know the risk of operating on patients with chronic pain. Anesthesiologists appreciate the importance of establishing patient rapport before and after surgery. Obstetricians communicate potential hazards of even "normal" deliveries. Family physicians look to three generations of relationships. Still, you know physicians in all fields who have been sued. Most are well-qualified, compassionate people who nevertheless "made a mistake." You also know that you are equally human, equally vulnerable. Despite this knowledge, the words, "You're being sued" strike home. As with the death of a loved one, you know that your life will change, change without your approval. As when walking a tightrope, you know that you can easily fall, yet are unsure of the net below.

"...Petitioner's estate expects to file an action..."

You quickly recall the half-dozen scenarios of your "worse cases." The child who coded after a routine umbilical hernia repair remains a vegetable with remarkably healthy organs. A seemingly certain malpractice case, where else does the mother vent fear, frustration, and anger at the medical establishment and the world? Then there was the case of the elderly man who died unexpectedly, the day before the planned discharge. There was no autopsy and no voiced family discontent. It seems strange for you to think of these cases now except to remember similar cases where lawyers were contacted months or years later. Many obstetric cases come to mind: several shoulder dystocias, postpartum hemorrhages, emergency C-section, preterm deliveries, a child with cerebral palsy. With or without disability, maternal and neonatal outcome expectations often conflict with imperfect nature of medicine and life. Both outcome expectations also coincide with the exponential rise in medical malpractice cases. Finally, there are the emergency room cases, thousands at least. With each encounter an unknown outcome, the odds for spontaneous untoward events are high. With every chest pain a potential MI, abdominal pain an aortic aneurysm, fever a meningitis, and vague fatigue a malignancy, you see a sea of uncertainty, sinking and floating.

"...A copy of said petition..."

With such events, you are advised two things: to contact your legal adviser and to discuss the case with no one else. While perhaps strong legal advice, spiritually the thought is divisive. The effects of mind-body separation are well known to those in psychiatry, and your patients frequently present with stress-induced problems. Are you any different or less vulnerable?

"...naming you as an expected adverse party..."

At work, you continue to see many patients, their illnesses sometimes manifest but often obscure. Most go home and improve, a few are hospitalized, and one even dies. While you continue to share the joy and sadness, health and disease, life and death, your vision changes. Some changes are no doubt beneficial: more courtesy, more sincerity, more explanation, fewer "mistakes." Other changes are not so clear-cut: more lab tests, more writing, more consultations, higher costs, less enjoyment. Fear, more of that too. Fear of failure, inadequacy, and judgment. Guilt over actions undone. You feel suspicion toward patients whose diseases do not conform; anger at a system that waits for the inevitable and then says, "I told you so", failure at yourself for not saving all patients from all diseases; frustration with a society that may forsake trust for technology, color for black and white, uncertainty for absolutes.

"...The petitioner's estate expects the witness to testify from personal knowledge and from medical record..."

At the end of the day, after your patients, staff, and colleagues have departed, you sit alone.

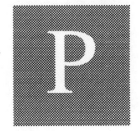

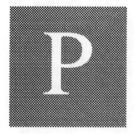

What began as a happy journey is now an uncertain destination. How will you feel after going home tonight and talking with your family and friends? Will you choose instead to remain silent and keep your routines apparently the same? Your mind seems open to many more questions than answers, raw emotions than concrete thoughts.

"...this petition having now been served."

Alliance of American Insurers
1501 Woodfield Road, Suite 400
Schaumburg, IL 60123
708/330-8500

American Insurance Agency
1130 Connecticut Ave, NW, Suite 1000,
Washington, DC 20036
202/828-7100

American Medical Assurance Co. (AMACO)
(only insures insurers)
303 E. Wacker Dr., Suite 1330, Chicago, IL 60601
312/565-6463

Insurance Information Institute
110 William St, New York, NY 10036
212/669-9200

"Physician Insurers Association of America:
Membership Directory"
Physician Insurers Association of America
Two Princess Rd., Lawrenceville, NJ 08648
609/896-4131 If busy, 609/896-2404 X258

Rebuttal to ATLA Report
"The Continuing Need for Legislative Reform of the Medical Liability System: A Response by the Medical Profession to Opponents of Tort Reform"

American Medical Association
Project on Professioanl Liability
312/464/4612

American Tort Reform Association
1212 New York Ave, Ste 515
Washington, DC 20005
202/682-1163

Professional Liability--History
Tracing the history of the liability problem

Not until the 1930s did professional liability suits begin to materialize in any significant numbers - a development that paralleled the birth of modern medicine and its sophisticated technology. There was an upswing in numbers of claims until World War II and then there was a temporary decline.

After World War II, the problem began to surface again, increasing in the 1960s. the rising volume of claims against physicians and hospitals, with their growing impact upon health care costs, health manpower and the delivery of health services -services increasingly paid for by the government - prompted President Richard Nixon in 1971 to direct the Secretary of Health, Education, and Welfare to create a Commission

on Medical Malpractice to gather current information on the problem and offer a set of recommendations.

In the introductory chapter of its final report issued in 1973, the Commission said, "The tempo of malpractice litigation again began to increase shortly after World War II. In part, this was due to the simple fact that many more people were able to afford, and received, medical care, automatically increasing the exposure to incidents that could lead to suits.

At the same time, innovations in medical science increased the complexities of the health care system. Some of the new diagnostic and therapeutic procedures brought with them new risks of injury; as the potency of drugs increased, so did the potential hazards of using them. Few would challenge the value of these advances, but they did tend to produce a number of adverse results, sometimes resulting in severe disability...(and) thus the number of malpractice claims and suits increased."

The Commission, in one of the first detailed examinations of medical liability claims on a nationwide basis, surveyed claims closed in 1970 taken from a universe representing approximately 90% of the total in the nation. The Commission found that there were 15,000 claim files closed in 1970, representing 12,000 incidents and patients and 22,000 defendants - physicians, hospitals, nurses, drug companies, and equipment manufacturers. An estimated 10.6% more claims were opened in 1970 than were closed in that year, which, the Commission pointed out, "indicates that direction and some of the magnitude of this change."

The claims increase was not surprising. Numbers of claims were growing steadily and the rate of increase was clearly accelerating. Some areas of the country, as is the case today, were affected more than others. The Commission's 1970 study showed Tennessee leading the list of states in the rate of increase - 40.9% - but that was partly due to the small base number of claims. California showed the greatest volume of change - up 26%. Upward blips were beginning to appear in Maryland, Texas and Missouri and in 11 other states, while a few, such as Minnesota, actually showed a downturn.

The Commission's 1970 analysis, however, merely underscored a developing trend.

"Between 1935 and 1975 - in that 40-year period - 80% of all medical malpractice lawsuits were filed in the final five years of that period," Elvoy Raines, professional liability expert with the American College of Obstetricians and Gynecologists, told the Senate Committee on Labor and Human Resources on July 10, 1984.(LIA)

Professional Liability in the 80s:
Education and community action. The following recommendations are made in this area:
- Take the professional liability issue to the public. The public has a vital stake in the professional liability problem, from the standpoints of cost, quality and access to medical care. The Task Force recommends that an intensive information campaign be conducted to improve public

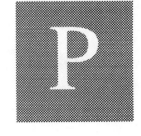

understanding and stress the need for legislative, judicial and other actions.

- Arm state, local and specialty medical societies with information to carry the professional liability message to the public. The Task Force will supervise the preparation of comprehensive informational materials, including background data, fact sheets, speech outlines and speeches, sample editorials, letters to the editor, display materials will be distributed throughout the federation and on request to individual members who will serve as advocates on this issue. AMA will also hold periodic briefings on professional liability activities for state, county, and specialty societies. The AMA's Washington Office will brief medical specialty organizations' Washington representatives. The innovative and aggressive risk management programs which the societies have developed deserve wide publication and should be incorporated into the broad-based national effort.

- Publish a pamphlet for individual patients. The pamphlet for patients will explain how the professional liability issue affects their own medical care, its costs, and its availability and will foster realistic expectations about medical care. It will be made available in quantity for distribution through physicians' offices.

- Develop an effective advocacy program on the professional liability problem. Physicians must have allies on this issue. An AMA action team composed of officers, trustees and staff representatives will carry the professional liability message to organizations and individuals that are, or should be, concerned with the issue. The exact nature of the professional liability crisis, objectively and persuasively documented, must be presented at every appropriate forum. Business groups, labor organizations, public interest groups, legislators, legal organizations, judicial conferences, academic centers, the, media, insurance groups, state and national agencies, organizations such as the American Association of Retired Persons (AARP), and others will be addressed at every opportunity. The reports of the Special Task Force will bound into one volume and distributed throughout the nation. In short, the AMA will intensify its role as the physician's national spokesperson on this issue.

- Enlist the cooperation of health care coalitions composed of opinion leaders and policy makers to address the professional liability problem. The support of health care coalitions, involved in efforts to contain health care costs by reducing the professional liability problem, will be recruited. The Task Force will develop a handbook with the AMA's Department of Health Care Coalitions for this purpose. The AMA will elicit support from groups such as the Chamber of Commerce, the Business Roundtable, and other professional and civic groups.

- Expand the AMA's clearinghouse role. The AMA can also fulfill an essential role as a national clearinghouse, assembling data, legislative information, materials form other organizations and other pertinent materials to share with physicians, medical organizations, legislators, policymakers and other interested individuals and groups. Plans to share information will be effected with organizations such as the Physician Insurers Association of America, the National Association of Insurance Commissioners, research centers such as the

Rand Corporation, and individual researchers actively involved on studies of professional liability. The Task Force will prepare and distribute to the federation, specialty societies and other groups, regular reports on new data, programs and developments.

- Maintain professional liability as a critical priority. The Special Task Force, with the resources of the AMA at its disposal, will be a permanent part of the AMA professional liability program. The research effort will not stop with the work already done and published by the Task Force. The Association's Center for Health Policy Research will focus on the effort to develop and publish reliable and current information on professional liability. AMA's Committee on Professional Liability will continue its studies of the costs and effects of professional liability of physicians, patients and the nation.

Commentary: An effective national information campaign is essential to generate action on the professional liability problem. The perception persists, perpetuated by those who stand to gain most from the existing system, that there is no professional liability crisis, only a "pocketbook" concern of physicians. A similar misconception, reinforced by repetition, is that insurance companies are accumulating huge profits at physicians' expense and ample funds are available to pay claims. Those who hold these misconceptions also are convinced that physician negligence - "malpractice" - is the only reason for the professional liability crisis.

These views are wrong and must be refuted. Objective data on the numbers of claims, severity of claims, rapidly climbing costs of insurance premiums, and growing losses of professional liability insurers document a crisis far more serious than past ones. For every premium dollar earned in 1984 in the professional liability insurance industry, $1.10 was paid out just for actual losses incurred, Best's Insurance Management Reports found in December 1984. When loss adjustment expenses and overhead costs are added in, the combined ratio rose to approximately $1.66 for every $1 of premium last year.

The public pays for a large portion of professional liability costs in pass-throughs for physicians' increased overhead, in the enormous costs of defensive medicine - the ordering of tests and procedures primarily to protect against lawsuits - and in the staggering waste of an inefficient legal system. The public also pays for a system that is encouraging, almost forcing, physicians to avoid high risk patients and specialties.

Physicians pay, too, not just in high insurance premiums, but in the personal anguish of claims and suits filed, especially if these actions are without merit. It is often not how the physicians practice, but the fact that they practice ever closer to the edges of technological frontiers that place them at greater legal risk. Physicians are among the nation's best and brightest - highly educated, motivated for the most part by humanitarian concerns, yet held accountable for complex judgments made under pressure of life-and-death considerations. No other professionals are held to such standards. Though negligence does occur, physicians are too often sued for adverse events - bad results - beyond their control. Even when

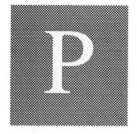

negligence exists, the system for compensating patients is being crushed by almost limitless awards and the costs of determining liability.

The realities of the professional liability situation must be brought to the public, to legislators, to lawyers, and to those in policy making positions. The record must be set straight - the situation put into proper focus.(LIA)

Tort Reform Glossary:

Ad damnum clauses - The ad damnum clause is that part of a plaintiff's initial pleadings which states the amount of monetary damages and other relief requested by the plaintiff in a court action. Most of the legislation on this subject provides for the elimination of the ad damnum clause altogether; legislation also often provides that the defendant be apprised of the precise amount sought by the plaintiff through the normal course of pre-trial discovery.

Arbitration - Arbitration statutes relate to voluntary procedures whereby patients and health care providers may enter into written agreements for the submission of any medical liability claims to binding arbitration. This procedure provides for limited judicial review of the arbitration decision.

Medical liability claims can currently be arbitrated in at least 30 states under the general arbitration statutes in those states. The chart only lists those states with arbitration legislation specifically for medical liability claims. Most of the medical liability arbitration statutes provide that written arbitration agreements may cover present and future medical injury claims. All of the statutes generally provide that a person's right to treatment shall not be prejudiced in any way by the decision whether or not to enter into an agreement for arbitration of medical liability claims. In other words, the agreement must truly be voluntary to be binding. Also, most statutes which permit arbitration agreements to cover future medical injury claims provide for a certain period of time, either following execution of the contract or provision of the services, in which the patient may reject the arbitration agreement.

Attorney fee regulation - The most common arrangement for payment of plaintiff attorney fees in medical liability cases is the "contingent fee." Under this type of arrangement the attorney receives as his fee an agreed upon percentage (commonly 30% to 50%) of any final award or settlement made to the plaintiff. Legislation enacted during the last few years regulating attorney fees in medical liability cases has taken several different approaches: a sliding scale for the plaintiff attorney fees in terms of a percentage of the award; court review of the proposed fees approval of what it considers to be a "reasonable fee", or limiting attorneys' fees to a certain percentage of the amounts recovered by the plaintiff.

Awarding costs, expenses and fees - A few states have provisions designed to deter the pursuit of frivolous medical injury claims. These statutes generally provide that where one party to the action has been found to have acted frivolously in bringing the suit, the party may be found liable for payment of the other party's reasonable attorney and expert witnesses fees and court costs. These provisions differ from the usual civil trial situation in which payment for attorney fees and expert witness fees are normally paid by the party who incurs them.

Collateral source provisions - The collateral source rule is a rule of evidence that prohibits the introduction into evidence at trial of any indication that a patient has been compensated or reimbursed for the injury from any source other than the defendant. Legislation modifying the collateral source rule has taken several approaches: permitting consideration of compensation or payments received from some or all collateral sources; requiring the mandatory offset against any award in the amount of some or all collateral source payments received by the plaintiff; or allowing the defendant to introduce evidence of the plaintiff's compensation from collateral sources. The jury is instructed to male a mandatory reduction of the award for economic loss by a sum equal to the difference between the total benefits received and the total amount paid by the plaintiff to secure such benefits.

Expert witness - Expert witnesses are required to explain many of the complex and difficult issues in a medical negligence case. Legislation affects the qualifications and use of expert benefits.

Limits on liability - Some states have enacted legislation that limits the liability of defendants in medical lawsuits. These statutes limit liability in one of several ways: limiting recovery of a particular type of damages; placing an absolute cap on the amount of damages recoverable; or placing an absolute cap on physician liability under a patient compensation fund.

Patient compensation fund - A patient compensation fund is a governmentally operated mechanism established to pay that portion of any judgment or settlement against a health care provider in excess of a statutorily designated amount. A fund may pay the remainder of the award or it may have a statutory maximum (e.g. one million dollars). Patient compensation funds are generally funded through an annual surcharge assessed against health care providers, with such surcharge often being a specified percentage of the provider's annual insurance premium. Patient compensation funds are also known as "excess recovery funds."

Periodic payments - In most states, unless otherwise agreed on by the parties or mandated by the court, judgments can only be lump-sum awards. Under a periodic payments system, the payments are made over the actual lifetime of the plaintiff or for the actual period of disability.

Pre-trial screening panels - Pre-trial screening panels are prerequisites to trial. Procedures for panels usually require a mandatory pre-trial to be conducted by a panel comprised of members as dictated by statute. In some states the pre-trial hearing is voluntary. The composition of the panel and its scope of inquiry vary greatly from state to state. All statutes establishing pre-trial screening procedures provide that the panel's decision is not binding on the parties and that it does not preclude a plaintiff from initiating a lawsuit. Although some states permit the decision of the panel to be introduced into evidence in a subsequent lawsuit, the panel's decision is not binding upon a judge or jury.

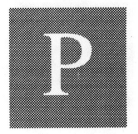

Res ipsa loquitur - Res ipsa loquitur ("the thing speaks for itself") is a common law doctrine which applies when a plaintiff can demonstrate that the injury occurred while the instrumentality causing the injury was under the exclusive control of the defendant and which, if operated in a non-negligent fashion, does not normally cause injury. In recent years, a number of state courts have expanded the application of res ipsa loquitur, and increased the effect of its applicability from that of a mere inference to that of a presumption, which if not rebutted, will allow the jury to reach no finding other than liability.

Legislation enacted in several states has codified the doctrine in regard to medical liability cases by delineating those circumstances when the doctrine may be applied, such as when a foreign object has been left in a body or the patient has suffered radiation burns. However, these statutes have sought to make it clear that the mere fact of injury is not sufficient to invoke the doctrine.

Standard of care - The standard of care in a medical negligence action is that level of care to which a health care provider is held accountable to a patient, and is based upon the prevailing level of care practiced within locality (community, state, or national).

Statute of limitations - A statute of limitations is a law that bars a cause of action after expiration of a specified time period. In many states the statute of limitations for medical liability actions begins to run only upon discovery of the injury. Injuries may be discovered several years after the treatment was provided, so the time period for filing an action may be uncertain. Some states have sought to eliminate the "long tail" by placing an absolute maximum time period within which medical liability suits may be brought. An exception to the time period is provided in some of these statutes where foreign objects are left in the body, or where the health care provider has fraudulently concealed the fact of injury. Most state statutes of limitations provide that if an injury is incurred by a minor, the statute is tolled (i.e., stops running) on the minor's cause of action until he reaches the age of majority. Changes in the statute of limitations for a minor's actions usually provide that the statute will begin running prior to the age of majority.(LIA)

Project Hope
Project HOPE
Health Science Education Center
Millwood, VA 22646
800/544-HOPE, 703/837-2100

Prostate Cancer
Us Too
(Information on support groups, diagnosis, and treatment options)
1120 N. Charles St, Suite 401
Baltimore, MD 21201
800/828-7866

Prosthetics
Prosthetist: Provides care to patients with partial or total absence of limb by planning fabrication of, writing specifications for, and fitting prosthesis under guidance of and in consultation with physician: Assists physician in formulation of prescription. Examines and evaluates patient's prosthetic needs in relation to disease entity and functional loss. Formulates design of prosthesis and selects materials and components. Makes casts, measurements, and model modifications. Performs fitting, including static and dynamic alignment. Evaluates prosthesis on patient and makes adjustments to assure fit, function, comfort, and workmanship. Instructs patient in prosthesis use. Maintains patient records. May supervise Prosthetic Assistants and other personnel. May lecture supervise laboratory activities relating to development of prosthesis. May lecture and demonstrate to colleagues and other professionals concerned with practice of prosthetics. May participate in research. May also perform functions of Orthotist.(DOT)

Prosthetics Assistant: Assists Prosthetist in providing care to and fabricating and fitting protheses for patients with partial or total absence of limb: Under direction of Prosthetist makes assigned casts, measurements, and model modifications. Performs fitting, including static and dynamic alignments. Evaluates prosthesis on patient to ensure fit, function, and quality of work. Repairs and maintains prostheses. May be responsible for performance of other personnel. May also perform functions of Orthotics Assistant (DOT)

American Academy of Orthotists and Prosthetists
717 Pendleton St, Alexandria, VA 22314
703/836-7118

American Board for Certification
in Orthotics and Prosthetics
717 Pendleton St, Alexandria, VA 22314
703/836-7114

Psychiatry
Psychiatrist: Diagnoses and treats patients with mental, emotional, and behavioral disorders: Organizes data concerning patient's family, medical history, and onset of symptoms obtained from patient, relatives, and other sources, such as Nurse, General Duty and Social Worker, Psychiatric. Examines patient to determine general physical condition, following standard medical procedures. Orders laboratory and other special diagnostic tests and evaluates data obtained. Determines nature and extent of mental disorder, and formulates treatment program. Treats or directs treatment of patient, utilizing variety of psychotherapeutic methods and medications. (DOT)

American Academy of Child
and Adolescent Psychiatry
3615 Wisconsin Ave., NW, Washington, DC 20016
202/996-7300

American Academy of Clinical Psychiatrists
PO Box 3212, San Diego, CA 92103
619/298-4782

American Academy of Psychiatry and the Law
1211 Cathedral St., Baltimore, MD 21201
301/539-0379

American Board of Psychiatry and Neurology
500 Lake Cook Rd., Suite 335, Deerfield, IL 60015
708/945-7900

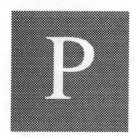

American Psychiatric Association
1400 K Street, NW, Washington DC 20005
202/682-6000

Black Psychiatrists of America
664 Prospect Ave., Hartford, CT 06105
203/236-2320

Psychoanalysis
Sigmund Freud: 1856-1939

JAMA. 1939 Oct 14; 113(16): 1494-5

On September 22, in his eighty-third year, Sigmund Freud, founder of psychoanalysis, died in London. Men in the future may evaluate fully his contribution to medicine. No doubt much of his teaching will be modified and some of it will be discarded. Certain, however, is the revolutionary influence he has had on psychiatry. Freud was born in 1856 in Freiberg, a small provincial town of Moravia, then belonging to the Austro-Hungarian Empire, a son of simple Jewish parents. His nationality and his race influenced his career. He became a physician though later confessing that his secret desire had been to become a novelist. He was destined to be a profound student of human nature.

In his medical studies Freud was stimulated far more by Charcot and Bernheim in France than by his Viennese teachers. The Vienna Medical School was dominated by the mechanistic attitude of Virchow's cellular pathology. In the light of that concept the unity of the human being as manifested in the functioning of the highest integrating centers (personality) was lost. Freud began his medical career as a neurologist, with contributions on aphasia and on infantile cerebral palsy. Like many of his contemporaries, he soon became aware of the sterility, ineffectiveness and fundamental inadequacy of current neurologic practice in the care of the neuroses. In a search for more light he went to Charcot, whose fame was then at its peak. Charcot had demonstrated experimentally that ideas can produce bodily symptoms. By hypnotic suggestions he had succeeded in reproducing artificially in his patients hysterical symptoms similar to those of which they complained spontaneously.

From Bernheim's and Liebeault's post-hypnotic experiments in Nancy Freud learned that unconscious psychologic processes may influence overt behavior. Next came the observations of Joseph Breuer in Vienna, with whom Freud collaborated after his return from France. The real discoverer of psychoanalysis was Breuer's famous patient Anna, who began to talk freely under hypnosis of forgotten experiences. This reminiscing while under hypnosis was not simple remembering. It involved a dramatic display and expression of repressed emotions. This verbal outburst of emotions in hypnosis, which had such a beneficial effect on Anna's hysterical symptoms, Freud and Breuer called "cathartic hypnosis"; Anna herself gave it the name "talking cure."

These two factors, remembering of forgotten traumatic emotional experiences and the expression of pent up emotions, have remained two important therapeutic factors in psychoanalysis. Cathartic hypnosis, however, lacked one important element of modern psychoanalytic technic: insight, the intellectual digestion of the repressed forgotten emotional experiences. Under hypnosis the conscious personality of the patient was entirely eliminated. Freud recognized this defect of hypnotic therapy. He tried to reproduce without hypnosis and during these attempts discovered the most fundamental dynamic fact of psychology - the fact of repression and resistance. In the waking state patients could not face these repressed emotions which came to the surface in hypnosis. Our resistance toward the recognition of emotions, wishes, and tendencies which are painful and in conflict with accepted standards Freud called repression. During patient experimentation between 1895 and 1900 Freud discovered the method of free association by which he was able to circumvent the emotional resistance of patients against facing and recognizing their unconscious motive forces. In free association, conscious control is eliminated. The patient gives free course to his ideas, which drift - now converging toward, now receding from, the pathogenic repressed material. During this procedure, more and more of the unconscious repressed material becomes conscious. The physician's role is not active. His influence on this process of self revelation consists mainly in increasing the patient's courage and confidence to face his real self. Now sexual matters, which had been shunned by physicians and patients but which are nevertheless a significant part of our lives, began to become apparent as determining factors in some psychologic disorders. Challenging the hypocritical attitude of his time, Freud described sexual phenomena objectively. The first rejection with which his views were met was mainly due to the publication of these discoveries.

The aim of psychoanalysis, as Freud conceived it, was not to tell people unpleasant truths about themselves but to cure patients by giving the integrative powers of their rational and conscious personality an opportunity to deal with those psychologic forces which were excluded from their conscious mind. Most important was the discovery that repressions may go back to early childhood, when the infantile ego is too weak to deal with the onslaught of violent emotions. Under certain conditions, when these repressions are too excessive, the repressed impulses find a morbid outlet in neurotic and psychotic symptoms: irrational fears and ideas, depressions, delusions and the whole gamut of psychopathologic phenomena. Psychoanalytic therapy is based on the principle that the mature conscious ego can deal with repressed emotions which the childish ego cannot tolerate.

Most shocking to contemporary attitudes was the discovery of what Freud called the "family tragedy." Naturally, the first emotional difficulties in which the child becomes involved concerns its parents. The typical combination of love and hate which the small child feels toward his parents Freud called the "Oedipus complex." More recently, the application of psychoanalysis to children had become a source of important information about early emotional and intellectual development.

The emotional reactions to the Freudian observations and formulations made objective evaluation extremely difficult. They permeated scientific discussions and developed strange accusations. Freud was accused of pansexualism, mysticism, dogmatism and unsound speculation. Moreover, Freud was held responsible for every vagary of his actual disciples and many a pseudoscientist who claimed to speak in his name. He was a pioneer working in an unknown territory - the dynamics of the mind; naturally his first generalizations were somewhat vague groping attempts. Nevertheless many of his observations have already passed the test of scientific scrutiny. The facts of repression, resistance, transference, infantile sexuality and its typical manifestations in family life, the unconscious emotional origin of psychoneurotic and many psychotic symptoms, the principal laws of psychodynamics as observed in such mechanisms as rationalization, projection and overcompensation form the basis of both normal and morbid psychology.

Sigmund Freud was 35 years old when he returned from Paris to Vienna and laid the foundations of psychoanalysis. Failing to be accepted and supported by his colleagues in Vienna, including at last even Breuer, he worked for ten years entirely alone. Gradually a few students began to gather around him. Among these early followers were Karl Abraham, Sandor Ferenczi, Max Eitingon, Karl Jung, Alfred Adler, Wilhelm Steckel, Otto Rank, Hans Sachs, Ernest Jones, and others whose names did not become so well known. Some of these pupils were unwilling to follow completely along the untrodden paths into which Freud was leading them. Chief among these dissenters were Jung, Adler and Rank. Yet already psychoanalysis has become firmly established in psychology, in education and in medicine. The technic of psychoanalytic therapy has become standardized and is taught to psychiatrists in psychoanalytic institutes. A number of well trained psychoanalysts are united in scientific societies. The effects of emotional factors on physiologic and pathologic processes are being studied by adequate methods. Such generalities as worry, fear, and overwork as causes of physical disturbances are being replaced by precise descriptions of the emotional factors. By this pathway Freud's influence on general medicine will be most felt in the future. But his influence on our times cannot be evaluated by restricting attention to the medical implications of his teachings alone. All the scientific fields which deal with man's relation to man and all the social sciences have received a new impetus from his dynamic psychology.

Correction:
Sigmund Freud's Age. - The Journal of the AMA, October 14, 1939, page 1494, stated that Sigmund Freud died Sept. 22, 1939, in his eighty-third year. Dr. Freud was born May 6, 1856, and was therefore at the time of his death in his eighty-fourth year. Dr. Freud died about 3 a. m. September 23, London time and, thus figured, would make the date of death here September 22. (Jour. AMA 1939 Oct 28;113(18))

American Academy of Psychoanalysis
30 E. 40th St Ste. 206, New York, NY 10016
212/679-4105

Psychology
American Board of Professional Psychologists
2100 E Broadway, Suite 313
Columbia, MO 65201
314/875-1267

American Psychological Association
1200 17th St., NW, Washington, DC 20036
202/955-7600

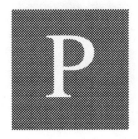

Psychosomatic Medicine
Academy of Psychosomatic Medicine
5824 Magnolia, Chicago, IL 60660
312/784-2025

Public Health
Nurse, Staff, Community Health alternate titles: public-health nurse Instructs individuals and families in health education and disease prevention in community health agency: Visits homes to determine patient and family needs, develops plan to meet needs, and provides nursing services. Instructs family in care and rehabilitation of patient, and in maintenance of health and prevention of disease for family members. Gives treatments to patient following physician's instructions. Assists community members and health field personnel to assess, plan for, and provide needed health and related services. Refers patients with social and emotional problems to other community agencies for assistance. Teaches home nursing, maternal and child care, and other subjects related to individual and community welfare. Participates in programs to safeguard health of children, including child health conferences, school health, group instruction for parents, and immunization programs. Assists in preparation of special studies and in research programs. Directs treatment of patient by Nurse, Licensed Practical And Home Attendant. Cooperates with families, community agencies, and medical personnel to arrange for convalescent and rehabilitation care of sick or injured persons. May specialize in one phase of community health nursing, such as clinical pediatrics or tuberculosis. (DOT)

Public-Health Dentist: Plans, organizes, and maintains dental health program of public health agency: Analyzes dental needs of community to determine changes and trends in patterns of dental disease. Instructs community, school, and other groups on preventive oral health care services. Produces and evaluates dental health educational materials. Provides clinical and laboratory dental care and services. Instigates methods for evaluating changes in dental health status and needs of community.(DOT)

Public Health Physician: Plans and participates in medical care or research program in hospital, clinic, or other public medical facility: Provides medical care for eligible persons, and institutes program of preventive health care in county, city, or other government or civic division. Gives vaccinations, imposes quarantines, and establishes standards for hospitals, restaurants, and other areas of possible danger. May conduct research in particular areas of medicine to aid in cure and control of disease. May be designated Medical Officer.(DOT)

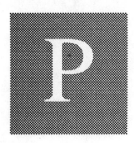

Legislation:

The Public Health Service Act of July 1, 1944 (42 U.S.C. 201), consolidated and revised substantially all existing legislation relating to the Public Health Service legal responsibilities have been broadened and expanded many times since 1944. Major organizational changes have occurred within the Public Health Service to support its mission to promote the protection and advancement of the Nation's physical and mental health. This is accomplished by:

- coordinating with the States to set and implement national health policy and pursue effective intergovernmental relations;
- generating and upholding cooperative in international health-related agreements, policies, and programs;
- conducting medical and biomedical research;
- sponsoring and administering programs for the department of health resources, prevention and control of diseases, and alcohol and drug abuse;
- providing resources and expertise to the States and other public and private institutions in the planning, direction, and delivery of physical and mental health care services; and
- enforcing laws to assure the safety and efficacy of drugs and protection against impure and unsafe foods, cosmetics, medical devices, and radiation-producing projects.

The Office of the Assistant Secretary for Health consists of general and special staff offices that support the Assistant Secretary for Health and the Surgeon General plan and direct the activities of the Public Health Service. (USG)

Contact county/state public health department for local programs and assistance

American Association of Public Health Physicians
Lexington-Fayette County Health Department
650 New Town Pike, Lexington, KY 40508
606/288-2486

American Public Health Association
1015 15th St. NW, Washington, DC 20005
202/789-5600

Association of the Schools of Public Health
1015 15th St. NW, Ste 404
Washington, DC 20005
202/842-4668

United States Public Health Service (USPHS)
200 Independence Ave. SW
Washington, DC 20201
202/245-7694

Public Health Departments, Statewide

Alabama Department of Public Health
State Office Bldg, 434 Monroe St.
Montgomery, AL 36130-1701
205/242-5052

Alaska Department of Health and Social Services
Alaska Office Bldg, Room 503, PO Box H,
Juneau, AK 99811
907/465-3090

Arizona Department of Public Health
1740 W. Adams, Phoenix, AZ 85007
602/542-1024

Arkansas Department of Public Health
4815 W Markham St, Little Rock, AR 72205
501/661-2243

California Health and Welfare Agency
Department of Health Services
Public Health Division
714 P St, No. 1253, Sacramento, CA 95814
916/445-2927

Colorado Department of Health
4210 E 11th Ave, Denver, CO 80220
303/320-8333

Connecticut Department of Health
150 Washington St, Hartford, CT 06106
203/566-2038

Delaware Department of Health
and Social Services
Division of Public Health, Jesse Cooper Bldg
802 Silver Lake Blvd, PO Box 637
Dover, DE 19903
302/739-4701

District of Columbia Department
of Human Services
Commission of Public Health
801 N Capitol St, NE, Washington, DC 20002
202/673-7700

Florida Department of Health
and Rehabilitative Services
Health Program Office, Bldg 2, Room 429
1317 Winewood Blvd.
Tallahassee, FL 32399-0700
904/487-2705

Georgia Department of Human Resources
Division of Public Health
878 Peachtree, Room 201, Atlanta, GA 30309
404/894-7505

Hawaii Department of Health
1250 Punchbowl St, PO Box 3378
Honolulu, HI 96813
808/548-6505

Idaho Department of Public Health
and Welfare
Division of Health
450 W State St, Boise, ID 83720
208/334-5945

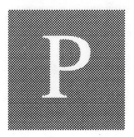

Illinois Department of Public Health
535 W Jefferson St, Springfield, IL 62761
217/782-4977

Indiana State Board of Health
1330 E Michigan St, PO Box 1964
Indianapolis, IN 46206
317/633-8400

Iowa Department of Public Health
Lucas State Office Bldg, Des Moines, IA 50319
515/281-5605

Kansas Department of Health and Environment
Division of Health, Landon State Office Bldg
901 SW Jackson St, Topeka, KS 66612
913/296-1500

Kentucky Human Resources Cabinet
Department for Health Services
275 E Main St, Frankfort, KY 40621
502/564-3970

Louisiana Department of Health and Hospitals
Office of Public Health Services
PO Box 60630, New Orleans, LA 70160
504/568-5052

Maine Department of Human Services
Bureau of Health
State House, Sta. 11, Augusta, ME 04333
207/289-3201

Maryland Department of Health
and Mental Hygiene
Office of Public Health Services
201 W. Preston St, 5th Floor, Baltimore, MD 21201
301/225-6525

Massachusetts Executive Office
of Human Services
Department of Public Health
150 Tremont St, 10th Floor, Boston, MA 02111
617/727-2700

Michigan Department of Public Health
3423 N. Logan, PO Box 30195, Lansing, MI 48909
517/335-8022

Minnesota Department of Health
717 Delaware St, SE, Minneapolis, MN 55440
612/623-5460

Mississippi Department of Public Health
PO Box 1700, Jackson, MS 39215-1700
601/960-7635

Missouri Department of Public Health
1730 Elm St, PO Box 570
Jefferson City, MO 65102
314/751-6001

Montana Department of Health
and Environmental Sciences
Division of Health Services
Cogswell Bldg, Room C-202, Helena, MT 59620
406/444-4473

Nebraska Department of Public Health
301 Centennial Mall S, 3rd Floor
PO Box 95007, Lincoln, NE 68509
402/471-2133

Nevada Department of Human Resources
Division of Health
505 E King St, Room 201, Carson City, NV 89710
702/687-4740

New Hampshire Department of Health and Human
Services
Division of Public Health Services
6 Hazen Dr, Concord, NH 03301
603/271-4501

New Jersey Department of Health
John Fitch Plaza, CN 360, Trenton, NJ 08625
609/292-7837

New Mexico Department of Health and
Environment
Division of Public Health, Harold Runnels Bldg
1190 St. Francis Dr, Santa Fe, NM 87501
505/827-2389

New York State Department of Health
Corning Tower, Empire State Plaza, Albany
NY 12237
518/474-2011

North Carolina Department of Environment,
Health, and Natural Resources
Office of Health Director, 513 N Salisbury St
PO Box 27687, Raleigh, NC 27611-7687
919/733-4984

North Dakota Department of Health and
Consolidated Laboratories
State Capitol, 2nd Floor
Judicial Wing, Bismarck, ND 585005-0200
701/224-2372

Ohio Department of Public Health
246 N. High St, PO Box 118
Columbus, OH 43266
614/466-3543

Oklahoma Department of Public Health
1000 NE 10th St, PO Box 53551
Oklahoma City, OK 73152
405/271-5600

Oregon Department of Human Resources
Division of Health
1400 SW 5th Ave, Portland, OR 97201
503/229-5032

Pennsylvania Department of Health
Health and Welfare Bldg, Box 90
Harrisburg, Pa 17108
717/787-6436

Puerto Rico Department of Public Health
Bldg A, Psychiatric Hospital Grounds
Call Box 9342, San Juan, PR 00908
809/767-6060

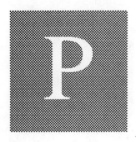

Rhode Island Department of Health
3 Capitol Hill, Providence, RI 02908
401/277-2231

South Carolina Department of Health and
Environmental Control
Office of Health Services, J. Marion Sims & R.J.
Aycock Bldg
2600 Bull St, Columbia, SC 29201
803/734-3900

South Dakota Department of Health
Division of Public Health
Foss Bldg, 523 E. Capitol, Pierre, SD 57501-3182
605/773-3364

Tennessee Department of Health and Environment
Health Services Bureau
344 Cordell Hull Bldg, Nashville, TN 37247-0101
615/741-7305

Texas Department of Health
1100 W. 49th St, Austin, TX 78756
512/458-7375

Utah Department of Health
288 North 1460 West, Salt Lake City, UT 84116
801/538-6111

Vermont Agency of Human Services
Department of Health
60 Main St, PO Box 70, Burlington, VT 05402
802/863-7280

Virgin Islands Department of Health
Government House, Charlotte Amalie,
St. Thomas, VI 00801
809/776-8311

Virginia Department of Health
James Madison Bldg, 109 Governor St,
Richmond, VA 23219
804/786-3561

Washington Department of Health
1300 SE Quince, EY-12, Olympia, WA 98504
206/586-5846

West Virginia Department of Health
and Human Resources
Public Health Bureau, State Capitol Complex
Bldg 3, Room 519, Charleston, WV 25305
304/348-2971

Wisconsin Department of Health
and Social Services
Division of Health
1 W Wilson St, PO Box 7850, Madison, WI 53707
608/266-1511

Wyoming Department of Health
Division of Health and Medical Services
117 Hathaway Bldg, Cheyenne, WY 82002-0710
307/777-7121

Pulmonary

American Association of Cardiovascular and
Pulmonary Rehabilitation
7611 Elmwood Ave, Suite 201
Middleton, WI 53562
608/831-6989

Board Certification in Pulmonary Disease
American Board of Internal Medicine
3624 Market St., Philadelphia, PA 19104
215/243-1500
800/441-ABIM (800/441-2246)

American College of Chest Physicians
3300 Dundee Road, Northbrook, IL 60062-2348
708/498-1400

Quality Assurance

Quality Assurance Coordinator Interprets and implements quality assurance standards in hospital to ensure quality care to patients: Reviews quality assurance standards, studies existing hospital policies and procedures, and interviews hospital personnel and patients to evaluate effectiveness of quality assurance program. Writes quality assurance policies and procedures. Reviews and evaluates patients' medical records, applying quality assurance criteria. Selects specific topics for review, such as problem procedures, drugs, high volume cases, high risk cases, or other factors. Compiles statistical data and writes narrative reports summarizing quality assurance findings. May review patient records, applying utilization review criteria, to determine need for admission and continued stay in hospital. May oversee personnel engaged in quality assurance review of medical records. (DOT)

American Board of Quality Assurance and Utilization Review Physicians
1777 Tamiami Trail, Ste 205,
Pt Charlotte, FL 33948
813/286-4411

JAMA Theme Issue: Quality of Medical Care
JAMA.1986 Aug 22/29;256(8)
JAMA's theme issue on quality of care includes background on the AMA initiative on Quality of Medical Care and Professional Self-Regulation, a discussion on the quality of care from the Council on Medical Service (defunct?), and a randomized trial of medical quality assurance and pelvimetry discussing applications of some of the ideas theorized in the essays in an educational setting.

Questionable Doctors

Public Citizen Health Research Group
2000 "P" St., N.W./Suite 700,
Washington, DC 20036
202/872-0320

Radiologic Technology

History: A long process of stabilizing standards of education and establishing qualifications for accreditation was culminated in 1944, when the AMA House of Delegates and the American Society of X-Ray Technicians (ASXT) adopted the first Essentials of an Accredited School of X-Ray Technology. These Essentials resulted from negotiations between the Council on Medical Education and Hospitals of the AMA and the Executive Committee of the ASXT. The ASXT, now the American Society of Radiologic Technologists (ASRT), subsequently contributed to the establishment and elevation of educational standards for radiologic technology through the varied activities of its educational committee, especially in the areas of curriculum development and instructor preparation.

The current Essentials of an Accredited Educational Program for the Radiographer were adopted in 1983 and revised in 1990 by the American College of Radiology (ACR), the American Medical Association (AMA), and the American Society of Radiologic Technologists (ASRT). The ACR and ASRT are the two organizations collaborating with the AMA Council on Medical Education in developing, revising, and adopting Essentials.

Radiation therapy technology has been recognized as a separate discipline within radiologic technology since 1964. The first set of Essentials for the radiation therapy technologist, adopted by the ACR, AMA, and ASRT in 1968, applied only to one-year programs. In 1972, the three groups provided for two-year programs by adopting Essentials for programs with a minimum entrance requirement of a high school diploma.

The current Essentials and Guidelines of an Accredited Educational Program for the Radiation Therapy Technologist were adopted by the ACR, AMA, and ASRT in 1988, and apply to all educational programs in radiation therapy technology, whatever the length or admission criteria.

In addition to their collaborative effort with regard to the Essentials, the ACR, a professional organization representing physician specialists, and the ASRT, a professional organization representing radiologic technologists, cooperate with CAHEA in the accreditation of allied health educational programs. The ACR and ASRT appoint representatives to the Joint Review Committee on Education in Radiologic Technology (JRCERT), which evaluates educational programs in radiography and radiation therapy technology for accreditation; forwards its accreditation recommendations to CAHEA; and provides consultation and guidance to educational programs. The JRCERT also plays a major role in developing and revising Essentials.

The American Society of Radiologic Technologists makes additional contributions to the development of radiologic technology by publishing the curriculum guide for radiography and radiation therapy technology educational programs; these comprehensive guides are revised regularly to reflect new areas of study for these disciplines. Upon request, the ASRT provides consultation in the areas of curriculum development and instructor preparation. Through the ASRT

Educational Foundation, numerous educational programs are provided for radiologic technologists during the annual ASRT meeting and throughout the year. In addition, various educational materials are compiled and distributed. Detailed information about the profession may be found in the professional history maintained by the organization.

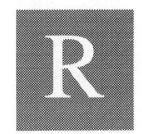

Radiation Therapy Technologist

Occupational Description: Radiation therapy technologists, under the supervision of radiation oncologists, administer radiation therapy services to patients. The radiation therapy technologist provides appropriate patient care, maintains pertinent records, and exercises judgment in the administration of prescribed courses of treatment, tumor localization, and dosimetry. The radiation therapy technologist is particularly concerned with the principles of radiation protection for the patient, self, and others while carrying out these duties.

Job Description: Professional competence requires that radiation therapy technologists apply knowledge of anatomy and physiology, oncology pathology, radiation oncology techniques, treatment planning procedures and dosimetry in the performance of their duties. They must also be able to communicate with patients, other health professionals and the public.

The radiation therapy technologist accepts responsibility for administering a prescribed course of treatment, observing the patient during treatment, and maintaining pertinent records of the treatment. Additional duties may include tumor localization, dosimetry, patient follow-up and patient education. Radiation therapy technologists must have a stable, self-assured personality and must display attributes of compassion, concern, and courtesy in meeting the special needs of the oncology patient.

Employment Characteristics: Radiation therapy technologists are employed in hospitals, free standing cancer centers, and private offices. Radiation therapy technologists employed on a full-time basis usually work 40 hours per week. Salaries and benefits vary with experience and employment location, but are generally competitive with other allied health specialties. Employment opportunities are available throughout the country, but may vary geographically.

According to the 1990 CAHEA Annual Supplemental Survey, entry level salaries average $27,804.

Radiographer.

Occupational Description: Radiographers provide patient services using imaging modalities, as directed by physicians qualified to order and/or perform radiologic procedures. When providing patient services, they continually strive to provide quality patient care and are particularly concerned with limiting radiation exposure to patients, self, and others. Radiographers exercise independent judgment in the technical performance of medical imaging procedures by adopting variable technical parameters of the procedure to the condition of the patient and by initiating lifesaving first aid and basic life support procedures as necessary during medical emergencies.

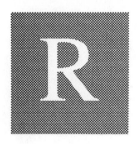

Job Description: Professional competence requires that radiographers apply knowledge of anatomy, physiology, positioning, and radiographic technique in the performance of their duties. They must also be able to communicate effectively with patients, other health professionals, and the public. Additional duties may include processing of film, evaluating radiologic equipment, managing a radiographic quality assurance program, and providing patient education relevant to specific imaging procedures. The radiographer displays personal attributes of compassion, courtesy and concern in meeting the special needs of the patient.

Employment Characteristics: Most Radiographers are employed in hospitals. However, there are also positions open to qualified professionals in specialized imaging centers, urgent care clinics, private physician offices, industry, and civil service and public health service facilities. Radiographers who are employed full-time usually work 40 hours per week. Salaries and benefits vary according to experience, ability, and geographic location, but are generally competitive with those of professions requiring comparable educational preparation. Employment opportunities are available throughout the nation, but may vary geographically.

According to the 1990 CAHEA Annual Supplemental Survey, entry level salaries average $21,033.

AMA Allied Health Department
312/464-4696

American Society of Radiologic Technologists
15000 Central Ave, Albuquerque, NM 87123
505/298-4500

Radiology

Radiologist Diagnoses and treats diseases of human body, using x-ray and radioactive substances: Examines internal structures and functions of organ systems, making diagnoses after correlation of x-ray findings with other examinations and tests. Treats benign and malignant internal and external growths by exposure to radiation from x-ray, high energy sources, and natural and manmade radioisotopes directed at or implanted in affected areas of body. Administers radiopaque substances by injection, orally, or as enemas to render internal structures and organs visible on x-ray films or fluoroscopic screens. May specialize in diagnostic radiology or radiation oncology. May diagnose and treat diseases of human body, using radioactive substances, and be certified in Nuclear Radiology or Nuclear Medicine. (DOT)

American Board of Radiology
2301 W. Big Beaver Road, Suite 625,
Troy, MI 48084
313/643-0300

American College of Radiology
1891 Preston White Drive, Reston, VA 22091
703/648-8900

American Roentgen Ray Society
1891 Preston White Dr., Reston, VA 22091
703/648-8992

American Society for Therapeutic
Radiology and Oncology
1891 Preston White Drive, Reston, VA 22091
703/648-8903

Radiological Society of North America
2021 Spring St., Oak Brook, IL 60521
708/571-2670

Rape
National Institute of Mental Health
Anti-Social and Violent Behavior Branch, DBAS,
Parklawn Bldg, Rm. 18-105,
5600 Fishers Lane, Rockville, MD 20857
301/443-3728

Rare Disorders
National Information for Orphan Drugs
& Rare Diseases
PO Box 1133, Washington, DC 20013-1133
800/336-4797

National Organization for Rare Disorders
PO Box 8923, New Fairfield, CT 06812
203/746-6518

Reference Criteria for Short Stay Hospital Review
Order from NTIS (U.S. Dept. of Commerce):
5285 Port Royal Rd., Springfield, VA 22161
703/487-4650 (Order #PB81-179889)

References
To effect greater uniformity in reference style among publications, the AMA has adopted a modified version of the format described in American National Standards Institute (ANSI) document Z39.29.1977. Each reference is divided by periods into the following bibliographic groups (listed in order): author(s), title, edition, imprint (place and name of publisher, date of publication, volume number, issue number, inclusive page numbers), physical description (physical construction or form), series statement, and supplementary notes (identifiers of the uniqueness of the reference or material necessary for added clarity). The period serves as a field delimiter, making each bibliographic group distinct and helping establish a sequence of bibliographic elements in a reference. The items within a bibliographic group are referred to as a bibliographic elements. They may be separated by a semicolon (if the elements are different or if there are multiple occurrences of logically related elements within a group; also, before volume identification data), a comma (if the items are sub-elements of a bibliographic element or a set of closely related elements), or a colon (before the publisher's name, between the title and the subtitle, and after a connective phrase [for example, "In," "Taken from," "Located at," "Accompanied by," "Available from"]).

The Uniform Requirements for Manuscripts Submitted to Biomedical Journals is also based on the ANSI document but, in some cases, has made modifications different from the ones described herein. Articles adhering exactly to the Uniform Requirements will be acceptable without challenge if accepted for publication in the AMA journal and

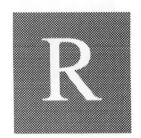

any necessary changes will be made by the AMA copy editors.

Because the reference style presented herein differs substantially from the previous AMA reference style, examples, where possible, will use the "old" example changed to the new style.

2.10.1 Listed References. - references to articles or books published or accepted for publication or to papers presented at professional meetings are listed in numerical order at the end of the communication (except as specified in 2.10.2, References, References Given in Text, and 2.10.6, References, Numbering). Each reference is a separate entry. References to mass circulation magazines or newspapers, material not yet accepted for publication, and personal communications (both oral and written) are not acceptable as listed references, except in unusual circumstances, and should be given parenthetically in the text (see References, References Given in Text, and , References, Unpublished Material).

2.10.2 References Given in Text. - In some circumstances, references may be included parenthetically in the text. Examples of forms are given here. Note that in the text (1) author(s) may or may not be named, (2) the title is not given, (3) the name of the journal is abbreviated only when enclosed in parentheses, and (4) inclusive page numbers are given.

The results were reported recently by West (Br Med J. 1981;282:355-357).
The results were reported recently in the British Medical Journal 1981;282:355-377).

References to publications not acceptable as listed references (see 2.10.1, References, Listed References) may be included parenthetically in the text. Use a concise form: name of periodical, date, initial page number.

The explanation is given in one recent account (Newsweek. March 17, 1980:102).
The Archives of Surgery article on surgeon glut was picked up by a local newspaper (Chicago Tribune. October 2, 1986:6).

2.10.3 Author's Responsibility for Accuracy. - Authors are responsible for the accuracy and completeness of the references in their communications. Any reference that appears to be inaccurate should be queried by the copy editor. Consult the bibliographic resources in the library or ask the author to verify and complete the reference.

2.10.4 Minimum Acceptable Data. - To be acceptable, a reference must include certain minimum data, as follows:

Journals: Author(s), article title, journal, year, volume, inclusive page numbers
Books: Author(s), title, place of publication, publisher, year

Enough information to identify and retrieve the material should be provided. More complete data (see 2.10.13, References to Journals, Complete Data, and 2.10.26, References to Books, Complete Data) should be used when available.

2.10.5 Number Permitted. - A good indication of the reliability of an author's work is the type and number of references selected. Too many references may indicate a lack of critical thinking; too few references may suggest the possibility of unwarranted speculation. References have two major purposes: documentation and acknowledgment. Acknowledgment references should be limited to reports that have contributed substantially to the author's own current work. Some journals suggest a limit for the number of references for a particular type of article. This will usually be described in the journal's instruction for authors. Exceptions to such limits may be permitted for special cases.

2.10.6 Numbers. - References should be numbered consecutively, using arabic numerals, in the order in which they are cited in the text. Unnumbered references are only occasionally used in AMA journals. In these exceptional cases, they usually appear alphabetically as a list of selected readings.

2.10.7 Citation. - Each reference should be cited in the text. Citation may also be made in tables, figures, and legends. Use arabic superscript numerals. These numerals appear outside periods and commas, inside colons and semicolons. When more than two references are cited at a given place in the copy, use hyphens to join the first and last numbers of a closed series; use commas without space to separate other parts of a multiple citation.

As reported previously,[1,3-8,19]
The derived data were as follows[3,4]
As reported previously,[*]

When a multiple citation involves more than 23 characters, use an asterisk in the text and give the citation in a footnote at the bottom of the page. Note that reference numerals in such a footnote are set full size, on line rather than as superscripts. Also note that the spacing is different from that in superscript reference citations.

[*]References 3,5,7,9,11,13,21,24-29,31.

If the author wishes to cite different page numbers from a single reference source at different places in the text, the page numbers are included in the superscript citation and the source appears only once in the list of references. Note that (1) the superscript may include more than one page number, citation of more than one reference, or both, and (2) all spaces are closed up. In listed references, do not use ibid or op cit.

These patients showed no sign of protective sphincteric adduction.[3(p21),9]
Westman[5(pp3,5),9] has reported eight cases in which vomiting occurred.

2.10.8 Authors. - Use the author's surname followed by initials without punctuation. In listed references, the names of all authors should be given unless there are more than six, in which case the names of the first three authors are used, followed by "et al." Note spacing and punctuation. Do not use and between names. (Abbreviations for Junior and Senior and Roman numerals follow author's initials.)

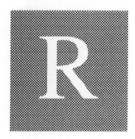

One author: Doe JF.
Two authors: Doe JF, Roe JP III.
Six authors: Doe JF, Roe JP III, Coe RT Jr., Loe JT Sr, Poe EA, van Voe AE.
More than six: Doe JF, Roe JP III, Coe RT Jr, et al.

When mentioned in the text, only surnames of authors are used. For a two-author reference, give both surnames. For references with more than two authors, give the first author's surname followed by "et al," "and associates," "and coworkers," or "and colleagues."

Doe[7] reported on the survey.
Doe and Roe[8] reported on the survey.
Doe et al[9] reported on the survey.

Note: Never use the possessive form *et al's*; rephrase the sentence.

The date of Doe et al[9] were reported.

2.10.9 Prefixes and Particles. - Surnames containing prefixes or particles should be spelled and alphabetized according to the preference of the persons concerned.

1. van Gylswyk NO, Roche CI.
2. Van Rosevelt RF, Bakker JC, Sinclair DM, Damen J, Van Mourik JA.

2.10.10 Titles. - In titles of articles, books, parts of books, and other material, retain the spelling, abbreviations, and style for numbers used in the original. Note, however, that all numbers are spelled out at the beginning of a title.

Articles and parts of books: In English-language titles, capitalize only the first letter of the first word, proper names, and abbreviations that are ordinarily capitalized (eg, DNA, EEG, VDRL). Do not enclose parts of books in quotation marks.

Books, journals, government bulletins, documents, and pamphlets: In English-language titles, capitalize the first and last words and each word that is not an article, preposition, or conjunction of less than four letters. In every language, italicize the title.

Genus and species: In all titles, follow AMA style for capitalization of genus and species and use of italics (see 8.1.7, Capitalization, Organisms, and 12.16.1, Nomenclature, Genus and Species). Use roman type for genus and species names in book titles.

2.10.11 Foreign-Language Titles. - Foreign language titles are usually not translated; if they have been, bracketed indication of the original language should follow the title.

1. Kojima M. Studies on the pathomechanism of solar urticaria [in Japanese]. Areugi 1984;33:224-230.
2. Abernathy JD. De la necessite de traiter l'hypertension moderee; une mauvaise interpretation des donnees de l'etude australienne. JAMA Suisse. 1987;7:237-241. Originally published, in English, in: JAMA.1986;256:3134-3137.

Reference to a foreign-language translation of an article should be permitted only when the original article is not readily available.

Foreign-language titles should be verified from the original when possible. Consult foreign-language dictionaries for accents, spelling, and other particulars.

Capitalization: For journal articles, follow the capitalization in Index Medicus. For books, pamphlets, and parts of books, retain the capitalization used in the original or consult the author or publisher. Note: In foreign-language titles, capitalization does not necessarily follow the rules given in 2.10.10, References, Titles. For example, in German titles (both articles and books), all nouns and only nouns are capitalized; in French, Spanish, and Italian book titles, capitalize only the first word, proper names, and abbreviations that are capitalized in English.

Foreign words of reference: Such words as tome (volume), fasciolo (part), Seite (page), Teil (part), Auflage (edition), Abteilung (section or part), Band (volume), Heft (number), Beiheft (supplement), and Lieferung (part or number) should be translated into English.

2.10.12 Subtitles - Style for subtitles follows that for titles (see 2.10.10, References, Titles) in regard to spelling, abbreviations, numbers, capitalization, and use of italics, except that for journal articles the subtitle begins with a lowercase letter. A colon separates title and subtitle. If the subtitle is numbered, use a roman numeral followed by a colon.

1. Milunsky A. "Prenatal detection of neural tube defects, VI: experience with 20,000 pregnancies." JAMA.1980;244:2731-2735.

References to Journals

2.10.13 Complete Data. - A complete journal reference includes (1) authors' names and initials; (2) title of article and subtitle, if any; (3) abbreviated name of journal; (4) year; (5) volume number; (6) part or supplement number, when pertinent, and issue month or number when pagination is not consecutive throughout a volume; and (7) inclusive page numbers.

2.10.14 Names of Journals. - Abbreviate and italicize names of journals. Use initial capital letters. Abbreviate according to the listing in the current Index Medicus (see 11.9 Abbreviations, Names of Journals). Include parenthetical designation of a city if it is included in the abbreviations given in List of Journals Index Medicus; for example, Acta Anat (Basel), J Physiol (Lond). In journals titles listed in Index Medicus, information enclosed in brackets should be retrained without brackets, eg, J Bone Joint Surg Br.

2.10.15 Page Numbers and Dates. - Do not omit digits from inclusive page numbers. The year, the semicolon following it, the volume number, the colon following it, and the page numbers are set with the spaces closed up.

1. Jones J Necrotizing Candida esophagitis. JAMA 1980;224:2190- 2191.

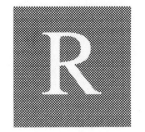

2.10.16 Serialized Article. - For a serialized article, the cited parts of which appear in the same volume, follow this example:

1. Lerner PI, Weinstein L. Infective endocarditis in the antibiotic era. N Engl J Med. 1966;274:199-206, 388-393.

2.10.17 Journals Without Volume Numbers. - In reference to journals that have no volume numbers or that have volume numbers but paginate each issue beginning with page 1, use one of the following styles:

1. Amar L. Cataracte et implant de Binkhorst. Bull Soc Ophthalmol Fr. 1976:351-356.
2. Shands KN, Fraser WA. Legionnaires' disease. Dis Mon. December 1980;27:1-59.
3. Abraham EP. The beta-lactam antibiotics. Sci Am. June 1981:76-97.

2.10.18 Parts of an Issue. - If an issue has two or more parts, the part cited should be indicated in accordance with the following example:

1. Border WA, Cohen AH. Renal biopsy diagnosis of clinically silent multiple myeloma. Ann Intern Med. 1980;93(pt 1):43- 46.

2.10.19 Issue Number. - Do not include the issue number or month except in the case of a special issue (see 2.10.20, References, Special Issue) or when pagination is not consecutive throughout the volume (ie, when each issue begins with page 1). In the latter case, the month or the date of the issue is preferable to the issue number.

Psychiatr Opinion. October 1973;10:34-38.

2.10.20 Special Issue. - References to all or part of a special issue of a journal should be given as follows:

1. Standards and guidelines for cardiopulmonary resuscitation (CPR) and emergency cardiac care (ECC). JAMA. 1986;255:2905- 2984.
2. McDonald WI. Attitudes to the treatment of multiple sclerosis. Arch Neurol. October 21, 1983;40(special issue):667-670.

(Note that the issue may be needed for identification.)

The following example shows the pagination in a supplementary special issue:

3. Hebert GA. Improved salt fractionation of animal serums for immunofluorescence studies. J Dent Res. 1976;55:A33-A38.

2.10.21 Supplements. - The following forms are used:

1. Gordon AS, chairman. Standards for cardiopulmonary resuscitation (CPR) and emergency cardiac care (ECC). JAMA 1974;277(suppl):833-868.

(Use this form whether or not pagination is consecutive with volume pagination and whether this is the only supplement to the volume or there are others.)

2. Blendon RJ. The prospects for state and local governments playing a broader role in health care in the 1980s. Am J Public Health. January 1981;71(suppl):9-15.

(Pagination is not consecutive with that of the volume; there may be several supplements to a volume, referred to by month.)

3. Keys A. Coronary heart disease in seven countries. Circulation. 1970;41(suppl 1):I-1-I-211.

(Supplements are published independently of volumes and are numbered; pagination in each is independent of that in others.)

4. Flodmark S. Clinical detection of blood-brain barrier alteration by mean of EEG: part 1. Acta Neurol Scand. 1965;41(suppl 13, pt 1):163-177.

(Volume 41 has multiple supplements; this supplement has two parts, each with independent pagination.)

5. Centers for Disease Control. Health information for international travel: including United States designated yellow fever vaccination centers. MMWR. September 1974;23(suppl):1S-76S.

(This refers to a supplement published in September, although there is an annual supplement [now called a summary] to the volume as well, which has an issue number.)

6. Centers for Disease Control. Vaccination certificate requirements for international travel. MMWR. 1973;22(suppl to No. 17):1S-54S.

(This is a supplement to No. 17, although there are both monthly and annual supplements as well.)

2.10.22 Abstracts. - Reference to an abstract of an article should be permitted only when the original article is not readily available (eg, foreign-language articles or papers presented at meeting but not yet published). If possible, references for both the original article and the abstract should be given. If the abstract is in the society proceedings section of a journal, the name of the society before which the paper was read need not be included unless the subject of the paper, the aims of the society, and the usual content of the journal are widely divergent.

1. Kremer H, Kellner E, Schierl W, Zollner N. Ultrasonic diagnosis in infiltrative gastrointestinal diseases [in German]. Dtsch Med Wochenschr. 1978;103:965-967. Taken from: JAMA. 1978;240:2784. English abstract.
2. Paillard M, Resnick N. Natural history of nosocomial urinary incontinence. Gerontologist. 1981;24:212. Abstract.

2.10.23 Special Department of a Journal. - When reference is made to material from a special department in a journal, the department should be identified only if the cited material has no byline or signature, or no page number. This is preferable to citing Anonymous.

1. How far to lower blood pressure. Lancet. 1987;2:251-252. Editorial.
2. Services for the mentally handicapped. Br Med J. 1981;282:489. News and Notes.
3. Interferon production by genetic engineering. Br

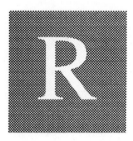

Med J. 1981;282:674-675. Leading article.
4. The development of scientific research in UK. Lancet. 1987;2:288. Notes and News.
5. Case records of the Massachusetts General Hospital: weekly clinicopathological exercises. N Engl J Med. 1981;304:831- 836. Case 14-1981.
6. Parsons GH, reviewer. West J Med. 1981;134:92-93. Review of: Grodin FS. Respiratory Function of the Lung and Its Control.

2.10.24 Other Material Without Author(s). - Reference may be made to material that has no author or is prepared by a committee or other group. The following forms are used:

1. Centers for Disease Control. Influenza - worldwide. MMWR. 1979;28:51-52.
2. Immunization Practices Advisory Committee. Influenza vaccine - recommendations of the ACIP. MMRW. 1979;28:231-238.
3. Council on Scientific Affairs. Scientific issues in drug testing. JAMA. 1987;257:3110-3114.
4. Oxford Cataract Treatment and Evaluation Team (OCTET). Long- term corneal endothelial cell loss after cataract surgery: results of a randomized controlled trial. Arch Ophthalmol. 1986;104:1170-1175.

2.10.25 Discussants. - If reference citation in the text names a discussant specifically rather than the author(s), eg, "as noted by Sachs,5" the following form is used (see also 2.10.40, References, Secondary Citations and Quotations).

1. Sachs W. In discussion: Baer RL, Andrade R, Seimanowitz VJ. Pemphigus erythematosus. Arch Dermatol. 1966;93:374-375.

References to Books

2.10.26 Complete Data. - A complete reference to a book includes (1) authors' surnames and initials; (2) surname and initials of editor or translator, or both, if any; (3) title of book and subtitle, if any; (4) number of editions after the first; (5) place of publication; (6) name of publisher; (7) year of publication; (8) volume number, if there is more than one volume; and (9) page numbers, if specific pages are cited.

1. Stryer L. Biochemistry. 2nd ed. San Francisco, Calif: WH Freeman Co; 1981:559-596.
2. Kavet J. Trends in the utilization of influenza vaccine: an examination of the implementation of public policy in the United States. In: Selby P, ed. Influenza: Virus, Vaccines, and Strategy. Orlando, FL: Academies Press Inc; 1976:297- 308.

2.10.27 Publishers. - the full name of the publisher should be given, abbreviated in accordance with AMA style, but without punctuation. If the name of a publishing firm has changed, use the name that was given on the work.

To verify names of publishers, consult *Books in Print*, the current issue of *Cumulative Book Index*, or *Publisher's Trade List Annual*.

2.10.28 Place of Publication. - Use the name of the city in which the main office of the publishing firm is located. Follow AMA style in the use of state names (see 11.5, Abbreviations, States, Territories, and Possessions). A colon separates the place of publication and the name of the publisher.

1. Barrows HS. Simulated Patients (Programmed Patients): The Development and Use of a New Technique in Medical Education. Springfield, Ill: Charles C Thomas Publisher; 1971.

In the case of overseas publishers with major US offices, use the US locations.

2. Fischer DH. Growing Old in America. New York, NY: Oxford University Press Inc; 1977:210-216.

2.10.29 Page, Volume, and Edition Numbers. - Use arabic numerals. Give specific page or pages if indicated by the author. The volume should be given if the work cited includes more than one volume. Do not indicate a first edition; if a subsequent edition is cited, the number should be given. (See also 2.10.41, References, Classical References.)

1. Spencer H. Pathology of the Lung. 3rd ed. Elmsford, NY: Pergamon Press Inc; 1976;2:980.
2. Fishbein M. Medical Writing: The Technic and the Art. 4th ed. Springfield, Ill: Charles C Thomas Publisher; 1978:46- 51.

2.10.30 Editors and Translators. - Names of editors, translators, translator-editors, or executive and section editors are given in accordance with the following forms:

1. Gray H; Goss CM, ed. Gray's Anatomy of the Human Body. 29th ed. Philadelphia, Pa: Lea & Febiger; 1973:1206.

(Gray is the author, Goss is the editor.)

2. Kuschinsky G, Lullmann H; Hoffmann PC, trans. Textbook of Pharmacology: Orlando, Fla: Academic Press Inc; 1973.

(Kuschinsky and Lullmann are the authors, Hoffmann is the translator.)

3. Plato; Taylor EA, trans-ed. The Laws. London, England: JM Dent & Sons Ltd; 1934:104-105.

(Plato is the author, Taylor is the translator-editor.)

4. Gaunt R. History of the adrenal cortex. In: Geiger SR, exec. ed. Handbook of Physiology: A Critical Comprehensive Presentation of Physiologic Knowledge and Concepts. Baltimore, Md: Williams & Wilkins; 1975;6:1-12.
5. Buege JA, Aust SD. Microsomal lip peroxidation. In Fleischer S, Packer L, eds. Methods in Enzymology. Orlando, Fla. Academic Press Ins; 1978;52:302.
6. MacLeod GK. Marketplace and regulatory trade-offs. In: MacLeod GK, Perlman M, eds. Health Care Capital: Competition and Control. Cambridge, Mass: Ballinger Publishing Co; 1978:1-6.

(MacLeod is the author of a chapter in a book of which he is also one of the editors.)

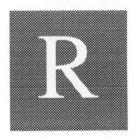

If a book has an editor but no author(s), the following form is used:

1. Boyer PD, ed. The Enzymes. 3rd ed. Orlando, Fla: Academic Press Inc; 1976;13:346.

When a book title includes a volume number, follow this example:

2. Walton WH, ed. Inhaled Particles, IV. Elmsford, NY: Pergamon Press Inc; 1975.

2.10.31 Parts of Books. - In some instances, reference is made to a part of a book that has a number of contributors as well as major authors or editors. In the title of the part (chapter or section), capitalize as for a journal title (see 2.10.10, References, Titles); do not enclose in quotation marks. Either inclusive page numbers or numerical designation of the part should be given, but not both.

1. Schulman JL. Immunology of influenza. In: Kilbourne ED, ed. The Influenza Viruses and Influenza. Orlando, Fla: Academic Press Inc; 1975:373-393.
2. Sencer DJ, Rubin RJ. Risk as the basis for immunization policy in the United States. In: International Symposium on Influenza Vaccines for Men and Horses, London 1972. New York, NY: S Karger AG; 1973;20:244-251.
3. Pinnell SR. Disorders of collagen. In: Stansbury JB, Wyngaarden JB, Fredrickson DS, eds. The Metabolic Basis of Inherited Disease. 4th ed. New York, NY: McGraw-Hill International Book Co; 1978: chap 57.

Special Materials

2.10.32 Governmental Bulletins. - References to bulletins published by departments or agencies of the US government should include the following information, in the order indicated: (1) name of author (if given); (2) title of bulletin; (3) place of publication; (4) name of issuing bureau, agency, department, or other governmental division; (5) date of publication; (6) page numbers, if specified; (7) publication number, if any; and (8) series number, if given.

1. Butler R. Alternatives to Retirement, Testimony Before the Subcommittee on Retirement Income and Employment. Washington, DC: House Select Committee on Aging; 1978. US Dept of Health, Education, and Welfare publication NIH 780- 243.
2. Melvin DM, Brooke MM. Laboratory Procedures for the Diagnosis of Intestinal Parasites. Atlanta, Ga: Centers for Disease Control; 1974. US Dept of Health, Education, and Welfare publication 75-8282.
3. Accommodating the Spectrum of Individual Abilities. Washington, DC: US Commission on Civil Rights; 1981:108-114.
4. Peanuts and Tea: A Selected Glossary of Terms Used by Drug Addicts. Lexington, Ky: National Institute of Mental Health Clinical Research Center; 1972.

2.10.33 Serial Publications. - If a monograph or report is one of a series, include the name of the series and the number of the publication.

1. McNulty JG. Radiology of the Liver. Philadelphia, Pa: WB Sanders Co; 1977:13. Saunders Monographs in Clinical Radiology.

2. Abbott MH, Folstein SE, Jensen BA, Pyeritz RE. Cognitive and psychiatric features of 68 persons with homocystinuria. In: Program and abstracts of the 34th annual meeting of the American Society of Human Genetics; October 30-November 2, 1983; Norfolk, Va. Abstract 217.

2.10.34 Theses and Dissertations. - Titles are given in italics. References to these should include the location of the university (or other institution), its name, and year of completion. If it has been published, the publisher's name and location should also be given.

1. Raymond CA. Uncovering Ideology: Occupational Health in the Mainstream and Advocacy Press, 1970-1982. Ithaca, NY: Cornell University; 1983. Thesis.
2. Van Praag HM. Monoamine Oxidase Inhibition as a Therapeutic Principle in the Treatment of Depression. Utrecht, the Netherlands: University of Utrecht; 1962. Thesis.

2.10.35 Special Collections. - References to material available only in special collections of a library take these forms:

1. Hunter J. An account of the dissection of morbid bodies: a monograph or lecture. 1757;(No. 32):30-32. Available in: Library of Royal College of Surgeons, London, England.

2.10.36 Congressional Record and Federal Register. - References to the Congressional Record and Federal Register take these forms:

1. Bregan PR. The return of lobotomy and psychosurgery. Congressional Record. February 24, 1972;118:E1602-E1612.
2. Federal Motor Vehicle Standard 213: child seating systems. Federal Register. March 26, 1970;35:5120; amended September 23, 1970;35:14778; April 10, 1971;36:6895-6896; June 29, 1971;36:12224-12226; March 23, 1973;38:7562
3. Inceptive grant criteria for state safety belt use laws (23 CFR 1213). Federal Register. April 11, 1974;39:13154.
4. Notice of proposed rule-making on Federal Vehicle Safety Standard 213: child seating systems. Federal Register. March 1, 1974;39:7959-7960.

2.10.37 Statutory Publications. - Occasionally, the need arises to cite a Congressional Act. The form for citation is as follows:

1. The Allied Health Profession Personnel Training Act of 1966. 42 USC 295h.

2.10.38 Audiotapes, Videotapes. - Occasionally, references may include citation of audiotapes or videotapes. The form for such references is as follows:

1. Blaustein AU, Gostein F, Demopoulos R. Pathology of the Cervix [tape/filmstrip]. Philadelphia, Pa. WB Saunders Co; 1974.
2. Platt WR. Color Atlas and Textbook of Hematology [slide presentation]. Philadelphia, Pa. JB Lippincott; 1975.
3. Ikeda S. Techniques of Flexible Bronchofiberscopy [videotape or 16mm film]. Baltimore, Md: University Park Press; 1974.

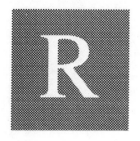

2.10.39 Unpublished Material. - References to unpublished material may include (1) articles that have been read before a society but not published and (2) material accepted for publication but not published. Date of publication and additional data should be added when they become known.

1. Reinarz JA. Percutaneous lung aspiration: a useful diagnostic adjunct in pneumonia. Presented at Ninth Interscience Conference on Antimicrobial Agents and Chemotherapy; October 19, 1974; Atlantic City, NJ.
2. Siegler M. The nature and limits of clinical medicine. In: Cassell EJ, Siegler M, eds. Changing Values in Medicine. Chicago, Ill: University of Chicago Press. In press.

In the list of references, do not include material that has been submitted for publication but has not yet been accepted. This material, with its date, should be noted in the text as "unpublished data," as follows:

These findings have recently been corroborated (Marman HE. January 1975. Unpublished data). Similar findings have been noted by Roberts and H. E. Marman, MD (unpublished data).

If the unpublished data referred to are those of the author, list as follows:

Other data (H.E.M., unpublished data, 1987)...

Do not include "personal communications" in the list of references. The following forms may be used:

In a conversation with H. E. Marman, MD (August 1966)....
According to a letter from H. E. Marman, MD, in August 1966....
Similar findings have been noted by Roberts and by H. E. Marman, MD (written communication, August 1966).

(Note that the author should give the date of the communication and indicate whether it was in conversation or in writing. Highest academic degrees should also be given.)

2.10.40 Secondary Citations and Quotations. - Reference may be made to one author's citation of, or quotation from, another's work. Distinguish between citation and quotation, ie, between work mentioned and words actually quoted. In the text, the name of the original author should be mentioned rather than the secondary source. (See also 2.10.25, References, Discussants.) The forms for listed references are as follows:

1. Hooper PJ. Cited by: Wilson CB, Cronic F. Traumatic arteriovenous fistulas involving middle meningeal vessels. JAMA. 1964;188:953-957.
2. Mitchell J. Quoted by: Goodfield GJ. Growth of Scientific Physiology. Mineola, NY: Dover Publication Inc; 1960:89.

2.10.41 Classical References. - These may deviate from the usual forms in some details. In many instances, the facts of publication are irrelevant and may be omitted. Date of publication should be given when available and pertinent.

1. Shakespeare W. Midsummer Night's Dream. Act II; scene 3; line 24.
2. Donne J. Second Anniversary. Verse 243.

For some classical references, The Chicago Manual of Style may be used as a guide, but use a period after an author's name.

3. Aristotle. Metaphysics. 3. 2.966b 5-8.

In biblical references, do not abbreviate the names of books. The version may be included parenthetically if the information is provided. References to the Bible are usually included in the text, but they may occasionally appear as listed references at the end of the article.

The story begins in Genesis 3:28.
Paul admonished against temptation (I Corinthians 10:6-13).
4. I Corinthians 10:6-13 (RSV).

2.10.42 Legal References. - A specific style variation is used for references to legal citations. Because the system of citation used is quite complex, with numerous variations for different types of sources and among various jurisdictions, only a brief outline can be presented here. For more details, consult A Uniform System of Citation (1986), frequently referred to as the Harvard "blue book" because of its cover.

Method of citation: A legal reference may be included in full in the text or in a footnote, or partially in the text and partially in a footnote.

In a leading decision on informed consent (Cobbs v Grant, 502 P2d 1 [Cal 1972]), the California Supreme Court state...
In a leading decision on informed consent,1 the California Court stated...
In the case of Cobbs v Grant (502 P2d 1 [Cal 1972])....
In the case of Cobbs v Grant....

Citation of cases: The citation of a case (ie, a court opinion) generally includes, in the following order, (1) the name of the case in italics (only the names of the first party on each side are used, never with "et al," and only the last names of individuals); (2) the volume number, name, and series number (if any) of the case reporter in which it is published; (3) the page in the volume on which the case begins and, if applicable, the specific page or pages on which is discussed the point for which the case is being cited; and (4) in parenthesis, the name of the court that rendered the opinion (unless the court is identified by the name of the reporter) and the year of the decision. If the opinion is published in more than one reporter, the citations to each reporter (known as parallel citations) are separated by commas. Note that v, 2d, and 3d are standard usage in legal citations.

Canterbury v Spence, 464 F2d 772,775 (DC Cir 1972).

(This case is published in volume 464 of the Federal Reporter, second series. The case begins on page 772, and the specific point for which it was cited is on page 775. The case was decided by the US Court of Appeals, District of Columbia Circuit, in 1972.)

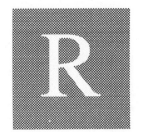

The proper reporter to cite depends on the court that wrote the opinion. Part H of *A Uniform System of Citation* contains a complete set of tables for all current and former state and federal jurisdictions.

US Supreme Court: Cite to US Reports (abbreviated as US). If the case is too recent to be published there, cite to Supreme Court Reporter (SCt) or US Law Week (USLW). If an author gives a citation to US Reports, Lawyer's Edition (LEd), ask for the citation to US Reports or Supreme Court Reporter. Do not include parallel citation.

US Court of Appeals (formerly known as Circuit Courts of Appeals): Cite to Federal Reporter, original or second series (F or F2d). These intermediate appellate-level courts heart appeals from US district courts, federal administrative agencies, and other federal trial-level courts. There are currently 13 US Courts of Appeals, known as circuits and referred to by number (1st Cir, 2d Cir, etc) except for the District of Columbia Circuit (DC Cir) and the new Federal Circuit (Fed Cir), which hears appeals from the US Claims Court and various customs and patent cases. Citations to the Federal Reporter must include the designation in parentheses with the year of the decision.

Wilcox v United States, 387 F2d 60 (5th Cir 1967).

US District Court and Claims Courts: Cite to Federal Supplement (F Supp). (There is only the original series so far.) These trial-level courts are not as prolific as the appellate courts; their function is to hear the original cases rather than review them. There are over 100 of these courts, which are referred to by geographical designations that must be included in the citation (eg, the Northern District of Illinois [ND Ill], the Central District of California [CD Cal], District of New Jersey [DNJ], as New Jersey has only one federal district).

Sierra Club v Froehlke, 359 F Supp 1289 (SD Tex 1973).

State Courts: Cite to the appropriate official (ie, state-sanctioned and state-financed) reporter (if any) and the appropriate regional reporter. Most states have separate official reporters for their highest and intermediate appellate courts (eg, Illinois Reports and Illinois Appellate Reports), but the regional reporters include cases from both levels. (State trial court opinions are generally not published.) Official reporters are always listed first, although as increasing number of states are no longer publishing them. The regional reporters are the Atlantic Reporter (A or A2d), Northeastern Reporter (NE or NE2d), Southeastern Reporter (SE2d), Southern Reporter (So or So2d), Northwestern Reporter (NW or NW2d), Southwestern Reporter (SW or SW2d), and Pacific Reporter (P or P2d). If only the regional reporter citation is given, the name of the court must appear in parentheses with the year of the decision. If the opinion is from the highest court of a state (usually but not always known as the supreme court), the abbreviated state name is sufficient (except for Ohio St); otherwise the full name of the court is abbreviated (eg, Ill App, NJ Super Ct App Div, NY App Div). A third, also unofficial, reporter is published for a few states; citation solely to these reporters must include the

court name (eg, California Reporter [Cal Rptr], Illinois Decisions [Ill Dec], New York Supplement [NYS]).

People v Carpenter, 28 Ill2d 116, 190 NE2d 738 (1963).
Webb v Stone, 445 SW2d 842 (Ky 1969).

When a case has been reviewed or otherwise dealt with by a higher court, the subsequent history of the case should be given in the citation. If the year is the same for both opinions, include it only at the end of the citation. The phrases indicating the subsequent history are set off by commas, italicized, and abbreviated (eg, aff'd [affirmed by the higher court], rev'd [reversed], vacated, appeal dismissed, cert denied [application for a writ of certiorari, ie, a request that a court hear an appeal, has been denied]).

Glazer v Glazer, 374 F2d 390 (5th Cir), cert denied, 389 US 831 (1967).

(This opinion was written by the US Court of Appeals for the Fifth Circuit in 1967. In the same year, the US Supreme Court was asked to review the case in an application for a writ of certiorari, but denied the request. This particular subsequent history is important because it indicates that the case has been taken to the highest court available and thus strengthens the case's value as precedent for future legal decisions.)

Citation of statutes: Once a bill is enacted into law by the US Congress, it is integrated into the US Code (USC). Citations of statutes include the title number (similar to a chapter number) and the section number.

33 USC 407.
(Section 407 of title of the US Code)
Environmental Quality Improvement Act of 1970, 42 USC 4371.
But: IRC 501 (c)(3).

(While it is part of the US Code, the Internal Revenue Code is commonly referred to by its own nomenclature. The section numbers in any act are not necessarily retained in the US Code.)

If a federal statute has not yet been codified, cite to Statutes at Large (abbreviated Stat, preceded by a volume number, and followed by a page number), if available, and the Public Law number of the statute.

Pub L No. 93-627, 88 Stat 2126.

Citation forms for state statutes vary considerably. The tables in part H of *A Uniform System of Citation* list examples for each state.

Ill Rev Stat ch 38, 2.
(Section 2 of chapter 38 of Illinois Revised Statutes)

Fla Stat 202.
(Section 202 of Florida Statutes)

Mich Comp Laws 145.
(Section 145 of Michigan Compiled Laws)

Wash Rev Code 45.
(Section 45 of Revised Code of Washington)

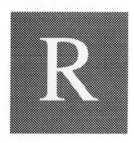

Cal Corp Code 300.
(Section 300 of California Corporations Code)

Citation of federal administrative regulations: Federal regulations are published in the Federal Register and then codified in the Code of Federal Regulations.

41 Federal Register 16950.
40 CFR 247.

(Section 247 of title 40 of the Code of Federal Regulations; title and section numbers for CFR do not necessarily correspond to those for USC.)

But: Treas Reg 1.52.

(Regulations promulgated by the Internal Revenue Service retain their unique format.)

Citation forms for state administrative regulations are especially diverse. Again, part H in A Uniform System of Citation lists the appropriate form for each state.

Citation of congressional hearings: Include the full title of the hearing, the subcommittee (if any) and committee name, the number and session of the Congress, the date, and a short description if desired.

Hearings Before the Consumer Subcommittee of the Senate Committee on Commerce, 90th Cong, 1st Sess (1965) (testimony of William Stewart, MD, surgeon general).

Citations to services: Many legal materials, including some cases and administrative materials, are published by commercial "services," often in looseleaf format. These services attempt to provide a comprehensive overview of rapidly changing areas of the law (eg, tax law, labor law, securities regulation) and are updated frequently, sometimes weekly. The citation should include the volume number of the service, its abbreviated title, the publisher's name (also abbreviated), the paragraph or section or page number, and the date.

7 Sec Reg Guide (P-H) 2333 (1984).
(Volume 7, paragraph 2333 of the Securities Regulation Guide, published by Prentice-Hall)

54 Ins L Rep (CCH) 137 (1979).
(Volume 54, page 137 of Insurance Law Reports, published by Commerce Clearing House)

4 OSH Rep (BNA) 750 (1980).
(Volume 4, page 750 of the Occupational Safety and Health Reporter, published by the Bureau of National Affairs)

Referrals, Physician
Public

Contact county medical society
To locate call:
local public library
local hospital
ask your doctor

Professional

Good Referral Habits
Physicians typically have many "markets" to which they must appeal if they are remain successful - patients, obviously, but also other physicians, third party payers, community agencies, etc. Specialists who rely on other physicians for the bulk of their patients must market themselves to these other physicians in the same way that primary care physicians must market themselves directly to patients.

Listed below are some of the things that you might do to build or maintain a healthy referral network.

Tips On How To Be a Good Referring Physician

1. When contacting a consultant, do so in a personal manner and with respect for that physician's convenience and self-respect. Writing an order and letting the nurse make the call is not sufficient.

2. If a physician initiates a call to a consultant,he or she should be on the line when that physician answers. Don't have a secretary call and then keep the other physician waiting. This is a sure way to cause resentment, usually unspoken but deeply felt.

3. Be sure that a clear distinction is made between a consultation and a referral. If the patient's return is desired, make sure the physician to whom the patient is referred knows that simply the problem is being referred and not the patient. It is not unethical to suggest to a patient that he or she may check with the physician for problems other than the specific problem they were referred to a consultant for.

4. Consultants should be given all the information which they need to do their best job. In emergency situations, all relevant medical facts should be discussed with the consultant in person or on the phone. When more time is available, a brief letter stating the patient's problem as well as all relevant notes, X-ray films, and lab results should be forwarded to the consultant, either through the mail or directly with the patient. Cryptic notes in the consultant's hospital box are not sufficient.

5. Don't wait until the last minute to refer patients for necessary treatment. A consultant should be given plenty of time to study the patient's history, conduct pre-op visits, etc.

6. Where appropriate, a patient's physician should use printed forms to inform consultants of exactly what is expected.

7. If appointments to consultants are made for patients by their regular physician, a referral

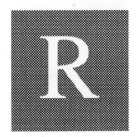

reminder notice should be used by that physician to insure that those patients keep their appointments. Having maps available illustrating the location of the consultant's office might also be helpful is assuring a patient's compliance.

8. If patients make their own appointments with a consultant, a physician should impress upon them the necessity of an early appointment. Also, make sure they can explain clearly to the consultant's appointment secretary the reason for their visits.

9. A referring physician should try to make sure that their patients know why they are being referred. They should be told exactly what to expect - what their treatment will likely entail and what the other physician is like. Make sure the patient acquiesces to the choice of a consultant, and remember that patients should not be left guessing who is in charge.

10. A referring physician should take pains not to create unreasonable expectations in patients about what a surgeon or specialist can do for them. In cases where diagnoses or surgery options have not yet been fully determined, patients should not be lead to believe that they have been determined. This could lead to friction between a referring physician and the consultant, and possibly cause a patient unnecessary confusion and consternation.

11. Don't dump troublesome patients on consultants just to get rid of them.

12. Some consultants may appreciate a report on the final disposition of a case in which they have played a part. If so, a referring physician should be prepared to provide such a report in the format which they find most useful.

13. A physician should keep track of all patients he or she has referred, and follow up with those consultants who are slow in communicating about the patient's progress.

Tips On How a Physician May Increase Referrals from Colleagues

1. Always remember that patients are the best source of referrals, whether they come to a physician directly or through a referring physician. Therefore:
- Patients shoudl be treated in such a way that they will be enthusiastic about recommending their physician's services to the physicians who referred them, or to their friends and acquaintances.
- Acknowledge patient referrals with a thank you, flowers, etc.
- Where appropriate, communicate to patients an openness for referrals (but don't solicit).

2. Colleagues obviously cannot refer patients to other M.D.s if they don't know them. Therefore, personal contact with potential referral sources should be made:
- Introducing oneself to the local hospital administrator and to key hospital personnel (both medical and non- medical).
- Making hospital rounds while other doctors are around.
- Eating breakfast and lunch at the hospital.

- Visiting the doctor's lounge at the hospital while other doctors are around.
- Introducing oneself to the Emergency Room physicians (check first and find out hospital policies on referring Emergency Room patients).
- If a doctor is new in town, introducing oneself to established colleagues in that area may also help. Do not pose a threat to these doctors, but offer help where appropriate.
- Physicians should take opportunities to recreate and socialize with other physicians.
- Attending meetings of local medical groups.
- Volunteering to serve on committees on local medical groups.

3. A Physician can build up a reputation among colleagues by:
- Giving scientific talks.
- Teaching in a hospital or medical school.
- Publishing scientific papers.

4. A physician should try to be listed in all of the referral services operated by local medical societies, local hospitals, etc.

5. A written information sheet detailing the goals, policies, and procedures by which referral patients are handled, and list of the various services offered as a referred physician for the colleagues who use the service is helpful.

6. Accommodating the needs of both the referring physician and the patient by seeing the patient promptly.

7. A physician may Install a private telephone line in the office that is connected to a recording device. Informing referring physicians of this private number and inviting dictated consultation requests or patient information at their convenience will only aid the process.

8. A physician should return patients to the referring physician. Do not steal patients. Cases where a referred patient subsequently chooses to remain under the referred physicians care should be discussed with the referring physician as honestly and tactfully as possible.

9. Reporting back promptly to a referring physician is helpful.
- Determine in what format a referring physician wishes to be informed of a patient's progress, then report to that physician using the desired format. In general, reports should be complete without verbosity.
- Even before the final report is drafted, a phone call or a brief preliminary report is often greatly appreciated. It aids the referring physician in dealing with an anxious patient or concerned relatives.
- In patient reports, the tone should inform without patronizing, educate without pontificating, direct without ordering, and solve the problem without disparaging the work of the referring physician.
- Where appropriate, let the referring physician decide how best to present the results of the consultant's efforts to the patient and his family.

10. Keep the referring physician apprised of the progress of his referred patient, or of any additional treatment that might be necessary.

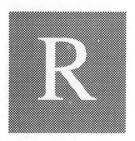

- Wherever feasible, the referring physician should be offered an active role in the case.
- The patient should not be referred to a third physician without first touching base with the physician who made the initial referral.
- The temptation to take over aspects of the patient's treatment that are not related to the immediate problem for which the patient was referred should be resisted, and any change in care should not be done without first conferring with the referring physician.
- If the referred physician wishes to make a diagnosis or prescribe a course of treatment different than that initiated by the referring physician, do so only after the matter has been discussed and explained to the referring physician. This discussion should take place out of earshot of the patient.

11. The treatment that the patient received from the referring physician should not be belittled. Any disagreements about diagnosis or treatment should be resolved with the referring physician, if possible, without involving the patient. When disagreement between physicians cannot be resolved, a frank and honest discussion of the matter with the patient, clearly explaining his options to him, is usually the best policy.

12. Do not repeat x-rays or lab tests that have already been done, unless there is a medical reason that dictates such additional studies. To do so might insult the referring physician.

13. Do not overcharge for your services. Complaints and resentments about excessive fees will be directed not only at you, but at the referring physician as well.

Tips On Keeping Your Referral Network Healthy

1. A physician should be aware of how every new patient enters his or her practice and by whom he or she was referred.

2. Express appreciation for every referral within a reasonable length of time.

3. Keep a rotary file of all referring doctors, with dated lists of referrals from each doctor.

4. A physician should keep track of all major referral sources, and periodically acknowledge in a personal manner their confidence in you.

5. Periodic surveys of major referral sources should be taken to assure satisfaction in their relationship with their choices and to get their suggestions on how to improve referral procedures.

6. Close attention to fluctuations in referral patterns should be noted by all physicians.

7. A physician should be aware of significant decreases in referrals from a major source. Call up and reestablish contact with a physician who has stopped referring patients .

8. Why patients leave a practice should be of interest to an MD. If the reason is because of deficiencies in office procedures or personnel, these deficiencies should be attended to immediately.

9. Good ethics and common sense should always be applied in dealing with referrals.

Physician Self-Referrals
Conflicts of interest. Physician ownership of medical facilities. Council on Ethical and Judicial Affairs, American Medical Association. JAMA.1992 May 6; 267(17):2366-9
In this report, the Council on Ethical and Judicial Affairs revisits the question of referral of patients to medical facilities in which physicians have financial interests ("self-referral"). The Council issued safeguards in 1986 to prevent abuses of self-referral and most recently updated the guidelines in 1989. Recent studies, however, have suggested that problems with self-referral persist; these problems undermine the commitment of physicians to professionalism. The Council has concluded that, in general, physicians should not refer patients to a health care facility outside their office practice at which they do not directly provide care or services when they have an investment interest in the facility. Physicians may invest in and refer to an outside facility if there is a demonstrated need in the community for the facility and alternative financing is not available.

Rehabilitation
American Academy of Physical Medicine and Rehabilitation
122 S. Michigan, Suite 1300, Chicago, IL 60603
312/922-9366

American Board of Physical Medicine and Rehabilitation,
21 First St. SW, Suite 674, Rochester, MN 55902
507/282-1776

American Congress of Rehabilitation Medicine
5700 Old Orchard Road, Skokie, IL 60077
708/966-0095

National Rehabilitation Information Center
8455 Colesville Rd., Suite 935,
Silver Spring, MD 20910
800/34-NARIC (800/346-2742)

Research
Computer Retrieval of Information on Scientific Projects(CRISP)
Research Documentation Section, Information Systems Branch,
Division of Research Grants, Westwood Bldg./Room 148,
5333 Westbard Avenue, Bethesda, MD 20895
301/496-7543

National Research Council, Office of Public Affairs
2101 Constitution, N.W., Washington, D.C. 20418
202/334-2000

Research Centers Directory 17th edition. ed.,
Piccirelli, Annette. (in two volumes)
Gale Research, Detroit. 1993.
ISBN 0-8103-7617-2 (set)

Research, Ethics

"Helsinki Report"
(Recommendations regarding biomedical research involving humans)
World Medical Association Handbook of Declarations, 1985
World Medical Association
(Association Medicale Mondiale-AMM)
28, Avenue des Alpes,
F-01210 Ferney-Voltaire, France.

Current update published in:
Bulletin of PAHO 24(4), 1990: Appendix, 606-9

To call from the United States, dial the following numbers: 011-33-50-40-7575; FAX 011-33-50-40-5937.

AMA Policy: Support of Biomedical Research: The AMA endorses and supports the following ten principles considered essential if continuing support and recognition of biomedical research vital to the delivery of quality medical care is to be a national goal: (1) The support of biomedical research is the responsibility of both government and private resources. (2) The National Institutes of Health must be budgeted so that they can exert effective administrative and scientific leadership in the biomedical research enterprise. (3) An appropriate balance must be struck between support of project grants and of contracts. (4) Federal appropriations to promote research in specifically designated disease categories should be limited and made cautiously. (5) Funds should be specifically appropriated to train personnel on biomedical research. (6) Grants should be awarded under the peer review system. (7) The roles of the private sector and of government in supporting biomedical research are complementary. (8) Although the AMA supports the principle of committed federal support of biomedical research, the Association will not necessarily endorse all specific legislative and regulatory action that affects biomedical research. (9) To implement the objectives of section 8, the Board will establish mechanisms for continuing study, review and evaluation of all aspects of federal support of biomedical research. (10) The AMA will accept responsibility for informing the public on the relevance of basic and clinical research to the delivery of quality medical care.

Residents

Internship:Preparation or Hazing?

Norman Cousins "A Piece of My Mind"
JAMA. 1981 Jan 23/30; 245(4): 377

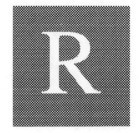

For the past two years, I have been privileged to visit medical schools and hospitals in various parts of the country. I have been able to meet with medical students and physicians at various stages in their training and their careers. The weakest link in the entire chain of physician training, it seems to me, is the ordeal known as the internship. More specifically, I refer to the theory that it is necessary to put medical school graduates through the meat grinder before they can qualify as full-fledged physicians. Putting it more delicately, the theory holds that anyone who wants to go into the medical profession must be given a rigorous and systematic exposure to the realities of the physician's life.

How does the internship prepare the physician for the "realities?" What if the "preparation" has the effect of dulling the sensitivities of the physician, or fostering feelings of resentment by an intern toward a patient who has a propensity for feeling his sharpest pains at 3 AM? What kind of judgment or scientific competence is it reasonable to expect of a physician who hasn't had any sleep for 32 hours? Is the workload at times not so much a sampling of later challenges as it is an exercise in what I can only describe only as disguised hazing at best and systematic desensitization at worst? Is it a good policy to subject seriously ill patients to treatment by physicians who are physically and emotionally exhausted? It was interesting and significant to me that the defense of the practice came from those who, having survived the experience, seemed determined not to permit others to escape. For the most part, however, I found that most physicians, on or off hospital staffs, saw little justification for the practice and, indeed, expressed serious reservations about it.

Some of the most productive discussions I had about the institution of the internship were in the open forums accompanying the grand rounds to which I was invited by various hospitals. Not infrequently, the subject of physician-patient relationship would come up. It wa recognized that the physician should take the initiative in this matter, to obtain the patient's full confidence as well as to promote confidence by the patient in his own healing system. Among the physician's useful attributes, it was generally agreed, was a supportive and compassionate attitude toward the patient.

It was at this point, however, that the discussion would break wide open. The physicians would generally say that the internship was hardly conducive to feelings of compassion toward patients. They pointed out that seeing patients under conditions of pressure and fatigue is no more satisfying for the physician than it is for the patient. One if the former interns would be certain to point out that having a man with a bloodstained knife come at you in the emergency room is enough to quiet the compassionate urgings in most doctors' souls. Another physician said he was ashamed to admit that he hoped (generally at 3AM) that his call-button-pressing patient would

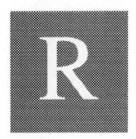

die before he got there. Compassion, apparently, is favored by circumstance.

In general, the most frequent question that was raised concerned public responsibility. How did the practice of 'round-the-clock medicine affect the patients themselves? One of the interns said it was difficult for him to see how medical administrators could defend themselves against charges of poor judgment by physicians on prolonged duty. At a time when the public is malpractice-suit prone, it would appear that the vulnerability of the hospital, medical school, or both to legal action would be sufficient to change the custom.

Over and above these specific problems is a matter I mentioned a moment ago: to what extent do the burdens placed on the interns come more under the heading of hazing than conditioning? Is a harsh and punitive attitude by some residents toward interns an essential part of the training of young physicians? Is it possible that some residents enjoy and exploit their power over the newcomers? Does hazing of this sort reflect credit on the profession? Is it really necessary?
The custom of overworking interns has long since outlived its usefulness. It doesn't lead to the making of better physicians. It is inconsistent with the public interest. It is not really worthy of the tradition of medicine.

National Association of Residents and Interns
292 Madison Ave., New York, NY 10017
800/221-2168

National Resident Matching Program
2450 N Street, NW, Suite 201,
Washington, DC 20037
202/828-0676

Intern: Historically "intern" was used to designate individuals in the first post-MD year of hospital training; less commonly it designated individuals in the first year of any residency program. Since 1975 the Directory of Graduate Medical Education Programs and the ACGME have not used the term, instead referring to individuals in their first year of training as residents.

Residents: An individual at any level of graduate medical education in a program accredited by the ACGME. Trainees in subspecialty programs are specifically included.

Fellow: A term used by some hospitals and in some specialties to designated trainees in subspecialty GME programs. The Directory of Graduate Medical Education Programs and the ACGME use of "resident" to designate all GME trainees in ACGME-accredited programs. (GME)

Statistics
JAMA Article of Note: Ration of First-year positions to Residents in Selected Larger Specialties for 1981, 1986 and 1991
JAMA.1992 Sept 2;268(9):1098

Respiratory Therapy
History: The occupation of respiratory therapist has experienced rapid growth. Prior to June 1972, the AMA evaluated and approved 18-month (two academic year) programs for the preparation of inhalation therapy technicians.

In the annual meeting in December 1972, the American Association for Inhalation Therapy (AAIT) changed its name to the American Association for Respiratory Therapy (AART). On July 1, 1974, the National Board for Respiratory Therapy (NBRT) assumed responsibility for credentialing qualified respiratory therapy technicians and respiratory therapists.

In the Essentials of an Approved Educational Program for the Respiratory Therapy Technician and the Respiratory Therapist adopted in June 1972, the requirements for a one-year technician program and a two-year therapist program were combined into a single document.

Experience after the Essentials were adopted in 1972 led to a differentiation between the two levels of occupation. Two separate sets of Essentials were drafted, one for the respiratory therapy technician and another for the respiratory therapist. The revisions of the 1972 document were developed under the leadership of the Joint Review Committee for Respiratory Therapy Education, in consultation with the four sponsoring organizations: American Association for Respiratory Therapy, American College of Chest Physicians, American Society of Anesthesiologists, and the American Thoracic Society. All of the organizations sponsoring the review committee subsequently adopted the revised document.

The AMA Council on Medical Education held two open hearings on the Essentials, in June and September of 1977, and the Essentials were widely distributed to assure adequate input from the community of interests. The Council on Medical Education adopted the Essentials at its September 1977 meeting.

In 1986, the Essentials for both occupations were once again consolidated in a single document, and the revision was adopted by all participating bodies.

Respiratory Therapist
Occupational Description: The respiratory therapist applies scientific knowledge and theory to practical clinical problems of respiratory care. The respiratory therapist is qualified to assume primary responsibility for all respiratory care modalities, including the supervision of respiratory therapy technician functions. The respiratory therapist may be required to exercise considerable independent clinical judgment, under the supervision of a physician, in the respiratory care of patients.

Job Description: In fulfillment of the therapist role, the respiratory therapist may:

1. Review, collect, and recommend obtaining additional data. The therapist evaluates all data to determine the appropriateness of the prescribed respiratory care, and participates in the development of the respiratory care plan.

2. Select, assemble, and check all equipment used in providing respiratory care.

3. Initiate and conduct therapeutic procedures, and modify prescribed therapeutic procedures to achieve one or more specific objectives.

4. Maintain patient records and communicate relevant information to other members of the health care team.

5. Assist the physician in performing special procedures in a clinical laboratory, procedure room, or operating room.

Employment Characteristics: Respiratory therapy personnel are employed in hospital, nursing care facilities, clinics, physicians' offices, companies providing emergency oxygen services, and municipal organizations.

According to the 1990 CAHEA Annual Supplemental Survey, entry level salaries average $23,116.

Respiratory Therapy Technician

Occupational Description: The respiratory therapy technician administers general respiratory care. Technicians may assume clinical responsibility for specified respiratory care modalities involving the application of well defined therapeutic techniques under the supervision of a respiratory therapist and a physician.

Job Description: In fulfillment of the technician role, the respiratory therapy technician may:

1. Review clinical data, history, and respiratory therapy orders.

2. Collect clinical data by interview and examination of the patient. This will include portions of the data by inspection, palpation, percussion, and auscultation of the patient.

3. Recommend and/or perform and review additional bedside procedures, x-rays, and laboratory tests.

4. Evaluate data to determine the appropriateness of the prescribed respiratory care.

5. Assemble and maintain equipment used in respiratory care.

6. Assure cleanliness and sterility by the selection and/or performance of appropriate disinfecting techniques, and monitoring their effectiveness.

7. Initiate, conduct, and modify prescribed therapeutic procedures.

Employment Characteristics: Respiratory therapy personnel are employed in hospitals, nursing care facilities, clinics, doctor's offices, companies providing emergency oxygen services, and municipal organizations.

According to the 1990 CAHEA Annual Supplemental Survey, entry level salaries average $19,254.

AMA Allied Health Department
312/464-4628

American Association for Respiratory Care
11030 Ables Lane, Dallas, TX 75229
214/243-2272

Retinitis Pigmentosa
National Retinitis Pigmentosa Foundation
1401 Mt. Royal Ave., 4th Floor,
Baltimore, MD 21217
800/638-2300; 301/225-9400 (in MD)

Retired Physicians
American Medical Association
Senior Physicians Services
(Formerly American Association of
Senior Physicians)
515 N. State Street, Chicago, IL 60610
312/464-2460

Retirement
American Association of Retired Persons
601 E Street, NW., Washington, DC 20049
202/434-2277

Review Courses
These programs are not affiliated with the AMA and their appearance in this directory does not constitute an endorsement nor an approval by the AMA.

ArcVentures, Inc.
Educational Services
820 W. Jackson Blvd, Chicago, IL 60607
312/258-5290

Sites available:
Chicago 312/258-5290
New Jersey 201/712-0897
Miami 305/530-1930
Los Angeles 213/258-5290

N.B.F.M. Review Course
Drew/UCLA School of Medicine
PO Box 66762, Los Angeles, CA 90066
213/563-5879 or 213/447-1262

National Medical School Review
c/o University of California, Irvine
Student Curricular Affairs, Med. Surg I - Room 125
Irvine, CA 92717
714/476-6282

Postgraduate Medical Review Education, Inc.
PO Box 414174, Miami Beach, FL 33141
800/433-3539

Stanley H. Kaplan
810 Seventh Ave, New York, NY 10019
212/492-5810, 800/527-8378

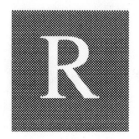

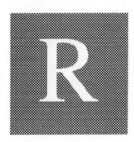

Reye's Syndrome

A rare disorder characterized by brain and liver damage following an upper respiratory tract infection, chicken-pox, or influenza. Reye's syndrome is almost entirely confined to children under age 15.

Causes

Evidence suggests that Reye's syndrome is often (but not invariably) related to taking aspirin for a viral infection. Physicians recommend that children be given acetaminophen instead of aspirin for viral infections or fever of unknown origin.

Symptoms and Signs

Reye's syndrome develops as the child is recovering from the infection, starting with uncontrollable vomiting, often with lethargy, memory loss, disorientation, or delirium. Swelling of the brain may cause seizures, deepening coma, disturbances in heart rhythm, and cessation of breathing. Jaundice indicates severe liver involvement.(ENC)

American Reye's Syndrome Association Disbanded (merged with National Reye's Syndrome Foundation)

National Reye's Syndrome Foundation
426 N. Lewis, Box 829, Bryan, OH 43506
800/233-7393 (outside OH)
800/231-7399 (in OH)

Rheumatism

American College of Rheumatology
17 Executive Park Dr. N.E., Suite 480, Atlanta, GA 30329
404/633-3777

Board Certification
American Board of Internal Medicine
3624 Market St., Philadelphia, PA 19104
215/243-1500
800/441-ABIM (800/441-2246)

Rhinology

American Rhinologic Society
Penn Park Medical Center
2929 Baltimore, Ste 105, Kansas City, MO 64108
816/561-4423

American Laryngological, Rhinological and Otological Society
PO Box 155, Bethesda Church Road, East Greenville, PA 18041
215/679-7180

Runaway Hotline

Missing Child Hotline
800/843-5678 9 a.m.-Midnight

National Center for Missing and Exploited Children
2101 Wilson Blvd. Suite 550, Arlington, VA 22201
703/235-3900

Runaway Hotline
800/231-6946

Rural Health

Daddy

William H. Hunter, MD "A Piece of My Mind"
JAMA. 1984 May 4: 251(17): 2184

Back in 1953 I had just begun my practice in the small town of Clemson at the foot of the Blue Ridge Mountains in South Carolina, In the beginning I spent a lot of time reading medical journals and waiting for the local people to find out I was in town.

One August evening near dusk, my wife, Jane, and I were sitting in the swing when two farmers approached the porch and asked: "You the new doctor?" I nodded.

"Well, Doc, Daddy's down and sick and the doctor we called isn't treating him right."

"What's the matter?"

"This here doctor wants to put Daddy in a hospital."

I asked what he'd been treating him for.

"He hadn't been treating him for nothin'. Last time Daddy had a doctor was in '33, when he fell out of the loft and broke his leg."

"Well, what did the doctor say was the matter?" I asked.

"He said Daddy was havin' a heart attack, and damned if he was gonna treat him at home. He wanted to take him down to the hospital in Anderson, Doc. That's 20 miles away. Are you comin' to see him or we just gonna stand here and talk?"

So, after going by my office and getting my new ECG machine that had never been used on a sick patient, I followed their truck up through the rolling hills toward the foot of the mountains.

This was the most beautiful country in the world, covered with small and middle-sized farms inhabited by very independent people. They'd come from Celtic stock and had been there since they drove out the Cherokee in 1781 (after the Indians came out for King George). They were fiercely loyal to each other, shared a common dislike for revenuers, voted Republican in a Democratic state, and yet were the most hospitable people I'd ever met. Pickens County, South Carolina, had produced more Congressional Medal of Honor recipients than any other in the United States, and while there's no record, they probably had more court-martialings as well.

"Daddy," whom I was going to see, turned out to be the patriarch of this part of the country. When we arrived, there were about 50 people standing around under the white oaks. Daddy raised himself from his bed, gasping a bit. He gave me a look that said: "Is this the best those boys could do? Guess I'll just have to put up with him."

He was 76 years old. The ECG confirmed a myocardial infarction with numerous PVCs, and there were wet rales in both lung bases. I was six weeks out of what I thought was a good internship in one of the best teaching hospitals in the

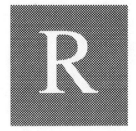

Carolinas, but I wasn't prepared for this. My looks must have betrayed me (Celtic types read a lot into looks), because Daddy gasped: "Doc, I was born in this house, lived here all my life, and I'm gonna die in this house. You just do the best you can."

I sent for an oxygen tank and sent Jane to the hospital for heparin. I used mercuhydrin intravenously and sat by his bed poking nitroglycerin into him and injecting Demerol until about 1 AM, when he was finally free of pain and his lungs began to clear. I went back out on the porch for some fresh air and saw more than 100 people had gathered under the trees. When I left at sunrise, many of them were still there.

I'm sure, deep down, that Daddy's recovery had more to do with his tough constitution, but I got the credit. There's never been a want of patients in my practice since then. And from that time, I was always invited to their family reunions, where the preacher would sit on one side of Daddy and I sat on the other.

National Rural Health Association
301 East Armour Blvd., Suite 420,
Kansas City, MO 64111
816/756-3140

National Health Service Corps Headquarters
(recruiting physicians for rural areas)
5600 Fishers Lane, Rockville, MD 20857
301/443-2900

Rural Information Center Health Services (RICHS)
National Agricultural Library
Beltsville, MD 20705
301/344-2547
800/633-7701

Safety

AMA Policy. Prevention of Deaths and Injuries From Automobile Accidents: The AMA supports legislation, such as that passed in many states, mandating the use of seat belts for occupants of motor vehicles and supports legislation requiring the passive restraint of infants and children in motor vehicles.
Motor Vehicle Accidents: The AMA (1) recognizes motor vehicle-related trauma as a major public health problem, the resolution of which requires a leadership role by physicians in concert with safety experts; and (2) strongly encourages other medical and health care organizations, as well as departments of health and transportation, to endorse the concept of motor vehicle related trauma as a public health problem, thereby lending its treatment to traditional public health measures.

Accomplices

Douglas S. Diekema, MD "A Piece of My Mind" JAMA. 1991 Feb 13;265(6): 802

The news coverage began with scenes of the tragedy, eerily illuminated by the flashing lights of emergency vehicles and the glow of floodlights that could not overcome the deeper shadows. A man, on top of the smashed vehicle, was trying to force his way into the wreckage.

Although disturbed by the scenes of the automobile accident, I was haunted most by a brief home video that immediately followed. Because it was shown on the 10-o'clock news by all the major television stations, I saw the home movie three times. I recognized two of its stars from the previous night, although I had known them only as dead bodies. My eyes fixed on the pretty young mother, smiling as her husband hammed in front of the camera. The scene shifted to a cheery bedroom, where the same man, the father, tickled his 6-week-old son. He made no effort to hide his pride in this recent addition to their young family. His wife sat quietly to the side until he playfully pulled her in front of the camera.

Each news program followed these images with a brief narrative of the tragedy - three people killed when their car was struck head-on by another vehicle whose driver was drunk. Each newscaster commented on the evils of drunk driving. But none seemed aware of the knowledge I held. None seemed to realize there had been accomplices.

I had difficulty clearing my mind as I picked up the telephone and tried to understand - a t 1 o'clock that morning - what the emergency room clerk was telling me. Slowly, some of her words began to penetrate. I was wanted downstairs. Fire rescue was six minutes away with two victims of a motor vehicle accident. Neither had a pulse. Neither was breathing. One was a baby. No other information was available. Could I please hurry. My nightmare.

Stumbling down the stairs, I began to review resuscitation medications and dosages. What size endotracheal tube would I need for the child? Anxiety greeted me in the faces of our small emergency room team. We don't see many babies with traumatic injuries.

I had two minutes to gather a few supplies, find an endotracheal tube I hoped would be small enough, and prepare myself for the worst. As I reached over to confirm that an intraosseous needle lay nearby, the emergency room entrance burst open. A frightened EMT ran through the door carrying a limp blue baby. He slid the small body onto a cart and backed away, apparently relived to be done with his part. The rest of us slipped into the rhythm of resuscitation: intubation, intraosseous line, large volumes of fluid, several rounds of drugs. Most of it is a blur to me now. As we waited for some response to the medications, the nurse to my left suggested I feel the head. Her eyes locked on mine as I touched the soft skin of this small child's head and felt the crushed skull. Holding back a rush of tears, I nodded. We had nothing more to offer.

My colleague had declared the father dead even before we ended our efforts. Word arrived that the mother, the driver, had died at the university hospital across town. The driver of the other car had a few bruises and cuts but would be fine. His intoxicated state had not prevented him from putting on his seat belt.

As I sat in the television's glow, tears of anger joined those of sadness. My frustration with the victims unnerved me. One small detail, provided us by the sheriff soon after our failed resuscitation attempt, greatly magnified this tragedy. He had found the infant's car seat 70 feet from the smashed vehicle. Obviously it has not been secured, nor had it carried the baby. Rescue workers had discovered the infant while removing his father from the car. The child had apparently been riding on his father's lap as the family returned from a visit with Grandpa and Grandma. Neither parent had been restrained. The baby had been crushed between his father and the passenger side of the dashboard.

The young family I had watched on television, so alive with joy and love, could have done nothing about the fact that a drunk driver would cross their path on cold December evening. But the truth was that they had failed to protect themselves and their baby from the encounter they couldn't prevent. If grieved me that they had been accomplices.

Physicians being asked to promote safety belt use

Rebecca Voelker AMNews4/15/91 p.3+

Ties linking medical, public health and law enforcement issues are taking new shape in the 1990s. One of the more prominent is about three inches wide with a silver buckle at its end.

Even though automobile safety belt use in the United States has risen drastically in the past decade, physicians are being urged to take a more active role in promoting their use.

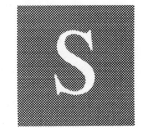

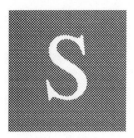

"This is still viewed as a safety matter, not a public health issue," said Kenneth Kizer, MD, MPH, director of the California Dept. of Health Services. "We need to push this farther into physicians' consciousness that it is not just a technical thing that cars have and that the highway patrol worries about."

In fact, Dr. Kizer wrote in last month's Western Journal of Medicine, safety belt promotion offers physicians one of the most economical and effective ways to boost the public's health and save lives.

According to the National Safety Council, injuries from motor vehicle accidents kill more than 47,000 people and disable another 1.8 million each year. The National Highway Traffic Safety Administration reports that motorists who wear safety belts are half as likely to be killed or seriously injured as those who don't. Similarly, belted motorists reduce by two-thirds the chances they will be hospitalized after a traffic accident.

Given the statistics, Dr. Kizer called safety belts "impressive prophylaxis," However, preventive measures do little good unless they are prescribed for those who need them most.

Dr. Kizer said physicians should direct special efforts toward teen-age drivers because they are at especially high risk of being injured in an automobile accident, and often have little contact with health care workers. He suggested speaking at schools, youth clubs and athletic groups to get the message across.

High-risk groups primarily are men younger than 25, individuals with low income and education levels, recent immigrants and some ethnic and minority groups, including blacks and hispanics.

One of the most effective ways for physicians to promote safety belt use is by asking in a health-risk assessment whether parents buckle up and use car seats with infants and children.

Not only should patients be reminded that safety belt use doubles their chances of surviving a car crash, Dr. Kizer advised that physicians reiterate the following truisms:

- Attempting to brace oneself in a 30-mph collision is the same as catching a 300-pound bag of cement dropping from a second-story window.
- Children held in arms or on laps are likely to be crushed against the dash or thrown from the vehicle in an accident.
- Even in fires and submersions, belted motorists are more likely to survive because they have a greater chance of remaining conscious.

In recent surveys physicians have ranked safety belt use high among health promotion habits they feel are important. In some of the literature, however, physicians have indicated they don't feel very effective in persuading patients to wear them.

Walter Larimore, MD, a family physician in Kissimmee, Fla., is trying to put that conflict into some perspective in a study with 13 physicians and their patients in rural areas of the Florida panhandle.

Eight of the 13 have gone through training and will employ interventions of no more than 40 seconds that encourage patients to use safety belts. Those 1,200 patients will be contacted at three months and six months to gauge their seat belt use. Their habits will be compared with those of 800 control patients.

"We want to know more about where physicians should focus their attention," said Dr. Larimore. "It's just a hypothesis, but it could be that our largest potential is, as organized medicine, to encourage federal and state laws" that would allow police to ticket drivers solely for failing to wear safety belts.

In the 37 states with mandatory safety belt laws, most are enforced as secondary violations in which motorists are stopped for more serious infractions. However, said Dr. Larimore, in nations where neglecting to buckle up is a violation in and of itself, compliance is often as high as 90%.

According to the National Highway Traffic Safety Administration, the 1989 compliance rate in this country was 46% overall, 50% in cities with safety belt laws and 33% in cities with no such law.

"Even though this doesn't seem very medical, it should be an important part of preventive medicine," said Gerald Keller, MD, a Mandeville, La., family physician and chairman of the American Academy of Family Physicians' (AAFP) Commission of Public Health and Scientific Affairs.

"Probably not enough physicians have taken notice of this, so we've got to make them more comfortable to say to patients, 'Do you smoke, drink, use seat belts?'" Dr. Keller said.

AAFP offers brochures, patient chart stickers, doorknob hangers and a comic book that promote safety belt use. For more information contact, AAFP, 8880 Ward Parkway, Kansas City. Mo. 64114.

Auto Safety Hotline
800/424-9393; 202/426-0123 (in Washington, DC)

Center for Safety in the Arts
5 Beekman St., New York, NY 10038
212/227-6220

Consumer Product Safety Commission
Washington, DC 20207
800/638-CPSC (800/638-2772)

National Child Safety Council
PO Box 1368, Jackson, MI 49204
800/222-1464

National Highway Traffic Safety Administration
HTS-10, US Department of Transportation
400 7th St., SW, Room 5130
Washington, DC 20590
202/426-9294

National Safety Council
1121 Spring Lake Drive, Itasca, IL 60143-3201
708/285-1121

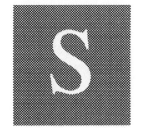

Sample Criteria

"Sample Criteria for Procedure Review:
Screening Criteria to Assist PSROS"
(#PB 81-179871)
"Reference Criteria for Short-Stay Hospital
Review" (#PB81-179889)

Order either from National Technical Information
Serivce (NTIS)
U.S. Dept. of Commerce
5285 Port Royal Rd., Springfield, VA 22161
703/487-4650

Sarcoidosis

Sarcoidosis Family Aid and Research Foundation
760 Clinton Avenue, Newark, NJ 07108
800/223-6429

School Health
School-Based Health Centers

In order to increase access to care, attention has
focused on using the school setting for health
centers. There are currently more than 120
school-based health centers that provide services
to adolescents who might not otherwise receive
such care[1].

The success of school-based health centers
reflects in part their flexibility, parent support, easy
access, no cost or low cost to students,
partnership with school staff and community
services, and student involvement.[2]

Controversy surrounding school-based health
centers revolves around issues of reproduction,
including counseling and the distribution of
contraception devices or prescription. However,
only 20% of total visits to school-based health
programs are for family planning services.[1]

Almost 9 of 10 (87%) physicians report that they
would refer adolescents to a clinic devoted strictly
to adolescent health services.[3]

A majority of physicians (63%) believe 15- to
17-year-olds should be able to consult a physician
privately without parents being informed of the
nature or outcome of the visit. Thirty-nine percent
approve of 12- to 14-year-olds visiting physicians
without parents being informed.

Highlights of AMA policy recommendations on
school-based health centers

The AMA recognizes the promise of school-based
health centers to provide health services to
adolescents, particularly in medically underserved
areas. Where school-based health services exist,
they should meet the following minimum
standards:

- Health services in schools must be supervised
  by a physician, preferably one who is
  experienced in the care of children and
  adolescents. Additionally, a physician should be
  accessible to administer care on a regular basis.
- On-site services should be provided by a
  professionally prepared school nurse or similarly
  qualified health professional. Expertise in child
  and adolescent development, psychosocial and
  behavioral problems, and emergency care is
  desirable. Responsibilities of this professional
  would include coordinating the health care of

students with the student, the parents, the
school, and the student's personal physician,
and assisting with the development and
presentation of health education programs in the
classroom.
- There should be a written policy to govern
  provision of health services in the school,
  developed by a school health council consisting
  of school and community-based physicians and
  nurses, school faculty and administrators,
  parents and (as appropriate) students,
  community leaders, and others.
- Before patient services begin, policies on
  confidentiality should be established with the
  advice of expert legal advisors and the school
  health council.
- Policies for ongoing monitoring, quality
  assurance, and evaluation should be
  established and executed.
- Health care services should be available during
  school hours. During other hours an appropriate
  referral system should be instituted.
- School-based health programs should draw on
  outside resources for care, such as private
  practitioners, public health and mental health
  clinics, and mental health and neighborhood
  health programs.
- Services provided should be coordinated to
  ensure comprehensive care. Parents should be
  encouraged to be intimately involved in the
  health supervision and education of their
  children.[1]

References:
1. AMA Council on Scientific Affairs. Providing medical
services through school-based health programs. JAMA
261() 1989: 1939-42.
2. Lear JG, Swerdlow J, Lewin ME, Van Wert J. Making
connections: A summary of Robert Wood Johnson
Foundation Programs of Adolescents. Princeton, NJ: The
Robert Wood Johnson Foundation.
3. Harvey, LK, Shubat SC. Physician and public attitudes
on health care issues, 1989 edition. Chicago: American
Medical Association. 1989. (ADL)

American School Health Association
P.O. Box 708, Kent, OH 44240
216/678-1601

Science

American Association for the
Advancement of Science
1333 H St., N.W., Washington, D.C. 20005
202/326-6400

National Science Foundation
1800 G Street, N.W., Washington, DC 20550
202/357-9498

Scleroderma

United Scleroderma Foundation, Inc.
PO Box 350, Watsonville, CA 95077
408/728-2202 (in CA)
800/722-HOPE (outside CA)

Scoliosis

National Scoliosis Foundation
P.O. Box 547, 93 Concord Ave.
Belmont, MA 02178
617/489-0880

The Scoliosis Association
P.O. Box 51353, Raleigh, NC 27609
919/846-2639

Scuba

Handicapped Scuba Association
116 W. El Portal, Ste 104
San Clemente, CA 92672
714/498-6128

Divers Alert Network (DAN) scuba accident hotline
Hall Laboratory for Environmental Science
Duke University Medical Center
Durham, NC 27710
919/684-8111

Second Opinion (For Patients)

Second Opinion Hotline
(Department of Health and Human Services)
800/638-6833
800/492-6603 (Maryland)

For free brochure, write:
Surgery Department
Department of Health & Human Services
Washington, DC 20201

Self Help

AMA Examines Roles of Self-Help Groups

Hannah L. Hedrick, PhD
adapted from "The Reporter" February 1992

For the past decade, the American Medical Association has been in the vanguard of associations willing to examine the benefits of self-help groups and has increasingly recognized them as one of many established helping methods. AMA policies, publications and activities have supported the study of self-help in educational programs and have increased the number of professional researchers and writers who understand groups and their role in the health care system.

At the corporate level, the AMA Employee Assistance Program refers employees, as appropriate, to self-help groups. The AMA has also sponsored support groups for smoking cessation, nutrition and weight loss, expectant mothers and the Persian Gulf conflict. These autonomous grassroots self-help groups, which operate without professional control and without a great deal of professional involvement, reflect the maturing of a movement that came of age during the 1980s.

Throughout that decade, the *Journal of the American Medical Association* and *American Medical News* were among the varied publications - including *Chicago Medicine, Good Housekeeping, New Woman, the New York Times, The New Yorker, Newsweek, Population*

Reports, Psychology Today, The Wall Street Journal The Washington Post and World Medical News - that featured articles on the benefits of self-help groups.

Phil Donahue, Ann Landers, Oprah Winfrey and other media figures refer frequently to the benefits provided by peer support groups in dealing with a multitude of problems. Almost all of the national and local docudramas on the "disease of the week," depicted people affected by AIDS, Alzheimer's disease, cancer, child abuse, domestic violence, mental illness, etc., involve and promote a successful self-help group.

Self-help groups typically exhibit the following characteristics and benefits:

Common Problem: Members immediately identify with one another.

Mutual Aid/Helper Therapy: Members benefit as much from giving help as from receiving it.

Network for Support: Members provide a network of emotional and social support through regular and special gatherings, telephone calls. newsletters, visits and computers.

Shared Information: Through the group process and written material, members capture and share their successful techniques for coping.

Low Cost: Expenses are shared through collections at meetings, minimal membership dues or fundraising projects.

Unconditional Acceptance: Members are usually encouraged to share their personal situations in a nonjudgmental, caring environment.

"Prosumer" Concept: Self-help group members frequently acquire a special ability to help, based on their development as both consumers and professionals ("prosumers") in the area of their problem.

Increasing Support in AMA Policies

Examination of and support for the self-help group movement has not been happenstance. An early blueprint for action vis-a-vis the contributions of self-help groups to public health appeared in the AMA report of The Health Policy Agenda for the American People (271 pages; 1987). The report emanated from a 5-year collaborative effort involving 172 health-related, business, government and consumer groups; the project was coordinated and largely financed by the AMA. Dissemination of information about self-help groups and regional coordination of self-help efforts was cited in conjunction with reducing disease and injury and promoting healthy behaviors. The report advised self-help groups to "make their presence known in the community through coalitions to develop and distribute regional directories" and establish clearinghouses "as a means of integrating these efforts at the state level."

This important policy was among the AMA contributions to the self-help movement reported by the AMA vice president for medical education, Carlos J.M. Martini, MD, at the 1989 Symposium on the Impact of Life Threatening Condition:

Self-Help Groups and Health Care Providers in Partnership, which was co-sponsored and co-chaired by the AMA. Martini summarized the many self-help group activities coordinated or supported by AMA staff at the national level, including:

- featuring self-help programs and open meetings at the National Leadership Conference, the National Conference for Impaired Professionals and other meetings;
- initiating and participating in the 1978 Surgeon General's Workshop on Self-Help and Public Health;
- using AMA publications to promote the involvement of health and human service providers in self-help groups; and
- providing leadership to the National Council on Self-Help and Public Health.

National Self-Help Clearinghouse
25 W. 43rd, Rm. 620, New York, NY 10036
212/642-2944

Self-Help Centers, Statewide

California Self-Help Center
UCLA. Department of Psychiatry
405 Hilgard Ave. Los Angeles, CA 90024-1563
1-800-222-LINK (CA only) or 310-825-1799

Connecticut Self-Help/Mutual Support Network
389 Whitney Ave. New Haven, CT 06511
203-789-7645

Illinois Self-Help Center
1600 Dodge Ave, #S-122, Evanston, IL 60201
708/328-0470

Iowa Self-Help Clearinghouse
Iowa Pilot Parents, Inc.
33 N. 12th St., P.O. Box 1151
Fort Dodge, IA 50501
1-800-383-4777 (IA only) or 515-576-5870

(Kansas) Self-Help Network
Campus Box 34
Wichita State University, Wichita, KS 67208-1595
1-800-445-0116 (KS only) or 316-689-3843

Massachusetts Clearinghouse of
Mutual Help Groups
Massachusetts Cooperative Extension
University of Massachusetts
113 Skinner Hall, Amherst, MA 01003
413-545-2313

Michigan Self-Help Clearinghouse
Michigan Protection and Advocacy Services, Inc.
106 W. Allegan #210, Lansing, MI 48933-1706
1-800-752-5858 (MI only) or 517-484-7373

(Minnesota) First Call for Help
166 E. 4th St., #310, St. Paul, MN 55101
612-224-1133

(Nebraska) Self-Help Information Services
1601 Euclid Ave., Lincoln, NE 68502
402-476-9668

New Jersey Self-Help Clearinghouse
St. Clares-Riverside Medical Center
25 Pocono Rd. Denville, NJ 07834
1-800-367-6274 (NJ only) or 201-625-9565

Texas Self-Help Clearinghouse
Mental Health Association in Texas
8401 Shoal Creek Blvd, Austin, TX 78758-7544
512-454-3706

Selling a Medical Practice

Sample Letter to Notify Patients of Practice Transfer

[Date]

Dear Patients [personalize if computer data base system permits]:

This letter is to inform you that I am leaving active practice on _____, 19____. I write this letter with mixed emotions because caring for you and all of my patients has been a great source of satisfaction and pleasure. I have made the decision because

_____

Since my concern for you is that you continue to receive the same kind of personal medical care that I have tried to provide you over the years, I am very pleased to announce that Dr. _____ will be taking over my practice. [Insert effective data if appropriate.

Doctor _____ comes to the practice with excellent credentials. [He/she] is a graduate of _____

medical school and received [his/her] residency training in _____ at _____. We share the same philosophies about the practice of medicine and it is reassuring to me to leave my practice in the hands of such a competent physician.

I am also happy to inform you that [office manager, medical assistant, nurse, etc.] will continue in the office. When you wish to make appointments just call the same telephone number _____and speak with_____.

I believe you will find Doctor _____ to be not only well trained but very compassionate and attentive to your needs.

You do not have an obligation to accept Dr. _____

as your physician. If you wish, you may request that your records be transferred to another physician. If so, we will need an authorization form from you. If you elect to be treated by Doctor _____, you can authorize the release of your records to [him/her] from my files on your next visit to our office.

Let me take this opportunity to thank you for your many years of loyalty and friendship. It has been a pleasure to serve as your personal physician. My [wife/husband], _____,

and I extend our best wishes to you for your future health and happiness.

Sincerely,

_____, MD
(BUY)

Decisions For Buyers And Sellers

The Selling Physician Must:

- conclude that he or she does want to sell the practice, weighing the pros and cons very carefully. This is not a decision to be made lightly or swiftly.
- establish appropriate, realistic values for both the tangible and intangible assets that collectively comprise the practice entity. This is not a simple task. Each medical practice is a unique enterprise. Many of the value judgments about intangible assets must necessarily be subjective. Other judgments about certain tangible assets can be made using different guidelines or formulae. The question is: What are these methods and which ones should be applied in given instances?
- market the practice properly to attract a willing buyer able to assume the financial obligations of purchase. The selling physician must carefully evaluate potential buying physicians to assure a good personal "fit" with the practice.

The selling physician also has some other important decisions to make. Does he or she want a clear "walk-away" sale or a more leisurely phase-out? If the physician opts for the second approach, then rather than finding a buyer to take over the practice immediately, the physician may need an associate. The associate could work with the senior physician for a period of time, usually from one to five years.

The same kind of arrangement may be worked out with a larger practice. An associate may join a practice that has more than one physician with the ultimate goal of replacing a retiring senior physician.

An arrangement of this type - a younger associate coming in to join an older one planning to retire - often has considerable appeal to both physicians. The new associate can consolidate a relationship with existing patients, become established, and reap full advantage of the retiring physician's goodwill. Ways of working out such a practice transfer are discussed in greater detail in Chapters 8,9, and 10, on negotiations, putting agreements into writing, and opportunities in groups and partnerships.

The Buying Physician Must:

- conclude that he or she does want to buy a practice. This is a highly involved process that must take into consideration a host of preferences about lifestyle, career goals, practice location, type of practice sought - solo, partnership, or group, the demographics of the practice location, and many other personal factors. Critical to the final decision is the buying physician's ability to finance a purchase.
- assess the potential practice from all possible angles, particularly its growth potential. Of great importance to buyer as well as to seller is the personal fit with the practice mentioned earlier.
- determine whether the values established by the seller for the various elements in the practice provide a reasonable and appropriate basis for price negotiations.

Both Buyer and Seller Must:

- work through a series of negotiation - sometimes adversarial in nature - as each tries to achieve the maximum desired advantage in the agreement.
- negotiate a complex legal agreement in which values are hammered out for tangible assets, such as equipment, furniture, supplies, accounts receivable, leases, and sometimes property, and for intangibles that are collectively dubbed "goodwill."
- handle tax allocations related to the buy/sell agreement.
- discuss and dispose of any liabilities in the practice, hidden or overt.
- agree on payment arrangements.
- effect transfer of the practice and its assets to the buyer.
- sometimes negotiate a covenant that the seller will not compete.
- specify conditions under which the selling physician will assist the buying physician in taking over the practice.

Obviously, buying or selling a practice is not simplistic. A great deal of money will ride on the final negotiations as will the future of the physician who buys the practice. A Physician involved in such negotiations would be well advised to accumulate all the information possible. He or she also would be wise to use the services of professionals familiar with buying and selling medical practices. It is a very special sale.(BUY)

Sex Education Report
"Guidelines for Comprehensive Sexuality Education"
National Guidelines Task Force
c/o Sex Information and Education
Council of the US(SIECUS)
130 W. 42nd, Suite 2500, New York, NY 10036
212/819-9770; FAX 212/819-9776

Sex and the Physician
Harold I. Lief, M.D.

Dealing with sexual problems of patients is an important part of medical practice and should be a significant concern of almost all physicians. When physicians are comfortable about inquiring into the sexual lives of their patients and when they take the initiative be asking appropriate questions, sexual problems are discovered in 15 to 50 per cent of patients, depending upon the type of practice.[1] Although sexual problems are rarely if ever fatal, many thousands of people are deeply troubled, anxious and depressed because of them. Marital disruption, even divorce, commonly results from untreated sexual problems.

Not all sexual problems confronting the physician are the usual sexual dysfunction, such as premature ejaculation and impotence in men or

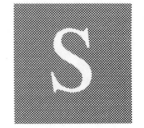

orgasmic dysfunction in women. Conflicts over sexual behavior, such as frequency, oral sex and coital positions, are even more common and sometimes more troublesome.[2] Sexual concerns resulting from illness and from medical procedures, such as hysterectomy, mastectomy and colostomy, also require counseling. Physical disorders may bring about sexual dysfunction; diabetes is the most common of these, but there are many others that may adversely affect sexual function. Medications, such as those used to treat hypertension, often cause sexual dysfunction.[3]

Unlike most other subjects in medical practice, sexuality often creates intense feelings in physicians. Because sex is a private and intimate subject, physicians are likely to be uncomfortable when taking a sexual history until they become experienced in treating patients with sexual problems.

Tendencies to regard sexual behavior as good or bad, important or unimportant - in short, values - are significant considerations. Probably more than in any other dimension of practice, values and ethics have to be taken into account - the physician's as well as the patient's. The physician must recognize that he has sexual values or preferences and that these may differ from those of the patient. The influences - intended and unintended - of these values will be discussed elsewhere in this volume.

In dealing with sexual problems, the physician has a splendid opportunity to practice preventive as well as therapeutic medicine. By assisting a young patient to overcome sexual anxieties and inhibitions, he helps prepare that person for satisfactory relationships throughout life, perhaps eventually for marriage. By counseling a married couple, enabling them to obtain greater mutuality and sexual pleasure, the physician reduces marital discord and may even prevent divorce and its emotional and physical sequelae for the couple and their children.

Marital unhappiness, separation and divorce have been implicated as causative factors in a variety of illnesses, especially depression, which, in turn, often contributes to many diseases. Somers quotes a report of the National Institute of Mental Health: "The single most powerful predictor of stress-related physical as well as emotional illness is marital disruption."[4] Helping patients with sexual problems is more than enriching, important as that is: It is good medical care because, by reducing one of the most common sources of human suffering, it helps prevent illness, the uprooting of families and the resultant social disorganization.

Most sexual problems brought to the attention of physicians, especially to family physicians, are those of couples. Some of these problems are primary causes of marital dysfunction. Most are consequences of other kinds of marital discord and, in turn, perpetuate and increase marital unhappiness. It seems reasonable, then, to make sex counseling and marriage counseling a "package" in the training of physicians and the delivery of medical care. Training in sex and marriage counseling is a logic requisite for primary care physicians - those practicing internal medicine, family medicine and obstetrics/gynecology. It is logical even in pediatrics, for it helps the practitioner to recognize

the connections between the parent's relationship and a child's sexual problems. An example of such a connection is the covertly seductive father of a teenage daughter, abetted by a sexually repressed wife, who interferes with the separation that is necessary for a girl in her early adolescence to transfer attachment from her father to male peers.

Sex counseling and couple counseling are not the only ways the physician can practice preventive medicine. Early intervention can occur in many other sexually related clinical situations, such as unwanted teenage pregnancies, premarital counseling, family-planning services during pregnancy, postpartum care and family-life education for teenagers and young adults. The pediatrician and obstetrician, dealing with children and adolescents or with young parents, have excellent opportunities to practice effective preventive medicine.

Physician's Attitudes

There is general agreement that the physician's capacity to help his patient is a result of three primary factors: attitudes, skill and knowledge (sometimes called the ASK formula). Attitudes can inhibit or enhance the acquisition of skills and even of knowledge from physician to patient. In few other aspects of medical practice are attitudes more important than in caring for patients with sexual problems.

Physicians have been socialized as boys and men or as girls and women before they become medical students. Sexual feelings, beliefs and values stemming from a particular religious, ethnic and social-class background are often intense and firmly held; therefore, physicians cannot learn about sex in the same relatively dispassionate way that they can study the Krebs cycle. In all of us, an interplay between our beliefs or ideas about sexual functions and dysfunctions on the one hand, and our values or preferences on the other, determines what our attitudes will be.

If a future physician grows up believing that masturbation is sinful, for example, he will retain the value judgment in practice that it is bad; thus he might react strongly and negatively to a patient's discussion of masturbation. If the physician believes that masturbation is normal for unmarried males and females but abnormal and bad in marriage, that judgment would influence the discussion of masturbation with a married partner.

Society impresses on its members many sexual values, some of them so gradually and covertly that they are absorbed and accepted without awareness. In addition, every person has life experiences that subtly leave marks largely outside his conscious recognition. The physician who is unaware of his own moral values may unwittingly impose them on the patient. On the other hand, some physicians who are fully aware of their values also try to impose them on patients.

A physician who cannot countenance premarital intercourse under any circumstance is clearly a poor choice for a single girl seeking contraceptive help. The physician who, because of strong religious beliefs, unconsciously regards out-of-wedlock pregnancy as justified punishment

for premarital coitus may find it impossible to prescribe a contraceptive even for a girl who has already had an out-of-wedlock pregnancy. It is thus that physicians may project their own values onto the clinical situation.

Similarly, personal attitudes may be held toward such sexual behaviors as oral-genital and anal-genital intercourse, extramarital sex, homosexual practices, sexual expression among the elderly and group sex. Even the idea that women may enjoy and actively pursue sex was strange to many gynecologists until the 1960s.[5] If a physician believes that women are essentially passive and submissive and should be paced by the husband's sexual interests, his attitude toward a woman who reports that she took the initiative sexually and that she actively enjoys it probably affects the way he deals with her.

Every physician who wishes to be a competent sex counselor must try to discern his patients' values and to become more aware of his own. It doesn't matter whether the physician's values are more conservative or liberal than the patient's. The patient may become threatened and respond with shame or anger if the physician attempts to change the patient's values abruptly. A good physician-patient relationship depends on the clarification of values and of possible conflicts between those of the patient and the physician.

Ethical Issues and Concerns in Sex Counseling

Ethical issues in sex counseling in many ways are like those in other aspects of medical care - professional competence, responsible care, informed consent and confidentiality. However, the intimate nature of sexual function, the self-esteem affected by it and the strong emotions associated with it intensify the significance of such issues. There are also unique aspects of sex counseling (e.g., the enhanced possibility of erotic feelings arising in the patient or the physician, the way in which the patient's and/or physician's erotic feelings are managed) that make accompanying ethical issues an even more important consideration for the physician than they are in medical care in general.

Imposing Standards (Values).

Although the general rule is not to impose sexual standards on patients, the patient's values are the most significant factors in sexual inhibitions or symptoms. An inhibited couple's puritanical ideas may have kept their sexual pleasure minimal; their values and those of the physician are the keys to successful therapy. Some attitude change toward greater tolerance and permissiveness often occurs, as the physician tries to modify an archaic conscience and rigid standards of behavior. When it happens, it happens slowly, often as a by-product of treatment, rather than by value confrontation and imposition. Occasionally, however, explicit reference to the differences in values of patient and physician is necessary.

In many sex counseling situations, the physician often must take a permission-giving role; e.g,., permission to a couple to experiment with new behaviors so that they can expand and enrich their sexual experiences. However, the physician must be sensitive to his patients' values and extremely careful not to jeopardize their trust in

him by demanding that they behave in ways that are inimical to their values. The correct timing of interventions is most important; decisions about how and when to offer recommendations should be made on the basis of sensitivity and experience.

Value conflicts between sexual partners are common. The physician's neutrality by no means precludes his making these conflicts as explicit as possible in an attempt to reach a satisfactory resolution.

Competence.

The physician must judge whether he has the competence to undertake therapy in a given situation. Certainly, it is unethical for him to promise to deliver more than is possible; even the most skillful practitioners have their share of failures. A physician's competence increases with experience in an ongoing process; yet he has to be reasonably certain that he is not only willing to help, but that his skills are equal to the clinical task. The levels of competence - diagnostician, educator, counselor, and skilled therapist - are discussed in by Lief and guidelines are given for judging one's own level.[6]

Exploitation.

Exploitation may be financial or sexual. Financial exploitation occurs when the physician continues to treat beyond his level of competence or uses inappropriate therapy merely to retain the patient. Financial exploitation is possible in any clinical situation. Sexual exploitation is more of a possibility in sex counseling than in other forms of counseling or psychotherapy. Patients with sex problems are particularly vulnerable to seduction, and sometimes they themselves use seduction as a magical means of reassurance about being worthwhile, of gaining power over a person perceived as more dominating, or of overcoming inhibitions of sexual desire, excitement or orgasm. The physician who actively or passively engages in erotic contacts with his patient is violating the patient's trust, and there is a very strong likelihood that the patient will be psychically damaged, if not by the contact then by the termination of an illusory love relationship with the therapist. The few authors who claim that sex between patient and therapist is helpful to the patient are unconvincing.[7,8]

There is a "gray area" in which affectionate touching, hugging even kissing - the "laying -on of hands" in a parental way - may be misinterpreted by the patient as erotic. Malpractice suits have been based on such misconceptions. Without duly restraining his warmth and affection, the physician must be cautious about the degree and the manner in which he displays affection for a patient.

Special Therapeutic Techniques. Special techniques, such as the sexological examination and the use of surrogate partners, raise ethical issues. Both techniques are controversial. The physician without special training should not carry out these procedures, but he should know about them and the pitfalls that are involved. Very few sex therapists actually watch their patients during sexual encounters; that procedure, too, is highly questionable, and the physician is advised not to refer to therapists who use it. It is not only ethically controversial, but it involves invasion of privacy and has potential legal complications.

Recommending sexually explicit books or films is ethical, provided the physician has first determined what his patient's attitudes toward such material are, and provided he does not impose his values in an authoritarian way.

Confidentiality and Informed Consent.

Confidentiality and informed consent raise ethical issues as they do in other aspects of medicine, but feeling about violation may be more intense. Many patients would not want others to know about their reason for seeking help or that they are even undergoing sex therapy. The charged feelings that most people have make it mandatory that the physician explain in detail the procedures and methods he intends to use.

There is a full discussion of the ethical issues in sex therapy and research in the publications on sex ethics by Masters, et al.[9,10]

Sexual health care is requested by many patients and needed by many more who are too embarrassed to ask for it. A sensitive, thoughtful, caring physician can be of enormous help to such patients. Sexual problems cannot be ignored. Even the physician who is disinterested or uncomfortable with his part of medical care must be willing to listen, to inquire and to refer tactfully and competently. The interested physician who gradually acquires greater competence as a sex counselor will derive a great deal of satisfaction from his efforts - usually short term and often effective. Helping patients with sexual problems can, in fact, be one of the most gratifying aspects of practice.

References

1. Burnap DW, Golden JS: Sexual problems in medical practice. J Med Educ 1967; 42:673-680.
2. Frank E, et al: Frequency of sexual dysfunction in 'normal' couples. N Engl J Med 1978; 299:111-115.
3. Reichgott MJ: Problems of sexual function in patients with hypertension. Cardivasc Med 1979; 3:149-156.
4. Somers AR: Marital status, health, and use of health services. JAMA 1979; 241:1818-1822.
5. Scully D, Bart P: A funny thing happened on the way to the orifice: Women in gynecology text books. Am J Sociol 1973; 78:1045-1050.
6. Lief H: Sex education in medicine: Retrospect and prospect in Rosenweig N, Pearsall FP (eds): Sex Education for the Health Professional. New York, Grune & Stratton, 1978.
7. McCartney J: Overt transference. J Sex Res 1966; 2:227-237.
8. Shepard M: The Love Treatment: Sexual Intimacy Between Patients and Psychotherapist. New York, PH Wyden, 1971.
9. Masters WH, et al: Ethical Issues in Sex Therapy and Research, Vol 1. Boston, Little, Brown and Company, 1977.
10. Masters WH, et al: Ethical Issues in Sex Therapy and Research, Vol 2. Boston, Little, Brown and Company.
(SMP)

Office Procedures

Robert C. Long, M.D.

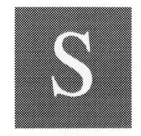

Leaders in the field of human sexuality commonly express the optinion that primary care physicians (family physicians, obstetrician-gynecologists and internists) should provide care to those couples who are experiencing sexual problems - even though these physicians, with infrequent exceptions, have had no specialized education in psychiatry, psychology, behavioral therapy or counseling beyond medical school. What is the justification for this belief which, on its face, does not seem to make much sense?

Physician-patient Relationship

Primary care physicians establish long-term relationships with many of their patients; these relationships may extend over two to three decades or even longer. No other health care practitioners are in such a unique position to intervene to prevent a self-perpetuating cycle of sexual anxiety. These physicians see patients at every stage of life and each encounter furnishes an opportunity to provide appropriate information on the varieties of normal sexual development and behavior. The opportunities to serve as a resource person, to practice preventive medicine, to maintain health, to treat illness and to counsel patients during times of stress are numerous. They occur daily.

In times of physical and emotional illness, most patients turn first to their family physician. Although most physicians perform creditably in response to their patients' health care needs, in the field of human sexuality they have failed. No physician, for example, would ignore mitral valve insufficiency or stenosis discovered on physical examination. He or she would either carry out appropriate diagnostic studies and therapy or refer the patient to an appropriate specialist. At the same time, however, this same otherwise competent physician ignores a specific sexual complaint. How can this behavior be explained?

There are several reasons. Many physicians separate sexual anxiety and dysfunction from the patient's general health status. This separation of sexual disease from other kinds of disease and activity is deeply rooted in our culture. Sex as a cause of illness has largely been ignored in medical education and practice. For example, most physicians, especially those in primary care, are familiar with the concept of psychosomatic medicine. Daily they encounter patients with somatic complaints whose origins lie in emotional stress. Yet all too infrequently do they recognize that how the patient feels about himself or herself as a sexual person and how he or she relates to others sexually provide a very common source of psychosomatic symptomatology. Fatigue, pelvic pain, mild depression, low back pain, headache, urinary tract symptoms, hyperacidity with or without ulcer formation and dyspareunia are commonly found in patients who lead sexual lives that they consider unsatisfactory.

Another reason for inattention to sexual problems by physicians is that many of them have never become comfortable with themselves as sexual persons. In this respect, they differ not a whit from the general population. Until recently it was

believed that the study of anatomy, physiology and pathology prepared a physician to deal with the sexual problems of others. This belief and the cultural tradition that sex is a taboo subject effectively blocked the teaching of human sexuality in medical schools until a decade or so ago. Lief reported that in 1961 only 3 of 82 medical schools offered courses in human sexuality;[1] today many of the 126 medical schools offer programs in this subject. This augurs well for the future, not only because primary care physicians will have a more solid academic background for treating sexual problems.

The point of all this is that most physicians are reared to believe that sex is evil, dirty or harmful. Consequently, the changing of attitudes that results in feeling comfortable about sex, and dealing comfortably with it in relation to ourselves and others, has to be a learned experience. A physician's inability to deal comfortably with sexual questions can have a devastating effect upon patients. Physician embarrassment blocks communication and further investigation, and the patient's belief that nothing helpful can be done is often reinforced.

Another reason given by primary care physicians for eschewing investigation of their patient's sexuality is a feeling of incompetence with the subject. In addition, many are fearful of doing harm. These reasons are legitimate but, for most physicians, the lack of competence can be rather easily overcome through participation in such continuing medical education courses as sexual attitude restructuring (SAR) and office management of sexual dysfunctions.

Management

Management encompasses four dimensions: time, adjunctive aids, record keeping and insurance.

Time. Time is said to be an important barrier to the inclusion of a marital-sexual history as part of the routine investigation of a person's health care status by primary care physicians. Although this may be true, I know of no data to substantiate the conclusion. I also believe that there is a general misconception concerning the amount of time needed to investigate sexual problems with patients.

The incorporation of a marital-sexual history as a routine part of the physical examination takes only a brief period of time. The determination of whether the sexual problem is primarily marital or primarily sexual takes a bit longer but should not present a real problem to those physicians who have made a commitment to the sexual health of their patients. Much can be accomplished even in a busy practice. The physician can spend five to ten minutes to determine whether the problem is primarily marital or sexual. The differentiation is not difficult. For those patients whose problems are primarily marital, referral to a marriage counselor can be made. For those who describe a good marital relationship but for whom sex has never met the couple's expectations in terms of pleasure, intimacy and response, a choice then arises. The physician can counsel the patient himself or refer the patient to an appropriate resource within the community, i.e., health professionals, most of whom are not physicians,

who are qualified sex therapists. It is essential, therefore, that physicians know the resources available within the community.

If the physician who engages in sex counseling or therapy undertakes specialized training based on the work of Masters and Johnson, Chaplain and others, special time must be alloted in his practice. There are probably as many models as there are individuals engaged in this therapy. As a solo gynecologist, I have evolved the following useful and practical model over a period of several years. The first four days of the week are engaged in the practice of general gynecology. The fifth day is devoted entirely to counseling couples whom I have carefully screened. The couples come directly from my practice or have been referred by other physicians.

Therapy in my office is confined to the diagnosis and treatment of the dysfunctions of the sexual response system: general sexual dysfunction (e.g., frigidity, lack of lubrication), anorgasmia and vaginismus in the female; premature ejaculation, retarded ejaculation and erectile incompetence in the male. Mental problems, homosexuality and deviant sexual behavior, e.g., fetishism, voyeurism, are referred. However, as a primary care physician, I often serve as a bridge in the referral of patients to other health professionals engaged in therapy in which I am not competent. This often requires two or three sessions. However, it has been my experience that after several sessions couples will accept referral more readily. Patients whom I treat are seen once a week or once every two weeks depending upon need and progress. The initial interview lasts one hour. Subsequent sessions last 25 to 40 minutes and charges are based on time.

Adjunctive Aids. Several aids are available to the primary care physician who has made a commitment to include an inquiry into the sexual health of his patient. For example, a preprinted form[2] can be given to the patient to complete prior to seeing the physician. This particular form consists of 49 questions that appear on separate cards and that the patient responds to with yes or no answers. The questions begin very generally (e.g., the existence of allergies, past serious illness or accident, immunizations, weight) and cover most of the organ systems. Those questions that concern marriage and sex appear near the bottom of list: marital problems, husband's attitudes, pregnancy, vaginal discharges, menstrual periods, problems about sex, questions about sex or birth control and a final question indicating whether the patient wishes to talk about a problem privately. My patients and I have found this very useful. They understand that discussion of almost any subject is acceptable and encouraged, although most patients will deny that they have serious marital/sexual problems. The physician receives much general information without spending a good deal of effort and time.

Another valuable aid in obtaining information and conserving time is a detailed questionnaire that evaluates sexual performance.

Audiovisual material also can be helpful. For example, I can describe sensate focus, the sine qua non of Masters and Johnson therapy, but illustrating this with three 10-minute audiovisual cassettes is much more effective.[3] The same applies to the "stop and go" or "stimulate/squeeze" exercises and to the employment of masturbation in cases of anorgasmia. Although I do not believe that audiovisual materials are essential to carry out sex therapy, they do serve to demonstrate and clarify, and they provide more time for dialogue in the exploration of other aspects of a problem. Such materials also increase my effectiveness and shorten therapy. The cassettes and the projector never leave my office and are used for no other purpose. I am not present in the room during the showing of the films, but there is a brief discussion about their contents immediately following.

Record Keeping. When personnel are interviewed for employment, they are apprised of the nature of the practice and the absolute necessity for confidentiality. No separate list of sex therapy patients is kept. That is, there is no cross filing. Employees are forbidden to extract charts from the files except for office visits, telephone calls, insurance purposes or other matters of absolute necessity. The objective is not to highlight the sexual aspect of my practice, but rather to regard it as an integral part no different than any other aspect. However, because of possible stigma, another precaution is taken. When a patient transfers from my practice to another physician's practice and later we receive a signed release form pertaining to her records, the patient is contacted and asked specifically whether record transfer is to include information regarding sexual, marital/sexual functioning and counseling. Those patients who instruct me to forward all material are then requested to sign a statement releasing this material.

Insurance. All patients are billed in accordance with fee-for-service based upon time. Sex therapy by physicians may be reimbursed by third-party payers if a DSM-III diagnosis, such as anxiety, generalized disorder state or depressive neurosis, can be made with respect to one of the spouses.

References:
1. LiefHI: Sex education of medical students and doctors. Pacif Med Surg 1965;72:52-8.
2. Data Sheets, Series 4000, Medical Practice Systems, Inc. 1970
3. EDCOA Productions, Inc, 310 Cedar Lane, Teaneck, New Jersey 07666.
(SMP)

Sexual misconduct in the practice of medicine. Council on Ethical and Judicial Affairs, American Medical Association.
JAMA. 1991 Nov 20; 266(19): 2741-5
The American Medical Association's Council on Ethical and Judicial Affairs recently reviewed the ethical implications of sexual or romantic relationships between physicians and patients. The Council has concluded that (1) sexual contact or a romantic relationship concurrent with the physician-patient relationship is unethical; (2) sexual contact or a romantic relationship with a former patient may be unethical under certain circumstances; (3) education on the ethical issues involved in sexual misconduct should be included throughout all levels of medical training; and (4) in the case of sexual misconduct, reporting offending colleagues is especially important.

Sexually Transmitted Diseases
American Social Health Association
P.O. Box 13827
Research Triangle Park, NC 27709
919/361-2742

National VD Hotline
American Social Health Association
800/227-8922; (CA 800/982-5883)

SIECUS (Sex Information
and Education Council of the US)
130 W. 42nd, Suite 2500, New York, NY 10036
212/819-9770
FAX 212/819-9776

JAMA Theme Issue: Sexually Transmitted Diseases (STD) JAMA. Apr 4, 1986. 255 (13) A full range of materials can be found in this theme issue of JAMA. Original contributions on sexually transmitted diseases and mortality, screeening for Chlamidia; special communications on treatment of various STDs and editorials on public support of STD clinical service are a sample of the subjects discusses. Book reviews also appear here, as well as a 'Questions and Answers' section on STDs.

Sick Building Syndrome
A collection of symptoms sometimes reported by people who work in modern office buildings; the symptoms include loss of energy, headaches, and dry, itching eyes, nose, and throat.

The cause of the syndrome is unknown, although it has been attributed to air conditioning, fluorescent lighting, loss of natural ventilation and light, and psychological factors, especially frustration at being unable to control physical conditions (such as temperature and ventilation) in the working environment. Some authorities believe that many outbreaks of sick building syndrome may be pseudoepidemics (conditions without physical causes that are thought to be a form of hysteria.(ENC)

National Safe Workplace Institute
1121 Spring Lake Drive, Itasca, IL 60143-3201
708/285-1121

Sickle Cell Anemia
Center for Sickle Cell Disease
Howard University
2121 Georgia Ave. NW, Washington, DC 20059
202/636-7930

National Association for Sickle Cell Disease
4221 Wilshire Blvd., Suite 360
Los Angeles, CA 90010
800/421-8453, 213/736-5455

Sjogren's Syndrome
Sjogren's Syndrome Foundation, Inc.
382 Main St., Port Washington, NY 11050
516/767-2866

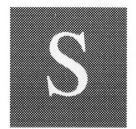

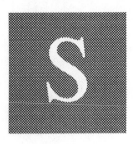

Sleep

American Sleep Disorders Association
604 Second St., SW, Rochester, MN 55902
507/287-6006

Smoking

The Toxic Effects of Tobacco Vapor With Report of Cases

JAMA. 1891 Oct 31; 17(18): 699

Dr. W. Carroll Chapman, of Louisville, said that usually the presence of tobacco poison in the systems of tobacco workers is manifested during the first day or two by violent vomiting, retching, purging and often a state of collapse, after which the system may become inured to it. Occasionally we find one whose constitution, even by contact and time, although there is a certain amount of toleration, refuses to receive it kindly, and emaciation begins, attended sooner or later by such symptoms as the following case illustrates:

Case I. - Willie C., aged 10 years, was found suffering extreme pain in the abdominal region, with the intensity centering at the umbilicus. Temperature, under the tongue, 100 degrees; pulse 108, small, wiry and irregular; respiration 20 to 22, but irregular - several short, shallow, respirations followed by one deep and gasping. Tongue glairy, red appearance and pointed. Patient constipated for the last several days; abdomen flat or rather depressed; urine scanty and slightly colored; skin dry, as were the hands and feet, the latter being a little cold. When near the patient the odor of tobacco was so pronounced that the doctor made inquiries regarding it and learned that he worked in a tobacco steamery and further, that he had slight attacks of similar pains at several different times except of a milder form.

As to the nicotianin, indications point strongly to its being a cause. According to Landerer it occurs only in dried tobacco leaves, and has the odor of that plant; a point strongly in its favor, as that odor was so distinct in every case the author had seen. It would seem further, that the basic substances and fatty acids were causative agents, because authors have proven, by physiological experiments, that these cause contraction of the pupil, dyspnea, abdominal pains, convulsions and death.

The author directs attention to two factors noticeable in all the cases, namely: the emaciation, and the time each one had followed the occupation, that is, from six weeks to three months. The three cases which he reports had not suffered from the vomiting and retching usually attendant upon young tobacco workers the first day or two. In the other, or milder cases, he neglected to inquire regarding that point.

The toxic effects of tobacco vapor and its treatment was a subject worthy of more consideration than the profession has accorded to it in the past, and he hoped that the next few years, aided by diligent and careful investigation, would place the matter in a more intelligent light.

AMA Policy: Smoking on Commercial Aircraft: (1) The AMA urges that careful investigation of the quality of air in passenger cabins of commercial aircraft be initiated to determine the levels of all cigarette smoke contaminants in smoking and non-smoking areas under present practices and under the conditions of any new practices that may be proposed for segregating smokers. (2) Until satisfactory data establish insignificant levels of such tobacco smoke contaminants, the AMA urges that: (a) cigar and pipe smoking be banned on all commercial aircraft; (b) cigarette smoking be banned on all scheduled flights of one hour or less and on all small planes of less than 60 passengers; (c) on longer flights, the smoking area continue to be delineated only after all non-smokers are accommodated; (d) smoking in multicompartment planes (e.g., B-747, DC-10) be limited to a single compartment; (e) the experiment on heavily traveled routes of scheduling some no-smoking flights for the convenience of the patient population, as well as some smoking and non-smoking flights, be encouraged; and that (f) special curtains or partitions between smoking and non-smoking areas be established.

Office on Smoking and Health, Technical Information Center
5600 Fishers Lane, Park Bldg, Room 1-16, Rockville, MD 20857
301/443-1690

JAMA Theme issue: Smoking
JAMA. 1991 Dec 11; 266(22)
Several issues have discussed the perils and controversies revolving around smoking (see also November 23/30, 1984; May 24/31, 1985; February 28, 1986; September 26, 1990). This current collection of materials contains articles regarding tobacco advertising and minors, the nicotine patch, smoking prevention, epidemiological reports from the CDC, and the AMA's most recent listing of publications without cigarette advertising (reproduced on the following pages).

Magazines Without Tobacco Advertising

JAMA 266(22) 1991 Dec 11; 3099-102
Since its first list appeared (JAMA. 262(10) 1989 Sept 8;1290-1291, 1295), the length has more than doubled. Credit for the idea of having only "smoke-free magazines" in physicians' reception rooms goes to DOC (Doctors Ought to Care), a group of physicians devoted to educating people about the causes of preventable illness. Publication of such a list in JAMA follows a resolution adopted by the American Medical Association's House of Delegates in 1987.

Accent on Living
PO Box 700, Bloomington, IL 61701

Adirondack Life
PO Box 97, Jay, NY 12941

Air & Space
370 L'Enfant Promenade SW
Washington, DC 20024

Alaska Magazine
808 E St, Anchorage, AK 99501

American Baby
475 Park Ave, New York, NY 10016-6999

American Health
28 W 23rd St, New York, NY 10010

American Heritage
60 Fifth Ave, New York, NY 10011

American History Illustrated
PO Box 822, Harrisburg, PA 17105

American Square Dance
PO Box 488, Huron, OH 44839

Americas
1889 F St NW, Washington, DC 20006

Animal Kingdom
185th St & Southern Blvd, Bronx, NY 10460

Antique Automobile
501 W Governor Road, Hershey, PA 17033

Arizona Highways
2039 W Lewis Ave, Phoenix, AZ 85009

Arthritis Today
1314 Spring St NW, Atlanta, GA 30309

Artist's Magazine
1507 Dana Ave, Cincinnati, OH 45207

Audubon
950 3rd Ave, New York, NY 10022

Aviation Week & Space Technology
1221 Avenue of the Americas
New York, NY 10021

Backpacker
33 E Minor St, Emmaus, PA 18049

Bicycling
33 E Minor St, Emmaus, PA 18049

Business Week
1221 Avenue of the Americas
New York, NY 10021

Byte
1 Phoenix Mill Lane, Peterborough, NH 03458

Cars & Parts
911 Vandermark Road, Sidney, OH 45365

Cat Fancy
PO Box 6050, Mission Viejo, CA 92690

Child
110 Fifth Ave, New York, NY 10011

Christian Herald
40 Overlook Drive, Chappaqua, NY 10514

Common Cause Magazine
2030 M St NW, Washington, DC 20036

Complete Woman
1165 N Clark St, Chicago, IL 60610

Consumer Reports
256 Washington St, Mt Vernon, NY 10550

Cooking Light
820 Shades Creek Parkway
Birmingham, AL 35209

Country Journal
2245 Kahn Road, Harrisburg, PA 17105-8200

Craftworks for the Home
70 Sparta Ave, Sparta, NJ 07871

Crafts
PO Box 1790, Peoria, IL 61656

Cyclist
20916 Higgins Court, Torrance, CA 90501

Dance Magazine
33 W 60th St, New York, NY 10023

Diabetes Forecast
1660 Duke St, Alexandria, VA 22314

Dog Fancy
PO Box 6050, Mission Viejo, CA 92690

Down Beat
180 W Park Ave, Elmhurst, IL 60126

Down East Magazine
PO Box 679, Camden, ME 04843

Elks Magazine
425 W Diversey Parkway, Chicago, IL 60614

Exceptional Children
1920 Association Drive, Reston, VA 22091

Exceptional Parent
1170 Commonwealth Ave, Boston, MA 02134

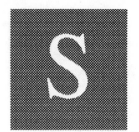

Farm Journal
230 W Washington St, Philadelphia, PA 19105

Final Frontier
2400 Foshay Tower, Minneapolis, MN 55402

Fishing Facts
N84 West 13660 Leon Road
Menomonee Falls, WI 53051

Florida Sportsman
5901 SW 74th St, Miami, FL 33143

Flying
1633 Broadway, New York, NY 10009

Flying Models
PO Box 700, Newton, NJ 07860

Freshwater & Marine Aquarium
144 W Sierra Madre Blvd, Sierra Madre, CA 91204

The Futurist
4916 Saint Elmo Ave, Bethesda, MD 20814

Garbage
435 Ninth St, Brooklyn, NY 11215

Garden
New York Botanical Garden, Bronx, NY 10458

Golf Illustrated
3 Park Ave, New York, NY 10016

Good Old Days
306 E Parr Road, Berne, IN 46711

Guideposts
39 Seminary Hill Road, Carmel, NY 10512

Hadassah Magazine
50 W 58th St, New York, NY 10019

Harvard Business Review
Teele Hall, Boston, MA 02163

Harvard Lampoon
44 Bow St, Cambridge, MA 02138

Harvard Medical School Health Letter
79 Garden St, Cambridge, MA 02138

Health
475 Gate Five Road, Sausalito, Ca 94965

Health News & Review
27 Pine St, New Canaan, CT 06840

Hippocrates
475 Gate Five Road, Sausalito, CA 94965

Historic Preservation
1785 Massachusetts Ave, Washington, DC 20036

Home Office Computing
730 Broadway, New York, NY 10003-9538

Horn Book Magazine
14 Beacon St, Boston, MA 02103-3704

Horse Illustrated
PO Box 6050, Mission Viejo, CA 92690

Horticulture
755 Boylston St, Boston, MA 02116

Income Opportunities
380 Lexington Ave, New York, NY 11382

Instructor
730 Broadway, New York, NY 10003

International Travel News
2120 28th St, Sacramento, CA 95818

Isaac Asimov's Science Fiction
380 Lexington Ave, New York, NY 10017

Itinerary
PO Box 2012, Bayonne, NJ 07002-2012

Journal of Irreproducible Results
PO Box 234, Chicago Heights, IL 60411

Kaleidoscope
326 Locust St, Akron, OH 44302

The Lion
300 22nd St, Oak Brook, IL 60521

MacUser
11 Davis Dr, Belmont, CA 94002-3001

MacWorld
501 Second St, San Francisco, CA 94107

MAD Magazine
485 Madison Ave, New York, NY 10022

Maine Fish & Wildlife
284 State St, Augusta, ME 04333

Maine Life Magazine
250 Center St, Auburn, ME 04210

Mature Outlook
Locust at 17th, Des Moines, IA 50336

Mayo Clinic Health Letter
Mayo Clinic, Rochester, MN 55905

Men's Fitness
21100 Erwin St, Woodland Hills, CA 91367

Men's Health
33 E Minor St, Emmaus, PA 18049

Midwest Living
1716 Locust St, Des Moines, IA 50336

Model Railroader
1027 N 7th St, Milwaukee, WI 53233

Modern Maturity
3200 E Carson St, Lakewood, CA 90712

Montana Magazine
PO Box 5630, Helena, MT 59604

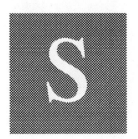

Mother Earth News
80 Fifth Ave, New York, NY 10011

Mother Jones
1663 Mission St, San Francisco, CA 94103

Ms.
230 Park Ave, New York, NY 10069

Muscle & Fitness
21100 Erwin St, Woodland Hills, CA 91367

Nation
72 Fifth Ave, New York, NY 10011

National Gardening
180 Flynn Ave, Burlington, VT 05401

National Geographic
1145 17th St NW, Washington, DC 20036

National Parks
1015 31st St NW, Washington, DC 20007

National Wildlife
1400 16th St NW, Washington, DC 20036

Natural History
Central Park West at 79th St, New York, NY 10024

The New Yorker
20 W 43rd St, New York, NY 10036

North American Review
1222 W 27th St, Cedar Falls, IA 50614

Nutrition Action Healthletter
1501 16th St NW, Washington, DC 20036

Oceans
2001 W Marin St, Stamford, CT 06902

Old House Journal
69A Seventh Ave, Brooklyn, NY 11217

Organic Gardening
35 E Minor St, Emmaus, PA 18049

Parenting
501 Second St, San Francisco, CA 94107

Parents Magazine
685 Third Ave, New York, NY 10017

PC Magazine
PO Box 2445, Boulder, CO 80322

PC World
PO Box 55015, Boulder, CO 80322

Personal Computing
PO Box 2492, Boulder, CO 80322

Petersen's Hunting
8490 Sunset Blvd, Los Angeles, CA 90069

Petersen's Photography
8490 Sunset Blvd, Los Angeles, CA 90069

Popular Communications
76 North Broadway, Hicksville, NY 11001

Popular Photography
1633 Broadway, New York 10009

Popular Woodworking
1320 Galaxy Way, Concord, CA 94520

Prevention
33 E Minor St, Emmaus, PA 18049

Railfan & Railroad
PO Box 700, Newton, NJ 07860

Reader's Digest
Pleasantville, NY 10570

Runner's World
33 E Minor St, Emmaus, PA 18049

Sail
Charleston Navy Yard, 100 First Ave,
Charlestown, MA 02129

Salt, Inc
PO Box 1400, Kennebunkport, ME 04046

Satellite Orbit
8330 Boone Blvd, Vienna, VA 22180

Saturday Evening Post
1100 Waterway Blvd, Indianapolis, IN 46202

Science
1333 H St NW, Washington, DC 20005

Science News
1719 N St NW, Washington, DC 20036

The Sciences
2 E 63rd St, New York, NY 10021

Scientific American
415 Madison Ave, New York, NY 10017

Sea Frontiers
4600 Rickenbacker Causeway, Miami, FL
33149-9900

Shape
21100 Erwin St, Woodland Hills, CA 91367

Sierra
730 Polk St, San Francisco, CA 94109

Single Parent
8807 Colesville Road, Silver Spring, MD 20910

Sixteen Magazine
157 W 57th St, New York, NY 10019

Skin Diver Magazine
8490 Suset Blvd, Los Angeles, CA 90069

Smithsonian
900 Jefferson Drive, Washington, DC 20560

Society
Rutgers University, New Brunswick, NJ 08903

Southern Accents
PO Box 10411, Birmingham, AL 35202

Sports Afield
250 W 55th Ave, New York, NY 10019

Stork
1100 Waterway Blvd, Indianapolis, IN 46206

Sunset Magazine
80 Willow Road, Menlo Park, CA 94025

Theatre Crafts
135 Fifth Ave, New York, NY 10010

Threads
63 S Main St, Newtown, CT 06470

Travel Holiday
Pleasantville, NY 10570

Travel & Leisure
1120 Avenue of the Americas
New York, NY 10036

Twins
6740 Antioch, Merriam, KS 66204

Utah Holiday
419 E First South, Salt Lake City, UT 84111

Vegetarian Times
PO Box 570, Oak Park, IL 60303

Venture Magazine
Christian Service Brigade
765 Kimberly Drive, Carol Stream, IL 60188

Vermont Life
61 Elm St, Montpelier, VT 05602

Vibrant Life
55 W Oak Ridge Drive, Hagerstown, MD 21740

Video Review
902 Broadway, New York, NY 10010

Walking Magazine
711 Boylston St, Boston, MA 02116-2616

The Washington Monthly
1711 Connecticut Ave NW
Washington, DC 20009

Weight Watchers Magazine
360 Lexington Ave, New York, NY 10017

West Coast Review of Books
5265 Fountain, Upper Terrace, Los Angeles, CA
90029

Westways
PO Box 2890, Los Angeles, CA 90051

Western Outdoors
3197 E Airport Loop Drive, Costa Mesa, CA 92626

Wildlife Conservation
New York Zoological Society, Bronx, NY 10460

Women's Sports & Fitness
1919 14th St, Boulder, CO 80302

Workbasket
4251 Pennsylvania Ave.
Kansas City, MO 64111-9990

Work Bench
4251 Pennsylvania Ave, Kansas City, MO
64111-9990

World Monitor
1 Norway St, Boston, MA 02115

Writer's Digest
1507 Dana Ave, Cincinnati, OH 45207

Yankee
Main St, Dublin, NH 03444

Zoogoer
National Zoological Park, Washington, DC 20008

For Children And Teenagers

Big Bopper
3500 W Olive Ave, Burbank, CA 91505

Black Beat
355 Lexington Ave, New York, NY 10017

Bop
3500 W Olive Ave, Burbank, CA 91505

Boy's Life
1325 Walnut Hill Lane, Irving, TX 75038-3096

Cricket
PO Box 300, Peru, IL 61354

Highlights for Children
PO Box 269, Columbus, OH 43272

Humpty Dumpty
1100 Waterway Blvd, Indianapolis, IN 46206

Jack and Jill
1100 Waterway Blvd, Indianapolis, IN 46206

Kid City
1 Lincoln Plaza, New York, NY 10023

Ladybug
PO Box 300, Peru, IL 61354

Ranger Rick's
1412 16th St NW, Washington, DC 20036

Right On!
355 Lexington Ave, New York, NY 10017

Sassy
230 Park Ave, New York, NY 10169

Sesame Street
1 Lincoln Plaza, New York, NY 10022

Seventeen
850 Third Ave, New York, NY 10022

Teen
8490 Sunset Blvd, Los Angeles, CA 90069

3-2-1 Contact
1 Lincoln Plaza, New York, NY 10023

YM
685 Third Ave, New York, NY 10017

Snake Bite
To locate anti-venom
Arizona Poison Control Center
602/626-6016
For exotic snakes
Also contact local zoo

Systematized Nomenclature of Medicine (SNOMED)
College of American Pathologists
325 Waukegan Road, Northfield, IL 60095
708/446-8800

Social Health
American Social Health Association
P.O. Box 13827
Research Triangle Park, NC 27709
919/361-2742

Socioeconomic Characteristics of Medical Practice
Gonzalez, ML. *Socioeconomic Characteristics of Medical Practice*
American Medical Association, Chicago. 1992
annual; 162pp. ISBN 0-89970-404-2/OP192692

Spanish
Spanish Speaking Physicians, list of:
Interamerican College of Physicians & Surgeons
212/599-2737

Speakers, Health-Related Issues
Speaker's Training

It is not enough for physicians to know the facts. They have to be able to communicate these facts to an audience and communicate them convincingly.

Jargon

Avoid sophisticated words the average person doesn't understand. Take a few moments to write down the words you were trained to use, the words specialists use, the words your professor used... and then the translation.

This should be a starting point in terms of finding your own weak spots when it comes to jargon.

For example...When you mean
Administer .. say .. Give
Facility .. say .. Hospital, daycare center, nursing home
Hypertension .. say .. high blood pressure
Malpractice .. say .. Professional Liability
Fee-for-service practitioner .. say .. Private practice doctor

HMOs, IPAs, PPOs - and their definitions
Cardiac arrest .. say ..Heart attack

And so on...

Keep in mind if the audience is the man or woman on the street. The people who work in the garage, drycleaners and supermarket.

People listening will realize you are an authority if they understand you, not if you talk above them. You always want to be perceived as a caring, communicative physician.

The Speaker's Voice

Speakers need to monitor their voices, especially:

Pitch - Changes in pitch are inflections. They give your voice luster, warmth and vitality. Your inflections can make you sound happy, sad, angry, pleased, dynamic or listless.

Rate - The best rate of speech depends on the vocal attributes of the speaker. Avoid speaking so quickly that your audience loses track of your ideas or so slowly that your listeners get bored.

Pauses - Pauses can signal the end of a thought unit, give an idea time to settle in and lend dramatic impact to a statement.

Vocal Variety - Vocal variety is the "spice" of speaking. Practice reading poetry to master vocal variety.

Pronunciation - Practice the correct pronunciation of all words out loud.

Articulation - Be aware of your speech pattern and regional dialects. Work on eliminating sloppy articulation, such as dropping last syllables of words.

Radio is perhaps the most difficult medium through which to convey your message. Recall tests indicate that people retain more information from the printed page than they do from television, and they recall even less from radio. Radio is immediate and intimate: no matter what activity one is engaged in, the sound fills the room. However, listeners can be easily distracted, as well. And so your voice is all you have to hold listeners' attention.

The important advantage of radio is that it offers frequent opportunities to get your message out. There may be dozens of radio stations in your community and each one has hours of airtime to fill. An interesting and compelling guest - which you can be - will be invited back again.

Interview

A physician being interviewed on the radio needs to:
• Be calm, be relaxed.
  Often the thought that thousands of people are listening causes stiffness and formality, Don't take on the tone of a graduation address. Remember that only one or two people are listening in any one place and they don't feel like part of a huge crowd. They're sitting in an armchair relaxing. Think of yourself as talking with a small group and be informal.

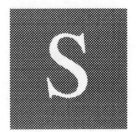

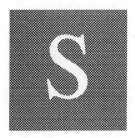

- Be succinct; be direct.
  Long, rambling answers can make your listeners tune out or turn off. On the other hand, don't let the interviewer cut you off if you haven't made your point. Answer as quickly as possible, but don't be reduced to "yes, but..." and "Well, maybe..." Be confident in your answers, and you'll sound confident to the listeners. Use anecdotes to help make your point most effectively.
- Relate the information to the folks at home. What is the interest to them? Will they realize it? How will it affect their lives? Even if you have a massive amount of information, you should stick to that which is of interest to the most listeners. Don't assume they understand how it concerns them. Don't' assume they understand or care about your "practice" or "problems."
- Beware of punch lines.
  They may work on the lecture circuit, but not with an absent audience. If you're not an experienced comedian, punch lines can fall flat.
- Be a good listener.
  You may hear a pre-planned question, but the most have changed it slightly. They may ask your opinion during someone else's segment. Hear out the question; don't run over the ends of lines. Don't assume you know what the host really means. Ask him or her to restate the question if you're not sure you heard it correctly.
- Be prepared.
  The key to a good interview is to be prepared and to simplify the answers. You are the expert and should speak accordingly. You don't have to be defensive and it isn't necessary to back up every statement with a scientific reference. You are the authority. Be prepared for different styles of interviews, also. Below are pointers for phone interviews and question-and-answer session, the most likely formats for a radio show using the HHS programming.
- It's okay to say "I don't know."
  Don't make up information - or guess at an answer - if you don't know. Tell the interviewer or caller that you'll get back to him or her with the correct information.
- Avoid these two phrases: "Off the record" and "No Comment."
  Under no circumstances should you tell an interviewer that something is "off the record." It often isn't. If you don't want to hear the information repeated or printed in the newspaper, you probably shouldn't be saying it to a reporter."No comment" will bring you no more calls from that interviewer. Usually, people mean they can't answer the question - whatever the reason - when they say "no comment." It's much better to explain why you can't answer the question: you don't know, or the information is confidential. This friendly explanation will help keep the interview going smoothly, rather than abruptly putting a stop to your host's questions.

More on Phone Interviews

- Respond warmly to an interviewer who is not in the room with you.
- Try to maintain a conversational quality with energy in your voice. Remember, your voice must convey the power of your message.
- Answer each question in concise statements. When you have completed your response, wait silently for the interviewer's next question.
- If you stumble on a word or deliver an unclear answer, don't hesitate to restate your answer.

- Although the reporter is the one asking the question, remember as you answer that you are talking to the general public.
- Always prepare a friendly closing statement, thanking the interviewer for the opportunity to have your message heard.

Question and Answer Sessions

Before you respond to any question, have your basic message/objective in mind:

- Anticipate any difficult questions. Is there an area of controversy involving the association or organized medicine that may arise? Practice your answer for content and style.
- Listen very carefully to the entire question - avoid interrupting the questioner.
- Make certain the question is appropriate. Before you answer, correct any misinformation, misstatements or incorrect assumptions.
- Don't hesitate to ask for clarification.
- Pause and think before answering questions.
- Break down multiple-part questions, answering each part separately.
- Don't respond negatively to the hostile questioner. You may have to use "bridging" techniques to get away from the hostile question and make your point. If your point is important information that the public needs to hear, say so, and you'll be allowed to make your point.
- Be personable and tactful.
- Finally, prepare your spokespersons for the unforseen. What if...
- Things get slow and boring. Some hosts are skilled at pacing and maintaining interest, but some are not. You then must take the ball. If things get slow, or the host doesn't seem to have any more questions, tell an anecdote, throw some questions back to the host, speak more vigorously, but don't just sit there and wind down. It's to your benefit to make the interview fly. Get excited and stay that way. Be colorful, but don't perform.
- Things Get Nasty or Hostile. Don't take direct questions too personally. The interviewer is performing a job by asking the most interesting and thought-provoking questions possible. In most cases, he won't attack you personally; if he does, of course, you can object. But in most cases, he is looking for a little controversy and an interesting exchange. Answer as honestly and candidly as you can. If the host persists too long or too far, make a simple request to move on. Remember one thing: it's you who is the medical expert and you have credible, important information to impart. Just keep providing answers as honestly and as often as you can. If you answer politely and remain calm, you will win where it counts: with the listeners.
- You and the Interviewer Know Each Other Already. Be careful not to get into old-times "in" talk or overdo the back-patting. Listeners will feel left out.
- The Interviewer is Very Nervous. Think it won't happen? It will! Remain calm and start talking. If you appear calm and ready to talk, it will help. Always have a specific message to deliver and you won't have any problem filling the time. (AMF)

Special Purpose Examination (SPEX)

Exam administered by individual
state licensing boards:
Federation of State Medical Boards of the U.S.
2626B West Freeway, Fort Worth, TX 76102
817/335-1141

Specialists, Board Certified

"Choosing a Medical Specialty"
Council of Medical Specialties
PO Box 70, Lake Forest, IL 60045
708/295-3456

ABMS Compendium of Certified
Medical Specialists
available annually revised from:
American Board of Medical Specialties
One Rotary Center, Suite 805, Evanston, IL 60201
708/491-9091

Directory of Medical Specialists
Marquis Who's Who, Macmillan Directory Division
3002 Glenview Road, Wilmette, IL 60091
708/441-2387
800/621-9669 (outside IL)

Specialty Boards

Medical Practice: Specialization
Lester S. King

Shortly after the middle of the 19th century,
specialization in medicine increased greatly. It
formed part of the vast expansion of knowledge
and the improvement in patient care that
characterized the era. However, there also
developed many internal strains whose study
provides an excellent approach to medical
practice and the sociology of medicine.

Central to the story of specialization is the
consultant, who could help the general practitioner
with a difficult case. In the 17th and 18th
centuries, in Great Britain, the physician, who held
an MD degree, would act as consultant for the
apothecary who did not have university training.[1]
In the United States, even though the distinction
of physician and apothecary did not obtain, the
consultant was qualified to give advice. When
called in consultation he could unearth new
evidence, or reinterpret the data already
amassed, to reach a diagnosis or evaluate
treatment. He was an expert who gave an opinion
and made recommendations but did not ordinarily
take over the conduct of the case.

In the larger cities, especially among medical
school faculty, a consultation practice was a much
sought goal, one that might accrue almost
automatically to the professor of medicine. Such
an honor, however, had to be earned, for such
men had to be better trained and more
knowledgeable than their colleagues. They
generally had a long apprenticeship in pathology,
and spent a great deal of time in teaching, as well
as in keeping up with current developments. The
paradigm of consultant was, perhaps, William
Osler. In the smaller and nonacademic
communities a consultant would have a less
exalted status. He would be a fellow practitioner
who engaged in regular medical practice in the
community. While not necessarily better trained

than his colleagues, he would have acquired a
reputation in some particular area and his opinion
would be received with respect.

In its annual meetings the American Medical
Association recognized a trend toward
specialization. The presentation of papers took
place in sections, where men with special interests
could meet to promote those interests. By 1859
six such sections were recognized for the annual
meeting: (1) anatomy and physiology; (2)
chemistry and materia medica; (3) practical
medicine and obstetrics; (4) surgery; (5)
meteorology, medical topography, and epidemic
diseases; and (6) medical jurisprudence and
hygiene. The first two groups comprehended what
we now call the basic sciences; group 3,
significantly enough, combined general medicine
and obstetrics; surgery, in group 4, remained by
itself. Infectious diseases were bracketed with
environmental data, an interesting sidelight on the
prebacteriologic era.[2]

Gradually the number of sections increased.
When the AMA decided to sponsor the
International Congress of Medicine, to be held in
Washington, DC, in 1887, the original plans called
for 18 separate sections at which papers might be
presented. The purely clinical sections embraced
the following areas: medicine, surgery, obstetrics,
gynecology, ophthalmology, otology, dermatology
and syphilis, nervous diseases and psychiatry,
laryngology, and diseases of children. These
subjects had thus received formal recognition as
approved specialties.[3]

The AMA, which served primarily the general
practitioner, crystallized its position in 1869.[4]
Specialism was certainly advantageous for the
science of medicine, but opinions differed
regarding "its benefits to the profession." There
was objection that the specialties "operate unfairly
toward the general practitioner, in implying that he
is incompetent to properly treat certain classes of
disease, and narrowing his field of practice." The
report went on, "It is natural that in any changes
from old-beaten paths, there should be some
temporary confusion, but...as soon as the relations
between special and general practice become
better adjusted...great advantages will accrue,
even to the general practitioner."

The AMA formally adopted the view that
specialties were a proper field of practice, that
specialists should obey the same rules of
professional "etiquette" as general practitioners,
and that "it shall not be proper for specialists
publicly to advertise themselves as such, or to
assume any title not specially granted by a regular
chartered college."[5]

The AMA had officially accepted specialism as a
major movement in medicine but was relatively
powerless to smooth out the conflicts between the
specialists and the general practitioners. The
dissensions between the two groups could not be
settled by official ukase and surfaced
progressively over the next 40 years. In the
medical literature during that time the specialties
at first showed a defensive posture. Later the
general practitioners were on the defensive. In
1874 an editorial pointed out14 that the previous
15 years had witnessed bitter opposition "against
the cultivation of specialties" but these
nevertheless had proved themselves

"indispensable to progress in medicine." The great problem was how to find the proper distinction between "general and special practice" to achieve the best interests of medicine and the greatest good of the patients.

The general practitioner was expected to treat the simpler affections and should be "competent" to judge between mild and serious conditions. As soon as special skill was required, the case should be 'gracefully resigned" to the specialist. Since this, the writer admitted, "is not the general custom," he offered a highly simplistic remedy. In medical schools the teachers should emphasize "the symptoms which should always demand the resignation of the case to the expert." The practitioner should be aware of his limitations. No practitioner "who has the best interests of his patient at heart" can ignore the claims of the experts. To do so is to "sacrifice the dearest of all professional obligations to the paltry and mean consideration of a few extra dollars in his own purse." This mixture of high moral principle and concrete economic consideration was a fairly constant ingredient of the entire controversy.

The people at large were showing an increasing demand for specialists, and often might bypass the family doctor and go directly to a specialist. The complaints against the specialists are delicately phrased and qualified, but when we analyze the rather long paper we find two main areas of discontent. The one involves status, and the other the monetary aspects of practice.

Frankly expressed is the practitioner's fear of losing the patient. The writer also feared that the specialist would disparage what had already been done for the patient. There existed, as well, a widespread feeling that the specialist was prompted by pecuniary considerations. The general practitioner "spends all his time looking after $3.00 ailments," while the specialist collects $5 and $10 a visit, or performs surgical operations for which he makes a substantial charge.

There was strong emphasis on the "commercialism" that the author saw as invading medicine and especially affecting specialists. He admitted, however, that the doctor "who deprives himself of many of the pleasures of life that he may minister to suffering humanity, should be properly remunerated so that he may have the ordinary comforts of life." We must realize that the physician - certainly the general practitioner - was not at that time really well-to-do, and that the problem of making a living loomed large in the first part of the 20th century.

Between 1866 and 1906 the same problems and complaints, variously phrased, recurred again and again. The literature shows quite a repetitive character. The general practitioner feared that he might lose patients, along with status. In the medical literature defense took the form partly of counterattack against the specialists, partly of recommendations toward self-improvement.

Counterattack was directed against the shortcomings of specialists. The general practitioner derived satisfaction from pointing to individual instances of bad practice. Specialists were criticized for inadequate training, rendering them prone to ignore whatever fell outside their own field of interest. There resulted diagnostic errors that no experienced general practitioner would make.

The fault was attributed chiefly to insufficient experience in general practice - premature specialism. One practitioner in 1887 noted the "rattlebrained person who, having tried general practice for a year or so and miserable failed, immediately takes up some sub-department of medicine...and becomes a specialist."[6] Of course, the better and more vocal specialists agreed that physicians who wanted to specialize should have extensive experience in general practice before limiting themselves to a particular field.

The specialists were also subjected to the charges of money-grubbing and commercialism. An important complaint declared that they were always able to find something to operate on. Such charges were directed particularly at gynecologists. "The older men are more conservative, but the younger men are making their reputation and are doing at the expense of the general practitioner."[7] While the gynecologists were commonly the subject of attack, specialists in eye, ear, nose, and throat came off fairly well.

Despite the various charges, specialism, was firmly established. The real problem was, how far would the process of subdivision go, and what effect would this have on the general practitioner -problems still oppressive today. With the growth of specialism general practitioners expressed a very real fear that they would sink to the level of mere referral centers, shunting patients to this or that specialist. One physician told of a woman who came to him, saying she did not want to consult him but wanted the name of "the best man in Pittsburgh on livers."[8] Patients would bypass their family doctor and go to some specialist they thought would be appropriate for their self-diagnosed condition.

Leaders in the profession might decry the overspecialization and brand it as absurd. F.C. Shattuck[9] said scornfully, in 1897, "We have an Association of Orificial Surgeons in this country. A few years ago a recent graduate asked me, apparently seriously, to give the name of a specialist in rheumatism. We can afford to laugh at these things." Later he declared, sarcastically, in discussing specialism, "Why not a chair in medical schools for the diseases of old age as well as for the diseases of children?"[10] Yet specialism did progress inexorably until the "absurdities" of 1900 have turned into the flourishing specialties of rheumatology and gerontology.

By way of a more positive approach, some generalists encouraged their fellow practitioners to have greater confidence in themselves. The general practitioners could assimilate the great progress that specialism had made and thus treat their patients more intelligently. Postgraduate courses would help so that the general practitioner could do for himself what formerly went to specialists. One practitioner declared[11] that the graduate from "any good hospital" should be able to perform creditably "such operations as tracheotomy, thoracentesis, and amygdalotomy, repair the recently lacerated perineum, attend to simple and many compound fractures, do minor gynecological work," as well as the work of the family physician, "and still leave enough for the specialist." A little self-confidence will often enable

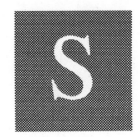

one to do as good work in such cases as the specialists, and at the same time advance his own professional and financial interests.

Another practitioner voiced his complaints against the "crazes" that derived from the work of specialists, particularly in gynecology. He encouraged his colleagues by saying, "The specialist is beginning to acknowledge his dependence on the practicing physician...The humble general practitioner is the real 'Ironsides' of the army of medical science."[12]

The struggle between specialists and general practitioners was merely one aspect of a much wider conflict, involving an elite group that claimed special knowledge and ability and expected corresponding rewards. These claims had to be hammered out on the anvil of experience - did in fact the special knowledge yield better results commensurate with the increased cost? Furthermore, were any advantages vitiated by compensatory drawbacks? In one or another form these conflicts had afflicted the medical profession for hundreds of years.

Medical practice had always involved competition for patients. The growth of specialism in the last third of the 19th century rendered the process more acute than ever. The struggle, however, was taking place in a constantly shifting environment. The entire culture was in flux, and the relation of physicians to each other and to their patients had to undergo severe and constant readjustments as the cultural and economic environment changed.

Bibliographic Notes:

1. Lester S. King, "The British Background for American Medicine," JAMA 1982;248:217-220; "Medical Education: The Early Phases," ibid, pp 731-734.
2. Trans AMA 1859;12:639.
3. JAMA 1884;3:671; see also Lester S. King, "The AMA Gets a New Code of Ethics," JAMA 1983;249:1338-1342.
4. "Report of the Committee on Specialties, and on the Propriety of Specialists Advertising," Trans AMA 1869;20:111-113.
5. Trans AMA 1869;20:28.
6. "The Relations of General Practice to Specialism," Med Rec 1874;9:597-598.
7. A particularly important source of opinion is the extensive discussion that followed several papers on specialism. The discussion is much more revealing than the actual papers and is found in Bull Am Acad Med 1899;4:186-199. The present reference is on page 195.
8. Ibid, p 191.
9. F.C. Shattuck, "Specialism, the Laboratory, and Practical Medicine," Boston Med Surg J 1897;136613-617.
10. Quoted in editorial, "Specialism in Medicine," Boston Med Surg J 1900;143:379-380.
11. Onslow Allen Gordon, "Specialists and General Practitioners," NY Med J 1896;63:601.
12. Woods Hutchinson, "Some of the Disadvantages of Specialism," Med Rec 1895;48:518-519.(AGE)

American Board of **Medical Specialties**
One Rotary Plaza, Suite 805
Evanston, IL 60201
708/491-9091

Council of Medical Specialty Societies
P.O. Box 70, Lake Forest, IL 60045
708/295-3456

American Board of **Allergy And Immunology**
U. City Science Ctr, 3624 Market St., Philadelphia, PA19104
215/349-9466
(Includes the subspecialty of Diagnostic Laboratory Immunology)

American Board of **Anesthesiology**
100 Constitution Plaza, Hartford, CT 06103
203/522-9857
(Includes the subspecialties of Critical Care Medicine and Pain Management)

American Board of **Colon And Rectal Surgery**
875 Telegraph Road, Suite 410, Taylor, MI 48180
313/295-1740

American Board of **Dermatology**
Henry Ford Hospital, Detroit, MI 48202
313/871-8739
(Includes the subspecialties of Dermapathology,Dermatological Immunology, and Diagnostic Laboratory Immunology)

American Board of **Emergency Medicine**
200 Woodland Pass, Suite D
East Lansing, MI 48823
517/332-4800
(Includes the subspecialty of Pediatric Emergency Medicine)

American Board of **Family Practice**
2228 Young Dr., Lexington, KY 40505
606/269-5626
(Includes the subspecialties of Geriatric Medicine and Sports Medicine)

American Board of **Internal Medicine**
U. City Science Ctr, 3624 Market St.
Philadelphia, PA 19104
215/243-1500
800/441-ABIM (800/441-2246)
(Includes the subspecialties of:
Cardiac Electrophysiology, Cardiovascular Disease, Critical CareMedicine, Diagnostic Laboratory Immunology, Endocrinology and Metabolism, Gastroenterology, Geriatric Medicine, Hematology, Infectious Disease, Medical Oncology, Nephrology, Pulmonary Disease, and Rheumatology)

American Board of **Neurological Surgery**
Smith Tower, Suite 2139, 6550 Fannin St.
Houston, TX77030-2701
713/790-6015
(Includes the subspecialty of Critical Care Medicine)

American Board of **Nuclear Medicine**
900 Veteran Ave., Rm. 12-200
Los Angeles, CA 90024
213/825-6787
(Includes the subspecialties of Nuclear Radiology, and Radioisotopic Pathology)

American Board of **Obstetrics And Gynecology**
4225 Roosevelt Way, NE, Ste. 305
Seattle, WA 98105
206/547-4884
(Includes the subspecialties of Critical Care
Medicine,Gynecologic Oncology, Maternal and
Fetal Oncology, and Reproductive Endocrinology)

American Board of **Ophthalmology**
111 Presidential Blvd., Suite 241
Bala Cynwyd, PA 19004
215/664-1175

American Board of **Orthopaedic Surgery**
737 N. Michigan Ave., Suite 1150
Chicago, IL 60611
312/664-9444
(Includes the subspecialty of Hand Surgery)

American Board of **Otolaryngology**
5615 Kirby Dr., Suite 936, Houston, TX 77005
713/528-6200

American Board of **Pathology**
5401 W. Kennedy Blvd., P.O. Box 25915
Tampa, FL 33622
813/286-2444
(Includes certification in Anatomic and Clinical
Pathology
as well as the subspecialties of
BloodBanking/Transfusion Medicine, Chemical
Pathology, Cytopathology, Dermatopathology,
Forensic Pathology, Hematology,
Immunopathology, Medical Microbiology,
Neuropathology,Pediatric Pathology, and
Radioisotopic Pathology)

American Board of **Pediatrics**
111 Silver Cedar Ct., Chapel Hill, NC 27514
919/929-0461
(Includes the subspecialties of Adolescent
Medicine, Diagnostic Laboratory Immunology,
Neonatal-Perinatal Medicine, Pediatric
Cardiology, Pediatric Critical Care,Pediatric
Emergency Medicine, Pediatric Endocrinology,
Pediatric Gastroenterology, Pediatric
Hematology-Oncology, Pediatric Infectious
Disease, Pediatric Nephrology,Pediatric
Pulmonary Disease, and Pediatric Sports
Medicine)
(See also American Board of Pathology - Pediatric
Pathology
American Board of Surgery - Pediatric Surgery)

American Board of **Physical Medicine And
Rehabilitation**
Suite 674, Norwest Center
21 First St., SW, Rochester, MN 55902
507/282-1776

American Board of **Plastic Surgery**
7 Penn Center, Suite 400
1635 Market St., Philadelphia, PA 19103
215/587-9322
(Includes the subspecialty of Hand Surgery)

American Board of **Preventive Medicine**
Dept. of Community Medicine
Wright State University,
P.O. Box 927, Dayton, OH 45401 513/278-6915
(Includes certification in Aerospace Medicine,
OccupationalMedicine,Public Health and
Preventive Medicine, as well as the subspecialty
of Underseas Medicine)

American Board of **Psychiatry And Neurology**
500 Lake Cook Rd., Suite 335, Deerfield, IL 60015
708/945-7900
(Includes certification in Psychiatry and Neurology
as well as the subspecialties of Child and
Adolescent Psychiatry,Geriatric Psychiatry, and
Clinical Neurophysiology)

American Board of **Radiology**
2301 W. Big Beaver Road, Suite 625
Troy, MI 48084
313/643-0300
(Includes certification in Diagnostic Radiology,
RadiationOncology, Radiological Physics, and
Radiology as well as the subspecialty of Nuclear
Radiology)

American Board of **Surgery**
1617 John F. Kennedy Blvd., Ste. 860,
Philadelphia, PA19103
215/568-4000
(Includes the subspecialties of General Vascular
Surgery,Pediatric Surgery, Surgical Critical Care,
and Surgery of the Hand)

American Board of **Thoracic Surgery**
1 Rotary Center, Suite 803, Evanston, IL 60201
708/475-1520

American Board of **Urology**
David C. Utz, Secy.
31700 Telegraph Rd., Ste. 150
Birmingham, MI 48010
313/646-9720

Speech

Speech Pathologist: alternate titles: speech
clinician; speech therapist: Specializes in
diagnosis and treatment of speech and language
problems, and engages in scientific study of
human communication: Diagnoses and evaluates
speech and language skills as related to
educational, medical, social, and psychological
factors. Plans, directs, or conducts habilitative and
rehabilitative treatment programs to restore
communicative efficiency of individuals with
communication problems of organic and
nonorganic etiology. Provides counseling and
guidance and language development therapy to
handicapped individuals. Reviews individual file to
obtain background information prior to evaluation
to determine appropriate tests and to ensure that
adequate information is available. Administers,
scores, and interprets specialized hearing and
speech tests. Develops and implements
individualized plans for assigned clients to meet
individual needs, interests, and abilities. Evaluates
and monitors individuals, using audio-visual
performance to modify, change, or write new
programs. Maintains records as required by law,

establishment's policy, and administrative regulations. Attends meetings and conferences and participates in other activities to promote professional growth. Instructs individuals to monitor their own speech and provides ways to practice new skills. May act as consultant to educational, medical, and other professional groups. May conduct research to develop diagnostic and remedial techniques. May serve as consultant to classroom teachers to incorporate speech and language development activities into daily schedule. May teach manual sign language to student incapable of speaking. May instruct staff in use of special equipment designed to serve handicapped. See Audiologist for one who specializes in diagnosis of, and provision of rehabilitative services for, auditory problems. (DOT)

American Speech-Language-Hearing Association
10801 Rockville Pike, Rockville, MD 20852
301/897-5700
800/638-TALK referrals to Speech-Language Pathologists

Sperm Bank
American Fertility Society
2140 11th Ave, S, Ste 200
Birmingham, AL 35205-2800
205/933-8494

Cryo Laboratory Facility
100 E. Ohio St., Chicago, IL 60611
312/751-2632

Spinal Cord Injury
American Spinal Injury Association
250 East Superior, Room 619, Chicago, IL 60611
312/908-3425

National Spinal Cord Injury Association
600 W. Cummings Park, Woburn, MA 01801
800/962-9629

Spinal Cord Injury Care Center
Northwestern Memorial Hospital
Rehabilitation Institute
312/908-6000
Learning Resource Center 312/908-2859

Spinal Cord Injury Hotline
800/526-3456; 800/638-1733(MD only)

Spinal Cord Society
Charles E. Carson, Ph.D. Pres.
2410 Lakeview Dr., Fergus Falls, MN 56537
218/739-5252

Sports Medicine
American College of Sports Medicine
P.O. Box 1440, One Virginia Ave.
Indianapolis, IN 46206
317/637-9200

American Orthopaedic Society for Sports Medicine
2250 E Devon, Suite 115, Des Plaines, IL 60018
708/803-8700

Board Certification
American Board of Family Practice
2228 Young Drive, Lexington, KY 40505
606/269-5626

Sports injuries hotline:
Women's Sports Foundation
342 Madison Ave, Suite 728, New York, NY 10173
212/972-9170
800/227-3988

State Medical Societies
Medical Association of the State of Alabama
19 S. Jackson St., P.O. Box 1900
Montgomery, AL 36102
205/263-6441

Alaska State Medical Association
4107 Laurel St., Anchorage, AK 99501
907/562-2662

Arizona Medical Association
810 W. Bethany Home Road, Phoenix, AZ 85013
602/246-8901

Arkansas Medical Society
P.O. Box 5776, 10 Corporate Hill Dr.,
Suite 300, Little Rock, AR 72215
501/224-8967

California Medical Association
221 Main St, P.O. Box 7690
San Francisco, CA 94120
415/541-0900

Colorado Medical Society
P.O. Box 17550, Denver CO 80217
303/779-5455

Connecticut State Medical Society
160 Saint Ronan St, New Haven, CT 06511
203/865-0587

Medical Society of Delaware
1925 Lovering Ave, Wilmington, DE 19806
302/658-7596

Medical Society of the District of Columbia
1707 L St, NW, Suite 400, Washington, DC 20036
202/466-1800

Florida Medical Association
760 Riverside Ave, P.O. Box 2411
Jacksonville, FL 32204
904/356-1571

Medical Association of Georgia
938 Peachtree St, NE, Atlanta, GA 30309
404/876-7535

Guam Medical Society
850 Governor Camacho Rd, Tamuning, GU 96911
671/646-5801

Hawaii Medical Association
1360 S. Beretania St, Honolulu, HI 96814
808/536-7702

Idaho Medical Association
P.O. Box 2668, 305 W. Jefferson, Boise, ID 83701
208/344-7888

Illinois State Medical Society
20 N Michigan Ave, Suite 700, Chicago, IL 60602
312/782-1654

Indiana State Medical Association
322 Canal Walk, Indianapolis, IN 46202
317/261-2060

Iowa Medical Society
1001 Grand Ave, West Des Moines, IA 50265
515/223-1401

Kansas Medical Society
1300 SW Topeka Blvd, Topeka, KS 66612
913/235-2383

Kentucky Medical Association
300 N Hurstbourne Ln, Suite 200
Louisville, KY 40222
502/426-6200

Louisiana State Medical Society
3501 N. Causeway Blvd, Sutite 800
Metairie, LA 70002
504/832-9815

Maine Medical Association
P.O. Box 190, Manchester, ME 04351
207/622-3374

Medical and Chirurgical Faculty
of the State of Maryland
1211 Cathedral St, Baltimore, MD 21201
301/539-0872

Massachusetts Medical Society
1440 Main St, Waltham, MA 02154
617/893-4610

Michigan State Medical Society
120 W Saginaw, East Lansing, MI 48823
517/337-1351

Minnesota Medical Association
2221 University Ave, SE, Suite 400
Minneapolis, MN 55414
612/378-1875

Mississippi State Medical Association
735 Riverside Dr, Jackson, MS 39202
601/354-5433

Missouri State Medical Association
P.O. Box 1028, 113 Madison St.
Jefferson City, MO 65102
314/636-5151

Montana Medical Association
2021 11th Ave, Helena, MT 59601
406/443-4000

Nebraska Medical Association
1512 Firs Tier Bank Bldg, Lincoln, NE 68508
402/474-4472

Nevada State Medical Association
3660 Baker Lane, #101, Reno, NV 89509
702/825-6788

New Hampshire Medical Society
7 N. State St, Concord, NH 03301
603/224-1909

Medical Society of New Jersey
2 Princess Rd, Lawrenceville, NJ 08648
609/896-1766

New Mexico Medical Society
7770 Jefferson, NE, Suite 400
Albuquerque, NM 87109
505/828-0237

Medical Society of the State of New York
420 Lakeville Rd, P.O. 5404
Lake Success, NY 11042
516/488-6100

North Carolina Medical Society
P.O. Box 27167, 222 N. Pearson St.
Raleigh, NC 27611
919/833-3836

North Dakota Medical Association
P.O. Box 1198, Bismarck, ND 58502
701/223-9475

Ohio State Medical Association
1700 Lake Shore Drive, Columbus, OH 43204
614/486-2401

Oklahoma State Medical Association
601 NW Expressway, Oklahoma City, OK 73118
405/843-9571

Oregon Medical Association
5210 SW Corbett Ave, Portland, OR 97201
503/226-1555

Pennsylvania Medical Society
777 E. Park Dr, P.O. Box 8820
Harrisburg, PA 17105
717/558-7750

Puerto Rico Medical Association
P.O. Box 9387, Santurce, PR 00908
809/721-6969

Rhode Island Medical Society
106 Francis St, Providence, RI 02930
401/331-3207

South Carolina Medical Association
P.O. Box 11188, Columbia, SC 29211
803/798-6207

South Dakota State Medical Association
1323 S. Minnesota Ave, Sioux Falls, SD 57105
605/336-1965

Tennessee Medical Association
2301 21st Ave South, P.O. 120909
Nashville, TN 37212
615/385-2100

Texas Medical Association
401 W 15th St, Austin, TX 78701
512/370-1300

Utah Medical Association
540 E Fifth South, Salt Lake City, UT 84102
801/355-7477

Vermont State Medical Society
136 Main St, Box H, Montpelier, VT 05601
802/223-7898

Medical Society of Virginia
4205 Dover Rd, Richmond, VA 23221
804/353-2721

Virgin Islands Medical Society
P.O. Box 5986, St. Croix, VI 00823
809/778-5305

Washington State Medical Association
2033 Sixth Ave, Suite 900, Seattle, WA 98121
206/441-9762

West Virginia State Medical Association
4307 MacCorkle Ave, SE, P.O. Box 4106,
Charleston, WV 25364
304/925-0342

State Medical Society of Wisconsin
P.O. Box 1109, 330 Lakeside St.
Madison, WI 53701
608/257-6781

Wyoming Medical Society
P.O. Drawer 4009, 1920 Evans Ave.
Cheyenne, WY 82003
307/635-2424

Statistics, Health-Related

The following essay presents some current examples of health policy issues for which physicians will likely encounter data and statistics in their medical practices. Selected examples include: variations in utilization of health care services; hospital mortality data; and utilization review, quality assurance and peer review.

Since the importance of these issues will likely increase in the coming years, it is essential that physicians understand the appropriate role of statistics in their evaluation. This is particularly true in those instances (e.g., release of hospital mortality data) where physicians may be called on by patients to explain the clinical meaning of published data.

Hospital Mortality Data

The Health Care Financing Administration (HCFA), which administers the Medicare program, has released selected statistical information on the performance of those hospitals which participated in the Medicare program in 1986.

The information to be released would include, for each hospital, the number of Medicare beneficiaries treated and the percentage of beneficiaries who died within 30 days of admission. This information is to be compared with an estimate of the number of deaths that would be expected at the same hospital

(calculated through a regression analysis) if that hospital's experience conformed to the national experience with patients of similar age, sex, incidence of complicating diseases, and prior hospitalization in 1986. HCFA has taken the position that a comparison of data drawn from the individual hospital with the estimate drawn from the population as a whole will give consumers useful information about the quality of care provided by individual hospitals.

Release of such data can, of course, have important implications. As such, it is essential that any information not be misleading to the public. However, there is at least one fundamental flaw in the design of this plan which may foster the proliferation of misleading statistics: In essence, the HCFA plan invites reviewers of these data to compare noncomparable populations.

The population that is subject to comparison consists of Medicare beneficiaries with a specific diagnosis in a hospital. Given the plan proposed by HFCA, the population to which comparisons will be made may differ from this population in several important ways. These include the following: '

1. Race. In drawing an estimate from the overall population, HCFA has ignored race as a factor that could influence the outcome of specific procedures. Thus a hospital that, because of location, has a preponderance of patients who are of one race may be compared with a hospital population that serves several races.

2. Medicare status. While each hospital's data are drawn from Medicare patients alone, the national population of citizens over the age of 65 includes people who are not on Medicare. Medicare covers those with prior social security coverage and their dependents. It does not include those who did not work, or who did not work in a covered occupation, such as federal employees without other jobs. In addition, while Medicare does cover some individuals under age 65, such as those with end-stage renal disease, these individuals are not comparable to members of the population as a whole who are in the same age group.

3. Severity of illness. No measure of the severity of illness is included in the estimate drawn from the national population. As a result, a hospital that may selectively receive patients whose condition is more critical, or that receives more terminally ill patients, will inevitably show mortality rates higher than those estimated.

Because of these deficiencies, questions have been raised about whether the methods being used by HCFA can produce valid predictions of mortality rates for specific hospitals. It has further been questioned as to whether it is appropriate to imply that differences between a hospital's mortality rate and an estimated national mortality rate are due solely to the quality of care provided by the hospital. The number of factors that could influence such an outcome (i.e., the mortality experience) is simply too great to permit inferences to be drawn about any one factor.

The limitations of the Hospital Mortality data, of course, center on outliers - cases where the actual mortality rate falls outside the range of predicted mortality rates. These data lead one to believe

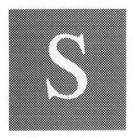

that there may be a quality problem whenever the actual mortality rate is above the upper end of the range of predicted mortality rate.

The key question that must be addressed is the reason that any such outlier might occur. An example may be in using diagnostic categories. An actual rate shown of 48% is above that predicted, 28 to 35%. This outlier could occur for several reasons including:

1. The normal random error that is expected in any statistical model. Some observations always lie above the regression line;

2. The exclusion of important explanatory variables from the predictive model (e.g., severity of illness, race, Medicare status of the hospital); and

3. A quality problem may actually exist in this diagnostic category in this hospital.

The problem is that there is no easy way for the public to discern which of the reason is the correct one. Accordingly, it is essential that physicians understand, and be able to inform their patients, as to what can be legitimately inferred from these data.

Geographic Variations in the Utilization of Health Care Services

A substantial and growing body of research has identified significant differences from one geographic are to another in the utilization of health care services. For example, tonsillectomies have been found to vary from 151 per 10,000 population in one area to as few as 13 per 10,000 in another. Hysterectomies have been found to be performed on 70 percent of women in one locality compared to 30 percent in another.

A key issue raised by these data is whether these differences in utilization can be explained by demographic or epidemiologic factors. (In other words, are these populations comparable?) Are there a greater number of elderly in one area than in another, for example? Is it possible that individuals requiring certain types of treatment are being referred from one geographic area into another? Statistical research indicates that often such area-to-area differences cannot be explained solely in terms of demographic or epidemiologic differences. Any number of other factors (e.g., variations in patient needs, differences in medical practice styles) may be important.

Another issued raised by such variations is whether certain health care services are being provided unnecessarily in some areas of the country. Simply because in one area there is a relatively high incidence of a specific procedure, it cannot be assumed that the procedure is being performed unnecessarily. It is equally possible that in an area with a relatively low rate of a given procedure, the procedure may not be performed often enough. Too little provision of medical services is as undesirable as too much.

Utilization Review, Quality Assurance, and Peer Review

The application of statistical concepts to medical practice data is a major component of utilization assurance processes. There is likely to be increasing use of such statistical applications in these areas, due to the greater amount of medical care data being generated by payment systems, and due to the increasingly sophisticated techniques for evaluating and comparing such data.

Nearly all medical review programs make use of the same statistical principles discussed earlier. For example, it is not at all uncommon for reviewing bodies to examine data that indicate specific hospitals or physicians who exhibit practice patterns that significantly deviate from the median level of care provided for a particular diagnosis. Such analysis can lead to the identification of utilization "outliers," i.e., hospitals or physicians who provide significantly more or less services to a particular kind of patient compared to other hospitals or physicians. The same analysis can be applied to mortality rates and other data that may be regarded as indicators of possible quality problems.

While definitive judgments concerning appropriate utilization and quality of care typically must await the review of the medical chart by a physician, a key component of review programs is the development of screening criteria that can be applied to all, or a sample, of cases as an administratively efficient means of detecting possible utilization or quality problems. Those flagged as possible problems can then be referred for further medical review to determine if a problem in fact exists.

The following sections describe some recent and emerging uses of extensive data analysis in the use of, as an example, severity of illness measures.

Severity of Illness Measures

In recent years there has been growing interest in the notion of "measuring quality." Researchers, as well as payors interested in obtaining maximum value for their health dollar, have explored a number of ways in which empirically-derived quantifiable indicators of the quality of medical care can be identified. One of the key components of quality assessment activities such as these is a mechanism for adjusting cases by the severity of illness of the patient on admission. This step is necessary because quality measurements systems use information contained on the patient medical record or insurance claim form indicating admitting diagnosis or disease category, yet there is a wide disparity in severity of illness among patients within a particular diagnosis or disease category. This disparity is often significant enough to distort outcome data which fails to take severity into account.

There are at least five leading systems used by hospitals to measure severity of illness that also are being used to assess quality of care. All of them employ to varying degrees the data and statistical analysis techniques discussed earlier. For example, MedisGroups, developed by MediQual Systems, classifies patients at

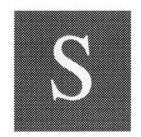

admission on the basis of severity of illness derived from objective clinical findings. Computerized software integrates severity information with hospital resource use data (length of stay and charges) so that analysis can be undertaken of the care being performed at the individual physician level. Another system, Apache II (developed by William A. Knaus of the George Washington University Medical Center), assesses severity of illness of intensive care unit patients based on objective clinical criteria and then assigns an empirically-derived probability of death based on that severity level. A provider whose patterns of treatment reflects a higher than predicted death rate would be subjected to further investigation. The other systems are Patient Management Categories (PMC) developed by Wanda Young of the University of Pittsburgh; Disease Staging, developed by SysteMetrics, Inc.; and CSI, computerized severity index, developed by Susan Horn of Johns Hopkins University.(MMP)

Accidents
National Safety Council
1121 Spring Lake Drive, Itasca, IL 60143-3201
708/285-1121

Diseases
National Center for Health Statistics
6525 Belcrest Road, Room 1140
Hyattsville, MD 20782
301/436-7016

Pharmaceutical Drugs
American Pharmaceutical Association
2215 Constitution Ave., N.W.
Washington, DC 20037
202/628-4410

Hospital Procedures
Healthcare Knowledge Resource
(Formerly Commission on Professional & Hospital Activities)
3853 Research Park, P.O. Box 303
Ann Arbor, MI 48106
313/930-7830

Hospital Statistics
American Hospital Association
840 N. Lake Shore Drive, Chicago, IL 60611
Statistics Center 312/280-6521

Medical Practice:
Professional expense information reported from the Socioeconomic Monitoring System refers to tax-deductible professional expenses from medical practice, not including contribution made for physicians into deferred compensation plans. Non-solo practitioners are asked to report only their share of their practices' total expenses. The major components of total expenses are defined as follows: (1) office expenses, including rent or mortgage for office space, telephones, and utilities; (2) total nonphysician payroll expenses, including fringe benefits; (3) medical materials and supplies, such as drugs, x-rays films, and outside expenses for laboratory work and other services; (4) depreciation, lease, and rent for medical equipment; and (5) professional medical liability insurance premiums. Other expenses are not separately itemized in the surveys.

Weeks and Hours of Practice

The time spent in practice is measured in weeks per year and hours per week. Three measures of total hours in practice can be distinguished. Total professional hours combines hours in patient care with those in other professional activities, such as teaching, research, and administration. Hours in patient care activities excludes other professional hours. Direct patient care hours includes only time spent directly seeing patient; time spent in patient-related activities, such as interpreting tests and telephone contacts with patients and their families, is excluded. Direct patient care hours are allocated by activity into hours spent seeing patients in the office, on hospital rounds, in surgery (operating and delivery rooms), and in other settings. The figure "Distribution of Average Direct Patient Care Hours per Week of All Physicians, 1984 and 1991", in *Socioeconomic Characteristics of Medical Practice* excludes physicians in psychiatry, radiology, anesthesiology, and pathology. The Table indicates that hours per week and the allocation of direct patient care hours by activity were relatively stable from 1984-1991(SCM)

Gonzalez, ML, Ed. *Socioeconomic Characteristics of Medical Practice.* Chicago, American Medical Association. 1992. Annual. 162 pp.
ISBN 0-89970-458-1/OP192690

Statistics, Physicians
Data Research
Center for Health Policy Research
American Medical Association
312/464-5022

Physician population:
Roback, G; Randolph, L; Seidman, B.
Physician Characteristics and Distribution in the U.S. 1992. Chicago, American Medical Association. Annual. pp. 283
ISBN 0-89970-456-5 /OP390292

Stroke
Damage to part of the brain caused by interruption to its blood supply or leakage of blood outside of vessel walls. Sensation, movement, or function controlled by the damaged area is impaired. Strokes are fatal in about one third of cases and are a leading cause of death in developed countries.(ENC)

National Institute of Neurological
Disorders and Stroke
9000 Rockville Pike, Bethesda, MD 20892
301/496-5751

National Stroke Association
300 E. Hampden Avenue, Englewood, CO 80110
303/762-9922

The Stroke Foundation
898 Park Avenue, New York, NY 10021
212/734-3461

Stuttering

National Center for Stuttering
200 E. 33rd St., New York, NY 10016
212/532-1460
800/221-2483 9 a.m.-5 p.m. EST

Stuttering Resource Foundation
123 Oxford, New Rochelle, NY 10804
800/232-4773

Sudden Infant Death Syndrome

American Sudden Infant Death Syndrome Institute
275 Carpenter Dr., Atlanta, GA 30328
800/232-SIDS (800-232-7437)
800/847-SIDS (GA only)

National Sudden Infant Death Syndrome
Foundation
10500 Little Patuxent Parkway
Columbia, MD 21044
301/964-8000
800/221-SIDS (800/221-7437)

Sudden Infant Death Syndrome Clearinghouse
8201 Greensboro, McLean, VA 22102
703/821-8955

Suicide
Overdose

L. Jeffry Price, MD "Poetry and Medicine"
JAMA. 1992 Mar 11; 267(10): 1304

Your life was neatly packaged
when you came to us,
all hopes and farewells
written in two looseleaf testaments.
You had taken the whole amount
and cast yourself on
the quiet barbiturate flood.
The hospital linen you
willed a winding sheet
and floated so much
at peace, I thought yours
the dreaming face of Gad,
uncreased by human care.
We kept you tethered
with I.V. line
and respirator tubing
throughout that long dream.
After a week, you lay
aground on the mattress,
your face awake and twisted
by the world again.
I wished for you
a modicum of peace,
short of that one
in which all souls cast
their perfect reflection.

American Association of Suicidology
2459 S. Ash, Denver, CO 80222
303/692-0985

Survivors of Suicide
(For family and friends of the deceased)
Send stamped self-addressed envelope
3251 N. 78th St, Milwaukee, WI 53222

Suicide, Medical Students
A Sensitive Subject

Elliott B. Oppenheim, MD "A Piece of My Mind"
JAMA. 1982 Apr 2: 247(13): 1875

When my medical school class began there were 64 eager students, and 64 students eventually finished four years later. I recall each year the story surrounding the one who did not make it and was replaced.

From the first day we were told how small our class size was; it was obvious to anyone who had come from the larger universities. One Berkeley graduate said, "I had more people than this in my organic lab!"

The newness of the school soon faded, but the excitement of histology, physiology, and courses I can no longer remember propelled us through the first quarter.

Tight groups of friends readily developed, but one person seemed to remain anonymous even within this small group of 64. It was the classics major, dark-haired, with round-rimmed tortoise-shell glasses, soft-spoken, who, when we were in social groups, was always alone. He did not play touch football, throw the Frisbee, or enter political discussions about the Vietnam situation.

As students we were thinking axons, glutamine transferase, and polysaccharides, but he was still marveling over Virgil, Cicero, and Chaucer. His father had wanted him to be a physician, and Ted took the requisite premedical courses, applied to medical school, and was accepted. Shortly after class began, he found his enthusiasm was simply not in pancreatic acini, loops of Henle, or intestinal villi. How could he ever hold his father's admiration if he left medical school?

He and I discussed this predicament one day at lunch. It was late in the southern California fall, just before finals, when we lunched and shared his secrets. I told him about my desire to become a novelist and he related his wish to translate the Greek classics. He did not want to be a physician.

Like a small boat at sea tossed in a storm, the class was overwhelmed by finals. After Christmas break, there we were, back again. This time it was anatomy, more histology, and physiology. I seem to remember we were learning about red blood cells in afternoon lab when our class president entered the room.

"Ted committed suicide last night. He overdosed on barbs," he said. "The parents want no remembrances."

We were shocked, but little was ever said. Few of us realized the loss. No one had known him! The administration made no effort to give us any understanding of the complex issues, and I don't think that the department of psychiatry even knew about it until years later. Classes went on without an ectopic beat, much less a run of ventricular tachycardia.

A student replaced Ted within a week and ultimately did well. He wanted to be a physician.

Despite our small class size and a number of small groups, Ted had remained a distant outsider. He was in every way unaffiliated and anonymous. He had a girl friend, but she was 300 miles away. His parents, with whom he had been both distant and close, made their goals and his need to achieve them a clear contingency.

The rugged medical students were concerned with new anatomy vocabulary and excluded their paternal role with a classmate. It was not an optimal time for class support since we, too, were new. We barely knew one another.

So there he was without an acceptable solution...except one.

The first days of medical school are like an angel food cake in the making. There is stress in the transition from lay person to medical student, and if a door is slammed prematurely, the cake can fall.

A small class does not guarantee closeness, but support systems do guarantee, at least, the probable identification of those of us with serious emotional problems. In our second year one professor invited small discussion sessions to his home. These groups of 12 ostensibly dealt with ethical issues in medicine, but the topics were far-ranging and allowed us an opportunity to interact.

The troubled student is usually identifiable if one looks carefully. Like rales in pneumonia, loneliness, anxiety, and drug use (including alcohol) are important signs in the presuicide.

I believe that medical schools should conduct "get-acquainted" groups led by faculty members with eight to 12 students meeting every four weeks. Most physicians who would volunteer to host such a group would be sensitive enough to spot a troubled student. The faculty person would also be seen as approachable in a time of need.

While it may be impossible to rework a medical student's life even with empathetic friends, for many, medical school is the beginning of psychotherapy or psychoanalysis that eventually does create a happier physician.

Physicians are fearful about approaching patients as people and worry, "If the patient has the same problem I do, how can I help if I have not helped myself?" We have an aversion to emotional turmoil as medical students that persists in the physician. But as we learn to approach our patients, we must also learn to approach our colleagues.

Parents wish success for their offspring, but it is the child who must be successful. Vicarious parental success is an inordinate and unfair burden for a medical student.

Faculty meetings and administrative sensitivity are important adjuncts to prevention of suicide in medical students, but as in many medical issues, the answer literally lies in our hands. We must knock on a door every once in a while, risk being intrusive, and learn to talk with our brethren about a sensitive subject.

Suntanning Salons

Harmful effects of ultraviolet radiation. Council on Scientific Affairs. JAMA. 1989 Jul 21; 262(3): 380-4 Tanning for cosmetic purposes by sunbathing or by using artificial tanning devices is widespread. The hazards associated with exposure to ultraviolet radiation are of concern to the medical profession. Depending on the amount and form of the radiation, as well as on the skin type of the individual exposed, ultraviolet radiation causes erythema, sunburn, photodamage (photoaging), photocarcinogenesis, damage to the eyes, alteration of the immune system of the skin, and chemical hypersensitivity. Skin cancers most commonly produced by ultraviolet radiation are basal and squamous cell carcinomas. There also is much circumstantial evidence that the increase in the incidence of cutaneous malignant melanoma during the past half century is related to increased sun exposure, but this has not been proved. Effective and cosmetically acceptable sunscreen preparations have been developed that can do much to prevent or reduce most harmful effects to ultraviolet radiation if they are applied properly and consistently. Other safety measures include (1) minimizing exposure to ultraviolet radiation, (2) being aware of reflective surfaces while in the sun, (3) wearing protective clothing, (4) avoiding use of artificial tanning devices, and (5) protecting infants and children.

Surgeon General
M. Joycelyn Elders MD
c/o Public Health Service
200 Independence Ave. SW
Washington, DC 20201
202/245-6467

Surgery
Surgeon: Performs surgery to correct deformities, repair injuries, prevent diseases, and improve function in patients: Examines patient to verify necessity of operation, estimate possible risk to patient, and determine best operational procedure. Previews reports of patient's general physical condition, reactions to medications, and medical history. Examines instruments, equipment, and surgical setup to ensure that antiseptic and aseptic methods have been followed. Performs operations, using variety of surgical instruments and employing established surgical techniques appropriate for specific procedures. May specialize in particular type of operation, as on nervous system, and be designated Neurosurgeon. May specialize in repair, restoration, or improvement of lost, injured, defective, or misshapen body parts and be designated Plastic Surgeon. May specialize in correction or prevention of skeletal abnormalities, utilizing surgical, medical, and physical methodologies, and be designated Orthopedic Surgeon. (DOT)

American Board of Surgery
1617 John F. Kennedy Blvd.
Philadelphia, PA 19103
215/568-4000

American College of Surgeons
55 E. Erie St., Chicago, IL 60611
312/664-4050

International College of Surgeons
1516 N. Lake Shore Dr., Chicago, IL 60610
312/787-6274

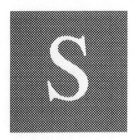

National Second Opinion Program
800/638-6833 (MD 800/492-6603)

Surgical Technologist

History: The profession of surgical technology was developed during World War II when there was a critical need for assistance in performing surgical procedures and a shortage of qualified procedures and a shortage of qualified personnel to meet that need. Individuals were educated specifically to assist in surgical procedures and to function in the operative theatre.

The era of development in education for the surgical technologist was initiated in 1959 when the Association of Operating Room Nurses (AORN) established a committee to work with representatives of the American College of Surgeons, the American Nurses Association, and the National League of Nursing in addressing the growing need for surgical technologists, the apparent lack of consistency in the way they were being educated, and the need to define the relationship of the surgical technologist with other members of the surgical team.

The Association of Surgical Technologists (AST) (until 1978 called the Association of Operating Room Technicians) was organized in July 1969, with an advisory board of representatives from AORN, the American College of Surgeons (ACS), the American Hospital Association (AHA), and the American Medical Association (AMA).

In December 1972, the AMA's Council on Medical Education adopted the recommended educational standards for this field and the Accreditation Review Committee on Education in Surgical Technology (ARC-ST) was formed. The ARC-CT is jointly sponsored by AST, ACS, and AHA in collaboration with the AMA.

The accreditation policies and processes of the ARC-ST comply with the standards for nationally recognized agencies established by the US Department of Education and the Council on Postsecondary Accreditation.

Occupational Description: Surgical technologists are integral members of the surgical team who work closely with surgeons, anesthesiologists, registered nurses, and other surgical personnel delivering patient care and assuming appropriate responsibilities before, during, and after surgery.

Job Description: Surgical technologists prepare the operating room by selecting and opening sterile supplies. Preoperative duties also include assembling, adjusting, and checking nonsterile equipment to ensure that it is in proper working order. Common duties include operating sterilizers, lights, suction machines, electrosurgical units, and diagnostic equipment.

When patients in the surgical suite, surgical technologists may assist in preparing them for surgery by providing physical and emotional support, checking charts, and observing vital signs. They have been educated to properly position the patient on the operating table, assist in connecting and applying surgical equipment and/or monitoring devices, and prepare the incision site by clearing the skin with an antiseptic solution.

Surgical technologists have primary responsibility for maintaining the sterile field, being constantly vigilant that all members of the team adhere to aseptic technique.

They most often function as the sterile member of the surgical team who passes instruments, sutures, and sponges during surgery. After "scrubbing," they don gown and gloves and prepare the sterile setup for the appropriate procedure. After other members of the sterile team have scrubbed, they assist them with gowning and gloving and with the application of sterile drapes that isolate the operative site.

In order that surgery may proceed smoothly, surgical technologists anticipate the needs of surgeons, passing instruments and providing sterile items in an efficient manner. They share with the circulator the responsibility for accounting for sponges, needles, and instruments before, during, and after surgery.

Surgery technologists may hold retractors or instruments, sponge or suction the operative site, or cut suture materials as directed by the surgeon. They connect drains and tubing and receive and prepare specimens for subsequent pathology analysis. They are responsible for preparing and applying sterile dressings following the procedure and may assist in the application of nonsterile dressings, including plaster or synthetic casting materials. After surgery, they prepare the operating room for the next patient.

Surgical technologists are most often members of the sterile team but may function in the nonsterile role of circulator. The circulator is not gowned and gloved during the surgical procedure but is available to respond to the needs of the individual providing anesthesia, keep a written account of the surgical procedure, and participate jointly with the scrubbed person in counting sponges, needles, and instruments before, during, and after surgery. In operating rooms where local anesthetics are administered, they meet the needs of the conscious patient.

Certified surgical technologists with additional specialized education or training may also act in the role of the first surgical assistant. The first surgical assistant provides aid in exposure, hemostasis, and other technical functions that will help the surgeon carry out a safe operation with optimal results for patient.

Surgical technologists also may provide staffing in postoperative recovery rooms where patients' responses are carefully monitored in the critical phases following general anesthesia.

Employment Characteristics: A majority of surgical technologists work in hospitals, principally in operating rooms and occasionally in emergency rooms and other settings which call for knowledge of an ability in maintaining asepsis. A much smaller number work in a wide variety of settings and arrangements including out-patient surgicenters, private employment by physicians or as self-employed technologists.

Those who work in hospital and other institutional settings are usually expected to work rotating shifts or to accommodate on-call assignments to assure adequate staffing for emergency surgical

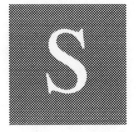

procedures during evening, night, weekend, and holiday hours. Otherwise, surgical technologists follow a standard hospital work day.

Salaries vary depending upon the experience and education of the individual, the economy of a given region, the responsibilities of the position, and the working hours. According to the 1990 CAHEA Annual Supplemental Survey, entry level salaries average $16,736.

Demand for technologists varies among communities and geographic regions. Prospective students are advised to assess the market for graduates within the region in which they would like to work before matriculating in an educational program. Such information is likely to be available through local employment offices, local accredited programs, and hospital councils or hospitals.(ALL) AMA Allied Health Department 312/464-4622

Association of Surgical Technologists 8307 Shaffer Pkwy, Littleton, CO 80127 303/978-9010

Surrogate Motherhood/Parents
Surrogate Parent Foundation
8383 Wilshire Blvd., Ste 750D
Beverly Hills, CA 90211
213/824-4723

Teaching Hospitals

Council on Teaching Hospitals
2450 N Street, N.W., Washington, DC 20037
202/828-0490

Technology Assessment

American Medical Association Diagnostic and
Therapeutic Technology Assessment (DATTA)
Program. For a list of DATTA Reports - see AMA
section

AHCPR Reports

US Department of Health and Human Services
Agency for Health Care Policy and Research
(AHCPR) Reports

Titles and Ordering Information (1981-1990)
U.S. Department of Health and Human Services
Public Health Service
Agency for Health Care Policy and Research
Parklawn Building, Room 18-12
Rockville, MD 20857

Foreword

The Office of Health Technology Assessment
(OHTA) is a component of the Agency for Health
Care Policy and Research (AHCPR). OHTA
evaluates the safety and effectiveness of new or
unestablished medical technologies that are being
considered for coverage under Medicare. These
assessments are performed at the request of the
Health Care Financing Administration (HCFA).
They are the basis for recommendations to HCFA
regarding coverage policy decisions under
Medicare.

Questions about Medicare coverage for certain
health care technologies are directed to HCFA by
such interested parties as insurers,
manufacturers, Medicare contractors, and
practitioners. HCFA formally refers those
questions of a medical, scientific, or technical
nature to OHTA for assessment.

The assessment process includes a
comprehensive review of the medical literature
and emphasizes broad and open participation
from within and outside the Federal Government.
A range of expert advice is obtained by widely
publicizing the plans for conducting the
assessment through publication of an
announcement in the Federal Register and
solicitation of input from Federal agencies,
medical specialty societies, insurers, and
manufacturers. The involvement of these experts
helps assure inclusion of the experienced and
varying viewpoints needed to round out the data
derived from individual scientific studies in the
medical literature.

After information is received from experts and the
scientific literature, the results are analyzed and
synthesized into an assessment report. Each
report represents a detailed analysis of the safety,
clinical effectiveness, and uses of new or
unestablished medical technologies considered
for Medicare coverage. These Health Technology
Assessment Reports form the basis for the Public
Health Service recommendations to HCFA and
are disseminated widely.

Health Technology Assessment Reports, 1990

1. Assessment of Liver Transplantation, 41 pp.,
PB90-101304.
2. Diagnosis and Treatment of Impotence, 22 pp.,
PB90-101411.
3. Surface/Specialty Coil Devices and Gating
Techniques in Magnetic Resonance Imaging, 23
pp., PB90-101437.
4. Electroencephalographic (EEG) Video
Monitoring, 14 pp., PB91-127100.
5. Carotid Endarterectomy, 13 pp., PB91-127118.
6. Extracranial-Intracranial Bypass to Reduce the
Risk of Ischemic Stroke, PB91-145748.

Health Technology Assessment Reports, 1989

Abstracts of Office of Health Technology
Assessment Reports 1988-1989, 9 pp.,
PB90-101429.

1. The Role of Speech-Language Pathologists in
the Management of Dysphagia, 10 pp.,
PB90-101205.
2. Thermography for Indications Other Than
Breast Lesions, 34 pp., PB90-101148.
3. Cardiac Output By Electrical Bioimpedance, 5
pp., PB90- 101197.
4. Real-Time Cardiac Monitors, 12 pp.,
PB90-101155.
5. Guidelines for Home Air-Fluidized Bed Therapy,
16 pp., PB90-101189.
6. Cardiac Catheterization in a Freestanding
Setting, 12 pp., PB90-101213.

Health Technology Assessment Reports, 1988

Abstracts of Office Health Technology
Assessment Reports 1988-1989. 9 pp.,
PB90-101429.

1. Reassessment of Cardiokymography, 4 pp.,
PB90-101122.
2. Reassessment of Transillumination Light
Scanning for the Diagnosis of Breast Cancer, 12
pp., PB90-101130.
3. Reassessment of Autologous Bone Marrow
Transplantation, 18 pp., PB90-101098.

Health Technology Assessment Reports, 1987

Compilation of 6 Reports, 100 pp. (Individual
reports also available), PB89-156681.

Abstracts of Office of Health Technology
Assessment Reports, 1987, 8 pp., PB90-101353.

1. Transurethral Urethroscopic Lithotripsy
Procedure for the Treatment of Kidney Stones, 13
pp., PB88-250113.
2. Radiographic Absorptiometry for Measuring
Bone Mineral Density, 35 pp., PB88-250139.
3. The Cardiointegram in the Diagnosis of
Coronary Artery Disease, 10 pp., PB89-101166.
4. Chemical Aversion therapy for the Treatment of
Alcoholism, 23 pp., PB90-101182.
5. Endoscopic Laser Photocoagulation in the
Treatment of Upper Gastrointestinal Bleeding, 27
pp., PB90-101338.
6. Cardiac Rehabilitation Services, 81 pp.,
PB90-101346.

Health Technology Assessment Reports, 1986

Compilation of 11 Reports, 391 pp. (Individual reports also available), PB88-250121. Abstracts of Office of Technology Assessment Reports, 1986, 12pp., PB88-209481.

1. Fully Automated Ambulatory Blood Pressure Monitoring of Hypertension, 22 pp., PB87-177838/AS.
2. Cochlear Implant Devices for the Profoundly Hearing Impaired, 44 pp., PB87-177820/AS.
3. Continuous Positive Airway Pressure for the Treatment of Obstructive Sleep Apnea in Adults, 19 pp., PB87-193074/AS.
4. Hemofiltration as a Substitute for Hemodialysis in the Treatment of End-Stage Renal Disease (ESRD), 19 pp., PB87- 214300/AS.
5. Laboratory Tests for the Management of End-Stage Renal Disease (ESRD) Dialysis Patients, 26 pp., PB87-214300/AS.
6. Dual Photon Absorptiometry for Measuring Bone Mineral Density, 71 pp., PB87-204020/AS.
7. Single Photon Absorptiometry for Measuring Bone Mineral Density, 37 pp., PB87-201489/AS.
8. Hemoperfusion in Conjunction with Deferoxamine for the Treatment of Aluminum Toxicity or Iron Overload in Patients with End-Stage Renal Disease, 20 pp., PB87-204012/AS.
9. Angelchick Anti-Reflux Prosthesis, 34 pp., PB87-202735/AS.
10. Endoscopic Electrocoagulation in the Treatment of Upper Gastrointestinal Bleeding, 26 pp., PB88-157797/AS.
11. The Reuse of Hemodialysis Devices Labeled "For Single Use Only," 61 pp., PB88-195763/AS.

Health Technology Assessment Reports, 1985

Compilation of 17 Reports, 376, pp., PB86-197803/AS. (Individual reports also available)

Abstracts of Office of Health Technology Assessment Reports, 1985, 20 pp., PB86-198132/AS.

1. Extracorporeal Shock Wave Lithotripsy (ESWL) Procedures for the Treatment of Kidney Stones, 13 pp., PB86-121811/AS.
2. Percutaneous Ultrasound Procedures for the Treatment of Kidney Stones, 19 pp., PB86-121829/AS.
3. Debridement and Other Treatment of Mycotic Toenails, 13 pp., PB86-121837/AS.
4. Transurethral Urethroscopic Lithotripsy Procedures for the Treatment of Kidney Stones, 11 pp., PB86-121845/AS.
5. 24-Hour Ambulatory Esophageal pH Monitoring, 14 pp., PB86- 121852/AS.
6. Thermography for Indications Other Than Breast Lesions. (Withdrawn)
7. Allogeneic Bone Marrow Transplantation (BMT) for Indications Other Than Aplastic Anemia and Leukemia, 24 pp., PB86- 121860/AS.
8. Autologous Bone Marrow Transplantation (ABMT), 20 pp., PB86- 121878/AS.
9. Stereotactic Cingulotomy as a Means of Psychosurgery, 31 pp., PB86-121886/AS.
10. Cardiokymography, 4 pp., PB86-133790/AS.
11. Patient Selection Criteria for Percutaneous Transluminal Coronary Angioplasty, 36 pp., PB86-133808/AS.
12. Bilateral Carotid Body Resection, 12 pp.,

PB86-133816/AS.
13. Magnetic Resonance Imaging, 106 pp., PB86-132131/AS.
14. Apheresis in the Treatment of Guillain-Barre Syndrome, 16 pp., PB86-151024/AS.
15. Portable Hand Held X-Ray Instrument (Lixiscope) (revised), 12 pp., PB86-151032/AS.
16. Implantable Automatic Cardioverter-Defibrillators, 20 pp., PB86-154671/AS.
17. Apheresis in the Treatment of Systemic Lupus Erythematosus (SLE), 18 pp., PB86-154663/AS

Health Technology Assessment Reports, 1984.

Compilation of 26 Reports, 455 pp., PB85-203784/AS. (Individual reports also available)

1. Transillumination Light Scanning for the Diagnosis of Breast Cancer, 16 pp., PB85-150712/AS.
2. Implantable Pump for Chronic Heparin Therapy, 9 pp., PB85- 150720/AS.
3. Electrotherapy for Treatment of Facial Nerve Paralysis (Bell's Palsy), 9 pp., PB85-150407/AS.
4. 13CO2 Breath Test for Diagnosing Bile Acid Malabsorption, 12 pp., PB85-154540/AS.
5. Noninvasive Method of Monitoring Cardiac Output by Doppler Ultrasound, 19 pp., PB85-151363/AS.
6. Ambulatory Electroencephalographic (EEG) Monitoring, 30 pp., PB85-150738/AS.
7. 13CO2 Breath Test for Diagnosing Fat Malabsorption, 16 pp., PB85-154094/AS.
8. Transcutaneous Electrical Nerve Stimulation for Acute Pain Treatment for Ambulatory Patients, 12 pp., PB85-153377/AS.
9. Apheresis Used in Preparation for Kidney Transplant, 8 pp., PB85-151371/AS.
10. Carbon Dioxide Lasers in Head and Neck Surgery, 8 pp., PB85- 151389/AS.
11. Hyperbaric Oxygen Therapy for Acute Cerebral Edema, 20pp., PB85-153385/AS.
12. Intraoperative Ventricular Mapping, 24 pp., PB85-152999/AS.
13. Apheresis in the Treatment of Chronic Relapsing Polyneuropathy, 9 pp., PB85-151397/AS.
14. Diagnostic Endocardial Electrical Stimulation (Pacing), 16 pp., PB85-151405/AS.
15. Neuromuscular Electrical Stimulation in the Treatment of Disuse Atrophy in the Absence of Nervous System Involvement, 13 pp., PB85-151413/AS.
16. Hyperbaric Oxygen for Treatment of Chronic Peripheral Vascular Insufficiency, 11 pp., PB85-152916/AS.
17. Hyperbaric Oxygen in Treatment of Severed Limbs, 12 pp., PB85-153393/AS.
18. External Counterpulsation, 15 pp., PB85-150399/AS.
19. Transplantation of the Pancreas, 30 pp., PB85-153724/AS.
20. Streptokinase Infusion for Acute Myocardial Infarction, 19 pp., PB85-157428/AS.
21. Nd:YAG Laser for Posterior Capsulotomies, 19 pp., PB85- 157428/AS.
22. External Open-Loop Pump for the Subcutaneous Infusion of Insulin in Diabetics, 34 pp., PB85-151439.
23. Laser Trabeculoplasty (LTP) for Open Angle Glaucoma, 20 pp., PB85-163111/AS.
24. Local Hyperthermia for Treatment of Superficial and Subcutaneous Malignancies, 27 pp., PB85-179554/AS.

25. Percutaneous Transluminal Angioplasty for Obstructive Lesions of the Aortic Arch Vessels, 20 pp., PB85-179539/AS.
26. Percutaneous Transluminal Angioplasty for Obstructive Lesions of Arteriovenous Dialysis Fistulas, 15 pp., PB85-179547/AS.

Health Technology Assessment Reports, 1983

Compilation of 22 Reports, 322 pp., PB85-121762/AS. (Individual reports also available)

1. EEG Monitoring During Open Heart Surgery, 17 pp., PB85- 192789/AS.
2.-3. Apheresis for the Treatment of Goodpasture's Syndrome and Membranous Proliferative Glomerulonephritis, 10 pp., PB85- 192797/AS.
4. Electroversion Therapy for the Treatment of Alcoholism, 4 pp., PB85-195261/AS.
5. Anti-Gastroesophageal Reflux Implantation, 6 pp., PB85- 195253/AS.
6. Closed-Loop Blood Glucose Control Device, 20 pp., PB85- 195256/AS.
7. Plasma Perfusion of Charcoal Filters for Treatment of Pruritis of Cholestatic Liver Disease, 7 pp., PB85-195238/AS.
8. Topical Oxygen Therapy in the Treatment of Decubitus Ulcers and Persistent Skin Lesions, 14 pp., PB85-192805/AS.
9. Fully Automated Ambulatory Blood Pressure Monitoring of Hypertension, 15 pp., PB85-191781/AS.
10. Hyperbaric Oxygen for Treatment of Actinomycosis, 11 pp., PB85-191773/AS.
11. Photokymography, 5 pp., PB85-192771/AS.
12. Cardiokymography, 14 pp., PB85-192813/AS.
13. Negative Pressure Respirators, 19 pp., PB85-206019/AS.
14. Diathermy as a Physical Therapy Modality, 21 pp., PB85- 206027/AS.
15. Hyperbaric Oxygen for Treatment of Crush Injury and Acute Traumatic Peripheral Ischemia, 12 pp., PB85-192763/AS.
16. Liver Transplantation, 47 pp., PB85-121747/AS.
17. Computer Enhanced Perimetry, 9 pp., PB86-127719/AS.
18. Lactose Breath Hydrogen Test for the Diagnosis of Lactose Malabsorption, 15 pp., PB86-127727/AS.
19. Implantable Chemotherapy Infusion Pump of the Treatment of Liver Cancer, 18 pp., PB86-127727/AS.
20. External Infusion Pump for Heparin, 7 pp., PB86-127743/AS.
21. Lactulose Breath Hydrogen Test for Small Bowel Bacterial Overgrowth and Small Bowel Transit Time, 16 pp., PB86- 127750/AS.
22. Thermography for Breast Cancer Detection, 24 pp., PB86- 127768/AS.

Health Technology Assessment Reports, 1982

Compilation of 26 Reports, 290 pp., PB85-121754/AS. (Individual report not available)

1. Electrotherapy for Treatment of Facial Nerve Paralysis (Bell's Palsy), 11pp.
2. Hyperbaric Oxygen Therapy for Treatment of Organic Brain Syndrome (Senility), 13 pp.
3. Hyperbaric Oxygen Therapy for Treatment of Multiple Sclerosis, 11 pp.

4. Gastric Freezing for Peptic Ulcer Disease, 20 pp.
5. Bolen's Test for Cancer, 7 pp.
6. Bendien's Test for Cancer and Tuberculosis, 3 pp.
7. Rehfuss Test for Gastric Acidity, 3 pp.
8. Rheumatoid Vasculitis Therapeutic Apheresis, 10 pp.
9. Home Blood Glucose Monitors, 20 pp.
10. Ambulatory Blood Pressure Monitoring in Hypertensives Using Semiautomatic, Patient-Activated Portable Devices, 10 pp.
11. Apheresis for Multiple Sclerosis, 11 pp.
12. Hyperbaric Oxygen Therapy for Treatment of Arthritic Diseases, 10 pp.
13. Plasmapheresis and Plasma Exchange for Thrombotic Thrombocytopenic Purpura, 14 pp.
14. Obesity and Protein Supplemented Fasting, 13 pp.
15. Serum Seromucoid Assay, 23 pp.
16. Percutaneous Transluminal Angioplasty for Treatment of Stenotic Lesions of a Single Coronary Artery, 23 pp.
17. Melodic Intonation Therapy, 12 pp.
18-20. Bone (Mineral) Density Studies, 15 pp.
21. Hyperbaric Oxygen Therapy for Treatment of Soft Tissue Radionecrosis and Osteoradionecrosis, 13 pp.
22. Hyperbaric Oxygen Therapy for Treatment of Chronic Refractory Osteomyelitis, 11 pp.
23. Carbon Dioxide Laser Surgery for Selected Conditions, 14 pp.
24. Percutaneous Transluminal Angioplasty in Treatment of Stenotic Lesions of the Renal Arteries, 15 pp.
25. Endothelial Cell Photography, 4 pp.
26. Photoplethysmography, 2 pp.

Health Technology Assessment Reports, 1981

(Compilation of 25 Reports, 260 pp., PB85-114049/AS. (Individual reports not available)

1. Alcohol Aversion Therapy, 13pp.
2. Hydrotherapy (Whirlpool) Baths for Treatment of Decubitus Ulcers, 5 pp.
3. Ultraviolet Light for Treatment of Decubitus Ulcers, 5 pp.
4. Transsexual Surgery, 18 pp.
5. Urine Autoinjection (Autogenous Urine Immunization), 4 pp.
6. Therapeutic Apheresis for Rheumatoid Arthritis, 13 pp.
7. Stereotaxic Depth Electrode Implantation Prior to Surgical Treatment of Focal Epilepsy, 6 pp.
8. Cytotoxic Leukocyte Test for the Diagnosis of Food Allergy, 10 pp.
9. Sublingual Provocative Testing and Neutralization Therapy for Food Allergies, 7 pp.
10. Intracutaneous (Intradermal) and Subcutaneous Provocative and Neutralization Testing and Neutralization Therapy for Food Allergies, 10 pp.
11. Intracranial Pressure Measurement, 8 pp.
12. B-Mode Scan in Peripheral Arterial Disease, 10 pp.
13. Tinnitus Maskers, 9 pp.
14. Percutaneous Transluminal Angioplasty in Treatment of the Lower Extremities, 14 pp.
15. Transcutaneous Electrical Nerve Stimulation for Acute Postoperative Incision Pain, 14 pp.
16. Shortwave Diathermy, 8 pp.

17. The Use of Human Tumor Stem Cell Drug Sensitivity Assays for Predicting Anticancer Drug Effects, 13 pp.
18. Ethylenediamine-Tetra-Acetic Acid (EDTA) Chelation Therapy for Atherosclerosis, 16 pp.
19. Ultraviolet Absorbing or Reflecting Spectacle Lenses for Aphakic and Pseudophakic Patients, 14 pp.
20. The Use of the Bentonite Flocculation Test in the Diagnosis of Rheumatoid Arthritis, 5 pp.
21. Desoxyribonucleic Acid-Bentonite Flocculation Test for the Diagnosis of Rheumatoid Arthritis, 5 pp.
22. The Use of the Mycoplasma Completion Fixation Test in the Diagnosis of Rheumatoid Arthritis, 6 pp.
23. The Kunkel Test for Estimating Total Serum Gamma Globulin Levels in Patients with Rheumatoid Arthritis, 6 pp.
24. The Role of Joint Scans Using Technetium-99m Pertechnetate in Diagnosing and Assessing Therapeutic Gain in Arthritis, 20 pp.
25. The Use of Anti-Inhibitor Coagulant Complex (Activated Prothrombin-Complex Concentrate) in the Treatment of Patients with Hemophilia A and Antibodies to Factor VIII, 16 pp.

Thermography
A technique in which temperature patterns on the surface of the skin are recorded in the form of an image.(ENC)

American Academy of Thermology
P.O. Box 1324, Vienna, VA 22180
703/938-6140

Thoracic
American Thoracic Society
1740 Broadway, New York, NY 10019-4374
212/315-8700

American Association for Thoracic Surgery
13 Elm St., Manchester, MA 01944
508/526-8330

American Board of Thoracic Surgery
1 Rotary Center, Suite 803, Evanston, IL 60201
708/475-1520

Society of Thoracic Surgeons
111 E. Wacker Drive, Ste. 600, Chicago, IL 60601
312/644-6610

Thyroid
American Thyroid Association
Mayo Clinic
200 First St. SW, Rochester, MN 55905
507/284-4738

Tinnitus
American Tinnitus Association
PO Box 5, Portland, OR 97207
503/248-9985

Tissue Banks
American Association of Tissue Banks
1350 Beverly Road, Ste 220-A, McLean, VA 22101
703/827-9582

Tourette Syndrome
Tourette Syndrome Association
42-40 Bell Boulevard, Bayside, NY 11361
800/237-0717

Transitional Year
Accreditation Council of
Graduate Medical Education
Transitional Year Review Committee
515 N. State St, Chicago, IL 60610
312/464-4920

Translations
Depository of Unpublished Translations
National Translation Center, Library of Congress
101 Independence Avenue, SE
Washington, DC 20540
202/707-0100

Transplantation
American Society of Transplant Surgeons
716 Lee St., Des Plaines, IL 60016
708/824-5700

Children's Transplant Association
PO Box 53699, Dallas, TX 75253
214/287-8484

Transplants, Liver (Experimental Status)
National Institutes of Health
301/496-5787

More transplants planned

AMNews 10/19/92 p.2

Pittsburgh - About 10 patients with life-threatening hepatitis B are being considered for a baboon-liver transplant, despite the Sept. 6, 1992, death of the first man to undergo the surgery, medical officials say. The first baboon-liver recipient, a 35-year-old man whose identity was never revealed, died 10 weeks after his transplant at Presbyterian University Hospital. A hospital spokeswoman says the new candidates are undergoing medical evaluations and discussing the possible risks and benefits with doctors.

Trauma
American College of Emergency Physicians
P.O. Box 619911, Dallas TX 75261-9911
214/550-0911

American Trauma Society
1400 Mercantile Lane, Ste 188
Landover, MD 20785
800/556-7890

Travel, International - Health Aspects
Centers for Disease Control
Center for Preventive Services, Atlanta, GA 30333
404/332-4559, 404/639-2779

Inoculations
Contact local/county health department
Chicago Department of Public Health
312/744-4340

International Association for Medical
Assistance to Travelers (IAMAT)
417 Center St., Lewiston, NY 14092
716/754-4883

Mobility International
(aid to handicapped people when traveling)
228 Borough High St, London, SEI 1JX, England
71 4035688

Mobility International, U.S.A
(North American affiliate of Mobility International)
P.O. Box 3551, Eugene, OR 97403
503/343-1284

"Yellow Book" or "Health Information for
International Travel"
Publication #017-023-00187-6
Superintendent of Documents
U.S. Government Printing Office
Washington, DC 20402
202/783-3238

Traveler & Immigrant Aid Societies, Statewide
Alabama
Traveler Aid Society of Birmingham
3600 Eighth Ave S, Suite 110-West
Birmingham, AL 35222
205/322-5426

Family Guidance Center of Montgomery, Inc
925 Forest Ave, Montgomery, AL 36106
205/265-0568

Arizona
Travelers Aid of Tucson
40 West Veterans Blvd, Tucson, AZ 85713
602/622-8900

California
Travelers Aid Society of Long Beach, Inc
947 East 4th St, Long Beach, CA 90802
310/432-3485

Travelers Aid Society of Los Angeles, Inc
566 South San Pedro, Los Angeles, CA 90013
213/955-9758

Travelers Aid Society of Alameda County, Inc
1761 Broadway, Oakland, CA 94612
510/444-6834

Travelers Aid Society of San Diego
1765 Fourth Ave, Suite 100, San Diego, CA 92101
619/232-7991

Colorado
Travelers Aid Services
1245 E Colfax Ave, Suite 408, Denver, CO 80218
303/832-8194

Connecticut
Travelers Aid Services of Hartford
Catholic Charities, 896 Asylum Ave.
Hartford, CT 06105
203/522-2247, 203/5222-8241

Family Counseling of Greater New Haven
1 State St, New Haven, CT 06511
203/865-1125

Delaware
Family & Children's Service of Delaware
2005 Baynard Blvd, Wilmington, DE 19802
302/658-5303

District of Columbia
Traveler's Aid Society of Washington, DC
512 C St, NE, Washington, DC 20002
202/546-3120

Florida
Travelers Aid of Daytona Beach
330 Magnolia Ave, Daytona Beach, FL 32114
904/252-4752

Community Service Council of Broward County
1300 S Andrews Ave, Fort Lauderdale, FL 33315
305/524-8371

Travelers Aid Society of Tampa, Inc
1005 N Marion St, Tampa, FL 33602
813/273-6506

The Center for Family Services
2218 South Dixie Highway
West Palm Beach, FL 33401
407/655-4483

Georgia
Travelers Aid of Metropolitan Atlanta, Inc
40 Pryor St, SW, Suite 400, Atlanta, GA 30303
404/527-7400

Travelers Aid of Savannah
PO Box 23975, Savannah, GA 31403-3975
912/233-2801

Illinois
Travelers & Immigrants Aid of Chicago
327 S LaSalle St, Room 1500, Chicago, IL 60604
312/435-4500

Travelers Aid
526 20th St, Rock Island, IL 61201
309/786-5424

Kentucky
Family and Children's Agency
1115 Garvin Place, PO Box 3784
Louisville, KY 40201
502/583-1741

Louisiana
Travelers Aid Society of Greater New Orleans
846 Baronne St, New Orleans, LA 70113
504/525-8726

Maryland
PATH: People Aiding Travelers and the Homeless
111 Park Ave, Baltimore, MD 21201
410/685-3569

Massachusetts
Travelers Aid Society of Boston, Inc
17 East St, Boston, MA 02111
617/542-7286

Michigan
Travelers Aid Society of Detroit
211 W Congress, 3rd Floor, Detroit, MI 48226
313/962-6740

Minnesota
Travelers Aid
404 S 8th St, Minneapolis, MN 55404
612/335-5000

Missouri
Mullanphy Travelers Aid
The Globe Bldg, 702 N Tucker Blvd.
St. Louis, MO 63102
314/241-5820

New York
Child and Family Services Travelers Aid Division
The Ellicott Square Bldg
295 Main St, Room 828, Buffalo, NY 14203
716/854-8661

Travelers Aid Services
2 Lafayette St, 3rd Floor, New York, NY 10007
212/577-3806

North Carolina
Travelers Aid of Charlotte, Inc
500 Spratt St, Charlotte, NC 28206
704/334-7288

Travelers Aid/Family Services of Wake County
401 Hillsborough St, Raleigh, NC 27603
919/821-0790

Family Services/Travelers Aid
PO Box 944, Wilmington, NC 28402
919/392-7051

Family Services of Winston-Salem
610 Coliseum Drive
Winston-Salem, NC 27106-5393
919/722-8173

Ohio
Travelers Aid--International Institute
707 Race St, Suite 300, Cincinnati, OH 45202
513/721-7660

Family Service Association/Travelers Aid
184 Salem, Room 790, Dayton, OH 45406
513/222-9481

Oklahoma
Travelers Aid Society of Oklahoma
412 NW 5th St, Oklahoma City, OK 73102
405/232-5507

Pennsylvannia
Travelers Aid Society of Philadelphia
311 S Juniper St, Suite 500-05
Philadelphia, PA 19107
215/546-0571

Travelers Aid Society of Pittsburgh
Greyhound Bus Terminal
11th and Liberty Ave, Pittsburgh, PA 15222
412/281-5466

Commission on Economic Opportunity
of Luzerne County
211-213 S Main St, Wilkes-Barre, PA 18701
717/826-0510

Puerto Rico
Travelers Aid of Puerto Rico, Inc
Luis Marin International Airport
San Juan, PR 00913
809/791-1034 or 1054

Rhode Island
Travelers Aid Society of Rhode Island, Inc
177 Union St, Providence, RI 02903
401/521-2255

Tennessee
Travelers Aid Society
46 N 3rd St, Suite 708, Memphis, TN 38103
901/525-5466

Nashville Union Mission
129 7th Ave S, Nashville, TN 37203
615/780-9471

Texas
Travelers Aid/American Red Cross
2630 Westridge, Houston, TX 77054-1510
713/668-0911

Utah
Travelers Aid Society of Salt Lake City
210 Rio Grande, Salt Lake City, UT 84101
801/328-8996

Virginia
Peninsula Family Services & Travelers Aid, Inc
1520 Aberdeen Road, PO Box 7315
Hampton, VA 23666
804/838-1960

Travelers Aid Society of Virginia
503 East Main, Richmond, VA 23219
804/643-0279

Wisconsin
Community Advocates/Travelers Aid
4906 W Fond du Lac Ave, Milwaukee, WI 53216
414/449-4774

Tropical Medicine
Walter Reed, MD 1857-1902

JAMA. 1902 Nov 29; 39(22): 1402

In the death of Dr. Walter Reed of the Army, which occurred November 23 (1902), scientific medicine has suffered a severe loss, and the profession has been bereft of a constant and enthusiastic student. Walter Reed was born in Virginia in 1857, was graduated from the Medical Department of the University of Virginia, Charlottesville, and from Bellevue Hospital Medical College, New York. He was appointed from Virginia to the Medical Department of the Army and was commissioned first-lieutenant and assistant surgeon, June 26, 1875; five years later he was made captain and assistant surgeon, and on Dec. 4, 1893, was promoted to the position of major and surgeon. At the time of his death he was at the head of the list of majors of the Medical Department of the Army. He made special studies in bacteriology at the Johns Hopkins Hospital, Baltimore, then was assigned to duty as attending surgeon at St. Paul, and from there was selected by the Surgeon-General as bacteriologist in his office, and was on duty there from 1893 until the outbreak of the Spanish-American War. During that time he was a member of the board of medical officers to investigate and report on the prevalence of typhoid fever in home camps and the commission recommended the plan of collecting excreta in galvanized iron tanks, which was afterwards successfully carried out at the U.S. General Hospital, Presidio, Cal., and was followed by cessation of the disease. His especial work was in the line of preventive medicine and military hygiene. His most notable services to the science of medicine were those connected with yellow fever. He was appointed president of the board the other members of which were Drs. Carroll and Agramonte of the Army, which met in Cuba for the study of yellow fever, and their discoveries in connection with the cause and prevention of this disease mark an epoch in medicine. Their reports have already been published in THE JOURNAL and show the highest degree of scientific accuracy combined with excellent discrimination. Dr. Reed was operated on for appendicitis on November 17, but did not rally from the operation, and died November 23.

Memorial to Major Walter Reed
JAMA 1903 Aug 15; 41(9):430

A meeting of the committees appointed by the American Medical Association and the American Association for the Advancement of Science has been called to meet at Bar Harbor, Me., August 15, to confer regarding the memorial in honor of the late Major Walter Reed, M.D. There are other committees beside the ones above mentioned, and the object is to secure immediate, concerted action and unanimity of purpose. The chairman of the committee representing the American Medical Association is Dr. W.W. Keen, Philadelphia, and Dr. Daniel C. Gilman, Baltimore, is chairman of the committee representing the American Association for the Advancement of Science. It is to be hoped that the various committees will be heartily supported by those whom they represent, and that in the immediate future a memorial worthy of the man and his work will be dedicated to Major Reed.

American Society of Tropical Medicine and Hygiene
8000 Westpark Drive, Suite 130
McLean, VA 22102
703/790-1745

Tuberous Sclerosis
National Tuberous Sclerosis Association
4351 Garden City Dr., Suite 660,
Landover, MD 20785
800/225-6872

Twins
Center for Study of Multiple Birth
333 East Superior St., Suite 476
Chicago, IL 60611
312/266-9093

National Organization of Mothers of Twins Club
12404 Princess Jeanne, N.E.
Albuquerque, NM 87112
505/275-0955

Twinline
2131 University Ave., Suite 234
Berkeley, CA 94704
415/644-0861

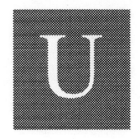

Ultrasound

American Institute of Ultrasound in Medicine
11200 Rockville Pike, Suite 205
Rockville, MD 20852
301/881-2486

Ultrasound task force/CSA reports the future of ultrasonography. Report of the Ultrasonography Task Force. Council on Scientific Affairs, American Medical Association. JAMA. 1991 Jul 17; 266(3): 406-9
Future advances in ultrasonography will undoubtedly occur in three major areas: diagnostic capability, instrumentation, and clinical applications. In the area of diagnostic capability, spatial and contrast resolution offer excellent opportunities for improvement. Continued research into tissue characterization is worthwhile, even though efforts to date have been more frustrating than fulfilling. Blood flow studies and new contrast agents are among the more promising areas for future development. New techniques of signal detection, analysis, and display in Doppler imaging may overcome some present limitations, including those in color flow imaging.

Gynecologic sonography. Report of the ultrasonography task force. Council on Scientific Affairs, American Medical Association. JAMA. 1991 Jun 5; 265(21): 2851-5
Sonography, because it is nonionizing, is the preferred imaging modality for the female pelvis. Traditionally, transabdominal, transcystic studies were performed However, development of transvaginal and transrectal transducers has led to enhanced imaging capabilities of the pelvis. These new technologies will likely improve our ability to understand gynecologic pathology. The clinical use of pelvic ultrasonography depends on a thorough understanding of normal anatomy and cyclical changes and on the relative limitations of the imaging modality in specifically characterizing pathologic processes. This article reviews the accepted role of pelvic sonography in gynecologic disease and provides a preview of some of the potential applications of recent advances in sonographic technology.

Doppler sonographic imaging of the vascular system. Report of the Ultrasonography Task Force. Council on Scientific Affairs, American Medical Association. JAMA. 1991 May 8; 265(18): 2382-7
Ultrasonic vascular imaging has been used for more than 20 years to define vascular anatomy, pathologic changes in vessel size, and perivascular abnormalities. In the last decade, development of duplex Doppler technology has permitted the evaluation of both anatomic vascular features and physiologic blood flow parameters in a variety of locations. Doppler "color flow" imaging promises to expand these applications. In many instances, duplex Doppler technology has replaced more invasive angiographic procedures for evaluation of suspected vascular abnormalities. Improved ultrasound duplex technology, combined with the relatively inexpensive, rapid, noninvasive aspects of ultrasonography has made it a valuable screening examination for suspected flow abnormalities.

Ultrasonic imaging of the abdomen. Report of the ultrasonography task force. Council on Scientific Affairs, American Medical Association. JAMA. 1991 Apr 3; 265(13): 1726-31
As new imaging modalities emerge and existing technologies improve, indications for a particular imaging method may change. This article examines current indications for abdominal and prostatic ultrasound examination and, where possible, compares ultrasound with other imaging techniques. This is not an attempt to list all possible ultrasound indications or examinations, but rather an attempt to serve as an aid to informed imaging selection based on current literature and equipment.

Medical diagnostic ultrasound instrumentation and clinical interpretation. Report of the ultrasonography task force. Council on Scientific Affairs. JAMA. 1991 Mar 6; 265(9): 1155-9
Over the past 20 years, there has been a dramatic increase in the use of ultrasonography as an imaging modality. The introduction of real-time ultrasonography and Doppler units for the measurement of blood flow in the 1970s, recent advances in transducer design, signal processing, and miniaturization of electronics, along with the lack of radiation exposure, have been primarily responsible for the increased use of ultrasound. However, although ultrasonography can provide diagnostic information safely and easily, interpretation of the information requires an understanding of the physics behind ultrasound, how that physics is translated into ultrasound instrumentation, recognition of artifacts that are associated with the various types of ultrasonography, and identification of these artifacts in specific anatomic locations.

Undersea Medicine

Board Certification
American Board of Preventive Medicine
Department of Community Medicine
Wright State University, P.O. Box 927
Dayton, OH 45401
513/278-6915

Undersea and Hyperbaric Medical Society, Inc.
9650 Rockville Pike, Bethesda, MD 20814
301/571-1818

Urinary Incontinence

HIP (Help for Incontinent People, Inc.)
PO Box 544, Union, SC 29379
803/585-8789

Simon Foundation
PO Box 815, Wilmette, IL 60091
800/23-SIMON (800/237-4666)

Urology

Urologist Diagnoses and treats diseases and disorders of genitourinary organs and tract: Examines patient, using x-ray machine, fluoroscope, and other equipment to aid in determining nature and extent of disorder or injury. Treats patient, using diathermy machine, catheter, cystoscope, radium emanation tube, and similar equipment. Performs surgery, as indicated. Prescribes and administers urinary antiseptics to combat infection. (DOT)

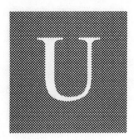

American Association of Clinical Urologists, Inc.
1120 N. Charles St., Baltimore, MD 21201
301/539-7168

American Board of Urology
31700 Telegraph Road, Suite 150,
Birmingham, MI 48010
313/646-9720

American Urological Association
1120 N. Charles St., Baltimore, MD 21201
301/727-1100

Valuing a Medical Practice

In general, reasons for valuing medical practices can be grouped into four major areas:

- Determining the value of the operating practice for purchase, sale, or merger
- Determining the value of physical assets for purchase or sale apart from or in addition to the operation practice
- Determining the value of the medical practice for the purpose of obtaining debt or equity financing, including the sale of stock or partnership interests to partners
- Determining the value of physical assets for reimbursement, tax, or insurance purposes

Where physical assets are being valued independent of an operating entity or business, the more traditional appraisal approaches to valuation are appropriate. Usually, however, the valuation of an operating entity includes certain physical assets. In such cases a more comprehensive, income-based approach to the medical-practice valuation would be more relevant and accurate. (ENH)

Buying and Selling Medical Practices: A Valuation Guide Chicago; American Medical Association. 1990. 99pp. ISBN 0-89970-383-6\OP370089

Vascular Surgery

Board Certification
American Board of Surgery
1617 John F. Kennedy Blvd.
Philadelphia, PA 19103
215/568-4000

Society for Vascular Surgery
13 Elm Street, Manchester, MA 01944
508/526-8330

Veterans Benefits Administration

Veterans Benefits Administration
Department of Veterans Affairs
810 Vermont Ave, NW, Washington, DC 20420
202/535-8619

Hotline for fraud, waste, and abuse
800/488-8244

Veterinary Medicine

Veterinarian: Diagnoses, and treats diseases and injuries of pets, such as dogs and cats, and farm animals, such as cattle or sheep: Examines animal to determine nature of disease or injury and treats animal surgically or medically. Tests dairy herds, horses, sheep, and other animals for diseases and inoculates animals against rabies, brucellosis, and other disorders. Advises animal owners about sanitary measures, feeding, and general care to promote health of animals. May engage in research, teaching, or production of commercial products. May specialize in prevention and control of communicable animal diseases and be designated Veterinarian, Public Health. May specialize in diagnosis and treatment of animal diseases, using roentgen rays and radioactive substances, and be designated Veterinary Radiologist. (DOT)

American Veterinary Medical Association
930 N. Meacham Rd., Schaumburg, IL 60196
708/605-8070

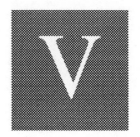

Video Clinics

"American Medical Television Video Digest"
(Monthly video subscription offers CME credit)
AMA Division of Television, Radio, and Film
800/933-4AMT (800/933-4268)

Network for Continuing Medical Education (NCME)
One Harmon Plaza, 7th Floor
Secaucus, NJ 07094
201/867-7600

Video Display Terminals

Health effects of video display terminals. Council on Scientific Affairs. JAMA. 1987 Mar 20; 257(11): 1508-12
About 15 million video display terminals are in use in the United States, and their numbers will continue to swell. Much concern has been raised by their users about possible adverse health effects. The extensive collection of research papers and state-of-the-art reports on this subject are reviewed in this article.

Statement on VDT and pregnancy:
American College of Obstetricians and Gynecologists
409 12th Street, SW, Washington, DC 20024-2188
202/638-5577

Vitamins

Vitamins and Their Sources in the Diet

Fat Soluable

Vitamin A/Good sources include: Liver, fish-liver oils, egg yolk, milk and dairy products, margarine, various fruits and vegetables (such as carrots and apricots)

Vitamin D/Good sources include: Fortified milk, oily fish (such as sardines, herring, salmon, and tuna), liver, dairy products, egg yolk

Vitamin E/Good Sources include: Vegetable oils (such as corn, soy bean, olive, and sunflower oils), nuts, meat, green leafy vegetables, cereals, wheat germ, egg yolk

Vitamin K/Good Sources include: Green leafy vegetables (especially cabbage, broccoli. and turnip greens), vegetable oils, egg yolk, cheese, pork, liver

Water-soluble

Thiamine/Good Sources include: Wheat germ, bran, whole-grain or (vitamin B1) enriched cereals and breads, brown rice, pasta, liver, kidney, pork, fish, beans, nuts

Riboflavin/Good Sources include: Liver, milk, cheese, eggs, green leafy (vitamin B2) vegetables, whole grains, enriched breads and cereals, brewer's yeast

Niacin/Good Sources include: Liver, lean meat, poultry, fish, whole (nicotinic acid) grains, enriched breads and cereals, peanuts, dried beans

Pantothenic acid/Good Sources include: Liver, heart, kidney, fish, egg yolk, skimmed milk, brewer's yeast, wheat germ, most vegetables

Pyridoxine/Good Sources include: Liver, chicken, pork, fish, whole (vitamin B6) grains, wheat germ, bananas, potatoes, dried beans, peanuts

Biotin/Good Sources include: Liver, kidney, peanuts, dried beans, egg yolk, mushrooms, cauliflower, bananas, grapefruit, watermelons

Folic acid/Good Sources include: Green leafy vegetables (such as spinach and broccoli), mushrooms, liver, nuts, dried beans, peas, egg yolk, whole-wheat bread

Vitamin B12/Good Sources include: Liver, kidney, chicken, beef, pork, (cycanocobalamin) fish, eggs, cheese, butter, yogurt, other dairy products

Vitamin C/Good Sources include: Citrus fruits, tomatoes, potatoes, green leafy vegetables, green peppers, strawberries, cantaloupe

Vitamin needs

A varied diet usually provides all vitamin needs. For vegans (who eat no animal products), vitamins B12 and D may be lacking; these vitamins can be obtained from supplements or, in the case of vitamin D, through adequate exposure to sunlight.(ENC)

Vitamin preparations as dietary supplements and as therapeutic agents. Council on Scientific Affairs. JAMA. 1987 Apr 10; 257(14): 1929-36
Healthy adult men and healthy adult nonpregnant, nonlactating women consuming a usual, varied diet do not need vitamin supplements. Infants may need dietary supplements at given times, as may pregnant and lactating women. Occasionally, vitamin supplements may be useful for people with unusual life styles or modified diets, including certain weight reduction regimens and strict vegetarian diets. Vitamins in therapeutic amounts may be indicated for the treatment of deficiency states, for pathologic conditions in which absorption and utilization of vitamins are reduced or requirements increased, and for certain nonnutritional disease processes. The decision to employ vitamin preparations in therapeutic amounts clearly rests with the physician. The importance of medical supervision when such amounts are administered is emphasized. Therapeutic vitamin mixtures should be so labeled and should not be used as dietary supplements.

Vitiligo
National Vitiligo Foundation
Texas American Bank Building, P.O. Box 6337, Tyler, TX 75711
214/561-4700

Volunteerism
Study: Two-thirds of doctors give charity care

Howard Larkin AMNews 3/9/92 p27-28

Nearly two-thirds of doctors surveyed said they recently had provided care free or at reduced rates based on patients' ability to pay.

Those 63.8% who provided charity care said they averaged about 6.6 hours doing so - about 10.6% of their medical and administrative time in the week before the survey, according to the American Medical Association, which conducted the survey.

Medicare and Medicaid services, which in many cases pay less than usual fees, as well as uncompensated care resulting from patients not paying their bills, were excluded from the estimates.

General and family practice physicians were most likely to give free or reduced fee care, with 71.2% saying they had in the week before the survey. Surgeons were the next most likely, with 70.2%, followed by radiologists at 65.7% and anesthesiologists at 63.7%

Pathologists were least likely to have given charity care at 52.2%, followed by "other specialties" at 53.6% and pediatricians at 53.9%.

About 2,100 physicians responded to the just-released survey, which was conducted in the fall of 1990 by the AMA Center for Health Policy Research. A similar survey of 4,000 physicians conducted by the center in 1988 had nearly identical results, said David Emmons, PhD, who analyzed the 1990 data.

The AMA survey does not explain differences among specialties in the proportion of physicians reporting charity care, Dr. Emmons said. But a spokesman for the American Academy of Family Physicians speculated that the nature of family practice may explain why general and family practice physicians reported the highest rates.

Family physicians are likely to see a wider variety of patients than most specialists, according to the spokesman. Also, general and family practice doctors are more likely to be located in rural areas, where a higher proportion of the population is poor and access to care outside a private doctor's office is limited.

Likewise, the nature of problems requiring surgery could account for high rates among surgeons, said Robert Brown, MD, a general surgeon in Midland, Mich. "A lot of what we do is emergent. You can't refuse care in an emergency."

Thomas Roe, MD, a Eugene, Ore., pediatrician, expressed surprise that the proportion of pediatricians reporting charity care was so low. Excluding Medicaid could be the culprit. "We see patients," said Dr. Roe, who estimates that 20% of his practice is public aid and another 5% no charge.

Dr. Roe also donates time to a free clinic for the homeless and helped set up a program through the local medical society promoting the acceptance of Medicare assignment for low-income elderly patients. Local physicians accept assignment for patients carrying "courtesy cards" issued by the program.

Dr. Brown agreed that excluding Medicaid diminishes physicians' true charity work. He said that Medicaid pays him as little as 25 cents on the dollar, and the cost of collecting it sometimes exceeds the payment.

"In our office we quite frankly prefer to do Medicaid patients for free," Dr. Brown said. He also helped establish one of the nation's first medical society courtesy card programs.

Both doctors said providing charity care is a part of their duty as physicians. As a matter of policy, the AMA urges all physicians to share in the care of indigent patients.

Beyond a humane and professional obligation to serve those unable to pay, there may be good business reasons to do so as well, Dr. Brown said. Continuing to treat patients who have lost jobs and health insurance may pay off when they return to work, he said.

"It's like the grocer who used to carry people in hard times. Maybe the supermarket won't do it now, but the guy on the corner would."

Physicians providing charity care: 1990
AMNews 3/9/92 pp27-8

Location:

Rural	72.6%
Small metropolitan	63.0
Large metropolitan	61.1
All Physicians	63.8

Specialty

General/family practice	71.2
Internal medicine	62.2
Surgery	70.2
Pediatrics	53.9
Obstetrics/Gynecology	61.7

Source: AMA Center for Health Policy Research

Most physicians give charity care

AMNews 9/14/92 p78

Nearly two thirds of physicians provide an average of 6.6 hours of charity medical care a week, according to an updated survey from the AMA Center for Health Policy Research. At the current cost of medical services, physicians contribute the equivalent of $6.8 billion a year to needy patients.

How to reap the benefits of volunteering

Mary Hegarty AMNews 5/4/92 p38

Veteran volunteers follow these guidelines to enrich the experience of working with the homeless:

- Don't be judgmental. "These are the disenfranchised," says David Freedman, MD, a Chicago family physician. "They don't have the wherewithal to go one mile get help. They are demoralized. But everyone needs health care."
- Find a clinic that takes care of the paperwork. "They should let doctors be doctors," says Pedro Jose Greer, Jr., MD, of Miami.
- Don't burn out. Volunteer consistently, but only as often as is comfortable for you, such as once a month. "One night every month is not something people can't do," says James Wallace, MD, a Bethesda, Md., internist, who volunteers at a shelter-based clinic.
- Don't volunteer on your day off. Take time from your work day, or volunteer in the evening. "Doctors work hard," Dr. Greer says. "We deserve that day off."

JAMA Article of Note: Physician Service Opportunities Abroad JAMA. 1990 Jun 27; 263(24): 3237-45

Care Medico
660 First Ave., New York, NY 10016
212/686-3110

"Doctors to all people"
(Physicians who help civilians in war areas.)
American Foundation
161 Cherry St., New Canaan, CT 06840
203/966-5195

Doctors of the World (Medicines du Monde)
(Maintain database of MD volunteers--matches to missions worldwide)
65 Broadway, New York, NY 10012
212/529-1556

Medecins Sans Frontieres
(Doctor's Without Borders)
8, rue St. Sabin, F-75544 Paris Cedex 11, France
1 40212929

New York Office
30 Rockefeller Plaza, Suite 5425
New York, NY 10112
212/649-5961

National Council for International Health
1701 K St, Ste 600, Washington, DC 20006
202/833-5900

Peace Corps
800/424-8580

Volunteer Programs, Adolescents

Amigos de las Americas (Friends of the Americas)
(For adolescents interested in the medical field; program visits Central and South America)
5618 Star Lane, Houston, TX 77057
713/782-5290
800/231-7796 (800/392-4580 TX)

Weight Chart
Height-Weight Tables for Adults:
Metropolitan Life Insurance Co.
Health and Safety Education Dept., 16W
1 Madison Ave., New York, NY 10010
212/578-2211

Wheelchair Exercise
National Handicapped Sports and
Recreation Association
P.O. Box 33141, Farragut Station
Washington, DC 20033
202/783-1441

National Wheelchair Athletic Association
2107 Templeton Gap Rd., Suite C
Colorado Springs CO 80907
303/632-0698

Women in Medicine
Equal, Not Really

Jane Marshall "A Piece of My Mind" JAMA. 1985
Aug 16; 254(7): 953

How can it be that at the age of 35, being an
accomplished, respected physician, a happily
married woman for 11 years, and a mother of two
beautiful children, I feel melancholy, inadequate,
and guilt-ridden? Ever since I can remember, my
goals have been similar to those of most men. I
have enjoyed competitive, physically demanding
sports and achieved multiple varsity letters in high
school. Excellence in general academics, and in
particular science, was more important to me than
even to my brother. The resultant conflicts of
being a competitive and feminine woman in our
society have been numerous. Nevertheless, I
have always managed. In my 20s I was able to
ride the early waves of "women's liberation." But
now, at 35, the waves have crashed into the shore
and eroded the sand.

My 6 1/2 year old gentle, vulnerable, and sensitive
son has developed a "mild-to-moderate stutter."
Stutter, stammer, and dysfluency are all different
words for basically the same problem. My
husband and I were recently called into our son's
private school for a conference with his first-grade
teacher, speech pathologist, director of the lower
school, and assistant headmaster. During our
hour together, we were informed that a probable
causative factor in this was my working. Not
enough mother-child time was the bottom line. It
was strongly recommended that I alter my
schedule if I felt "it was worth it." Worth it! Of
course it was worth it!

Our initial response to this conference was anger.
Both my husband and I were negatively
impressed with our perception of these educators'
lack of sensitivity to the plight of the "working
mother" and "working couple." However, after
serious review of our pressured and rushed
lifestyle, I arranged an extended overdue vacation
that corresponded with my son's school vacation.
During this more relaxed intimate time together,
his speech pattern became significantly more
fluent. A partial solution to my child's stutter
obviously included a more permanent change in
my working schedule to increase our time
together.

But what about my career and all the years of
social deprivation to afford me more time to study?
The years of "investing for my future" would now
be set aside for something certainly more "worth
it"! Worst of all there was my guilt. Why was I at
fault? I have spent more time with my children
than many nonworking mothers. My husband and
I have almost completely eliminated our social and
athletic activities in order to spend our free time
with our children. This obviously was not enough
for our more vulnerable eldest child!

I will, of course, alter my work load. I will curtail
teaching and publishing activities. I have a mind
full of ideas that will not be written by me but by
others.

Every time I hear my son speak, I feel his pain and
frustration. I am filled with sorrow and guilt. I now
know I am not equal to my male colleagues. In
many ways I am better. However, I may not be
allowed to show you or them because first I am a
mother and wife and then I am a physician. I
suppose I may continue to cry myself to sleep for
many years. And when my daughter comes to me
for career advice - what should I tell her?

Rumble in the Ranks
Sexism may be a fact of medical life, but
women are fighting back

Janice Perrone AMNews 10/7/91 p41

There is a growing chorus of women doctors who
accuse the profession of gender-related bias and
harassment, and who are effectively fighting back.
Their stories have emerged in the wake of the
widely publicized resignation in May of
neurosurgeon Frances Conley, MD, from the
faculty at Stanford University School of Medicine.
Dr. Conley alleged that she had tolerated
demeaning and inappropriate behavior from some
male colleagues for more than two decades. After
a summer of intense publicity she won
concessions from Stanford, and last month she
withdrew her resignation.

Medicine's attention to sexism in its rank follows a
sharp rise in the number of women physicians.
More than 98,000 physicians in the United States
now are women; they account for about 17% of all
U.S. physicians, up from 8% in 1970. But about
40% of medical students now are female; by the
year 2010, some 30% of all physicians are
expected to be women.

"People who have done research on minority
groups say that when a subgroup constitutes
about 30% of the work group, they can start to talk
about their issues," says Dr. Lenhart, a clinical
instructor in psychiatry at Harvard Medical School,
who heads a subcommittee on gender-equity
issues for the American Medical Women's Assn.
"There are enough women in medicine that that's
what's happening now."

Gender bias in medicine ranges from subtle
slights to overt sexual harassment and
discrimination. AMWA's hot line ([703] 838-0500)
receives about 35 calls per year. Most calls are
"about the subtle things - being addressed in
demeaning terms, being put down, left out of
collegial communications," Dr. Lenhart says.

Mary Rowe, PhD, an ombudsman and adjunct professor of management at Massachusetts Institute of Technology, has coined the term "microinequities" to describe the subtle yet unfair and inappropriate behaviors that female professionals frequently encounter. She calls them "small in nature but not trivial in effect."

Examples include: having negative presumptions made about your professional capabilities or dedication; having your suggestions ignored, then praised when a man offers them; being assigned to positions that don't provide opportunities for advancement; and being the recipient of disrespectful comments.

"Microinequities are fiendishly efficient in perpetuating unequal opportunity because they are in the air we breathe, in the books we read, in television we all watch, and because we cannot change the personal characteristic that leads to the inequity," writes Dr. Rowe.

Janet Shepherd, MD, former editor of Balance, a magazine for women physicians that ceased publication last year, says the most blatant sexism occurs in academic medicine. "Nobody can stop you from taking care of patients once you're in private practice, and in that setting you're not seeking promotions. In academics, your whole advancement is political."

But Dr. Lenhart says that women physicians in some private practice groups also face significant discrimination. "Another group complaining a lot are those in half-time positions in HMOs, which are frequently held by women with children. The benefit packages and opportunities are disproportionately low in part-time positions in some organizations."

Dr. Lenhart's AMWA committee offers moral support to hot-line callers and advice on how to respond to gender bias. Combatting discrimination also was a discussion topic at a national conference for women physicians held in August near Denver. In workshops there and in subsequent interviews. Dr. Dodson and other speakers outlined successful strategies.

Key among those was the importance of developing allies. "One thing women might learn to do better is to polit on an individual basis," says Holly Atkinson, MD, senior vice president of programming and medical affairs for Lifetime Medical Television and medical correspondent for NBC's "Today" show. "Nothing works like directly asking for help."

Seeking alliances was an important part of Dr. Lenhart's advice to the angry Midwestern residents. She suggested they first meet with the dean. As a result, "When they went to the residency director to complain, they already had the dean's support. I also advised them to ask for something specific, which they did: They asked for a formal policy that all fellowships be advertised. I also told them to give themselves time to calm down."

When lining up allies, Dr. Dodson stresses the valuable role that male colleagues can play. "Some of the male doctors in the hospital have been my biggest supporters." Named pediatrics chairman after the division she headed became a

department, she speculates that the administration didn't want her for the job, but she had five years' tenure and her division was running smoothly, so they promoted her while downplaying her role in hospital affairs.

In addition to helping her get a seat at hospital board meetings, some male colleagues worked with her almost weekly on how to deal with the hospital administration and how to develop management and administrative skills. On one occasion, she was excluded from a session to photograph the department chairmen for the hospital's annual report. But the other six chairmen - all about 15 years her senior - refused to allow the photo to be taken without her and waited 20 minutes until she could get there.

Letting those who are respected by the power structure go to bat for you clearly can help, but it's also important at times to directly confront the discriminating individuals, Dr. Dodson says. She used this approach in response to another slight.

The same year she became chairman, two male department chairmen also were appointed. "They were announced. I wasn't. It could not have been an oversight because we have a hospital newspaper that talks about the janitor's granddaughter's birthday.

"When I confronted the administration, I was told I had an ego problem."

Instead of getting angry, Dr. Dodson took a tip from a communications course she had taken and emphasized to the administration how their behavior was hurting the hospital.

"I told them I didn't have an ego problem, I had a recognition problem, and that when they recognized the other chiefs and not me, they made it difficult for me to do my job. I told them I needed their support to make pediatrics a better department for their hospital."

It's important to conclude such confrontations on a congenial note, as men usually do, and not to take them personally or hold a grudge, Dr. Dodson says. "I've had several confrontations like this, and they were most unpleasant. But at the end of it, we end up shaking hands. Women tend to think about these things when they're over and take the attitude of, 'I'm taking my ball and bat away and I'm not going to play with you anymore.' That doesn't help. It makes things worse."

Dr. Atkinson and others at the women's conference echoed this view. "We should take it as a compliment when another person will spar with you," Dr. Atkinson says. "It shows that the other person respects your position. If you look at it that way, it's a real esteem-enhancer."

At the conference and in interviews with women physicians, several additional suggestions for fighting sexism emerged:
- Choose your battles. "Ask yourself, 'If I win this battle, will it improve my working situation or my career?'" Dr. Atkinson advises.
- Meet with other women physicians to solve problems. "That way women see that they're not the only ones this is happening to, and you can get each other to calm down before you take any action," Dr. Lenhart says.

- Refine your arguments on women's issues when confronting your superiors. "There's been a lot of debate in academic medical centers about what it's going to cost to have maternity leave, flex time and job sharing," Dr. Atkinson says. "We need to start talking about the costs of male behaviors in our society." For example, alcoholism is more common among men but its costs are not calculated as male-related costs of business, she says.

- Change your own attitude, if you want to change others'. Dr. Atkinson compares the situation to pulling on one string in a mobile; the others will be forced to move as well. "If a woman has a contract and the terms are not equal to a man's, she can go along and smolder or she can change her behavior. She can hire a lawyer, confront the administration, learn negotiating skills or get training for leadership positions. Whatever she does is going to necessitate a change in those she interacts with."

- Emphasize your professional self. "Looking young and being soft-spoken can be a disadvantage," admits Dr. Dodson. "When I need to meet with the administration, I frequently make the appointment for a time when I've been on call for 24 hours. I show up in my scrubs with my stethoscope. Somehow that reminds me and them that I am a physician and this is what I'm here for, not for something like Mickey Mouse."

- Use humor effectively. Says Dr. Bernstein, "Over the years I have stood up for myself in a way that was funny and not antagonistic. People ceded the point to me because I wasn't confrontational. Yet I could walk away with my self-esteem in good shape because I hadn't let myself be humiliated."

- Learn to negotiate salaries and contracts. "Women physicians make less money across the board than male physicians," Dr. Atkinson says, and studies have shown that the contracts women physicians practice under are "lousy" by and large. "The agreements allow a practice to fire the woman, and then they bring in a younger person for much less money. This is an important point because most women are employed by group practices and HMOs."

All these strategies are designed to help women score victories against gender bias. But in some situations, resigning, not fighting, may be the best course. Dr. Atkinson suggests performing a cost-benefit analysis.

"If the situation stays the same, what's the cost? You might pay a price like no promotion, low salary or self-esteem. Then ask yourself, 'If I get what I want, what's the benefit and what are the costs?' They might ask you to pay with isolation or hostility.

"But a key question here is, 'Are the costs irrevocable or are they short-term?' If you eventually win their respect, it may be worth it."

Sometimes, however, you lose even when you win.

"The advantages of putting up a fight and winning are that women have achieved chairmanship and success in medicine," Dr. Shepherd says. "The drawbacks are that many are perceived as bitches on the way there, while men who get to that level are just seen as having achieved success.

"There are a lot of women doctors who just can't handle being thought of that way. They need people to like them."

Women in Medical Practice
Activity and Specialty Choice

In 1970, there were 25,401 female physicians in the United States. By 1988, that number had nearly quadrupled to 98,446, while the overall physician population grew by 80%. During the same period, the number of female doctors rose from 7.7% to 16.4% of the physician population. Tables 2.1-2.3 give some background information on the number of females in the medical profession and their activity status.

In 1988, about one in four women physicians was still in residency or fellowship training. Table 2.3 shows that 45.9% were in office-based practice, and 10.4% were in hospital-based practice. Compared to 1970, women physicians were more likely to be in hospital-based practice in 1988. However, women still represented just 12.9% of all office-based physicians, (see Table 3.2, *Women in Medical Practice*) Only a small percentage of women were primarily engaged in research, teaching, or administrative activities in 1988. (WIM)

Women in Medicine in America

For the second time in the history of the United States, women are thriving in the medical profession. The first time was in the last quarter of the 19th century, soon after Elizabeth Blackwell and her sister, Emily, opened the pioneering Woman's Medical College of the New York Infirmary in 1869 because no other regular medical school in the city would accept women. Over 20 years before, in 1848, Elizabeth Blackwell had been the first American woman to receive a medical degree. Women's medical schools flourished in the latter half of the 1800s - another 16 existed - and it was not unheard of, 100 years ago, for women physicians to combine the dual demands of career and family. A year before Abraham Flexner published his watershed report on medical education in 1910, all but three of these schools had closed.

In the last quarter of this century there has been another renaissance for women entering the medical field. The number of women physicians more than quadrupled between 1970 and 1990, from 25,401 to over 100,000. (Table 1.1) Projections suggest that 30% of physicians will be female by the year 2010.

With the publication *Women in Medicine in America*, the American Medical Association's (AMA) Women in Medical Services is responding to a continuing desire for information about women physicians. It includes both a discussion of the issues facing women in medicine today and over 60 statistical tables reflecting all parts of a woman's career, from medical school through practice.

In recent years, the American Medical Association has been overwhelmed with requests for the type of information found in *Women in Medicine*. This pursuit of information corresponds both with the

growing representation of women in medicine and the questions raised when members of a formerly small minority in a profession assume a major place in its ranks.

The earlier era of prosperity for women in medicine may contain some lessons for today. Prevented from entering male medical schools, women founded their own - theirs was, of necessity, a separatist movement. The numbers were encouraging: women represented only .8% of the physician population in 1870,but 6% by the turn of the century. The 6% representation was a peak not attained again by women until the second half of this century.

Most female physicians were clustered in New York, Boston, and Philadelphia where the first women's medical schools and hospitals were founded. By 1900, women were more than 18% of Boston's physicians. Two surveys done on graduates of their own medical schools in the late 1800s revealed that women typically worked in private practice as general practitioners or ob/gyns, or in women's institutions. The surveys differ on marital status: One found that 47% of its graduates married, the other discovered that less than 20% had done so.

As the century ended, more opportunities for coeducational training unfolded, and women welcomed the attainment of their long-term goal in medical training - integration. In 1894, women made up at least 10% of the study body at 18 medical schools run by men. And when the Woman's Medical College of the New York Infirmary was absorbed by Cornell University Medical School in 1899, Emily Blackwell, one of the Infirmary's founders, said that Cornell's acceptance of women made "a separate medical school for women unnecessary." Seventy women from the women's medical school entered Cornell in 1900. But by 1903 that number had been reduced to ten.

The fall of that women's medical school and the corresponding reduction of places for women echoed elsewhere. In 1910, more than half the medical schools in America did not accept women. The lack of acceptance persisted. In 1946 the dean of a large medical school in the East admitted to limiting the enrollment of women to 6%. Even in the 1960s, women still faced small quotas when trying to enter medical schools. However, despite the quotas and the then small number of women in medicine, women were in the profession to stay. The American Medical Association opened membership to women in 1915.

Perhaps the lessons to be learned from those more difficult times are about parity and the need within the profession for a view which fully integrates, rather than excludes, those whose gender raises uncomfortable issues about training and practice. Women must be allowed to thrive in any institution and in any specialty in which they can make a contribution. As discussed in various chapters of Women in Medicine in America, almost two-thirds of women physicians are found in five specialties: pediatrics; psychiatry; family practice; internal medicine; and obstetrics/gynecology. It is not that women must become surgeons; rather, that they must be able to comfortably pursue that specialty and secure

acceptance if they are to achieve parity in medicine. They must be found at all levels of administration, as heads of medical schools, clinical departments and medical societies.

The normative patterns of training and work for physicians that now exist are often difficult for women who want to have families and have a career in medicine. Approximately 75% of female physicians are married, and 85% of those married or previously married have children. Again, the point is that all women physicians should have the option to have children and still have tenured positions, be heads of departments, and pursue specialties that require many years of training - just as do male physicians with children.

Medicine has changed women, but women are changing medicine, too. Residency programs can no longer treat a pregnant resident as an oddity; it simply happens too often. And new decisions and opportunities that reflect the needs of today's female and male physicians are being made. Maternity and paternity leave policies, expanding the time track to tenure, reducing the hours that residents are allowed to work, shared positions, child care programs in hospitals - the fact that these exist and are increasing is evidence that women are being better served as physicians. As Nancy Dickey, MD, a member if the Board of Trustees at the AMA, says, "There are still barriers, but there are very few hurdles that can't be leaped by women who are energetic and dedicated." If the extraordinary strides women in medicine have made thus far are indicative of future successes, Dr. Dickey will be proven correct. (WIM)

Physicians by Gender

	1970 #/%	1980 #/%	1990 #/%
total MDs	334,028	467,679	615,421
Men	308,627/92.4	413,395/88.4	511,227/83.1
Women	25,401/ 7.6	54,284/11.6	104,194/16.9

Source: American Medical Association Physician Masterfile

Women in Medical Practice
Net Income
Mean income data for 1981 and 1988 in Table 3.28 (see Women in Medicine) show that female physicians averaged $96,397 in net income after expenses but before taxes in 1988, only 63.5% of the male average income of $151,853. However, the growth rate for female earnings between 1981 and 1988 was 82.1%, while male earnings grew just 66.7%. For comparison, the average price level increased 30.5% over this seven year period, so both male and female physicians experienced significant real earnings growth (WIM)

American Medical Women's Association
801 N. Fairfax, Alexandria, VA 22314
703/838-0500

Women's Health
Women's Health, Public Welfare

Bernadine Healy, MD JAMA 1991 Jul 24/31; 266(4), 566-8

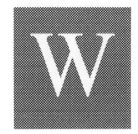

While leafing through a pile of the press clippings that regularly cross my desk at the National Institutes of Health (NIH), I was struck particularly by two headlines in the Philadelphia Inquirer (May 31, 1991;sect A:1) that said, "Menopause Becoming 'Au Courant' as It Hits Women of Baby Boom" and, as the article continued on another page, "Menopause Comes of Age as Medical and Social Issue." Indeed, women's health, in general - in terms of research, services, and access to care - has come of age and become a priority medically, socially, and politically.

The Article "Gender Disparities in Clinical Decision Making,"[1] the report of the Council on Ethical and Judicial Affairs of the American Medical Association in this issue of THE JOURNAL, is to be applauded for its important contribution to answering the question of why women's health research and care demand such particular attention and vigor. The report documents the disparity between genders in regard to access to certain critical diagnostic and therapeutic interventions - specifically, kidney dialysis and transplantation, diagnosis lung cancer, and catheterization for coronary bypass surgery. And it asks each of us to acknowledge and consider the fact that clinical decision making is based not only on scientific indications, but also on "myriad social, economic, and cultural factors" that may result in gender disparities in the provision of health care. One sentence in the report is the anthem of its message: "The medical community cannot tolerate any discrepancy in the provision of care that is not based on appropriate biological or medical indications."

This credo has two implications: first, that we possess the knowledge that allows us to undertake scientific evaluation; and second, that we are able to dismiss and invalidate other subtle factors that allow discrimination.

Research alone cannot correct the disparities, inequities, or insensitivities of the health care system, but it makes a critical contribution. Because much of our current knowledge is based, as the report indicates, on research in which the study populations were predominantly men, our responsibility now is to establish the science base that will permit reliable diagnoses, as well as effective treatment and prevention strategies, to provide care to women, based on "appropriate biological or medical indications." The NIH is committed to meeting this challenge directly and to addressing the important recommendations of this report. Indeed, in the NIH's mission to use the methods of science toward the interests of public health and welfare, women's health research must figure prominently.

In September 1990, the NIH established the Office of Research on Women's Health, a major step forward for women's health concerns. Charged with ensuring that research conducted and supported by the NIH appropriately addresses issues regarding women's health, it sees that women particularly fully and appropriately in clinical research, including clinical trials.

The new office vigorously responded to the concerns and recommendations of the General Accounting Office report and implemented a strengthened and revitalized NIH policy on the inclusion of women in study populations (published in the NIH Guide to Grants and Contracts, August 24, 1990, and February 2, 1991). The seriousness of purpose with which the NIH has addressed this policy is already evident. All NIH staff responsible for review and scientific management of research grants and contracts attended training sessions; NIH peer review groups and all of the institute and center advisory councils received formal briefings on these policies; and the NIH has revised its grant application forms to require information about the composition of study populations in proposed clinical research. The NIH has taken the position that no applications will be funded in which women and minorities are not adequately represented in planned clinical research populations, as appropriate, unless compelling scientific justification is provided.

Although the major portion of research conducted or supported by the NIH benefits both men and women, there are areas of special need for new knowledge that are unique to women. Accordingly, another of the report's recommendation has already been embraced by the NIH: "More medical research on women's health and women's health problems should be pursued." The NIH has embarked on two major efforts that will dramatically affect research regarding women's health.

First, through a series of activities in 1991 - including an invited scientific conference and a public hearing to gather the viewpoints of women's health advocates - the NIH Task Force on Opportunities for Research on Women's Health will assess the current status of such research, identify research opportunities and gaps in knowledge, and recommend a comprehensive NIH plan for future directions for research on women's health during the next 10 to 20 years. Experts in the fields of basic and clinical sciences, practitioners interested in women's health, and women's health advocates are being asked to recommend a research agenda focusing on diseases, disorders, and conditions unique to women, more serious in women, or having different risk factors or interventions in women. This agenda will recommend research priorities across each stage of life and will help guide such research into the next century.

Second, we have recently launched a new initiative that will be the most definitive, far-reaching study of women's health ever undertaken. The Women's Health Initiative will examine heart disease and stroke, cancer, and osteoporosis - the major causes of death, disability, and frailty in women of all races and socioeconomic strata. Comprising three components - a large prospective surveillance study, a nationally based community intervention and prevention study, and randomized clinical trials - the study will examine the effects of menopause on disease in older women, as well as diet modification, smoking cessation, use of hormones, and physical exercise. Seven NIH

institutes will be involved, and coordination by the Office of Research on Women's Health will ensure that the institutes contribute their knowledge, expertise, and wisdom to an integrated, productive research program.

The Office of Research on Women's Health is also undertaking an evaluation of the medical, social, and legal barriers to inclusion of women of childbearing potential in clinical research, a project that will benefit all researchers in designing and implementing research protocols. Broader policy questions pertaining to women's health are also being investigated: Should guidelines be developed to indicate when a study should be designed specifically to evaluate gender differences? Is it feasible to develop guidelines to evaluate an intervention over the course of the menstrual cycle? Can issues such as potential fetal damage, the liability for fetal damage, and possible adverse effects on fertility be overcome in designing studies to include women? The answers to these questions are critical to progress in research on women's health.

An additional goal of the NIH and its Office of Research on Women's Health is to set an agenda for nurturing women in leadership roles in biomedical research. We applaud the recommendation in the report that "awareness of and responsiveness to sociocultural factors that could lead to gender disparities may be enhanced by increasing the number of female physicians in leadership roles and other positions of authority in teaching, research, and the practice of medicine."[1] It is our plan in 1992 to host a conference that will address on a national scale how we can better encourage, recruit, maintain, and promote women in scientific and medical careers.

Over the past years, the number of women entering medical schools has increased steadily, and the federal government now has women in two of the highest jobs in the Department of Health and Human Services - as Surgeon General and as director of the NIH. However, I would suggest that there may be one omission from the report's discussion. Progress in addressing the gender discrepancies that have been documented cannot depend alone on swelling the ranks of female researchers and physicians or on physicians who "examine their practices and attitudes for influence of social or cultural biases."[1]

Here, more may be needed. Namely, we must train all medical students, male and female, to understand the biological differences between the sexes, to take the time to listen to their patients, to respect their patients' concerns and anxieties, and, most of all - as so many women have consistently written to me - to take them seriously.

Just as the NIH had been forced to rethink and revamp its research agenda and policies regarding women, so too must other institutions reconsider their processes, philosophies, and training curricula that have contributed to gender disparities in health care. The NIH plans to work with institutional review boards and other administrators to assist in this process.

The Journal has tackled some thorny and difficult issues in the past several issues, including its recent discussions of the future of the American

health care system. Access to care, access to appropriate interventions and diagnosis, and access to participation in clinical trials are all important concerns for women.

The report adopted by the House of Delegates of the American Medical Association, while providing important recommendations for change, documents a situation that cannot persist. The NIH is committed to conducting and supporting the research that will provide the important foundation on which clinical decision making depends. But solutions to the subtle factors that have allowed discrepancies in the provision of care that is not based on appropriate biological or medical indications lie not only in research, training, and education, but also within each of us.

References
1. Council on Ethical and Judicial Affairs, American Medical Association. Gender disparities in clinical decision making. JAMA.1991;266:559-562.

Center for Research on Women and Gender
University of Illinois College of Medicine
1640 W. Roosevelt Road, Chicago, IL 60612
312/413-7752

Worker's Compensation
Federal
230 S. Dearborn, Chicago, IL 60604
312/353-5656

Alabama Workers' Compensation Division
Department of Industrial Relations
602 Madison Ave, Montgomery, AL 36130
205/242-2868

Alaska Division of Workers' Compensation
Department of Labor
P.O. Box 25512, Juneau, AK 99802
907/465-2790

Arizona State Compensation Fund
3031 North Second St, Phoenix, AZ 85012
602/631-2000

Arkansas Workers' Compensation Commission
Justice Bldg, 2nd Floor, Little Rock, AR 72201
501/682-3930

California Department of Industrial Relations
Wing A, 5th Floor
395 Oyster Point Blvd, S
San Francisco, CA 94080
415/737-2600

Colorado Department of Labor and Employment
1120 Lincoln St, 13th Floor, Denver, CO 80203
303/894-7530

Connecticut Workers' Compensation Commission
1890 Dixwell Ave, Hamden, CT 06514
203/789-7783

Delaware Division of Industrial Affairs
Department of Labor
820 N French St, Wilmington, DE 19801
302/571-2877

District of Columbia Office
of Workers' Compensation
Department of Employment
1200 Upshur St, NW, 3rd Floor
Washington, DC 20011
202/576-6265

Florida Division of Workers' Compensation
Labor and Employment Security Department
301 Forest Bldg, Tallahassee, FL 32399
904/488-2514

Georgia State Board of Workers' Compensation
1 CNN Center, Suite 1000, Atlanta, GA 30303
404/656-2034

Hawaii Disability Compensation Division
Labor and Industrial Relations Department
830 Punchbowl St, Honolulu, HI 96813
808/548-5414

Idaho State Insurance Fund
1215 W State St, Boise, ID 83720
208/334-2370

Illinois Industrial Commission
100 W Randolph St, Suite 8-272
Chicago, IL 60601
312/814-6555

Indiana Worker's Compensation Board
402 W Washington St, W196
Indianapolis, IN 46204
317/232-7103

Iowa Division of Industrial Services
Department of Employment Services
1000 E Grand, Des Moines, IA 50319
515/281-5934

Kansas Division of Workers' Compensation
Department of Human Resources
600 Merchants Bank Tower, Topeka, KS 66612
913/296-3441

Kentucky Workers Claims
The 127 Bldg, U.S. 127 S, Frankfort, KY 40601
502/564-3070

Louisiana Office of Labor
PO Box 94094, Baton Rouge, LA 70804
504/925-4221

Maine Workers' Compensation Commission
State House Station #27, Augusta, ME 04333
207/289-3751

Maryland Workers' Compensation Commission
6 N. Liberty St, Room 940, Baltimore, MD 21201
410/333-4775

Massachusetts Industrial Accident Board
600 Washington St, 7th Floor, Boston, MA 02111
617/727-4300

Michigan Bureau of Workers' Compensation
Department of Labor
PO Box 30016, Lansing, MI 48909
517/373-3480

Minnesota Workers' Compensation Division
Department of Labor and Industry
444 Lafayette Road, Saint Paul, MN 55101
612/296-6490

Mississippi Workers' Compensation Commission
1428 Lakeland Drive, Jackson, MS 39216
601/987-4200

Missouri Division of Workers' Compensation
Labor and Industrial Relations Department
722 Jefferson St, PO Box 58
Jefferson City, MO 65102
314/751-4231

Montana State Compensation and
Mutual Fund Insurance
Department of Administration
5 S Last Chance Gulch, Helena, MT 59601
406/444-6518

Nebraska Workmen's Compensation Court
State Capitol, 13th Floor
PO Box 94967, Lincoln, NE 68509
402/471-2568

Nevada State Industrial Insurance System
515 E Musser St, Carson City, NV 89714
702/687-5220

New Hampshire Workmen's
Compensation Division
Department of Labor
19 Pillsbury St, Concord, NH 03301
603/271-3174

New Jersey Division of Workers' Compensation
Department of Labor
John Fitch Plaza, CN 381, Trenton, NJ 08625
609/292-2414

New Mexico Workmen's
Compensation Administration
Labor and Industrial Commission
180 Randolph SE, Albuquerque, NM 87106
505/841-6000

New York Workers' Compensation Board
180 Livingston St, Brooklyn, NY 11248
718/802-6666

North Carolina Industrial Commission
Department of Economic and
Community Development
430 N Salisbury St, Raleigh, NC 27603
919/733-4820

North Dakota Workers' Compensation Bureau
4007 N State St, Bismarck, ND 58501
701/224-3800

Ohio Workers' Compensation Bureau
246 N High St, Columbus, OH 43266
614/466-1935

Oklahoma Workers' Compensation Committee
1915 N Stiles, Oklahoma City, OK 73105
405/557-7600

Oregon Workers' Compensation Division
Department of Insurance and Finance
Labor and Industries Bldg, Salem, OR 97310
503/378-3304

Pennsylvania Bureau of Workers' Compensation
Department of Labor and Industry
3607 Derry St, 4th Floor, Harrisburg, PA 17120
717/783-5421

Rhode Island Workers'
Compensation Commission
One Dorrance Plaza, Providence, RI 02903
401/272-0700

South Carolina Workers'
Compensation Commission
PO Box 1715, Columbia, SC 29202
803/734-5744

South Dakota Division of Labor and Management
Department of Labor
Kneip Bldg, Pierre, SD 57501
605/773-3681

Tennessee Workers' Compensation
Department of Labor
501 Union Bldg, Nashville, TN 37243
615/741-2395

Texas Workers' Compensation Commission
200 E Riverside Drive, Austin, TX 78704
512/448-7900

Utah Industrial Commission
160 E 300 S, Salt Lake City, UT 84111
801/530-6800

Vermont Department of Labor and Industry
7 Court St, Montpelier, VT 05602
802/828-2286

Virginia Workers' Compensation Commission
PO Box 1794, Richmond, VA 23214
804/367-8666

Washington Department of Labor and Industries
234 General Administration Bldg
M/S: HC-901, Olympia, WA 98504
206/753-6307

West Virginia Division of Workers' Compensation
PO Box 3051, Charleston, WV 25332
304/344-2580

Wisconsin Division of Workers' Compensation
Industrial Labor and Human Relations
PO Box 7901, Madison, WI 53707
608/266-6841

Wyoming Workers' Compensation Division
Department of Employment
122 W 25th St, Cheyenne, WY 82002
307/777-7441

American Samoa Workmen's
Compensation Commission
Legal Affairs, Pago Pago, AS 96799
684/633-5520

Guam Department of Labor
PO Box 9970, Tamuning, GU 96911
671/646-9241

Northern Mariana Islands
Civil Service Commission
Personnel Management Office
Office of the Governor, Saipan, MP 96950
670/234-6925

Puerto Rico State Insurance Fund
PO Box 365028, San Juan, PR 00936
809/781-0122

U.S. Virgin Islands Department of Labor
PO Box 890, Christiansted, Saint Croix, VI 00820
809/773-1994

World Health Organization
The World Health Organization (WHO)
was established in 1948 as an agency of the
United Nations with responsibilities for
international health matters and public health. Its
headquarters is in Geneva, Switzerland; there are
also regional offices for Europe, Africa, North
America, South America, Southeast Asia, the
Eastern Mediterranean, and the Western Pacific
(including Australia).

The WHO has campaigned effectively against
certain infectious diseases, notably smallpox
(which was officially declared as eradicated
throughout the world in 1980), tuberculosis, and
malaria. Its other functions include sponsoring
medical research programs, organizing a network
of collaborating national laboratories, and
providing expert advice to its 160 member states
on matters such as health service organizations,
family health, the use of medicinal drugs, the
abuse of drugs, and mental health. The
organization's current strategy is described in its
campaign "Health for all by the year 2000." The
plan gives specific targets for basic public health
measures, such as the provision of piped water
supplies and other basic sanitation, the universal
provision of immunization of children against
infectious diseases, and reductions in the use of
tobacco and alcohol.(ENC)

Headquarters
World Health Organization
CH-1211, Geneva 27, Switzerland 91 21 11

Regional Office for the Americas
525 Twenty-Third St. NW, Washington, DC 20037
202/861-3200

WHO Publications Center
49 Sheridan Ave., Albany, NY 12221
518/436-9686

World Medical Association
World Medical Association
(Association Medicale Mondiale-AMM)
28, Avenue des Alpes
F-01210 Ferney-Voltaire, France
Telephone 50 40 7575
FAX 50 40 5937

World Medical Journal
Editorial information available through:
World Medical Association
Executive Editor
Dr. C.A.S. Wink,
100 Wigmore St., London W1H 9DR, England

Co-editor
Walter Burkhart
Hädenkampstr 5, 5000 Köln 41 Germany

Writers

Good Scientific Writing
Charles G. Roland, M.D.

"If you know, you can utter it in English." - Martin H. Fischer

In this essay I shall try to answer three questions. One is the query my readers will expect to have answered: "What is good scientific writing?" The second, both more difficult and more important, can be posed thus: "Does the goodness of scientific writing, or its badness, really matter?" Finally, and logically, the question arises, "How does one learn to write well?" Any of my editor-writer colleagues who have wrestled with these problems will perhaps sympathize with my diffidence when I admit that I cannot answer my own questions. But then, many important questions are not truly answerable. The thought which invests a seriously proposed answer justifies the attempt.

Before proceeding I must make one comment. Any definition of good scientific writing must, for reasons which will become evident, be subjective. Readers will find areas of disagreement. I hope these areas will be small, but their existence is inevitable and should not invalidate the general concepts.

What is good scientific writing?

Scientific writing is a phenomenon. It is not itself science. Rather, it is art applied to the task of describing science. The appropriateness of the heavy emphasis on medical writing, in the sections that follow, lies in the fact that medicine is a classic example of the interdependence of art and science. And this relation leads me to suggest a close analogy between scientific writing and laboratory practice, for I have no doubt that much art is required to experiment productively, but my background in the laboratory is too slight to leave me comfortable in pursuing the analogy in detail.

Medical practice demands both art and science. Whether the physician practices well or practices badly depends, of course, upon both his acquisition of the art and his mastery of the science. But in this discussion, both of medical practice and of scientific writing, I propose that we consider the science invariable; the hypothetical physicians of my essay shall all know the same "amount" of science, and the writing will all be equally "true" or "valid" scientifically. The variables then are artistic, in the broadest sense.

Now I have established the rules. By doing so I have simplified the analogy to the point where it is elemental. When Dr. Smith, a "good" physician, practices he melds his scientific knowledge with

the art of medicine. If Dr. Smith is a good writer also - by no means an inevitable combination - then he presents his scientifically valid information (or hypothesis) melded with literary artistry.

Because I have used the words art, artistic, and artistry, perhaps I should make clear an important differentiation. Literary ability, in my discussion of scientific writing, does not mean literary genius. What it does mean is the ability to write clearly, unequivocally, concisely, and pleasingly. Most of us who write are merely adequate practitioners. Literary genius I know nothing about. If a physician who had literary genius came to me asking for instruction in writing, I hope I would have the good sense to leave him alone. Genius finds, or makes, its own ways.

Good writing is not necessarily the absence of error; strictly correct writing can be dreadfully dull and, therefore, bad. Nevertheless science would be vastly improved if two categories of faults - errors and infelicities - could be eliminated. The first, and the most obvious, is the true error: the non-sentence, the incorrect subject reference, the use of the passive voice, boring repetitiveness of sentence structure. These last infelicities cause more difficulty, simply because they are relative rather than absolute faults.

By the time a medical article is published, most of the true errors will have been eliminated by the journal's editorial staff, if it has one; so the major difficulty with the published literature is infelicitous presentation. Nevertheless, every effort to improve scientific writing must direct itself to both kinds of error

All writing is literary activity. But science has become dissociated from the humanities, and physicians seem to think that scientific writing is not a literary form; the very word "literary" frightens many, who believe that science is objective while literature is subjective. They pursue this belief to its questionably logical conclusion by supposing that science is only objective, and that therefore it must be antiliterary. And from this belief, rarely expressed but common, comes a contempt for good-writing - not for writing, but for doing it well.

Does Good Writing Matter?

The attitude I have just described does exist. How common it may be, I do not know. But to anyone who has this attitude of contempt, the answer to the question "does good writing matter?" is "No." Nevertheless they are wrong, on several counts.

It does matter to write well. Good writing has been described as good manners. Those who can not or will not write well epitomize bad manners. Moreover, they forget that writing unread, or read but not understood, is irrelevant trivia, totally worthless. So both good manners and good sense should lead the physician to want to write better.

The aim of science is not just to discover new facts and create new hypotheses: the aim is to discover fact, make hypotheses, and disseminate these to the rest of the scientific world for study, evaluation, acceptance, and incorporation into Science. Good scientific writing is clear and unequivocal, and thus good writing will be more easily read, understood, and evaluated than will

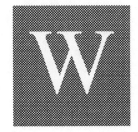

W

bad writing. Indeed, this fact occasionally makes the reader suspicious that a badly written article may have been so prepared deliberately, to disguise the scientific deficiencies of the work. Richard Asher, writing in the Lancet (August 27, 1949), remarked that "obscurity is bad, not only because it is difficult to understand but also because it is confused with profundity, just as a shallow muddy pool may look deep."

There is another reason to write well, a completely practical one. In these days when we are being overwhelmed by the burgeoning mass of the literature, attention to its dimensions has largely been limited to considering the number of journals, and the number of articles each contains. Not usually considered is the number of words in an article. But consider this passage, published in a major scientific periodical in this country.

The thesis herein offered is that woman (like man) is a biologic, social, and cultural creature, and as such is dependent for health on the acceptance, approval, support, and encouragement of significant individual members of the social group to which she belongs. In other words, her self-evaluation is determined, in the last analysis, on how she perceives and symbolizes this attitude, behavior, expectations, etc., of the group of which she is a member. Intimate human relations and interactions are so essential to health that one's sanity and potential for self-fulfillment are jeopardized for the most part by the perceived threat of disapproval, rejection, devaluation, or loss of security.

Just to read the passage, without spending any additional time trying to understand it, takes me 36 seconds. I am a reasonably rapid reader, but no means a speed reader. Let me assume that the time I take to read this passage is the average time for physicians. Let me further suppose that this passage would be read by 50,000 readers. (Considering the journal in which this passage was published, that is a highly conservative estimate.) I can edit the passage in many ways, one of which I show here.

Woman is a biologic, social, and cultural creature, dependent for health on the acceptance and encouragement of members of her social group. Her self-evaluation is determined by her perceptions and symbolizations of the attitudes of her group. Interactions are so essential to health that one's sanity and potential for self-fulfillment are jeopardized by perceived threats of disapproval, rejection, devaluation, or loss of security.

Without question this version is shorter. I hope you will agree that it is easier to read and understand than was the original. I would further propose that it says the same thing that the original says (which incidentally turns out to be not very much, when some of the sanctifying jargon is removed). I can read this passage in 22 seconds. And if I subtract the time is takes to read the edited version from the time to read the original, and multiply the answer by our hypothetical 50, readers, it appears that the author has wasted 8 days of time of his combined readership. And this calculation is based on only one paragraph, not the entire lengthy paper.

Authors complain especially bitterly about delays between acceptance and publications by journals. Yet in many published articles the author could have removed redundancies and compressed language to shorten the material by 25 to 50%. Taking the lower figure, 25% and applying that to a monthly which published 1200 pages a year, it would require 300 fewer pages to publish the same number of articles; that is, editor could publish 30 more 10-page papers per year than he can now. Just think what this means to the backlog of material that seems to hang like a millstone around the neck of many an editor. The possibilities are intoxicating. Furthermore, at a time when so many scientific periodicals are instituting or have already instituted page charges, and when the complaints about payment of such page charges are increasing rapidly, editing such as I have suggested provides a way for the journal to decrease the amount of charge to an individual author while maintaining the same level of income for the journal.

Finally, a quite different reason why good writing does matter: the pursuit of excellence. This pursuit has been a sorry casualty of our age. Although many individuals feel the urge to excel intellectually, the desire is far from universal. Yet I am sufficiently old-fashioned to believe that every person has a responsibility to do everything he does as well as he possibly can. And for the physician and the scientist this means that each has a responsibility to report his scientific observations as well as he possibly can.

How to Learn to Write Well

After the acceptance of this responsibility - one I would boldly call a moral responsibility - you naturally ask next, how can the conscientious author learn to write more skillfully? There is no simple response, no easy way. But I shall attempt to provide a few brief directions.

First, you learn to write by writing. Or perhaps I should say, you cannot not learn to write if you do not do it. So the author or potential author must devote much time to this chore. Writing is not easy. It is hard work. The urge to avoid the effort is great. The man who says he is too busy to write often means that he contrives to be too busy to write. As every sensible person knows, he can find time for anything that is important to him. Finding time for writing means finding a distraction-free locale, and keeping it free of distractions. Most of these come from within - the urge to do something else, write a letter, read a journal, clean shoes, take out the garbage, knit, anything but write - that is the urge to battle against. When I suggest that you must write, I do not mean that you must publish. Writers need to practice their art, and at least occasionally they should do so as an exercise in itself.

Whether or not the work is destined to appear in print, you should try to have it criticized by someone whose judgment you respect. Ideally this critic should have exemplary patience and unlimited time, as well as some expertise in your area of knowledge and considerable literary good sense. Seek his candid comments - but skip the whole exercise if you find that you can not react calmly and productively to candid comments.

In addition to your self-preceptorship, which is the most important part of any writer's training, you may supplement your education by attending courses on medical writing and by reading books on the subject. "Courses" that are merely series of lectures do little for the student. Workshops, on the other hand, can be most useful, and these I recommend highly. As for books about writing, they can be useful but only to supplement the hard work of writing itself.

However, one kind of reading can help the writer immeasurably. This is the reading of well written books and articles, both in your field (if you can find them) and in general literature. A process analogous to osmosis seems operative, so that some of the techniques of skillful writers insensibly become part of the reader's writing skills - but only if he reads deeply and carefully and often.

I have found useful, books by Hemingway and Orwell as examples. But every reader must find his own exemplars; I am sufficiently prejudiced to suggest that there is little likelihood of finding, in the current best-seller lists for fiction, an author whose style one would wish to use as a guide.

As far as reading well written prose in your field is concerned, that is what *Good Scientific Writing* about. I began to collect the examples because participants in writing workshops asked me to direct them to well written scientific articles and books. From this request came the series on "Good Scientific Writing," which has appeared in *Archives of Internal Medicine*. Each part of the series appeared under a motto by Lord Chesterfield that epitomizes the rationale for the project and for the book: "We are more than half what we are by imitation. The great point is to choose good models and to study them with care." (WRT)

American Medical Writers Association
9650 Rockville Pike, Bethesda, MD 20814
301/493-0003

American Medical Association

Mission Statement: to promote the science and art of medicine and the betterment of public health.

515 North State Street, Chicago, IL 60610
312/464-5000
Fax--312/464-4184

History: The Founding of the American Medical Association
Lester S. King, MD

A medical society is not a philanthropic or altruistic organization. It exists for the sake of its members, to help them gain certain benefits. Societies come into existence when a group of individuals, having aims in common, feel that they can achieve their aims more readily by joint action than by individual effort. If other members of the community also benefit, this will be a plus value that will promote general goodwill and induce more ready acceptance of the society's goals.

The American Medical Association, whose origins are well documented, is a prime example of this total process. At its birth in 1846 (under a different name), the reasons for its existence were clearly stated: "Resolved, That it is expedient for the Medical Profession of the United States, to institute a National Medical Association, for the protection of their interests, for the maintenance of their honour and respectability, for the advancement of their knowledge, and the extension of their usefulness."[1] To understand the origins of the AMA, we must understand the terms of this resolution and the factors that led up to it.

The enumerated goals fall into two clearly separable groups: the first bears directly on the welfare of the physician - promoting his interests, honor, and respectability; the second has a broader application - the advancement of knowledge and extension of usefulness. These aid the community as well as the physician, since he can thus offer better service.

The National Medical Association, later the AMA, came into being not in a vacuum but in response to urgent needs that, in turn, reflected the whole environment in which medicine found itself. This environment, however, had been undergoing continuous change, and without the awareness of these changes the actual events of 1846 and 1847 are rather meaningless.

The national association developed naturally out of the numerous state and local medical societies that had been founded over the preceding decades. In the formation of such local groups, a major impetus was the need to protect the trained practitioner from the competition of the untrained, the empirics, and the quacks. The local societies could exert pressure on legislatures for measures that would restrict competition. A society as a pressure group, seeking restrictive legislation, is a time-honored manifestation of the guild spirit. In the first decades of the 19th century, the moves toward the licensing of practitioners, with resulting monopolistic benefits, were reasonably

successful, although different parts of the country offered different responses.

The medical profession could readily unite their opposition to quacks and pretenders. Other groups, with different interests, exerted counterpressures to blunt any monopolistic trends and to allow greater freedom in matters of health. In part, these counterpressures were formalized through well-organized sects, as we found in the discussion of Thomsonianism. But in large part the objections reflected the general climate of opinion in the Jacksonian era, diffuse popular reaction against monopoly, a reaction indefinite but powerful and widespread.

Until the later 1830s, the state societies in the aggregate enjoyed a modest success against the quacks and pretenders. The physicians could work together against a common foe. However, new internal strains were developing within the medical profession, and by the 1840s threatened a polarization. Physicians might agree that only a "regular" training fitted a man to practice medicine, and, furthermore, that the right to practice should be formalized with a license. But then the question arose, who would control the granting of licenses?

This problem, more acute in some states than in others, reflected the changes in medical education that were developing over a 30- to 40- year period. Originally, when medical schools were few and training took place through the apprenticeship, license examinations were conducted by county societies, whose membership represented the medical establishment. The societies appointed censors who examined the candidates. However, as already noted, medical school graduates enjoyed special privileges, specifically, that their diplomas exempted them from examination - they could legitimately practice merely by registering their diploma. Here we have a threat to the establishment, and the growth of a potential new power within the profession.

Some available statistics tell an interesting story. In 1800, when the country had five medical schools, only 20 men had received the MD degree, while for the quinquennium 1796 to 1800 the total number had been only 80. By 1849, when there were some 38 active medical schools, the total number of graduates was about 1,370.[2] We also want to know how many practitioners qualified by examination. Overall statistics are not available, but fairly reliable data exist for New York State. In 1820, thirty-eight students received the MD degree from medical schools in the state, while "three times that number were examined and licensed by censors of the state and county societies." In 1830, the comparable figures were 56 medical degrees and about 117 licensed by examination. The proportion was changing, but only slowly. By 1846, however, there was a marked reversal, with 246 graduates from schools within the state and only eight or ten licensed through examination.[3] Conventry[4] offered slightly different figures for 1845 and 1846. According to his data, the graduates of medical colleges in the state "averaged" 225, while those who took the

American Medical Association

examination numbered only 13 and 18, respectively.[4] The county medical societies, which originally determined the fitness to practice, were clearly being shorn of the power so to do. This change in power structure was producing tensions, and the loss of licensing fees, which went to the examiners, was also a factor in producing dissatisfaction among society members.

It would seem that too many persons were practicing medicine. The total number of practitioners could be divided into two groups: the "regular" physicians who followed the long-standing medical traditions, and the "irregulars" who included the empirics, sectarians, and quacks. Were there, in fact, too many practitioners of all types? The regulars would say yes, and would remedy the trouble by eliminating all the irregulars. The latter, however, would say no, and to a large extent the general public agreed with them. Presumably, legislation reflects the popular will. The legislatures of the several states had granted only limited privileges to the regular physicians, and, furthermore, through the second quarter of the century, these privileges were gradually being eroded. Equality was being extended to the irregular practitioners.

Were there too many regular physicians? One faction, the better trained and the more conservative, maintained the affirmative, claiming an excess of poorly trained physicians. If the standards of medical education were to be sharply raised, this would reduce the number of men entering the medical schools and, consequently, the number who would enter practice. On the other hand, a small but powerful group of educators, who had founded duly chartered medical schools and derived financial support therefrom, wanted to increase the number of medical student and, hence, the eventual number of practicing physicians. This opposition the irregulars, caused great difficulty in the new organization.

These differences within the regular medical profession gradually strengthened the concept of elitism that ever since the time of John Morgan had never laid far below the surface. In the turmoil of the late 1840s, this trend showed itself more and more and became a dominant factor later in the century.

All the problems varied in intensity among the several states, and each state, taking account of its own environmental and social circumstances, attempted its own remedies. But the powers of the states were too localized, and the problems too complex. The inability of any single state society to deal competently with them soon became apparent to the more farsighted physicians. Over a period of 20 years, from about 1826, there were many efforts to form some sort of national medical society, excellently summarized by Stookey,[5] all proved abortive. There is no need to repeat here the story of these numerous frustrated attempts.

Cooperation had never been a prominent American trait, for "rugged individualism" more nearly expressed the American character. The earlier attempts at a national organization, in Vermont, New York, Georgia, Ohio, and New Hampshire, all came to naught. The historian naturally asks the question, Why did the earlier attempts to achieve some sort of joint cooperation all fail, until the final success of 1845-1846? The answer, I suggest, lay in an overall worsening of the situation that by 1844 had come to a climax. In that year, as we have seen, any special legal privileges enjoyed by the medical profession were generally withdrawn, and the era of "free trade" in medicine had begun.

For some authors, the founding of the AMA represents primarily a reform movement in medical education. This view stems largely from the aggressive rhetoric of Nathan Smith Davis, the "father of the AMA," whose narrative account is important source material for the period. Davis himself was especially interested in education, and he strongly emphasized the need for improved standards. The question of educational reform, however, must be placed in a broader perspective that will take account of the complexities of the situations.

The AMA came into existence under the impetus provided by the New York State Medical Society, which had been severely shaken by the legislative events of 1844. The legislature, influenced by the Thomsonians and by a populist tide, had revoked the special privileges of the regular medical profession. Although the medical license remained available, it lost all force and meaning. Anyone could practice, even without a license, and could collect any debts stemming from such practice. Free trade in medicine became a fact of life in New York (and, actually, in the rest of the country as well). The immediate reaction of the regular physicians in New York gives us a rare insight into the "embryology" of the AMA and the way that physicians perceived the changing functions of a medical society.

The new legislation was passed in May 1844. In June 1844, the Albany County Medical Society, in a special meeting, heard a report that analyzed the situation and recommended the course the society should take. The report[6] first gave a version of the way the societies came into existence. Originally, the county society provided a means whereby the members "may readily be recognized by each other and by the public, may exercise a general supervision over each other, and cooperated to promote the common welfare." A student, after being taught "the science and art of Medicine" and passing the examination, is "admitted into the profession as one worthy of its honors and fitted to assume its duties." The society was a body of physicians "presenting certain guarantees of capacity and character...so that its members may be readily recognized by the public."

The law had thus recognized "education physicians" and gave the public "the means of recognizing them." Supposedly, it was the height of absurdity for anyone to consult "an ignorant person when it is possible to procure the services of an educated physician." Nevertheless, some persons did commit this absurdity, and to protect the public from such "folly," the law prohibited irregular practice, under penalties. It has seemed proper to protect "a few silly persons" from "their own bad judgment."

But, the report continued, "a large portion of the public think that education and science are not necessary to qualify men for medical practice." Numerous sects sprang up that attracted a substantial public following. The authors modestly admitted that "we have not...the right to impose on them [the public] our ideas of wisdom" - if anyone who knows the facts is foolish enough to consult with quacks, he must suffer the consequences. Furthermore, the authors admitted, restrictive legislation was hard to enforce. It created a "cry of persecution," and might seem to place the medical profession in a false position, as if selfishly fighting for its own privileges rather than "defending the public against their own rashness and folly." The authors did not want to engage in controversy with special sects, "with ignoble adversaries."

Regarding the laws of 1844, the proper response of the medical society was not to seek restoration of privileges, but rather to put its house in order. "We ought to endeavor to infuse more spirit into our County societies, to have more frequent meetings, and to promote cordiality of feeling among the members. The rules of medical ethics should be scrupulously observed." Now that the law was changed, "it will be practicable to raised the standard of admission into the County Societies...into which those who find the requirements too high need not enter...The dignity and respectability of our profession is to be promoted not by asking for legal privileges, but by an increase of individual zeal and a more cordial cooperation." The barrier that separates the physician from the quacks is formed, not by legislation, but "by the high attainments and honorable deportment" of the physicians, and it is this barrier that "depends on us to make higher and stronger."

The report ended with a resolution, that "it would not be conducive to the interest or respectability of the medical profession" to seek any remedial legislation on "any medical subject whatsoever." The report and the resolution were unanimously adopted. The society seemed willing to stand by itself, without legislative help.

The whole report shows a remarkable mixture of resignation to the course of events, bitterness over what has transpired, and continued arrogance. Equally important, it showed a sensible recognition that the future can be salvaged through revitalizing the medical societies, and raising their standards and their level of discipline. Yet, at that time, the members of the society did not look further than their own local society.

I suggest that after the initial shock had passed, men of greater vision looked to a broader scene. They could perceive an overall solution through a national rather than a local society.

In 1839, the New York State Medical Society had passed a resolution recommending a meeting of nationwide delegates, three from each state medical society and one from each regularly constituted medical school. Although invitations had been sent out, no one responded and no meeting took place. In 1844, at the state society meeting, the topic again came up for discussion, especially in reference to raising the standards of medical education. Dr. Davis, a newly appointed delegate, only 27 years old, had been deeply concerned with this aspect. The debate continued into the meeting of 1845. At that time a resolution was passed, urging the convocation of delegates from "medical societies and colleges in the whole Union,"[7] to meet in Philadelphia, in 1836, to consider the problem of elevating the standards of medical education. A committee was appointed to implement the resolution, with Dr. Davis as chairman. A forceful and indefatigable correspondent, he, more than any other single person, deserves the credit for bringing the convention into existence.

Davis' own account of the convention emphasized quite exclusively the educational aspects and ignored other important facets. The indispensable document for studying the founding of the AMA is the official Proceedings of the conventions of 1846 and 1847, containing the minutes and the committee reports. When we study these we gain a somewhat different perspective.

At the initial meeting on May 5, 1846, there was some difficulty in determining the status of the various persons who attended and just what they represented, but these problems were not of serious import. After the election of officers, a maverick resolution to adjourn the convention sine die was decisively rejected, and the delegates settled down to the main business. A committee, of which Davis had been the chairman, brought in six resolutions that were "adapted to fulfill the immediate objects contemplated by the Convention."[8]

The first resolution indicated the purpose of the Association, already quoted. The second proposed a committee to plan the organization of the next meeting, and the third proposed an invitation to all "regularly organized Medical Societies, and chartered Medical Schools" to attend the next meeting in Philadelphia, in 1847. The remaining resolutions have to do directly with the goals of the Association and their implementation, and form the essence of the proceedings. Thus, the fourth resolution recommended a "uniform and elevated standard" for the MD degree; the fifth, "a suitable preliminary education" for all who would study medicine; and the sixth a uniform code of medical ethics for the entire medical profession in the United States.

American Medical Association

American Medical Association

A further resolution, from the floor rather than the steering committee, recommended the separation of the teaching of medicine from the licensing to practice. This really meant that a diploma should not be an automatic license. Instead of multiple licensing bodies - local societies and medical facilities - there should be only a single licensing board for each state. This resolution engendered much debate but was finally referred to a committee. Other resolutions passed at the convention are not relevant for our purpose.

The president of the convention appointed committees to consider these various resolutions and to report at the next meeting in 1847. Dr. Davis was appointed only to the committee on organization, and the final framework of the Association owes much to him and to his remarkable energy. However, he did not serve on any of the other committees that hammered out the doctrinal points. These committee reports, presented at the 1847 meeting, embody the representative thinking of the convention.

To appreciate the problems of the convention, we must recognize the essential guild structure, comparable to the British guilds such as the Royal College of Physicians or the Society of Apothecaries. Obviously, the overall environment in the United States in the 1840s differed markedly from that of Great Britain a century earlier. The goals, however, have much in common and include some basic components of all guild structures.

At the same time there was an important difference. Traditionally, a guild, in promoting the interest of its members, tries to establish a monopoly through appropriate legislative action. In the United States of the 1840s, the social and political climates effectively prevented any hope that legislation would approve monopolistic privileges. However, there remained scope for a voluntary organization that could promote the interests of its members through other than special legal privileges. For effectiveness, such an organization would depend on may factors, but the two most important elements come directly from essential and traditional guild practice: first, the control over apprentices (ie, over those would want to enter the guild); and second, a disciplinary control over those who were already in.

The concept of apprenticeship, for a long time traditional in American medicine, had by the mid-19th century been largely superseded by newer modes of medical education. A medical guild had to maintain standards, and this it could do, over the long run, only by controlling the entrance into the profession. If a centralized voluntary association wanted to control new admissions into the cadre of practicing physicians, there would need to be an agreement between medical societies and medical faculties. As we have already seen, there was considerable tension between these groups.

A guild would also need to exert control over those members who had finished their training and were actually engaged in their profession. In classical guild terminology, this would include all who had finished their apprenticeship to become journeymen or masters. The code of professional ethics was an instrument of control - transgression of the code would permit expulsion of the erring member from the guild.

The code, a weapon for keeping members in line and maintaining discipline, gave rise to a vast array of problems that will be treated later. We have a voluntary organization designed to further the interests of the medical profession (with subsidiary benefits overflowing to the general public); a firm organization was needed to pursue its goals; such a pursuit required a control over admission to the profession and control over the members already in practice - this would be accomplished by regulating medical education and establishing a code of ethics; and, furthermore, a voluntary organization must rely on itself and on public opinion, and not on specific legislative support. This interpretation is, of course, ex post facto, derived entirely by inference from the documents of the period and the whole course of events. The course of events proceeded as if these views were implicit at the time of the first convention, though they were not explicitly spelled out.

The convention of 1846 tried to face, squarely and honestly, the problems that affected the whole medical profession in the mid-1840s. The key to these problems (and the proposed solutions) lies in the committee reports, presented and discussed at the 1847 meeting and adopted as the framework for the AMA. I need not enter into the parliamentary aspects of the convention, nor the change in title from National to American Medical Association, that took place at the end of the 1847 meetings. I will restrict my analysis to three topics - the impact of the code of medical ethics, the problems of medical education, and the concept of elitism. We will see how these topics affected the course of the AMA throughout the entire 19th century.

Bibliographic Note
The most readily available account of the founding of the AMA is Morris Fishbein's History of the American Medical Association, 1847-1947 (Philadelphia, WB Saunders Co, 1947). For more detailed discussion of special aspects, with abundant references, two helpful texts are Martin Kaufman's Homeopathy in America (Baltimore, The Johns Hopkins University Press, 1968) and William G. Rothstein's American Physicians in the Nineteenth Century (Baltimore, The Johns Hopkins University Press, 1972). An essential primary source is The Proceedings of the National Medical Conventions Held in New York, May 1846, and in Philadelphia, May 1847, Philadelphia, value is N.S. Davis' History of the American Medical Association From Its Organization up to January, 1855 (Philadelphia, Lippincott Grambo & Co, 1855).

References

1. Proceedings of the National Medical Convention, p 17.
2. Transactions of the American Medical Association 1849;2:299.
3. N.S. Davis, History of Medical Education and Institutions in the United States, Chicago, SC Griggs & Co, 1851, pp 116-117.
4. Charles B. Coventry, "Remarks on Some of the Proceedings of the New York State Medical Society," NY J Med 1846;7:192-199.
5. Byron Stookey, "Origins of the First National Medical Convention, 1826-1846," JAMA 1961;177:133-140.
6. NY J Med 1844;3:281-286.
7. Davis, History of the AMA, p 23.
8. The remaining quotations come from the Proceedings, pp 16-22. (AGE)

American Medical Association Presidents 1847-1992

1847

47-48	Nathaniel Chapman-University of Edinburgh (Great Britain)
48-49	Alexander H. Stevens-University of Pennsylvania
49-50	John C. Warren-Harvard University
50-51	Reuben D. Mussey-Medical Institute of Darmouth College
51-52	James Moultrie-University of Pennsylvania
52-53	Beverly R. Wellford-University of Maryland
53-54	Jonathan Knight-Yale College
54-55	Charles A. Pope-University of Pennsylvania
55-56	George B. Wood-University of Pennsylvania
56-57	Zina Pitcher-Middlebury College, Vermont
57-58	Paul F. Eve-University of Pennsylvania
58-59	Harvey Lindsly-Columbia Medical College
59-60	Henry Miller-Transylvania University
60-61	Eli Ives-Yale College
61-62	No Session Held
62-63	No Session Held
63-64	Alden March-Brown University, Providence, Rhode Island
64-65	Nathan Smith Davis-College of Physicians and Surgeons of Western New York at Fairfield
65-66	Nathan Smith Davis-College of Physicians and Surgeons of Western New York at Fairfield
66-67	D. Humphreys Storer-Harvard College
67-68	Henry F. Askew-University of Pennsylvania
68-69	Samuel D. Gross-Jefferson Medical College
69-70	William O. Baldwin-Transylvania University
70-71	George Mendenhall-University of Pennsylvania
71-72	Alfred Stille-University of Pennsylvania
72-73	David Wendell Yandell-University of Louisville
73-74	Thomas Muldrop Logan-Medical College of South Carolina
74-75	Joseph Meredith Toner-Vermont Medical College
75-76	William K. Bowling-Ohio Medical College
76-77	James Marion Sims-Jefferson Medical College
77-78	Henry I. Bowditch-Harvard Medical College
78-79	Tobias G. Richardson-University of Louisville
79-80	Theophilus Parvin-University of Pennsylvania
80-81	Lewis Albert Sayre-College of Physicians and Surgeons, Columbia University
81-82	John Thompson Hodgen-University of Missouri at St. Louis
82-83	Joseph J. Woodward-University of Pennsylvania
83-84	John Light Atlee-University of Pennsylvania
84-85	Austin Flint-Harvard Medical College
85-86	Henry Frazer Campbell-Medical College of Georgia
86-87	William Brodie-College of Physicians and Surgeons, Columbia University
87-88	Elisha Hall Gregory-St. Louis University
88-89	Alexander Y.P. Garnett-University of Pennsylvania
89-90	William Wirt Dawson-Medical College of Oho
90-91	Edward Mott Moore-University of Pennsylvania
91-92	William T. Briggs-Transylvania University
92-93	Henry Orlando March-Harvard Medical College
93-94	Hunter Holmes McGuire-Winchester Medical College
94-95	James Farquhar Hibberd-College of Physicians and Surgeons of Columbia University
95-96	Donald MacLean-University of Edinburgh
96-97	Richard Beverly Cole-Jefferson Medical College
97-98	Nicholas Senn-Chicago Medical College (Northwestern University Medical School)
98-99	George M. Sternberg-College of Physicians and Surgeons, Columbia University

American
Medical
Association

American
Medical
Association

99-00   Joseph M. Mathews-University of Louisville

1900

00-01   William Wilson Keen-Jefferson Medical College

01-02   Charles Alfred L. Reed-Cincinnati College of Medicine

02-03   John Allen Wyeth-University of Louisville Medical School

03-04   Frank Billings-Chicago Medical School (Northwestern University Medical School)

04-05   John Herr Musser-University of Pennsylvania

05-06   Lewis Samuel McMurtry-Tulane University

06-07   William James Mayo-Indiana Medical College of LaPorte/University of Missouri

07-08   Joseph Decatur Bryant-Bellevue Hospital Medical College

08-09   Herbert Leslie Burrell-Harvard Medical School

09-10   William C. Gorgas-Bellevue Medical College

10-11   William Henry Welch-College of Physicians and Surgeons in New York

11-12   John Benjamin Murphy-Rush Medical College (Chicago)

12-13   Abraham Jacobi-University of Bonn (Germany)

13-14   John A. Witherspoon-University of Pennsylvania

14-15   Victor C. Vaughan-University of Michigan

15-16   William Lewis Rodman-Kentucky Military Institute

16---   Albert Vander Veer-Columbian Medical College (George Washington University)

16-17   Rupert Blue-University of Maryland

17-18   Charles Horace Mayo-Chicago Medical College (Northwestern University)

18-19   Arthur Dean Bevan-Rush Medical College(Chicago)

19-20   Alexander Lambert-College of Physicians and Surgeons of Columbia University

20-21   William C. Braisted-College of Physicians and Surgeons of Columbia University

21-22   Hubert Work-University of Pennsylvania

22-23   Geo. E. De Schweinitz-University of Pennsylvania

23-24   Ray Lyman Wilbur-Cooper Medical College of San Francisco

24-25   William Allen Pusey-Medical College of New York University

25-26   William D. Haggard-University of Tennessee Medical Department

26-27   Wendell C. Phillips-University Medical College of New York

27-28   Jabez North Jackson-University Medical College of Kansas City

28-29   William Sydney Thayer-Harvard Medical School

29-30   Malcom LaSalle Harris-Rush Medical College(Chicago)

30-31   William Gerry Morgan-University of Pennsylvania

31-32   Edward Starr Judd-University of Minnesota School of Medicine

32-33   Edward Henry Cary-Bellevue Hospital Medical College

33-34   Dean DeWitt Lewis-Rush Medical College(Chicago)

34-35   Walter L. Bierring-University of Iowa at Iowa City

35-36   James S. McLester-University of Virginia

36---   James Tate Mason-University of Virginia Medical School

36---   Charles Gordon Heyd-University of Buffalo

37-38   John H.J. Upham-University of Pennsylvania

38-39   Irvin Abell-Louisville Medical College

39-40   Rock Sleyster-University of Illinois School of Medicine

40-41   Nathan B. Van Etten-Bellevue Hospital Medical School

41-42   Frank H. Lahey-Harvard University Medical School

42-43   Fred Wharton Rankin-University of Maryland Medical School

43-44   James Edgar Paullin-Johns Hopkins University School of Medicine

44-45   Herman L. Kretschmer-Northwestern University/Marquette University

45-46   Roger Irving Lee-Harvard Medical School

46-47   Harrison H. Shoulders-Nashville Medical College

47-48   Edward L. Bortz-Harvard Medical School

48-49   R. L Sensenich-Rush Medical School

49-50   Ernest E. Irons-Rush Medical School

50-51   Elmer L. Henderson-University of Louisville Medical School

51-52   John W. Cline-Harvard Medical School

52-53   Louis H. Bauer-Harvard Medical School

53-54   Edward J. McCormick-St. Louis University

54-55   Walter B. Martin-Johns Hopkins University School of Medicine

55-56   Elmer Hess-University of Pennsylvania

56-57   Dwight H. Murray-Indiana University School of Medicine

57-58   David B. Allman-Jefferson Medical College of Philadelphia

58-59   Gunnar Gundersen-Columbia University

59-60   Louis M. Orr-Emory University Medical School

60-61   E. Vincent Askey-University of Pennsylvania

61-62   Leonard W. Larson-University of Minnesota School of Medicine

62-63   George M. Fister-Rush Medical School

63-64   Edward R. Annis-Marquette University School of Medicine

64-65   Norman A. Welch-Tufts College Medical School Donovan F. Ward-University of Iowa College of Medicine

65-66   James Z. Appel-University of Pennsylvania

66-67   Charles L. Hudson-University of Michigan

67-68   Milford O. Rouse-Baylor University Medical School

68-69   Dwight L. Wilbur-University of Pennsylvania

69-70   Gerald D. Dorman-Columbia University

70-71   Walter C. Bornemeier-Northwestern University

71-72   Wesley W. Hall-Tulane University

72-73   C. A. Hoffman-University of Cincinnati

73-74   Russell B. Roth-Johns Hopkins University School of Medicine

74-75   Malcolm C. Todd-Northwestern University

75-76   Max H. Parrott-University of Oregon

76-77   Richard E. Palmer-George Washington University

77-78   John H. Budd-Dalhousie University of Halifax N.S.

78-79   Tom E. Nesbitt-University of Texas, Southwestern-Dallas

79-80   Hoyt Gardner-University of Louisville

80-81   Robert B. Hunter-University of Pennsylvania

81-82   Daniel T. Cloud-University of Illinois

82-83   William Y. Rial-University of Pittsburgh

83-84   Frank J. Jirka Jr.-Universitiy of Illinois

84-85   Joseph F. Boyle-Temple University

85-86   Harrison L. Rogers-Emory University

86-87   John J. Coury-Case Western Reserve University

87-88   William S. Hotchkiss-University of Texas-Galveston

88-89   James E. Davis-University of Pennsylvania

89-90   Alan R. Nelson-Northwestern University

90-91   C. John Tupper-University of Nebraska

91-92   John J. Ring-Georgetown University

92-93   John L. Clowe-Albany Medical College

American

Medical

Association

Office of the General Counsel

- Health Law and Ethics
- Corporate Law

The AMA is the law firm of the profession. The AMA's legal activities are conducted to ensure that the AMA complies with applicable laws, court decisions, and other medicolegal developments that affect the practice of medicine; and that the interests of the Association and the medical profession are represented in the courts through the initiation of health policy litigation or intervention in litigation that concerns important health policy issues.

Other key ongoing and planned activities include implementing the AMA/Specialty Society Medical Liability Project, providing timely advice on ethical issues to physicians through the Council on Ethical and Judicial Affairs, and helping physicians compete and prosper in their medical practices by providing the most comprehensive clearinghouse of information on medicolegal developments in the area of health care economics and regulation available to physicians. The Physician Negotiation Advisory Office will continue to educate physicians on antitrust laws and improve their ability to bargain with payers. An annual fellowship in medical ethics and health policy is offered.

Office Publications include:

Reports of the Council on Ethical and Judicial Affairs
Annotated Current Opinions of the Council on Ethical and Judicial Affairs
Current Opinions of the Council on Ethical and Judicial Affairs, 1992
Practice Parameters: A Physician's guide to their Legal Implications
Legal Implications of Practice Parameters
Medico-Legal Forms with Legal Analysis
The Citation

Guidebook on Medical Society Grievance Committees The purpose of this guidebook is to provide comprehensive direction to county and state medical grievance committees for the enforcement of professional medical ethics. This guidebook demonstrates how the disciplinary bodies of the state and county medical societies can properly and effectively enforce ethical standards of conduct. It also clarifies the legal rules implicated by ethical guidelines and ethics enforcement, so that state and county medical societies can proceed with their ethics enforcement program without fear of legal liability.

Health Law and Ethics

Council on Ethical and Judicial Affairs is responsible for interpreting principles of medical ethics.

History-The AMA Gets a New Code of Ethics

In the celebrations that marked the centennial year 1876, medicine shared in the general self-congratulation; yet despite the rhetoric, a note of caution made itself heard. The president of the American Medical Association commented, in 1876, on the code of ethics. This he called "the best ever given for the government of medical men," and he observed that most of the members might think it "as perfect as the Decalogue, and as incapable of improvement." Nevertheless, it did not seem to work very well. Even eminent physicians, sticklers for the "inviolability of the Code," tried to find the "easiest way of getting round its provisions without a flagrant violation of them." Such physicians "feel that they are hampered by the rules that are unjust and oppressive." The code of ethics was violated every day, "not only by the rank and file, but by men high in the profession." He pointed out that sooner or later modification would be necessary to keep up with the changing times.[1]

The AMA delegates disregarded the cautionary note of their President, but some New York physicians, in their State Society meeting, took direct and forceful action that produced a major schism. The root of the problem was the consultation clause. The president of the State Society indicated, in 1881, the need for change and appointed a special committee to present suggestions at the next annual meeting.

When the committee reported in 1882, it recommended a completely new and much abbreviated code. In reference to the consultation clause, it declared, quite simply, that members of the Medical Society of the State of New York "may meet in consultation legally qualified practitioners of medicine."[2] Gone were the stipulations regarding a "regular medical education" or the disability incurred by an "exclusive doctrine." In effect, regular physicians would be able to consult freely with homeopaths. This accorded with the laws of New York, which recognized no legal distinction between homeopaths and regulars.

After the report was moved and seconded, the parliamentary maneuvers began. Dr D. B. St John Roosa (1838-1908) wanted to abolish the code entirely and substitute a simple declaration that the only ethical offenses were "those comprehended under the commission of acts unworthy of a physician and a gentleman." This statement, he thought, was adequete to cover the ordinary friction of practice, for no written formula could make a man a gentleman unless he was so by nature.

American

Medical

Association

American Medical Association

The state convention thus faced three choices - the "old code," the "new code," and the "no code." Long speeches reflected the irreconcilable differences. The "no code" proposal failed to carry, so the original proposition - the adoption of a new code - was again before the meeting. After futile attempts to send the matter back to committee, or to postpone consideration, the new code was adopted, 52 to 18, more than the two-thirds majority needed.

All this took place in February 1882. Over the next several months, various medical societies and journals deplored the action.[4] When the AMA held its annual meeting in May 1882, Samuel D. Gross, unable to attend, wrote an excoriating letter. He called the action "an outrage which every member of the profession should consider as a deep personal insult, and which the Association should rebuke in a most stern and uncompromising manner."[5] Indeed, the AMA had definite retaliatory powers. It refused to seat the delegates of the State Society, so that the adoption of the new code had brought about the expulsion of the State Society from the AMA.

In the New York State Society there was now a great political activity. In the meeting of February 1883, many conservatives tried unsuccessfully to get the new code repealed, and the next year the whole situation finally boiled over. Before the state convention actually met in 1884, the supporters of the old code, who wanted to maintain affiliation with the AMA, devised a bold strategy. Since the new code had become part of the bylaws, there seemed to be little hope of mustering the two-thirds majority needed to repeal it. The supporters of the old code planned a totally new rival organization to be called the New York State Medical Association, which would reaffiliate with the AMA.

This old group code met the night before the regular State Society and unanimously passed a resolution to create this new State Association. There was a proviso that first the members should attend the Society meeting the next morning. If the Society did reenact the old code, the resolution creating the new Association would be void. The rump session was thus a threat, a saying in effect to the Society, either reenact the old code or we will form a rival association that will adhere to the old code.

The meeting the next morning was a mass of impassioned oratory, but the motion to repeal was defeated 105 to 124. As a result, the Association went ahead to complete its organization and then held its first annual meeting in November 1884.[6] For a number of years New York had two medical organizations. The "Society" was the original State organization that held to the new code and remained independent of the AMA. The "Association" was the freshly created rival that maintained the old code and affiliated with the AMA. The schism was not healed until 1903.

Of the some 5,000 physicians in the state, a considerable majority probably favored the old code. The new-code adherents came mostly from New York City, while the old-code adherents were preponderantly upstate. The adoption of the new code was probably a carefully planned political group. Certainly, the total vote 52 to 18, was extremely small considering the importance of the issue. All attempts to secure a reconsideration or to postpone definite action until the subject was referred to the grass roots were defeated. Once the code was changed it was firmly locked in. Quite probably the new-code faction had deliberately used surprise tactics to attain its objective.

A frequently voiced complaint indicted the new-code men for acting arbitrarily and not referring the matter to the AMA as a whole. The reasons for not doing so were simple. The supporters of the new code "knew the history of the American Medical Association too well to expect for a moment that it would listen to any proposition looking toward the liberalization of the profession." The "practical management and the dictation of its policy have been in the hands of one man," who used his power "as an obstacle to the scientific and political advancement of the profession."[7] The reference pointed to Nathan Smith Davis. In the meetings of the AMA he invariably opposed any liberalization and, we shall see, actual reforms took place only shortly before he died, when he was far too old to exert any further influence.

The old-code supporters charged that the drive for a new code had as it motivation the desire of urban specialists to make more money by getting referrals from homeopaths and this tapping into their extensive practice. This charge, in any crude sense, is not tenable. Actually, the new code reflected the changing total environment. It recognized the complex interactions of emerging social, economic, and scientific factors, and of elements not operative in the 1840s, when the old code was propounded. A new era was well under way, with a broad socioeconomic base and an irresistible momentum. The proponents of the new code, aware of the coming changes, felt that the old code had outlived its usefulness, but the AMA needed 20 more years to become officially aware of the fact.

As part of their objections to the new code, the conservatives note the sharp opposition between the homeopaths and the regulars and emphasized the total incompatibility of doctrines. "Physicians who consent to consult with persons who differ from them as light from darkness, whose views can not mingle any more than oil can mingle with water, are guilty of perpetrating fraud, and a robbery in taking a fee for it." The author later declared, "This so-called code...encourages a spirit of lawlessness and sanctions fraud...its adoption sent a thrill of joy through the heart of every quack in the land and gave pain to the wisest and best of our associates in the regular profession."[8]

Supporters of this attitude drew comfort from the repeated assertions that homeopaths were not "scientific," and as evidence they pointed to the extravagant claims of Hahnemann's original writings earlier in the century. Particularly objectionable was the use of incredible dilutions, often to the 20th or 30th decimal dilution. Actually, however, in the 1880s homeopathic practice was a far cry from the extravaganzas that Hahnemann had recommended 50 to 75 years earlier. A hard core of homeopaths did indeed maintain the infallibility of Hahnemann's tenets, but a strong movement of liberalization had been under way, dividing the "high-potency" faction (holding to the efficacy of fantastic dilutions) from the "low-potency" practitioners who held to modest dilutions. A physician commented in 1883 that although homeopathy still included "some so-called high dilutionists, its leaders have long since ceased to insist upon infinitesimal dosage as an essential principle of treatment."[9] The homeopaths themselves were in the throes of conflict[10] and, except for the extremists, were narrowing the differences between themselves and the regulars.

In 1878, the Homeopathic State Society indicated that their members could "make use of any established principle in medical science or any therapeutic facts founded on experiment and verified by experience."[11] The "exclusive dogma" that the AMA had condemned in 1847 was no longer exclusive. Then, too, the education of the homeopaths was approximately that of the regulars, and liberal physicians were recognizing the similarities.

For many physicians, the major objection to homeopathy was not so much the special details of its doctrines as the name, which set its practitioners apart from the regular profession. According to Austin Flint, Sr, a stalwart among conservatives, what really bothered the profession was not the special teachings of the homeopaths but their opposition to the regulars. The homeopaths were refused fellowship because of "a name and an organization distinct from and opposed to the medical profession." There would be no restriction on consultation if only the homeopaths "abandon the organization and the name."[12] Apparently, the homeopaths needed only to cease publicizing any opposition to regular medicine.

The rupture between the Society of Medicine of New York and the AMA tended to polarize the medical profession. The direct and most dramatic result of this conflict was the quarrel over the International Congress of Medicine of 1887.

As international congress, held every three years, had become a powerful force in promoting international communication and general good will. The eighth such congress was held in Copenhagen in the fall of 1884. A few months earlier, when the AMA met in May 1884, President Austin Flint, Sr, suggested that the ninth Congress be invited to meet in Washington, DC, in 1887. The AMA convention authorized a "committee of seven" (that actually became eight) to extend the invitation at the Copenhagen meeting. If this was accepted, the appointees would then "act as the Executive Committee, with full power to fix the time and make all necessary and suitable

arrangements." The committee was empowered to add to its membership and "perfect its organization."[13] The Congress in Copenhagen accepted the invitation.

When the "original committee" (the nomenclature will prove to be important) returned to the United States in 1884, it added to itself 18 additional members; then this enlarged committee, known as the general committee, promptly set to work. It established a permanent organization, made rules for membership and selection of delegations, and set up 18 sections for the presentation of papers. Later, for each section a preliminary list of officers and council members was announced. The listings included the outstanding physicians in their respective fields, such as Francis Delafield, William Pepper, T. M. Prudden, William Welch, Christian Fenger, Reginald Fitz, George Sternberg, and James Tyson. It was truly a list to be proud of.[14]

All this vast and effective preliminary work was completed, published, and generally circulated. Then, at the annual meeting of the AMA in New Orleans, (April 28-May 1, 1885) it was presented as a report. At this point there began an episode that had a major impact on American medicine.

At the convention in New Orleans, the reactionary component of American medicine was clearly in control. When Dr John S. Billings (1838-1913), as Secretary General of the Congress, presented the report of his committee, the AMA refused to accept it. The delegates were piqued that it had already been published prior to AMA approval. Clearly, the Committee had considered itself empowered to make all arrangements, but the AMA convention thought differently. A resolution was introduced whose preamble indicated the root objections, namely, that "The committee have proceeded, without authority from this body, to appoint the several officers of section and committees" (emphasis added). The AMA "declined to indorse or accept these appointments."[15]

What was wrong with the appointments? In the parliamentary jockeying, before any actual resolution was passed, a substitute motion was introduced that showed the real objection. A Dr Saunders, of Ohio, proposed that the actions of the Committee, "so far as they have gone, be approved by this body, provided all new-code men be left out." This was a clear indication that the convention would not tolerate the presence, whether on the general committee or among the officers of the special section, of any physician who had rejected the AMA code and embraced the new code. This substitute motion of Dr Saunders, with its blunt statement and even more blunt implications, failed to pass, 88 to 129. There were more subtle ways of accomplishing the same end.

The AMA convention reorganized the whole mechanism for conducting the Congress. It provided for a new committee that would include one member for each state. The new general committee thus consisted of the original eight

American
Medical
Association

American Medical Association

members appointed in 1884, plus 38 new men selected by the state delegations. The first general committee had become a non-entity, and the new general committee was charged to repair the work already done.[16]

Disturbed by the rapidly mounting adverse comment, the editor of JAMA, Nathan Smith Davis, tried to justify the actions of the convention. The original general committee, he said, had selected section officers "solely on account of their reputation at home and abroad, without regard to their membership in medical societies." As a result, the committee had included "some who has placed themselves in organizations of the profession, by openly repudiating the national Code of Ethics." The reference, of course, was to the members of the New York State Society. A second alleged error was the failure "to appreciate the importance of so distributing the officers of Sections as to represent...the members of the profession in all the leading geographical divisions of our country."

The AMA in New Orleans had aimed "only to correct these alleged errors," and for this purpose gave the newly enlarged committee the right to review, alter, and amend" what had already been done. This was a polite way of saying, to eliminate all heretics. The AMA had the right to alter the personnel of the committee, and the new committee, "men of sound conservative qualities...will be found disposed to make no unnecessary changes in the work already done."[17]

The new general committee promptly met on June 24. It did not want "to make any revolutionary or radical changes" in the appointments, and it removed "only four" of the section chairmen. Most notable was Dr Abraham Jacob of New York, the outstanding pediatrician in the United States but also a leader of the new-code adherents. The Committee also changed the rules for membership in the Congress. The American members, it decreed, "shall consist of delegates from the American Medical Association, and from Medical Societies in affiliation with the American Medical Association." As the Medical News commented, this reduced membership in the Congress to the constituency of the AMA.

The independent physicians began a vigorous counterattack. In Philadelphia, 29 outstanding men signed a resolution condemning the changes as "detrimental to the interests of the medical profession" and declined to hold "any office whatsoever in connection with the said Congress." The signers included such internationally recognized leaders as D. Hayes Agnew, J. M. De Costa, Louis Duhring, Samuel W. Gross, S. Weir Mitchell, William Osler, William Pepper, and Alfred Stille. In other cities, prominent physicians quickly added their remonstrances. The signatories in Boston, for example, included Henry P. Bowditch, Reginald Fitz, Francis Minot, J. Collins Warren, O. W. Holmes, David Cheever, and James C. White.[18]

JAMA reacted quite intemperately. The editor, N. S. Davis, criticized the signatories for not suggesting improvements that would have aided the committee. Had they done so, he continued, they would then have shown "more regard for the honor and interests of the profession than for their own personal prejudices and dislikes; in other words they would have acted like men, and not like half-grown school boys."[19] The implication that William Osler, O. W. Holmes, or S. Weir Mitchell were acting like half-grown school boys suggests what a raging fury must have overtaken Davis.

The New York State Medical Association - the group that adhered to the AMA code - suggested that there be two types of members: those who might take part in both the business meetings and the scientific proceedings, and those who might participate only in the scientific sessions. All voting privileges would be limited to members and affiliates of the AMA, but any physician, regardless of affiliation, could take part in the scientific sessions. JAMA, however, felt that all this was too cumbersome and that simpler means might guard against the admission of delegates who had "repudiated the National Code of Ethics."[20]

On Sept. 3, 1885, the new general committee, apparently heeding the swelling protests, capitulated in regard to membership and made a simple rule: The Congress shall consist of members of the regular profession of medicine," with no mention of adherence to the AMA or its code of ethics.[21] Then the Committee, having already driven away the leaders in American medicine, tried to woo back some of the prominent men who had previously been dismissed or who had refused to participate. The attempt to bring back the dissidents as officers of the Congress was not successful.

Nevertheless, by early 1886 the excitement was pretty well over. The Committee did put together a list of appointments. Austin Flint, who had been president of the Congress, died and N. S. Davis was appointed in his place. The roster of officers was presented to the AMA at its annual meeting in May 1886 and duly accepted.[22] Many foreign dignitaries were included in the final list, but the Americans made a sorry aggregate when compared with the list that Billings and his committee had put together in 1885. Only rarely did a prominent name appear.

The Congress itself was held in Washington, Sept. 5-10 , 1887. It was generally accounted a success. After the event, JAMA, in several editorials, expressed its satisfaction. The British journal, The Lancet, had declared the Congress "worthy of its predecessors." Davis hoped that now the medical press, "instead of nursing old prejudices...will henceforth labor for the unity and advancement of the profession as a whole" - clear call to the medical profession to accept the AMA viewpoint.[23]

With the Congress out of the way, the road might have seemed clear to a unification of the warring factions. Certainly, each side had made a point. The AMA had succeeded in mounting a well-attended and generally satisfactory international congress, in spite of the damaging publicity and the condemnation of leading medical figures.

The image of the AMA was undoubtedly somewhat tarnished. As one result, the outstanding physicians were turning away from the AMA toward their own specialty societies, as the focus of their professional attention. Such specialty groups assumed increasing prominence in the 1880s. There were many reasons for the expansion, and dissatisfaction with the AMA was certainly one of them. There did not result an increase of scientific knowledge, but another result was the weakening of the AMA in public esteem.

Forty years had elapsed since the code was devised, and much had changed. The homeopaths, for example, had established medical schools, were studying anatomy, physiology, and chemistry, were using textbooks written by regular physicians, and were no longer practicing an "exclusive system of medicine." In the Hahnemann Medical College, at least two thirds of the textbooks were "unquestionably orthodox." The practitioners no longer taught an exclusive system, and the most prominent homeopathists "publicly deny that their practice is based exclusively upon" such a doctrine, Although the writer was kindly disposed to homeopaths, other physicians continued to excoriate them and pointed to the claims that Hahnemann made as "utterly irreconcilable with the principles and practice of medicine and with the sciences upon which medicine is founded."[24]

Neither side was taking a balanced view. Certainly, some homeopaths were still adhering to the worst possible absurdities of Hahnemann, obviously incompatible with the medical sciences. Other homeopaths were extremely well educated and well versed in the sciences. And there were all stages in between. Then, of course, among the regular practitioners some were unbelievably ignorant of the medical sciences and were incomparably worse practitioners than were homeopaths.

The real question was, should the old hostility be perpetuated, or should there be a gradual accommodation? Whatever determined the answers had little to do with the amount of scientific knowledge that the homeopath might or might not possess, but rather with the personalities of the physicians themselves. The conservatives were looking more to the past; the liberals, more to the future.

The AMA convention in 1892 took cognizance of the problem and tried to defuse the situation by "interpreting" relevant passages in the code of ethics. The real point at issue was the question of consultations. An "explanatory declaration" tried to please everyone. Mere differences in "doctrine of belief" did not exclude anyone from "professional fellowship" and nothing in the code would interfere with the "most perfect liberty of individual opinion of practice." However, anyone who adopted a

name indicating some sectarian system, or who belonged to an association "antagonistic to the general medical profession," would be considered to have made "a voluntary disconnection or withdrawal from the medical profession proper." Nothing would make it proper "to enter into formal professional consultations with those who have voluntarily disconnected themselves from the regular medical profession," as defined previously.[25]

This interpretation showed the real point at issue. Any form of practice, especially in therapeutics, was acceptable if only it did not openly proclaim opposition to regular medicine. The type of treatment was secondary, but using the name of homeopath was unforgivable.

In the convention of 1892 there had been enough doubts to impel two relevant steps. Reexamination of the code seemed in order. The president appointed a committee of five to study the code and recommend any changes deemed wise. Then, in the hope of settling the New York dissension, another committee was appointed, of which Davis was chairman. This had the task of conferring with suitable committees from each of the two New York medical groups, the Society and the Association, "for the purpose of adjusting all questions of eligibility of members of said State Medical Society of New York to membership in this association."[26]

Preliminary reports were rendered at the AMA convention of 1893. The Committee to examine the Code of Ethics rendered only a partial statement and needed more time for a definite report, but meanwhile the chairman indicated in part what the majority of the committee had in mind. They advised a new interpretation of the word consultation. The term would properly apply only when two physicians jointly shared the management of a case. It would not apply when a practitioner transferred to a specialist the entire responsibility for the care of the patient. Such an interpretation would seem to clear the way for a specialist to accept referrals from homeopaths, who would then drop out of the picture.

The majority of the Committee also proposed some verbal changes. The importance of a "thorough medical education" was recognized. The committee suggested the statement, "No intelligent practitioner, who has a license to practice from some medical board of known and acknowledged legal authority...and who is in good moral and professional standing in the place in which he resides, should be refused consultation, when it is requested by the patient."[27]

Only four out of the five members signed this provisional statement. The fifth, Dr Didama, who had led the old-code faction in New York, filed a minority report. The existing code, he said, "is explicit, liberal, broad, humane, and founded on truth, justice, and reason," and has no "superfluous details."[28]

In 1893, Davis also reported. The New York Medical Society refused to appoint a committee to

American
Medical
Association

American Medical Association

meet with him until the AMA had removed the differrences that prevented "Cordial relations." This meant, said Davis, "a deliberate abolition of the national code of ethics," which of course he rejected. His report, the minutes stated, was received with great applause."[29]

The issues were clear. The New York Society would not rejoin the AMA until the code was revised. The special committee appointed to study the question, by a majority of four to one, wanted to change the code; however, Didama and Davis had strongly resisted changes.

Since the Committee had not made its definitive report until 1894, the actual vote on a new code could not take place until 1895. When the proposed changes did come up for a vote, the minutes give little information. We learn that the motion to adopt the new code of ethics, as recommended by the majority report, was "indefinitely postponed." The move to liberalize the code was dead. Didama and David had acted as principal executioners, but they had the support of the convention.[30]

Nevertheless, the separation of New York physicians into two distinct organization had become unendurable. After the turn of the century, the New York Medical Journal pointed out that unification could "readily be brought about if reason should prevail." The 13,000 physicians in New York "fail to find any underlying principle of sufficient importance to justify the existing division" - an elliptic way of saying that the question of consultation with homeopaths no longer held its former significance.[31] Any unification would, of course, require a vast amount of behind-the-scenes work with the AMA. Since N. S. Davis no longer exerted any active influence, the chances for revising the code were for the first time really bright.

Negotiations between the AMA and the State Association must have begun shortly after the turn of the century. In the AMA meeting of 1902, a resolution offered a whole new code that had already been approved by the council of the New York Medical Association. The new code was referred to a special committee of the AMA, to report for the final action the following year.

Meanwhile, tortuous negotiations were going on between the two state organizations. The State Association wanted the two groups to combine as a new entity, with a new charter. The State Society flatly refused. It had a continuous existence since 1806, and under no circumstances would it accept any plan that would interrupt its legal continuity even for an instant. The State Association had to yield, and the plans called for the two to unify into the Medical Society of the State of New York. The State Medical Association was thus rejoining the State Society from which it had seceded in 1884.

However, before the union could take place the AMA had to adopt a new code of ethics. This it did at the annual meeting of 1903. The minutes declared that the resolution moving the new code

"was unanimously unanimously amid tumultuous applause."

Only a small part of this new code concerns us here. The articles on consultation contained no statement at all concerning who may properly consult with whom, but there was a bland statement relative to sects. The new version declared, "It is incompatible to designate their practice as based on an exclusive dogma or a sectarian system of medicine."[32] In a sense, this was inviting the homeopaths to stop calling themselves homeopaths and to throw their lot in with the regular profession.

After the AMA adopted the new code, the union of the two state organizations was a formality, but not without emotion, barely hinted at in the minutes. The motion for union was passed unanimously and was received with enthusiastic applause.

Actually, some legal technicalities caused delay, and the final judicial order consolidating the two groups was not signed until Dec 9, 1905. The unification then became effective. In January 1906, the New York State Journal of Medicine, which had been the official journal of the State Association, now carried on its masthead, "Published Monthly by the Medical Society of the State of New York." The Association, a product of secession, had ceased to exist. There was again unity among the New York physicians, and the AMA had a new Code of Ethics.

Bibliographic Notes
For the detailed story behind the code of ethics the primary sources must be consulted. These include the Transactions of the American Medical Association, of the Medical Society of the State of New York, and later of the New York State Medical Association. The contemporary journals, especially the *New York State Medical Journal*, the *Boston Medical and Surgical Journal of the American Medical Association*, and the *Medical Record*, are indispensable.

References:
1. Trans AMA 1876;27:96.
2. Trans Med Soc State NY, 1882, p 75.
3. Ibid, pp 26-50.
4. The reactions of medical societies, quotations form their resolutions, and letters from physicians are extensively presented in Medical News for the year 1882, vol 40, passim.
5. Trans AMA 1882;33:3.
6. Trans NY State Med Assoc 1884;1:505-528. See also Trans Med Soc State NY 1884, pp 36-62
7. Henry G. Piffard, "The Status of the Medical Profession in the State of New York," fifth article, NY Med J 1883;37:589-592.
8. Trans Med Soc State NY, 1883 pp 49, 91.
9. R. O. Beard, "The Schools of Medicine," Pop Sci Monthly, 1883;22:535-539.
10. Piffard, "Status," third article, NY Med J 1883;37:484-487. See also Martin Kaufman's Homeopathy in American (Baltimore, Johns Hopkins Press, 1971, pp 116-124).
11. Quoted by Piffard, op cit, p 486.

12. Austin Flint, "Medical Ethics and Etiquette," fourth article, NY Med J 1883;37:369-376.
13. JAMA 1885;4:605.
14. JAMA 1884;3:499, 632, and 1885;4:415-419.
15. JAMA 1885;4:605-607. The editorial summaries the "official" view promulgated at the AMA convention in New Orleans.
16. JAMA 1885;4:548-552. See also 1885;5:136-138.
17. JAMA 1885;4:605-607, emphasis added.
18. Medical News, 1885;47:26, 27, 53, 83.
19. JAMA 1885;5:71.
20. Ibid, p 155.
21. Ibid, p 443.
22. JAMA 1886;6:602-603, and 1886;7:192-194.
23. JAMA 1887;9:497-498.
24. Edward Jackson, "Against Sectarianism in Medicine," Medical News 1889;55:425-427; Solomon Solis-Cohen, "An Ethical Question," Ibid, 427-435.
25. JAMA 1892;19:611-612.
26. JAMA 1893;20:693. See also JAMA 1892;18:1803
27. JAMA 1893;20:691-692; also 1894;22:508.
28. JAMA 1893;20:591-593, and 1894; 22:556-558.
29. JAMA 1893;20:693.
30. JAMA 1895;24:761-762.
31. NY Med J 1903;77:259-264.
32. JAMA 1903;40:1379-1381.
(AGE)

Council on Constitution and Bylaws functions as a fact-finding and advisory committee on matters pertaining to the AMA Consitution and Bylaws. The council's primary responsibility is to maintain effective and efficient governing documents to permit the officers, trustees, delegates and staff to conduct the business and affairs of the Association.

Constitution
Article I - Title And Definition

The name of this organization is the American Medical Association. It is a federacy of its state associations.

Article II - Objects

The objects of the Association are to promote the science and art of medicine and the betterment of public health.

Article III - State Associations

Constituent or state associations are those recognized medical associations of states, commonwealths, territories or insular possessions which are, or which may hereafter be, federated to form the American Medical Association.

Article IV - Component Societies

Component societies are those county or district medical societies contained within the territory of and chartered by the respective state associations.

Article V - Members

The American Medical Association is composed of individual members of states associations and others as shall be provided in the Bylaws.

Article VI - House Of Delegates

The legislative and policy-making body of the Association is the House of Delegates composed of elected representatives and others as provided in the Bylaws. The House of Delegates shall transact all business of the Association not otherwise specifically provided for in this Constitution and Bylaws and shall elect the general officers except as otherwise provided in the Bylaws.

Article VII - General Officers

The general officers of the Association shall be a President, President-Elect, Immediate Past President, Secretary-Treasurer, Speaker of the House of Delegates, Vice Speaker of the House of Delegates and fourteen Trustees, including a Resident Physician member and a medical student member. Their qualifications and terms of office shall be provided in the Bylaws.

Article VIII - Trustees

The Board of Trustees is composed of seventeen members, thirteen Trustees elected by the House of Delegates, including a Resident Physician member, a medical student trustee elected by the Medical Student Section Assembly, and the President, President-Elect and Immediate Past President of the Association. It shall have charge of the property and financial affairs of the Association and shall perform such duties as are prescribed by law governing directors of corporations or as may be prescribed in the Bylaws.

Article IX - Scientific Assembly

The Scientific Assembly of the American Medical Association is the conviction of its members for the presentation and discussion of subjects pertaining to the science and art of medicine.

Article X - Conventions

The House of Delegates shall meet annually and at such other times as deemed necessary or as provided in the Bylaws, in cities or places selected by the Board of Trustees. The Scientific Assembly shall meet at such times as the Board of Trustees deems necessary, or as provided in the Bylaws, in cities or places selected by the Board of Trustees.

Article XI - Funds, Dues And Assessments

Funds may be raised by annual dues or by assessment on the Active Members on recommendation by the Board of Trustees and after approval by the House of Delegates, or in

American
Medical
Association

American

Medical

Association

any other manner approved by the Board of Trustees as provided in the Bylaws.

Article XII - Amendments

The House of Delegates may amend this constitution at any convention provided the proposed amendment shall have been introduced at the preceding convention and provided two-thirds of the voting members of the House of Delegates registered at the convention at which action is taken, vote in favor of such amendment.

Administration

- Strategic Planning and Information Resources
- Marketing
- Financial Services
- Human Resources
- Library and Information Management

Strategic Planning and Information Resources

This activity develops plans for key health policy issues identified by the Board of Trustees and Senior Management. The goals for this area include strategies for managing the various issues, including key activities to be performed and results to be achieved. As the issues are developed, the success of their implementation is monitored and assessed. Divisions other than those defined below include that of Corporate Planning and of Information Planning and Automation Services, and Automation Consulting.

Division of Information Planning and Automation Services

The Division of Information Planning and Automation Services is responsible for developing and managing the enterprise computing environment that supports the AMA's Information Systems. This division constructs this strategic business tool, consisting of mainframe and minicomputers, operating systems, teleprocessing systems, and data communications through planning, evaluation, hardware and software implementation and support, consultation, and other data processing services in the support of the AMA's business and publishing units. Departments that fall under this division include that of Computer Operations, Electronic Publishing Services and Technical Support

Division of Systems and Programming

The major activities of the Division of Systems Programming are designed to ensure that all administrative and business systems are available to the AMA throughout the business day and to ensure that the corporate data are integral, secure, and accurate. The division also seeks to identify emerging business technologies and leverage them against the AMA's and Federation's growing need for information. Through expanded access to information, the AMA can better serve the Association's members and target/tailor its marketing activities and products.

Department of Data Resource Development

provides information on physicians for several different groups. The health care profession, when looking to verify credentials on MDs, should contact the AMA National Physician Credentials Verification Service (NCVS). Established as a life-long personal AMA member benefit, the AMA/NCVS collects, verifies, and maintains portfolios of primary-source verified information for use by physician subscribers throughout their careers when applying for licenses and privileges. This is a lifetime career service for physicians, which is particularly of interest to residents and International Medical Graduates (IMGs). Widespread use of the AMA/NCVS by hospitals, medical licensing boards, and others to evaluate physician applicants promotes professionalism. This, in turn, has a positive effect on the quality of care provided to the public. This office primarily answers credentialing information for hospitals, and hiring physicians.

Contact the National Physician Credentials Verification Service (NCVS): 800/677-NCVS (800/677-6287)

Department of Physician Data Services
provides physician biographies for businesses, hospitals, and others with a need for them in the form of a "Physician Profile". A "Physician Profile" is a computerized printout of biographical information on individual physicians that is used by health care organizations to verify physician credentials. In response to continued demand for more rapid information by users and to improve productivity, this service will implement more efficient automated processing systems. In addition to current FAX service, Profiles are to be offered via an electronic bulletin board service. Information on recently deceased physicians is also available through Physician Data Services. Contact them at 312/464-5199

The department services the public need, however, through the mail: To recieve a free biography of an MD, (the requests **must** be in writing) an interested party should send stamped self-addressed envelope to:

Physician Profile
Department of Physician Data Services
American Medical Assiciation
515 N. State, Chicago, IL 60610

Departmental publications include:
U.S. Medical Licensure Statistics

Department of Database Licensing Services
maintains and provides the systems that create specified mailing lists. This department also controls the information in the master file from which free current awareness periodicals "Throw-away" journals are distributed to defined specialists.

Department of Physician Biographic Records
maintains the database from which mailing and subscription lists are drawn. Physician's address changes to the system are directed to this department

American
Medical
Association

American
Medical
Association

Department of Masterfile Information

Programs includes the data services provided to various health-related organizations that provide data to the AMA Physician Masterfile and others. Current and historical data are made available to meet the data needs of these organizations for health manpower planning, policy development, research studies, and other purposes. AMA Insurance Agency, Inc. currently receives data tapes for insurance solicitations.

Department of Physician Professional

Activities maintains records regarding the type of practice, employment, primary, secondary and tertiary self-designation practice specialties, hospital and group affiliation used in the masterfile. Information on the number of hours worked, routinely updated by the department, is often used as the primary basis for classifying physicians.

Marketing

Division of Marketing Services

The primary thrust of the AMA's product marketing function is to ensure that the identified needs of AMA members and others are met with products and services that are developed, priced, promoted, and distributed according to conventional marketing standards for quality, customer satisfaction, and product performance as identified by market needs analysis. This is accomplished by providing support services such as market analysis and product planning, product development, promotional execution, customer service, and telemarketing. Critical activities include creation of a true product development process and refinement of the new fulfillment /customer service program. Departments included in this division are the departments of Marketing Management and Development, Marketing Services, Printing Services, Marketing Fulfillment, and Member and Customer Services.

Division of Market Research

Market Research assists the AMA in understanding and meeting the needs of members, potential members, and other publics by planning, conducting, and presenting the results of qualitative/quantitative research that supports development and evaluation of Board-approved issue plans. Emphasis will be placed on membership development, product development, and AMA communications that support advocacy, professionalism, and health of the public.

Division of Marketing Information

Several initiatives make up this division. AMA Product Marketing designs the product catalog of materials the AMA distributes. AMA Customer Services is there to help callers obtain AMA materials. To check on problems with orders, begin a subscription to a journal, or to order a back issue of a AMA publication that is no older that 18 months.

***Contact AMA Subscriber Services at:
312-670-7827 or 800-262-2350***

AMA Book Source is a member benefit that aids members in locating and purchasing medical books. The Book Source has more than 25,000 titles in stock and has access to most titles available in print.

***Contact the AMA Book Source at:
1851 Diplomat Road, Dallas, TX 75234
800/451-2262***

Financial Services

Financial Services is responsible for the accounting, budgeting, corporate taxation, and internal audit functions of the Association. The activities of these functions include the safeguarding of Association assets through the establishment of a sound system of internal controls; providing timely and accurate financial information; insuring compliance with generally accepted accounting principles, government regulations, and sound business practices; and establishing a financial reporting frame work to allow meaningful measurement of financial performance. Efforts are directed to the continued development of the financial control process to improve investment and operating returns through the careful analysis of costs and productivity. The Divisions of Budgets and Financial Accounting and Corporate Accounting and Real Estate are included in this area.

Human Resources

The objective of this program is to provide systems and services that assure that the Association attracts, develops, and retains competent, motivated staff for its present and future needs. Major Human Resources functions include employee relations and training, compensation, placement, employee communications, planning, and corporate security. Increased attention will be placed on making the AMA more attractive to current and potential staff and increasing the motivation of staff through targeted recruiting programs, tuition reimbursement and other compensation strategies. Specific projects include the implementation of programs and compensation strategies related to performance planning, benefits, cost containment, total compensation, staffing analyses, affirmative action, and community service activities.

Division of Library and Information Management

The activities of the AMA Division of Library and Information Management support the needs of the profession and related fields for medical and socioeconomic information. This is accomplished by providing timely and reliable information services and by developing information databases and publications. Research services and references include a clearinghouse of information on professional liability and other socioeconomic issues, specialized fee-for-service computer-assisted literature searching, and documents delivery on topics in medicine and on the history of the AMA and American medicine. The division also promotes the dissemination of scientific information by indexing JAMA, the specialty journals, AMnews and other AMA publications. In addition, the Department of Serials and Technical Services maintains control over the library's journal and monograph collection by making them available to other libraries through established library networks. The Archives at AMA Headquarters is a closed collection that holds several specialized collections.

Health Fraud collection is a unique archival resource for research on medical fraud, quackery, proprietary and "patent" medicine, and alternative medicine.

The collection is useful to a wide variety of researchers:

- **medical and legal historians** interested in the history, regulation, and prosecution of quackery and health fraud;
- **social historians** concerned with the societal role of medicine and the healing arts;
- **antiquarians** wishing background information on health-related items such as medicine bottles, devices, and promotional brochures;
- **genealogists** researching persons who engaged in fraudulent or questionable health promotions.

One of the goals of the AMA since its founding in 1847, has been to educate the public regarding health care fraud. In general, primary and secondary source data related to health fraud is scarce and difficult to locate because of its ephemeral and transient nature. Fraudulent promoters, needless to say, rarely kept detailed records on themselves; nor were such records often collected by academic centers or historical and medical societies.

In 1913 the AMA established the Propaganda Department, later the Department of Investigation, to gather and disseminate information concerning health fraud and quackery. The Department answered inquiries from physicians, Better Business Bureaus, the news media and members of the general public. In the course of preparing answers to these inquiries, the Department also corresponded with federal and state regulatory agencies, state and county medical societies, and experts in the field, to verify the legitimacy of promoters' claims. The record of these activities now forms the heart of the Historical Health Fraud Collection, which constitutes a primary source not only on quackery in medicine, but also on the social history of remedies sought by consumers during the past century.

The Collection contains...

- approximately 370 cubic feet of material (equivalent to about 185 file drawers) on more than 3500 fraudulent or alternative health practitioners, products, and practices which were the subjects of inquiries to and/or investigations by the AMA.
- The core of the Collection consists of letters of inquiry, together with responding letters from the AMA. Supplementing these are...

- correspondence with the practitioners themselves, government agencies, state and county medical societies, and other correspondents;
- newspaper clippings and magazine articles;
- advertisements, circulars, books, posters, testimonials, and other promotional materials;
- product and packaging samples; copies of legal and government documents produced during proceedings involving alleged health fraud and quackery.

The holdings range from single folders on many minor subjects, to files of several cubic feet on topics of great interest, such as alcoholism, cancer, and obesity "cures." The Collection spans the years 1880 through 1990. Most of the holdings begin in 1906 and end in 1975, when the Department of Investigation was abolished.

The recently published *Guide to the American Medical Association Historical Health Fraud and Alternative Medicine Collection* helps researchers and interested parties alike to become familiar with this collection due to its subject-based catagorization of the materials there.

Within the Archives is also the **AMA Policy Library**. Its holdings include AMA policy materials, copies of Board of Trustees reports and other actions by the AMA House of Delegates.

Another unit of this Division is the AMA Office of Permissions which grants permission to use materials published in AMA journals. Permissions are not granted over the phone, written requests to use AMA journal material should be sent to the attention of:

Laslo Hunyady
Permissions Office
515 N. State St., Chicago, IL 60610
FAX 312/464-5832

The Department of Scientific and Socioeconomic Indexing in addition to fulfilling its role in indexing AMA publications, has been involved in several genealogical projects. Information on physicians deceased before 1969 is available through this area due to a collection of records on physicians dating back to the mid-1800's. This area also provides current organizational information on the AMA by creating a yearly *Directory of Officials and Staff.*

Divisional publications include:
Directory of Deceased Physicians
AMA Library Serials Holdings List
Directory of Officials and Staff
American Medical News Index

American
Medical
Association

Medical Education and Science

- Science Technology and Public Health
  Council on Scientific Affairs
  Technology Assessment/DATTA program
- Medical Education

Medical Education and Science at the AMA, along with the Communications area, identifies needs among the medical and scientific communites, channeling the AMA's resources to find effective solutions to meet those needs. This is accomplished by developing and nurturing inter-organizational and inter-professional liaisons, including those with the nursing community and other related health professions, by encouraging support for AMA policies and activities among the scientific and academic elements of the profession; and by providing leadership and administrative support for the AMA Education Research Foundation (ERF); and by professionally directing and administering the AMA's scientific and medical education activities.

The **Office of Foundations and Administration** includes the AMA Education Research Foundation (ERF). Founded in 1951 as an initiative to help medical schools meet expenses, the AMA-ERF makes grants to medical schools to support excellence in medical education and to help medical students. Funding for biomedical research and experimental health care projects has also been granted from this foundation.

Science, Technology and Public Health

Division of Drugs and Toxicology

The AMA's involvement in the area of drugs and toxicology is aimed at identifying existing and emerging issues, developing appropriate responses for such issues, and creating a leadership presence for the Association in this arena. Key activities include providing information on drugs, drug policy, nomenclature, and toxicology; demonstrating leadership in the national effort to reduce the diversion and abuse of prescription drugs; expanding and formalizing the consultative database for AMA's *Drug Evaluations*; providing physicians with reliable information related to substance abuse; and creating and formalizing the approval of nonproprietary names for single entity drugs. Included within this Division are the Departments of Drugs, Clinical Toxicology and of Immunology and Infectious Disease.

Divisional publications include:

Drug Evaluations provides physicians and other health professionals with comprehensive, up-to-date, unbiased, consenus-driven information on the clincial use of drugs. *Drug Evaluations* is available in three formats: looseleaf subscription (which includes a newsletter), an annual text, and in CD-ROM as part of a product package.

Division of Health Science

The AMA health science activities are designed to establish a responsible role for the AMA in mental health, geriatric health, nutrition, preventive medicine and public health, adolescent health, and HIV infection and AIDS. This includes the identification of existing and emerging issues in each of these areas and the development of appropriate AMA responses including publications, proposed policies, conferences, and reports.

Department of Mental Health: A National Coalition of Physicians Against Family violence has been established for physicians interested in learning more about the various abuses constituting family violence, through the AMA department of Mental Health. A National Advisory council of physicians representing more than 49 specialty and medical societies has been developed to continue to guide the development of the campaign. Diagnostic and treatment guidelines on child abuse, child sexual abuse, domestic violence and elder abuse have been developed and disseminated.

HIV/AIDS Office is an area that will continue to receive major focus with planned activities such as a national primary care physician's survey and additional professional education activities. The AMA Task Force on AIDS, an official task force designated as such by the House of Delegates operates inherently with this office to assure activities in support of the many issues raised by the AIDS epidemic are addressed by the Association.

Office publications include:
HIV Infection and Disease: Monographs for Physicians and Other Health Care Workers (16 monographs in one volume)
HIV Early Care: Guidelines for Physicians

Department of Adolescent Health was created in 1988 to provide leadership to the AMA's efforts to improve the health status of youth. Current activities include the development of the AMA National Coalition on Adolescent Health, which consists of 34 national organizations, foundations, and government agencies directly concerned with adolescents; Guidelines for Adolescent Preventive Services project, which has developed a set of recommendations for clinical preventive services for adolescents; Healthier Youth by the Year 2000 Project, which was implemented to promote awareness of the national health objectives related to adolescents and has included the development of a national network of adolescent health professionals and publication of the Target 2000 newsletter; A school and community demonstration project, in conjunction with the National Association of State Boards of Education, to implement recommendations of the 1990 report of the National Commission on the role of the School and Community in Improving Adolescent Health.

American
Medical
Association

American
Medical
Association

Departmental Publications include
*The AMA Profiles of Adolescent Health series:
America's Youth: How Healthy are They? &
Adolescent Health Care: Use, Costs and
Problems of Success*

**Department of Preventive Medicine and Public
Health** pursues activities in the areas of smoking
cessation, women's health, and environmental
health.

Departmental Publications include:
*Guides to the Evaluation of Permanent Impairment
Occupational Health Services and First Aid Guide*

The **Council on Scientific Affairs** provides
advice and counsel to the Board of Trustees and
House of Delegates and recommends policy
positions on important issues in science and
medicine

Reports Of The Council On Scientific Affairs
Published Reports by year:

1993

- Diet and Cancer Report of the Council on
  Scientific Affairs: Diet and Cancer: Where do
  matters stand?. Arch-Intern-Med 153(1) 1993
  Jan 11. 50-6
  During the past decade, the scientific literature base on the
  putative but elusive relationship between diet and cancer
  expanded enormously. Increased emphasis by funding
  agencies, fueled in turn by broadening public interest in the
  topic, led to this growth. The laboratory and epidemiologic
  research conducted in the past decade has shown that a
  simple solution does not exist. The key to the diet/cancer
  puzzle may lie in nutrient interactions and in individual
  response to dietary factors, determined in turn by genetic,
  physiologic and life-style factors. Given the rapid strides
  being made in furthering the understanding of the
  biochemistry and molecular biology of cancer, it may be
  possible to look forward to the day when optimal dietary
  and life-style guidelines can be tailored to a specific
  individualized basis.

1992

- Clinical Ecology. Council on Scientific Affairs.
  JAMA. 1992 Dec 23-30; 268(24): 3465-7.
- Induced Termination of Pregnancy Before and
  After Roe v Wade: Trends in the Mortality and
  Morbidity of Women. Council on Scientific
  Affairs, American Medical Associaition JAMA
  1992 Dec 12;268 (22): 3231-39
  The mortality and morbidity of women who terminated their
  pregnancy before the 1973 Supreme Court decision in Roe
  v Wade are compared with post-Roe v Wade mortality and
  morbidity. Mortality date before 1973 are from the National
  Center for Health Statistics; data from 1973 through 1985
  are from the Centers for Disease Control and The Alan
  Guttmacher Institute. Trends in serious abortion-related
  complications between 1970 and 1990 are based on data
  from the Joint Program for the Study of Abortion and from
  the National Abortion Federation. Deaths from illegally
  induced abortion declined between 1940 and 1972 in part
  because of the introduction of antibiotics to manage sepsis
  and the widespread use of effective contraceptives. Deaths
  from legal abortion declined fivefold between 1973 and
  1985 (from 3.3 deaths to 0.4 death per 100,000
  procedures), reflecting increased physicians education and
  skills, improvements in medical technology, and, notably,
  the earlier termination of pregnancy. The risk of death from

legal abortion is higher among minority women and
women over the age of 35 years, and increases with
gestational age. Legal-abortion mortality between 1979
and 1985 was 0.6 death per 100,000 procedures, more
than 10 times lower than the 9.1 maternal deaths per
100,000 live births, between 1979 and 1986. Serious
complications from legal abortion are rare. Most women
who have a single abortion with vacuum aspiration
experience few if any subsequent problems getting
pregnant or having healthy children. Less is known about
the effects of multiple abortions on future fecundity.
Adverse emotional reactions to abortion are rare; most
women experience relief and reduced depression and
distress.

- Assault weapons as a public health hazard in
  the United States. Council on Scientific Affairs,
  American Medical Association. JAMA. 1992 Jun
  10; 267(22): 3067-70
- Violence against women. Relevance for medical
  practitioners. Council on Scientific Affairs,
  American Medical Association.
  JAMA. 1992 Jun 17; 267(23): 3184-9
  Evidence collected over the last 20 years indicates that
  physical and sexual violence against women is an
  enormous problem. Much of this violence is perpetrated by
  women's intimate partners or in relationships that would
  presumably carry some protective aura (eg,
  father-daughter, boyfriend-girlfriend). This violence carries
  with it both short- and long-term sequelae for women and
  affects their physical and psychological well-being.
  The high prevalence of violence against women brings
  them into regular contact with physicians; at least one in
  five women seen in emergency departments has symptoms
  relating to abuse. However, physicians frequently treat the
  injuries only symptomatically or fail to recognize the injuries
  as abuse. Even when recognized, physicians are often
  without resources to address the needs of abused women.
  This report documents the extent of violence against
  women and suggests path that the physician community
  might take to address the needs of victims.

1991

- Health effects of radon exposure. Report of the
  Council on Scientific Affairs, American Medical
  Association. Arch-Intern-Med. 1991 Apr; 151(4):
  674-7
  The consensus of scientists is that exposure to radon is
  hazardous, but disagreement exists about the effects of
  lower radon concentrations. Studies of underground miners
  have indicated that the risk of lung cancer increases in
  proportion to the intensity and duration of exposure to
  radon, and a recent authoritative report (BEIR IV) has
  concluded that estimates based on those studies are
  appropriate for estimating risks for occupants of homes.
  The BEIR IV report concluded that smoking cigarettes
  increases the risk of lung cancer associated with radon.
  Average radon levels in US homes range from 0.055 to
  0.148 Bq/L (1.5 to 4 pCi/L), depending on the
  circumstances of measurement. Few studies have
  investigated health outcomes in occupants of homes with
  high radon levels. In advising patients about reducing the
  risks associated with radon, physicians should consider the
  costs, as well as the benefits, of remedial actions, and they
  should emphasize that, by far, the best way to avoid lung
  cancer is to stop smoking.
- Biotechnology and the American agricultural
  industry. Council on Scientific Affairs, American
  Medical Association [see comments] JAMA.
  1991 Mar 20; 265(11): 1429-36
  To meet the needs of a rapidly growing population and
  minimize the toxic influences of traditional farming practices
  on the environment, the American agricultural industry has
  applied molecular technology to the development of food
  crops and livestock. By placing genes specific for highly
  desirable phenotypes into the DNA of plants, animals, and

bacteria, farmers have increased crop and livestock survival, enhanced the nutritional quality of foods, increased industry productivity, and reduced the need for toxic pesticides and herbicides. However, introduction of genetically modified foods into the marketplace has raised a spectrum of public health issues. Physicians, as the most proximal scientific resource for most individuals, are uniquely positioned to address patient concerns regarding the safety of genetically altered foods. This report provides an overview of the inherent risks and benefits of "agrogenetics" and offers a series of recommendations designed to promote the education of the medical community and dispel public misconception regarding genetic manipulation.

- **Medical diagnostic ultrasound instrumentation and clinical interpretation. Report of the ultrasonography task force. Council on Scientific Affairs. JAMA. 1991 Mar 6; 265(9): 1155-9**
Over the past 20 years, there has been a dramatic increase in the use of ultrasonography as an imaging modality. The introduction of real-time ultrasonography and Doppler units for the measurement of blood flow in the 1970s, recent advances in transducer design, signal processing, and miniaturization of electronics, along with the lack of radiation exposure, have been primarily responsible for the increased use of ultrasound. However, although ultrasonography can provide diagnostic information safely and easily, interpretation of the information requires an understanding of the physics behind ultrasound, how that physics is translated into ultrasound instrumentation, recognition of artifacts that are associated with the various types of ultrasonography, and identification of these artifacts in specific anatomic locations.

- **Doppler sonographic imaging of the vascular system. Report of the Ultrasonography Task Force. Council on Scientific Affairs, American Medical Association. JAMA. 1991 May 8; 265(18): 2382-7**
Ultrasonic vascular imaging has been used for more than 20 years to define vascular anatomy, pathologic changes in vessel size, and perivascular abnormalities. In the last decade, development of duplex Doppler technology has permitted the evaluation of both anatomic vascular features and physiologic blood flow parameters in a variety of locations. Doppler "color flow" imaging promises to expand these applications. In many instances, duplex Doppler technology has replaced more invasive angiographic procedures for evaluation of suspected vascular abnormalities. Improved ultrasound duplex technology, combined with the relatively inexpensive, rapid, noninvasive aspects of ultrasonography has made it a valuable screening examination for suspected flow abnormalities.

- **Ultrasonic imaging of the abdomen. Report of the ultrasonography task force. Council on Scientific Affairs, American Medical Association. JAMA. 1991 Apr 3; 265(13): 1726-31**
As new imaging modalities emerge and existing technologies improve, indications for a particular imaging method may change. This article examines current indications for abdominal and prostatic ultrasound examination and, where possible, compares ultrasound with other imaging techniques. This is not an attempt to list all possible ultrasound indications or examinations, but rather an attempt to serve as an aid to informed imaging selection based on current literature and equipment.

- **Report of the Council on Scientific Affairs: ultrasonic imaging of the heart: report of the Ultrasonography Task Force. Sahn-D; Kisslo-J. Arch-Intern-Med. 1991 Jul; 151(7): 1288-94**
The use of ultrasonography in cardiology has progressed so dramatically that not only is anatomic information available but information can also be derived about cardiac hemodynamics. Applications range from intravascular ultrasonic imaging of coronary atherosclerosis to

predictions of the severity of fetal valvular pulmonic stenosis detected in utero. We reviewed cardiac ultrasonography as utilized in B-mode imaging, pulsed and continuous-wave spectral Doppler, and Doppler color flow mapping. We reviewed specialized areas, including stress echo for wall motion analysis, valvular and congenital heart disease applications, and new applications in intraoperative, transesophageal, contrast echography, coronary imaging, and fetal echocardiography. Finally, future applications of quantitative flow mapping and intraluminal and interventional ultrasonography were considered along with the required technological advances.

- **The future of ultrasonography. Report of the Ultrasonography Task Force. Council on Scientific Affairs, American Medical Association. JAMA. 1991 Jul 17; 266(3): 406-9**
Future advances in ultrasonography will undoubtedly occur in three major areas: diagnostic capability, instrumentation, and clinical applications. In the area of diagnostic capability, spatial and contrast resolution offer excellent opportunities for improvement. Continued research into tissue characterization is worthwhile, even though efforts to date have been more frustrating than fulfilling. Blood flow studies and new contrast agents are among the more promising areas for future development. New techniques of signal detection, analysis, and display in Doppler imaging may overcome some present limitations, including those in color flow imaging.

- **Medical Informatics: an emerging medical discipline. Council on Scientific Affairs and Council on Long Range Planning and Development of the American Medical Associaition. J Med Syst. 1990 Aug; 14(4): 161-79**

- **Educating physicians in home health care. Council on Scientific Affairs and Council on Medical Education [corrected] [published erratum appears in JAMA 1991 May 8;265(18):2340] JAMA. 1991 Feb 13; 265(6): 769-71**
A growing proportion of health care, especially long-term care, should best and most appropriately be provided in the home setting. Physicians have largely remained on the periphery of this reemerging area of health care. Yet if home health care is to reach its full potential, physicians must fulfill their essential role as members of the home health team. Direct physician input and participation are needed to ensure that home health care is safe and medically appropriate. Physician involvement will enhance the supervision of medical care in the home, and physicians' expertise is also much needed for home health care quality assurance and clinical research. Role models and training experiences must be developed for new physicians so that they can integrate home health care skills and values into their future practices. Although most of the usual physician objections to home health care involvement can be addressed by education, the problem of inadequate reimbursement is substantive and must be addressed by policy change.

- **Use of animals in medical education. Council on Scientific Affairs, American Medical Association. JAMA. 1991 Aug 14; 266(6): 836-7**
The use of animals in general medical education is essential. Although several adjuncts to the use of animals are available, none can completely replace the limited use of animals in the medical curriculum. Students should be made aware of an institution's policy on animal use in the curriculum before matriculation, and faculty should make clear to all students the learning objectives of any educational exercise that uses animals. The Council on Scientific Affairs recognizes the necessity for the responsible and humane treatment of animals and urges all medical school faculty members to discuss this moral and ethical imperative with their students.

American
Medical
Association

American
Medical
Association

- Hispanic health in the United States. Council on Scientific Affairs. JAMA. 1991 Jan 9; 265(2): 248-52
Hispanics are the fastest growing minority in the United States. Typically, they are divided into five subgroups: Mexican American, Puerto Rican, Cuban American, Central or South American, and "other" Hispanics. Risk factors for morbidity and mortality vary among these subgroups. Use of health care services is affected by perceived health care needs, insurance status, income, culture, and language. Compared with whites, Hispanics are more likely to live in poverty, be unemployed or underemployed, and have little education and no private insurance. Hispanics are at an increased risk for certain medical conditions, including diabetes, hypertension, tuberculosis, human immunodeficiency virus infection, alcoholism, cirrhosis, specific cancers, and violent deaths. Proportionate to their representation in the population, there are few Hispanic health providers, emphasizing the need for all medical personnel to be knowledgeable about Hispanic health care needs.

- Asbestos removal, health hazards, and the EPA. Council on Scientific Affairs, American Medical Association. JAMA. 1991 Aug 7; 266(5): 696-7
Resolution 193 (A-90), which was adopted by the House of Delegates of the American Medical Association, called on the Council on Scientific Affairs to study the situation regarding asbestos abatement, the risks to health, and the appropriateness of Environmental Protection Agency regulations, policies, and control measures. This report reviews the current status of asbestos abatement as applied to schools and public buildings, which currently accounts for the major expenditure of public funds.

- Gynecologic sonography. Report of the ultrasonography task force. Council on Scientific Affairs, American Medical Association. JAMA. 1991 Jun 5; 265(21): 2851-5
Sonography, because it is nonionizing, is the preferred imaging modality for the female pelvis. Traditionally, transabdominal, transcystic studies were performed. However, development of transvaginal and transrectal transducers has led to enhanced imaging capabilities of the pelvis. These new technologies will likely improve our ability to understand gynecologic pathology. The clinical use of pelvic ultrasonography depends on a thorough understanding of normal anatomy and cyclical changes and on the relative limitations of the imaging modality in specifically characterizing pathologic processes. This article reviews the accepted role of pelvic sonography in gynecologic disease and provides a preview of some of the potential applications of recent advances in sonographic technology.

1990

- The worldwide smoking epidemic. Tobacco trade, use, and control. Council on Scientific Affairs. JAMA. 1990 Jun 27; 263(24): 3312-8
- Health status of detained and incarcerated youths. Council on Scientific Affairs. JAMA. 1990 Feb 16; 263(7): 987-91
Youths who are detained or incarcerated in correctional facilities represent a medically underserved population that is at high risk for a variety of medical and emotional disorders. These youths not only have a substantial number of preexisting health problems, they also develop acute problems that are associated with their arrest and with the environment of the correctional facility. Although the availability of medical services varies by the size of the institution, established standards are, in general, not being met.

- Saturated fatty acids in vegetable oils. Council on Scientific Affairs. JAMA. 1990 Feb 2; 263(5): 693-5

Concern has been expressed about the "atherogenicity" of coconut and/or palm oil in food products. Saturated fatty acids are found primarily in animal products and in "tropical oils" (coconut, palm, and palm kernel oils). Composition of the total diet over an extended period determines nutritional status and contribution to health. Specific foods and/or food ingredients need to be evaluated within the context of a person's total dietary pattern over time. Persons attempting to limit saturated fatty acid intake should be aware of the high content of saturated fatty acids in tropical oils. The American Medical Association is on record as supporting fatty acid labeling when cholesterol content is declared and cholesterol labeling when fatty acid content is declared. The American Medical Association has supported, and continues to support, voluntary efforts to increase public awareness of the composition and nutritional value of foods.

- Medical applications of fetal tissue transplantation. Council on Scientific Affairs and Council on Ethical and Judicial Affairs JAMA. 1990 Jan 26; 263(4): 565-70
Fetal tissue transplantation has been attempted for a limited number of clinical disorders, including Parkinson's disease, diabetes, immunodeficiency disorders, and several metabolic disorders. Fetal tissue has intrinsic properties--ability to differentiate into multiple cell types, growth and proliferative ability, growth factor production, and reduced antigenicity--that make it attractive for transplantation research. At this time the results from fetal tissue grafts for Parkinson's disease and diabetes have not demonstrated significant long-term clinical benefit to patients with these disorders. Further research will be necessary to determine the potential value of fetal tissue transplantation. For these clinical investigations to proceed, specific ethical guidelines are needed to ensure that fetal tissue derived from elective abortions is used in a morally acceptable manner. These guidelines should separate, to the greatest extent possible, the decision by a woman to have an abortion from her consent to donate the postmortem tissue for transplantation purposes. Such ethical guidelines are offered in this report.

- Persistent vegetative state and the decision to withdraw or withhold life support. Council on Scientific Affairs and Council on Ethical and Judicial Affairs. JAMA. 1990 Jan 19; 263(3): 426-30
Persons with overwhelming damage to the cerebral hemispheres commonly pass into a chronic state of unconsciousness (ie, loss of self-awareness) called the vegetative state. When such cognitive loss lasts for more than a few weeks, the condition has been termed a persistent vegetative state, because the body retains the functions necessary to sustain vegetative functions. Recovery from the vegetative state does occur, but many persons in persistent vegetative states live for months or years if provided with nutritional and other supportive measures. The withdrawal of life support from these persons with loss of higher brain function is a controversial issue, as highlighted by public debates and judicial decisions. This article provides criteria for the diagnosis of permanent unconsciousness and reviews the available data that support the reliability of these criteria. Significant legal decisions have been made with regard to withdrawal of life support to patients in persistent vegetative states, and the trends in this area are discussed.

- American Medical Association white paper on elderly health. Report of the Council on Scientific Affairs [published erratum appears in Arch Intern Med 1991 Feb;151(2):265] Arch-Intern-Med. 1990;150:(12): 2459-72

- Home care in the 1990s. Council on Scientific Affairs JAMA. 1990 Mar 2; 263(9): 1241-4
Home care is a rapidly growing field that is beginning to attract greater physician interest and participation. Cost-containment pressures have led to reduced institutionalization in hospitals and nursing homes and to

more patients, both acutely and chronically ill, being cared for in their own homes. Undergraduate and graduate medical education programs are developing home care curricula, and academic medicine is beginning to develop a research agenda, particularly in the area of clinical outcome measurements. Medical care in the home is highly diversified and innovative. The areas of preventive, diagnostic, therapeutic, rehabilitative, and long-term maintenance care are all well represented as physicians develop new practice patterns in home care.

- Education for health. A role for physicians and the efficacy of health education efforts. Council on Scientific Affairs. JAMA. 1990 Apr 4; 263(13): 1816-9
Health education efforts have grown dramatically over the past decade and seek to improve the health of individuals by providing them with information that will lead to behavioral changes and thereby result in improved health. There is now substantial evidence to support the idea that health education activities can alter health behaviors, even though the mechanisms by which health education efforts succeed are largely unknown. Physicians could add to the success of health education efforts by incorporating preventive services into their patient encounters, particularly patients in high-risk situations. There are many examples of successful physician-based interventions, and a new emphasis on preventive services in primary care is emerging.

- A permanent US-Mexico border environmental health commission. Council on Scientific Affairs. JAMA. 1990 Jun 27; 263(24): 3319-21:
Public health officials, physicians, and politicians have long been aware of the squalid environmental conditions existing along the US-Mexico border. Some attempts have been made to improve the environmental pollution and causes of human disease, beginning as early as the 1930s with the IBWC, established in 1889. More recent agreements and legislation have called for US and Mexico cooperation by way of each nation's corresponding environmental agency (ie, the EPA and Mexico's SEDUE) and their agencies of foreign affairs (ie, the IBWC). Nevertheless, environmental monitoring and disease incidence data continue to point out that public and environmental health along the border--the result of uncontrolled air and water pollution and lack of disease vector control--is rapidly deteriorating and seriously affecting the health and future economic vitality on both sides of the border. Many prominent public health professionals and environmental organizations are concerned that the present working relationship between the United States and Mexico is not functioning well and cannot adequately cope with existing environmental conditions; for one thing, the efforts of the EPA and SEDUE are reviewed no more frequently than once a year by a staff quartered in Washington and Mexico City. Some projects to improve these conditions have been undertaken by the EPA and SEDUE and the IBWC; at present, the prospects for success do not appear promising. Consequently, these individuals and organizations have urged creation of a US-Mexico border environmental health commission. Congress did see fit last year to give responsibility for the environment to the IBWC in the form of Public Law 100-465. This law, however, does not address the full severity of environmental and public health degradation along the border; it does not address the pollution of the New River, Agua Prieta, the San Pedro River, or the Pacific Ocean, neither does it offer remedial control of hazardous waste sites, rabies, and other disease vectors. Moreover, the IBWC is only a deliberative body, not an implementing one.

- Medical and nonmedical uses of anabolic-androgenic steroids. Council on Scientific Affairs. JAMA. 1990 Dec 12; 264(22): 2923-7
Recent trends in the use, abuse, and diversion of steroids

for nonmedical purposes illustrate a growing problem that not only imposes health risks but presents ethical dilemmas as well. Concern over the known adverse effects, the limited research into the long-term effects, and the ethics of engineering body size and performance through anabolic-androgenic steroid use has led to legislative, legal, and education responses. Increased penalties for distribution to minors and stricter controls in prescribing practices have been enacted through state legislation and federal initiatives. Government, some health professional organizations, and some sports groups have denounced the nonmedical use of anabolic-androgenic steroids and have developed materials to educate their members, other professionals, athletes, educators, and the public at large.

- The IOM report and public health. Council on Scientific Affairs JAMA. 1990 Jul 25; 264(4): 503-6
A recent Institute of Medicine report defined "public health" as what society must do to keep people healthy and further defined it as involving the collection of data, assessment of problems, and assurance of health protection. Public health professionals include physicians, nurses, sanitarians, biostatisticians, engineers, and administrators, and epidemiology is public health's basic science. Past successes in the United States, such as increases in longevity and decreases in infant mortality and cardiovascular death rates, demonstrate that progress is possible; however, inequalities persist, for example, in infant mortality rates and availability of medical care to lower socioeconomic groups. The major responsibilities of public health departments include leading and coordinating public health efforts, controlling epidemics, carrying out disease and injury surveillance, collecting vital statistics, ensuring good medical and dental care for the indigent, environmental control, health education, and laboratory services.

- Conflicts of interest in medical center/industry research relationships. Council on Scientific Affairs and Council on Ethical and Judicial Affairs. JAMA. 1990 May 23-30; 263(20): 2790-3

- Societal effects and other factors affecting health care for the elderly. Report of the Council on Scientific Affairs. AMA Council on Scientific Affairs. Arch-Intern-Med. 1990 Jun; 150(6): 1184-9
With advances in medical care, life expectancy of Americans has increased dramatically. The increase in the size of the elderly population has had a major impact on health care provision and will have an even greater impact on our health care system over the next several decades. Although today's medical students will spend nearly half of their collective careers caring for the elderly, insufficient numbers of students show an interest in geriatrics. American society has become in many ways less traditional, and age is no longer seen as "a pathway to wisdom." Since we are now a more mobile society, extended families tend to scatter, and the elderly are frequently alone. We examine the effects of our rapidly changing, youth-oriented society on health care for the elderly.

American
Medical
Association

American
Medical
Association

1989

- Providing medical services through school-based health programs. Council on Scientific Affairs [see comments] JAMA. 1989 Apr 7; 261(13): 1939-42

  Resolution 162, which was adopted at the 1987 Annual Meeting by the Board of Trustees, called on the American Medical Association to study the efficacy of school-based health clinics. Recent data show that a significant number of school-aged youth are in need of an adequate source of health care. School-based health programs constitute a promising avenue for providing health services to adolescents, particularly in medically underserved areas. Although there are insufficient data to support universal establishment of school-based health programs, small-scale studies suggest that such programs are a viable means to increase access to health care for youth.

- Formaldehyde. Council on Scientific Affairs. JAMA. 1989 Feb 24; 261(8): 1183-7

  In response to Resolution 195 (A-87), the medical literature on the adverse health effects of formaldehyde was reviewed, and the potential cancer risk to anatomists and other related health professionals from exposure to the chemical is described. Though the evidence in humans is limited and controversial, both the Environmental Protection Agency and the Occupational Safety and Health Administration, in their consideration of available epidemiologic and toxicological studies, now regard formaldehyde as a possible human carcinogen and will regulate it accordingly.

- Dyslexia. Council on Scientific Affairs. JAMA 1989 Apr 21; 261(15): 2236-9

  Experts disagree on the etiology and definition of dyslexia. Neurological research is ongoing but is not yet conclusive. Specific educational techniques for diagnosis and remediation are available. Physicians can serve on multidisciplinary diagnostic teams and can act to support and provide informational resources to affected families.

- Mammographic screening in asymptomatic women aged 40 years and older. Council on Scientific Affairs. JAMA. 1989 May 5; 261(17): 2535-42

  Currently, age-specific recommendations for screening mammograms in asymptomatic women that have been developed by professional, voluntary, and governmental organizations differ. While there is strong epidemiologic evidence that mammographic screening in asymptomatic women aged 50 years or older reduces breast cancer mortality, the evidence for mortality reduction is not as clear for women aged 40 to 49 years. However, as described in this report, findings of further mortality and survival follow-up of subjects in earlier studies, as well as observations from more recent studies, suggest reductions in mortality and better survival in younger women as well. While mammography is currently the most effective method for detecting early breast cancers, some breast cancers may develop during the intervals between screening mammograms. The costs of mammographic screening also require consideration in the process of making national screening recommendations.

- Dietary fiber and health. Council on Scientific Affairs. JAMA. 1989 Jul 28; 262(4): 542-6

  During the last 18 years, considerable research has been conducted on the role of dietary fiber in health and disease. Interest was stimulated by epidemiologic studies that associated a low intake of dietary fiber with the incidence of colon cancer, heart disease, diabetes, and other diseases and disorders. Dietary fiber is not a single substance. There are significant differences in the physiological effects of the various components of dietary fiber. A Recommended Dietary Allowance for dietary fiber has not been established. However, an adequate amount of dietary fiber can be obtained by choosing several servings daily from a variety of fiber-rich foods such as whole-grain breads and cereals, fruits, vegetables, legumes, and nuts.

- Magnetic resonance imaging of the head and neck region. Present status and future potential. Council on Scientific Affairs. Report of the Panel on Magnetic Resonance Imaging. JAMA. 1988 Dec 9; 260(22): 3313-26

  Magnetic resonance imaging (MRI) has many bona fide applications in the head and neck region. The major strengths of its current conventional use include excellent soft-tissue contrast, multiplanar capabilities, noninvasiveness, and lack of ionizing radiation. Newer advances, including gradient-echo techniques, three-dimensional fourier transformation, paramagnetic contrast, and more efficient receiver coils, will improve images and expand indications for MRI. The technology, however, remains relatively expensive, and the additional information compared with that of other techniques might not always justify the difference in cost. Moreover, MRI's insensitivity to calcifications, lack of depiction of fine bone detail, and, in some areas, degradation caused by motion and other artifacts make computed tomography and other noninvasive studies more appropriate as a primary imaging tool in many circumstances. Continued careful clinical research should clarify the relative role of MRI and other imaging tools during the next several years.

- Magnetic resonance imaging of the abdomen and pelvis. Council on Scientific Affairs. JAMA. 1989 Jan 20; 261(3): 420-33

  Magnetic resonance imaging (MRI) of the abdomen presents greater inherent difficulties than other anatomic regions. However, new techniques now allow imaging comparable in quality to computed tomography (CT). Magnetic resonance imaging offers the advantages of greater tissue contrast, multiplanar imaging, and lack of ionizing radiation or risk of toxic reactions from iodinated contrast media. Its use remains limited by high cost, limited availability, lack of a bowel contrast agent, and long imaging time, which some patients cannot tolerate. In many areas of abdominal imaging, MRI is now comparable to CT, but because of the greater availability and lesser cost, CT remains the procedure of choice. Magnetic resonance imaging is more accurate for staging neoplasms of the liver, adrenal glands, kidneys, bladder, prostate, uterus, and cervix and may aid in diagnosis of hepatic, adrenal, and uterine masses. In selected patients, especially those in whom CT is inconclusive or those who cannot tolerate iodinated contrast material, MRI can provide valuable information. Development of faster scanning techniques and MRI contrast agents and wider availability will probably increase the usefulness of abdominal MRI. At this time, MRI complements other abdominal imaging procedures. In a small number of patients, however, it can provide unique information in a virtually risk-free manner.

- Low-level radioactive wastes. Council on Scientific Affairs. JAMA. 1989 Aug 4; 262(5): 669-74

  Under a federal law, each state by January 1, 1993, must provide for safe disposal of its low-level radioactive wastes. Most of the wastes are from using nuclear power to produce electricity, but 25% to 30% are from medical diagnosis, therapy, and research. Exposures to radioactivity from the wastes are much smaller than those from natural sources, and federal standards limit public exposure. Currently operating disposal facilities are in Beatty, Nev, Barnwell, SC, and Richland, Wash. National policy encourages the development of regional facilities. Planning a regional facility, selecting a site, and building, monitoring, and closing the facility will be a complex project lasting decades that involves legislation, public participation, local and state governments, financing, quality control, and surveillance. The facilities will utilize geological factors, structural designs, packaging, and other approaches to isolate the wastes. Those providing medical care can reduce wastes by storing them until they are less radioactive, substituting nonradioactive compounds, reducing volumes, and incinerating. Physicians have an important role in informing and advising the public and public officials about risks involved with the wastes and about effective methods of dealing with them.

- Infectious medical wastes. Council on Scientific Affairs. JAMA. 1989 Sep 22-29; 262(12): 1669-71

A number of recent incidents involving improper handling and disposal of hospital waste have prompted the demand for more stringent legislation to cover the management of infectious hospital waste. Resolution 53 (December 1987 Interim Meeting) called for the American Medical Association to promote the passage of federal legislation for the proper disposal of infectious hospital waste. This resolution has prompted a Council on Scientific Affairs report on the current status of infectious hospital waste management and of state and federal regulations to control such waste. The Council has concluded that existing federal and state regulations for the management of hazardous waste--in conjunction with the accreditation program of the Joint Commission on Accreditation of Healthcare Organizations and the guidelines of the Environmental Protection Agency and the Centers for Disease Control, if adhered to and properly enforced--should be adequate to ensure that the public and environment are not endangered. Therefore, the Council does not favor additional federal legislation at this time and recommends that this report be accepted in lieu of Resolution 53.Quality assurance in cervical cytology. The Papanicolaou smear. Council on Scientific Affairs. JAMA. 1989 Sep 22-29; 262(12): 1672-9

- Health care needs of homeless and runaway youths. Council on Scientific Affairs. JAMA. 1989 Sep 8; 262(10): 1358-61

Large numbers of homeless adolescents can be found in this country, with estimates of their numbers ranging from 500,000 to more than 2 million. Some are runaways while others are involuntarily without shelter, often having been forced out of their homes. Most receive no help from social service agencies and their lack of skills forces them into a marginal existence, leaving them vulnerable to abuse and victimization. Health problems are numerous and health care is generally inadequate for several reasons, including a lack of treatment facilities, the behavior of the adolescents themselves, the ability of providers to deal with such youths, and the questionable legal status of homeless adolescents. The Council on Scientific Affairs urges that reliable and up-to-date data on the extent of homelessness among adolescents and the nature of their needs be generated and that guidelines for the medical care of such youths be developed.

- Medical perspective on nuclear power. Council on Scientific Affairs. JAMA. 1989 Nov 17; 262(19): 2724-9

- Harmful effects of ultraviolet radiation. Council on Scientific Affairs. JAMA. 1989 Jul 21; 262(3): 380-4

Tanning for cosmetic purposes by sunbathing or by using artificial tanning devices is widespread. The hazards associated with exposure to ultraviolet radiation are of concern to the medical profession. Depending on the amount and form of the radiation, as well as on the skin type of the individual exposed, ultraviolet radiation causes erythema, sunburn, photodamage (photoaging), photocarcinogenesis, damage to the eyes, alteration of the immune system of the skin, and chemical hypersensitivity. Skin cancers most commonly produced by ultraviolet radiation are basal and squamous cell carcinomas. There also is much circumstantial evidence that the increase in the incidence of cutaneous malignant melanoma during the past half century is related to increased sun exposure, but this has not been proved. Effective and cosmetically acceptable sunscreen preparations have been developed that can do much to prevent or reduce most harmful effects to ultraviolet radiation if they are applied properly and consistently. Other safety measures include (1) minimizing

exposure to ultraviolet radiation, (2) being aware of reflective surfaces while in the sun, (3) wearing protective clothing, (4) avoiding use of artificial tanning devices, and (5) protecting infants and children.Science Literacy and Educational Standards

- Animals in research. Council on Scientific Affairs. JAMA. 1989 Jun 23-30; 261(24): 3602-6

- Musculoskeletal applications of magnetic resonance imaging. Council on Scientific Affairs [published erratum appears in JAMA 1990 Jul 25;264(4):456] [see comments] JAMA. 1989 Nov 3; 262(17): 2420-7

Magnetic resonance imaging provides superior contrast, resolution, and multiplanar imaging capability, allowing excellent definition of soft-tissue and bone marrow abnormalities. For these reasons, magnetic resonance imaging has become a major diagnostic imaging method for the evaluation of many musculoskeletal disorders. The applications of magnetic resonance imaging for musculoskeletal diagnosis are summarized and examples of common clinical situations are given. General guidelines are suggested for the musculoskeletal applications of magnetic resonance imaging.

1988

- Magnetic resonance imaging of the cardiovascular system. Present state of the art and future potential. Council on Scientific Affairs. Report of the Magnetic Resonance Imaging Panel. JAMA. 1988 Jan 8; 259(2): 253-9

State-of-the-art magnetic resonance imaging (MRI) generates high-resolution images of the cardiovascular system. Conventional MRI techniques provide images in six to ten minutes per tomographic slice. New strategies have substantially improved the speed of imaging. The technology is relatively expensive, and its cost-effectiveness remains to be defined in relation to other effective, less expensive, and noninvasive technologies, such as echocardiography and nuclear medicine. The ultimate role of MRI will depend on several factors, including the development of specific applications such as (1) noninvasive angiography, especially of the coronary arteries; (2) noninvasive, high-resolution assessment of regional myocardial blood flow distribution (eg, using paramagnetic contrast agents); (3) characterization of myocardial diseases using proton-relaxation property changes; and (4) evaluation of in vivo myocardial biochemistry. The three-dimensional imaging capability and the ability to image cardiovascular structures without contrast material give MRI a potential advantage over existing noninvasive diagnostic imaging techniques. This report analyzes current applications of MRI to the cardiovascular system and speculates on their future.

- Report of the organ transplant panel. Corneal transplantation. Council on Scientific Affairs. JAMA. 1988 Feb 5; 259(5): 719-22

Corneal transplantation is the most common form of organ transplantation practiced in the United States. Two procedures for transplantation are utilized. Penetrating keratoplasty is used in about 90% of the cases, with lamellar keratoplasty being utilized in the remaining situations. Demand for corneal transplantation exceeds the available supply of corneas. Advances in procurement and preservation must continue to meet this demand. Finally, these procedures are not without complications, and these are discussed to provide a clear risk-benefit analysis.

- Magnetic resonance imaging of the central nervous system. Council on Scientific Affairs. Report of the Panel on Magnetic Resonance Imaging. JAMA. 1988 Feb 26; 259(8): 1211-22

This report reviews the current applications of magnetic resonance imaging of the central nervous system. Since its introduction into the clinical environment in the early 1980s, this technology has had a major impact on the practice of

American

Medical

Association

American

Medical

Association

neurology. It has proved to be superior to computed tomography for imaging many diseases of the brain and spine. In some instances it has clearly replaced computed tomography. It is likely that it will replace myelography for the assessment of cervicomedullary junction and spinal regions. The magnetic field strengths currently used appear to be entirely safe for clinical application in neurology, except in patients with cardiac pacemakers or vascular metallic clips. Some shortcomings of magnetic resonance imaging include its expense, the time required for scanning, and poor visualization of cortical bone.

- Instrumentation in positron emission tomography. Council on Scientific Affairs. Report of the Positron Emission Tomography Panel. JAMA. 1988 Mar 11; 259(10): 1531-6
Positron emission tomography (PET) is a three-dimensional medical imaging technique that noninvasively measures the concentration of radiopharmaceuticals in the body that are labeled with positron emitters. With the proper compounds, PET can be used to measure metabolism, blood flow, or other physiological values in vivo. The technique is based on the physics of positron annihilation and detection and the mathematical formulations developed for x-ray computed tomography. Modern PET systems can provide three-dimensional images of the brain, the heart, and other internal organs with resolutions on the order of 4 to 6 mm. With the selectivity provided by a choice of injected compounds, PET has the power to provide unique diagnostic information that is not available with any other imaging modality. This is the first of five reports on the nature and uses of PET that have been prepared for the American Medical Association's Council on Scientific Affairs by an authoritative panel.

- Drug abuse in athletes. Anabolic steroids and human growth hormone. Council on Scientific Affairs. JAMA. 1988 Mar 18; 259(11): 1703-5
This report, the first in a three-part series on drug abuse by athletes, responds to adopted Resolution 4 (1984 Annual Meeting) and to Resolution 57 (1986 Annual Meeting), "Human Growth Hormone," which was referred to the Board of Trustees for action. Subsequent reports will cover other classes of abused drugs.(Resolution 57, A-86)

- Cyclotrons and radiopharmaceuticals in positron emission tomography. Council on Scientific Affairs. Report of the Positron Emission Tomography Panel. JAMA. 1988 Mar 25; 259(12): 1854-60
Positron emission tomography (PET) can probe biochemical pathways in vivo and can provide quantitative data; for that purpose, tracers labeled with positron-emitting radioisotopes are essential. This report describes the tracers that are being used or that may have future use, their production by cyclotrons, and other needed resources for PET imaging. Current routine and automated methods for convenient production of labeled compounds, coupled with simple computer-controlled accelerators, can support the creation of clinical PET centers in any large medical institution, obviating the need for in-depth research teams. An alternate approach involves the development of regional centers that provide in-house service and that supply fluorine 18- and carbon 11-labeled compounds to nearby hospitals with PET machines.

- Positron emission tomography in oncology. Council on Scientific Affairs. JAMA. 1988 Apr 8; 259(14): 2126-31
This report describes the current and potential uses of positron emission tomography in clinical medicine and research related to oncology. Assessment will be possible of metabolism and physiology of tumors and their effects on adjacent tissues. Specific probes are likely to be developed for target sites on tumors, including monoclonal antibodies and specific growth factors that recognize tumors. To date, most oncological applications of positron emission tomography tracers have been qualitative; in the

future, quantitative metabolic measurements should aid in the evaluation of tumor biology and response to treatment.

- Application of positron emission tomography in the heart. Council on Scientific Affairs. Report of the Positron Emission Tomography Panel.. JAMA. 1988 Apr 22-29; 259(16): 2438-45
This report discusses experimental and clinical applications of positron emission tomography to the heart, including measurements of blood flow to the myocardium and studies of metabolism and experimental injury. Most initial clinical studies have concentrated on ischemic heart disease, but the technique also has potential for investigation of cardiomyopathies, studying the neural control of the heart, and evaluating the effects of drugs on cardiac tissues.

- Positron emission tomography--a new approach to brain chemistry. Council on Scientific Affairs. Report of the Positron Emission Tomography Panel [published erratum appears in JAMA. 1989 Jun 16;261(23):3412] JAMA. 1988 Nov 11; 260(18): 2704-10
Positron emission tomography permits examination of the chemistry of the brain in living human beings. Until recently, positron emission tomography had been considered a research tool, but it is rapidly moving into clinical practice. This report describes the uses and applications of positron emission tomography in examinations of patients with strokes, epilepsy, malignancies, dementias, and schizophrenia and in basic studies of synaptic neurotransmission.

- Cancer risk of pesticides in agricultural workers. Council on Scientific Affairs. JAMA. 1988 Aug 19; 260(7): 959-66
This report discusses some of the inherent limitations of cancer studies in animals and humans and presents a qualitative carcinogen risk assessment of a number of pesticides based on the judgment of national and international authorities who have reviewed the available experimental and epidemiologic evidence. A large number of pesticidal compounds have shown evidence of genotoxicity or carcinogenicity in animal and in vitro screening tests, but no pesticides--except arsenic and vinyl chloride (once used as an aerosol propellant)-definitely have been proved to be carcinogenic in man. Resolution 94 (1-86), which was referred to the Board of Trustees, calls for the American Medical Association, through its scientific journals and publications, to alert physicians to the potential hazards of agricultural pesticides, to provide physicians with advice on such hazards for their patients, and to urge that these substances be appropriately labeled. This report addresses the potential carcinogenicity of pesticides by review of the available literature.

- Treatment of obesity in adults. Council on Scientific Affairs. JAMA. 1988 Nov 4; 260(17): 2547-51
Concern with weight control should begin sufficiently early in life to reduce the risk of developing obesity. The complex etiology of obesity is, in part, responsible for the difficulty physicians encounter in treating this condition. Prevention is the "treatment" of choice. Early identification of individuals genetically at risk can be helpful in targeting those most likely to gain excess weight. Numerous dietary regimens have been devised in an attempt to achieve progressive weight loss in obese individuals. Since the ultimate goal of a weight-reduction program is to lose weight and maintain the loss, a nutritionally balanced, low-energy diet that is applicable to the patient's life-style is most appropriate. Increasing energy expenditure through physical activity, in addition to decreasing energy intake, generally improves results in the management of obesity. Major changes in eating and exercise behaviors are necessary to ensure long-term weight control. Diet, exercise, and behavior modification are interdependent and mutually supportive. A comprehensive weight-reduction program that incorporates all three components is more likely to lead to long-term weight control.

- Evaluation of the health hazard of clove cigarettes. Council on Scientific Affairs. JAMA. 1988 Dec 23-30; 260(24): 3641-4
Resolution 43 (1987 Annual Meeting), adopted by the House of Delegates, resolved that the American Medical Association study the dangers associated with clove cigarettes, that policy recommendations regarding regulation of clove and other tobacco additives be developed, and that this information be made available to physicians and the public. Clove cigarettes are tobacco products. They therefore possess all the hazards associated with smoking all-tobacco cigarettes. In addition, inhaling clove cigarette smoke has been associated with severe lung injury in a few susceptible individuals with prodromal respiratory infection. Some individuals with normal respiratory tracts have apparently suffered aspiration pneumonitis as the result of a diminished gag reflex induced by a local anesthetic action of eugenol (the active component of cloves), which is volatilized into the smoke. The American Medical Association has an existing policy vigorously opposing the use of any tobacco product; no exemption from this policy is made for clove-containing cigarettes.

1987

- Aversion therapy. Council on Scientific Affairs. JAMA. 1987 Nov 13; 258(18): 2562-6
Aversion therapy is a series of techniques designed to reduce unwanted or dangerous behaviors. The most common applications of these techniques are to obesity, tobacco smoking, sexuality, oral habits, self-injurious and aggressive behaviors, and substance abuse. Most enthusiastic reports suffer from lack of control groups and control procedures. At this time, the best accepted application is for the treatment of chronic self-injurious behavior.
- Results and implications of the AMA-APA Physician Mortality Project. Stage II. Council on Scientific Affairs [published erratum appears in JAMA 1987 Aug 7;258(5):614] JAMA. 1987 Jun 5; 257(21): 2949-53
In response to several House of Delegates resolutions and Council on Scientific Affairs recommendations, the American Medical Association and the American Psychiatric Association have completed a joint study on physician suicide. Comprehensive interviews were conducted with surviving relatives and friends of 142 physicians who died by suicide and 101 physicians who died of causes other than suicide. The latter group, matched to the suicide group according to sex and age, served as a control sample. Bivariate relationships were found between several variables and risk for suicide, and all were examined in a multivariate framework. A preliminary profile of the physicians who took their own lives showed that they more often made prior suicide attempts, verbalized suicidal intentions, self-prescribed psychoactive drugs, and suffered financial losses.
- Preventing death and injury from fires with automatic sprinklers and smoke detectors. Council on Scientific Affairs. JAMA. 1987 Mar 27; 257(12): 1618-20
Resolution 2 (Annual Meeting 1985), which was referred to the Board of Trustees, asked the American Medical Association to urge government officials to require all new residential and nonresidential buildings to be equipped with rapid-response automatic water sprinklers and smoke detectors and to require their installation in existing high-rise buildings within three years unless existing code requirements are more stringent. This response to the resolution is a summary of the literature up to June 1986.

- Elder abuse and neglect. Council on Scientific Affairs. JAMA. 1987 Feb 20; 257(7): 966-71
Estimates of elder abuse approximate 10% of Americans over 65 years of age; obtaining accurate incidence and prevalence figures is complicated by factors including denial by both the victim and perpetrator and minimization of complaints by health professionals. Broad agreement exists in categorizing elder abuse as physical, psychological, and financial and/or material, despite lack of uniformity in definitions. Systematic scientific investigation provides limited knowledge about the causes of elder abuse. Most experts, however, believe that family problems and conflict are a major precipitating factor. Preliminary hypotheses for elder abuse include dependency, lack of close family ties, family violence, lack of financial resources, psychopathology in the abuser, lack of community support, and certain factors that may precipitate abuse in institutional settings. This report presents potential indicators of physical and psychological abuse, along with classification of elderly individuals at high risk, to assist the health professional in identification and prevention of elder abuse.
- Introduction to the management of immunosuppression. Council on Scientific Affairs. JAMA. 1987 Apr 3; 257(13): 1781-5
Advances in solid-organ allograft have depended in great measure on the development of improved means of suppressing the immune system of the recipient. This article presents an overview of the major forms of immunosuppression used in organ transplantation, specifically corticosteroids, azathioprine, antilymphocyte and antithymocyte globulin and cyclosporine, monoclonal antibody to the T3 receptor on lymphocytes, and blood transfusions.
- Vitamin preparations as dietary supplements and as therapeutic agents. Council on Scientific Affairs. JAMA. 1987 Apr 10; 257(14): 1929-36
Healthy adult men and healthy adult nonpregnant, nonlactating women consuming a usual, varied diet do not need vitamin supplements. Infants may need dietary supplements at given times, as may pregnant and lactating women. Occasionally, vitamin supplements may be useful for people with unusual life styles or modified diets, including certain weight reduction regimens and strict vegetarian diets. Vitamins in therapeutic amounts may be indicated for the treatment of deficiency states, for pathologic conditions in which absorption and utilization of vitamins are reduced or requirements increased, and for certain nonnutritional disease processes. The decision to employ vitamin preparations in therapeutic amounts clearly rests with the physician. The importance of medical supervision when such amounts are administered is emphasized. Therapeutic vitamin mixtures should be so labeled and should not be used as dietary supplements.
- Radioepidemiological tables. Council on Scientific Affairs. JAMA. 1987 Feb 13; 257(6): 806-9
In 1983, the Federal Orphan Drug Act was passed. This act included a rider intended as a foundation for compensating individuals with cancers allegedly caused by radiation exposures during certain nuclear events. In response, a National Institutes of Health working group was established that prepared the National Institutes of Health Radioepidemiological Tables. The tables permit computation of a "probability of causation" (otherwise known as "assigned share") that an individual's cancer was caused by earlier estimated exposure to radiation. However, several limitations have been noted in the accuracy of the computations and in the conditions under which the computations are applicable. These limitations have caused the Council on Scientific Affairs of the American Medical Association to recommend that the probability of causation approach not be applied to occupational radiation exposures or to diagnostic or therapeutic exposures in medicine.
- Health effects of video display terminals. Council on Scientific Affairs. JAMA. 1987 Mar 20; 257(11): 1508-12

American

Medical

Association

American Medical Association

About 15 million video display terminals are in use in the United States, and their numbers will continue to swell. Much concern has been raised by their users about possible adverse health effects. The extensive collection of research papers and state-of-the-art reports on this subject are reviewed in this article.

- Autopsy. A comprehensive review of current issues. Council on Scientific Affairs. JAMA. 1987 Jul 17; 258(3): 364-9
This report reviews the effects of decreased utilization of autopsy (less than 15% in 1985) on medical education and research, quality assurance programs, insurance claims processing, and cost containment. Recommendations to promote change include the innovative integration of postmortem examinations with new technology for education and research and the promotion of standards of accreditation of programs that include autopsy for graduate and undergraduate medical education. The use of autopsy to assess technological methods of diagnosis seems to be a reasonable expectation. Methods of reimbursement to validate autopsy as a medical act should be sought, and voluntary and government regulation to assure the role of autopsy in quality assurance programs is suggested.(Resolution 86, I-85)

- Radon in homes. Council on Scientific Affairs [published erratum appears in JAMA 1988 Jan 1;259(1):47] JAMA. 1987 Aug 7; 258(5): 668-72
Radon 222 and its radioactive decay products can enter buildings and, through inhalation, expose the inhabitants' pulmonary tissues to ionizing radiation. Studies of radon levels in the United States indicate that variations of 100-fold or greater exist among private dwellings. In one region, 55% of homes had levels exceeding 4 pCi/L (0.15 Bq/L), which is the guidance level recommended by the US Environmental Protection Agency. Ventilation and tightness of construction are important determinants of radon levels. In some instances, fans or heat exchangers can reduce excessive concentrations, but in others more elaborate remedial measures may be required. Physicians may obtain information about radon through Environmental Protection Agency regional offices and state radiation control programs. The risk of radiogenic cancer is believed to increase with exposure to ionizing radiation. According to some estimates, concentrations of radon decay products in US homes could be responsible for several thousand cases of lung cancer per year. Studies of radon levels in representative buildings and guidelines are needed to ensure safe, effective, and cost-effective countermeasures. Architects, contractors, designers, building code administrators, health physicists, and biomedical investigators can help with solutions.

- Scientific issues in drug testing. Council on Scientific Affairs. JAMA. 1987 Jun 12; 257(22): 3110-4
Testing for drugs in biologic fluids, especially urine, is a practice that has become widespread. The technology of testing for drugs in urine has greatly improved in recent years. Inexpensive screening techniques are not sufficiently accurate for forensic testing standards, which must be met when a person's employment or reputation may be affected by results. This is particularly a concern during screening of a population in which the prevalence of drug use is very low, in which the predictive value of a positive result would be quite low. Physicians should be aware that results from drug testing can yield accurate evidence of prior exposure to drugs, but they do not provide information about patterns of drug use, about abuse of or dependence on drugs, or about mental or physical impairments that may result from drug use.

- In vivo diagnostic testing and immunotherapy for allergy. Report I, Part I, of the allergy panel. Council on Scientific Affairs JAMA. 1987 Sep 11; 258(10): 1363-7
The diagnosis and treatment of allergic disease constitute a particularly difficult and complex field in medicine, a field

that has been complicated further by the promulgation and the use of unproved procedures and/or the inappropriate use of proved procedures. This report is the first in a series of reports prepared by a multidisciplinary panel appointed by the Council on Scientific Affairs of the American Medical Association. It discusses the necessity for proper clinical trials to generate reproducible results under similar conditions to adequately prove the validity of various diagnostic and therapeutic procedures. In vivo immunologic tests have been shown to be reliable and valid diagnostic tools and include skin tests with standardized allergenic extracts by prick, puncture, and intradermal techniques, skin end-point titration, and patch testing for contact allergic dermatitis. Other clinically useful physiologic tests include the exercise tolerance test, methacholine and/or histamine inhalation challenge test, and other inhalation tests utilizing either nasal or bronchial delivery. Oral challenge testing has also been utilized and includes open, single-blind, or double-blind techniques, depending on the requirements of the patient being studied. The second article is a continuation of the first report, and describes other challenge tests and unproved procedures. The third report of this series evaluates in vitro tests for allergy.

- In vivo diagnostic testing and immunotherapy for allergy. Report I, Part II, of the Allergy Panel. Council on Scientific Affairs [published erratum appears in JAMA 1987 Dec11;258(22):3259] JAMA 1987 Sep 18; 258(11): 1505-8
The first article in this series discussed the importance of properly designed clinical trials to validate various diagnostic and therapeutic procedures and also described clinically accepted and proved tests. This article discusses other challenge tests and unproved procedures. The value of provocation-neutralization procedures has been controversial; two promising clinical models have been developed that may allow definitive trials of efficacy. Immunotherapy with allergenic extracts has been shown to be a safe and effective procedure in carefully selected patients treated with potent, well-standardized antigens administered in adequate dosage. It has been proposed that many nonspecific signs or symptoms could be caused by exposure to Candida albicans or low-dose environmental substances. The cause-and-effect relationships between exposure to C albicans or other environmental substances and the disorders that are alleged to be associated with them are, for the most part, unproved.

- In vitro testing for allergy. Report II of the Allergy Panel. Council on Scientific Affairs. JAMA. 1987 Sep 25; 258(12): 1639-43
This report is the third of a series of reports prepared by a multidisciplinary panel appointed by the Council on Scientific Affairs of the American Medical Association. This report reviews the current status of in vitro tests available in the evaluation of immunologic and/or allergic diseases. A discussion of the large number of tests available to measure IgE is followed by an overview of the status of complement assays and tests being developed for evaluation of immune complexes. Cellular assays involving polymorphonuclear cells (basophils, eosinophils) and lymphocytes have increased in use; their appropriate indication and current worth are evaluated, as well as the therapeutic monitoring of theophylline serum concentrations. In the view of the panel, the rapidly proliferating number of in vitro diagnostic tests has great potential for the enhancement of the practice of allergy, but also a potential for misuse. Appropriate use of these tests is the focus of this report.

- Issues in employee drug testing. Council on Scientific Affairs. JAMA. 1987 Oct 16; 258(15): 2089-96

- Magnetic resonance imaging. Prologue. Council on Scientific Affairs. JAMA. 1987 Dec 11; 258(22): 3283-5
- Fundamentals of magnetic resonance imaging. Council on Scientific Affairs. JAMA. 1987 Dec 18; 258(23): 3417-23
Medical imaging methods traditionally have depicted variations in one or two simple physical variables in tissues, eg, physical density, atomic number, acoustic velocity, and radioactivity concentration. Magnetic resonance images reveal differences in several variables, with the prominent variables reflecting complex energy transfer mechanisms that occur at the atomic and nuclear levels. Furthermore, the relative contributions of these variables to the image are readily altered by changing the pulse sequence and the pulsing times within the sequence. These changes dramatically affect the image and its characterization of normal and abnormal anatomy. Hence, magnetic resonance images and their contributions to diagnostic medicine can be properly appreciated only if one has some understanding of the procedures by which they are produced.

1986

- Alcohol and the driver. Council on Scientific Affairs. JAMA. 1986 Jan 24-31; 255(4): 522-7
Scientific investigations have produced 50 years of accumulated evidence showing a direct relationship between increasing blood alcohol concentration (BAC) in drivers and increasing risk of a motor vehicle crash. There is scientific consensus that alcohol causes deterioration of driving skills beginning at 0.05% BAC or even lower, and progressively serious impairment at higher BACs. Drivers aged 16 to 24 years have the highest representation of all age groups in alcohol-related road crashes; young drivers involved in alcohol-related fatal crashes have lower average BACs than older drivers. Alcohol impairs driving skills by its effects on the central nervous system, acting like a general anesthetic. It renders slower and less efficient both information acquisition and information processing, making divided-attention tasks such as steering and braking more difficult to carry out without error. The influence of alcohol on emotions and attitudes may be a crash risk factor related to driving style in addition to driving skill. Biologic variability among humans produces substantial differences in alcohol influence and alcohol tolerance, making virtually useless any attempts to fix a "safe" drinking level for drivers. The American Medical Association supports a policy recommending (1) public education urging drivers not to drink, (2) adoption by all states of 0.05% BAC as per se evidence of alcohol-impaired driving, (3) 21 years as the legal drinking age in all states, (4) adoption by all states of administrative driver's license suspension in driving-under-the-influence cases, and (5) encouragement for the automobile industry to develop a safety module that thwarts operation of a motor vehicle by an intoxicated person.(Resolutions l8, 64, 83, A-84)
- Polygraph. Council on Scientific Affairs. JAMA. 1986 Sep 5; 256(9): 1172-5
The American Medical Association (AMA) Council on Scientific Affairs has reviewed the data on the validity and accuracy of polygraphy testing as it is applied today. The use of the control question technique in criminal cases is time honored and has seen much scientific study. It is established that classification of guilty can be made with 75% to 97% accuracy, but the rate of false-positives is often sufficiently high to preclude use of this test as the sole arbiter of guilt or innocence. This does not preclude using the polygraph test in criminal investigations as evidence or as another source of information to guide the investigation with full appreciation of the limitations in its use. Application of the polygraph in personnel screening, although gaining in popularity, has not been adequately validated. The few

limited studies that have been performed suggest no greater accuracy for the types of testing done for this purpose than for the control question polygraph testing used in criminal cases. The effect of polygraph testing to deter theft and fraud associated with employment has never been measured, nor has its impact on employee morale and productivity been determined. Much more serious research needs to be done before the polygraph should be generally accepted for this purpose. (Resolution 64, A-83)

- Dementia. Council on Scientific Affairs. JAMA. 1986 Oct 24-31; 256(16): 2234-8
Dementia has emerged as a national health concern. The demographics of our aging population suggest that this concern can only become more acute. For families that have a member with a primary dementing illness, this concern often becomes an all-consuming one. At present, our understanding of the primary dementias, especially Alzheimer's disease, is incomplete, and thus, most cases of primary dementia progress irreversibly. Nevertheless, there is much in the way of treatment, care, and support that can be provided by the practicing medical community to sustain the viability and vitality of patient and family.
- Autologous blood transfusions. Council on Scientific Affairs. JAMA. 1986 Nov 7; 256(17): 2378-80
Blood collected from a patient for retransfusion at a later time into that same individual is called "autologous blood." When the guidelines established by the American Association of Blood Banks are followed, autologous blood is the safest type of blood for transfusion. It also decreases the demand for banked blood and eliminates the risk of infection and alloimmunization from a transfusion. Autologous transfusions are becoming widely available; since 1974 the number of institutions providing autologous transfusion programs has increased more than fourfold. The Council on Scientific Affairs endorses the use of autologous blood transfusions. (Resolution 84, A-85)
- Health effects of smokeless tobacco. Council on Scientific Affairs. JAMA. 1986 Feb 28; 255(8): 1038-44
Tobacco in various forms has been used for centuries. Using snuff and chewing tobacco was popular in the United States during the 18th and 19th centuries, but current data on their use are limited. Pharmacologic and physiologic effects of snuff and chewing tobacco include the gamut of cardiovascular, endocrinologic, neurologic, and psychological effects that are associated with nicotine. A review of studies appearing in the scientific literature involving various populations and approaches indicates that the use of snuff or chewing tobacco is associated with a variety of serious adverse effects and especially with oral cancer. The studies suggest that snuff and chewing tobacco also may affect reproduction, longevity, the cardiovascular system, and oral health. One group estimated that the relative risk of oral cancer in longtime users of snuff varied from 1.8 to 48 times that of its occurrence in nonusers. But few of the studies have fully utilized accepted scientific and epidemiologic methods. The Council on Scientific Affairs concludes there is evidence demonstrating that the use of snuff or chewing tobacco is associated with adverse health effects such as oral cancer, urges the implementation of well-planned and long-term studies that will further define the risks of using snuff and chewing tobacco, and recommends that the restrictions applying to the advertising of cigarettes also be applied to the advertising of snuff and chewing tobacco.
- Lasers in medicine and surgery. Council on Scientific Affairs. JAMA. 1986 Aug 15; 256(7): 900-7
Clinical applications have been found for lasers in a number of medical and surgical specialties. New applications in current areas of use and extension of laser technology to other medical and surgical specialties will continue to occur as investigational uses are pursued. Lasers produce

American
Medical
Association

American Medical Association

medical and surgical effects in target tissues by heating them to the point of coagulation or vaporization, by ionizing molecular tissue, and by inducing photochemical effects through a mediating photosensitizer. Increased ability to transmit certain laser beams via fiber optics further extends areas of clinical application. Laser safety programs are essential to safeguard physician operators, ancillary personnel, and patients. Federal regulation, under two laws, deals with the laser radiation safety of devices and controls to ensure that devices reaching the market are reasonably safe and effective for their intended use.

1985

- Xenografts. Review of the literature and current status. Council on Scientific Affairs. JAMA. 1985 Dec 20; 254(23): 3353-7
  In response to growing public and legislative interest in organ transplantation, the American Medical Association's Council on Scientific Affairs has convened an advisory panel to prepare state-of-the-art monographs on several of the central topics. The first report of the panel, approved by the Council in February 1985, reviews the experimental work with xenografts. This report summarizes the published experience with animal and human xenografts to date and discusses the mechanisms of xenograft rejection. The report concludes that the process of xenograft rejection qualitatively resembles allograft rejection, involving both cellular and humoral immune mechanisms, but differs quantitatively depending on the genetic disparity between donor and recipient. Relative beneficial effects of various immunosuppression regimens, including cyclosporin on xenograft survival in donor recipient models with varying genetic disparity, have not yet been studied in a critical fashion.
- Status report on the acquired immunodeficiency syndrome. Human T-cell lymphotropic virus type III testing. Council on Scientific Affairs. JAMA. 1985 Sep 13; 254(10): 1342-5
- The use of cardiac pacemakers in medical practice. Excerpts from the report of the Advisory Panel. Council on Scientific Affairs. JAMA. 1985 Oct 11; 254(14): 1952-4
- Guidelines for reporting estimates of probability of paternity. Council on Scientific Affairs. JAMA. 1985 Jun 14; 253(22): 3298
- Effects of toxic chemicals on the reproductive system. Council on Scientific Affairs. JAMA. 1985 Jun 21; 253(23): 3431-7
  In an effort to make physicians more aware of the hazards of the workplace to pregnant workers, the Council on Scientific Affairs' Advisory Panel on Reproductive Hazards in the Workplace prepared this third and final report reviewing the effects of chemical exposure. A total of 120 chemicals were considered for reviews based on an estimation of their imminent hazard, ie, widespread use and/or inherent toxicity. Following a brief introduction, which sets out general principles, clinical applications, and aids to the recognition of a human teratogen, the report presents reviews and opinions for three representative chemicals. Information concerning the remaining 117 compounds is available upon request.
- Guidelines for handling parenteral antineoplastics. Council on Scientific Affairs. JAMA. 1985 Mar 15; 253(11): 1590-2 (Resolution 104, I-83)
- SI units for clinical laboratory data. Council on Scientific Affairs. JAMA. 1985 May 3; 253(17): 2553-4

- AMA diagnostic and treatment guidelines concerning child abuse and neglect. Council on Scientific Affairs. JAMA. 1985 Aug 9; 254(6): 796-800
  Child maltreatment is a serious and pervasive problem. Every year, more than a million children in the United States are abused, and between 2,000 and 5,000 die as a result of their injuries. Physicians are in a unique position to detect child abuse and neglect and are mandated by law to report such cases. These guidelines were developed to assist primary care physicians in the identification and management of the various forms of child maltreatment. A brief historical introduction and specific information about vulnerable families and children are presented. The physical and behavioral diagnostic signs of physical abuse, physical neglect, sexual abuse, and emotional maltreatment are delineated. Information about specific techniques for interviewing the abused child and family, case management objectives, reporting requirements, and trends in treatment and prevention are also provided.
- Current status of therapeutic plasmapheresis and related techniques. Report of the AMA panel on therapeutic plasmapheresis. Council on Scientific Affairs. JAMA. 1985 Feb 8; 253(6): 819-25
- Scientific status of refreshing recollection by the use of hypnosis. Council on Scientific Affairs. JAMA. 1985 Apr 5; 253(13): 1918-23
  The Council finds that recollections obtained during hypnosis can involve confabulations and pseudomemories and not only fail to be more accurate, but actually appear to be less reliable than nonhypnotic recall. The use of hypnosis with witnesses and victims may have serious consequences for the legal process when testimony is based on material that is elicited from a witness who has been hypnotized for the purposes of refreshing recollection.
- Saccharin. Review of safety issues. Council on Scientific Affairs. JAMA. 1985 Nov 8; 254(18): 2622-4
  This report reviews the experimental and epidemiologic data related to the carcinogenicity of saccharin. The results of animal studies suggest a species and organ effect. In single-generation studies in rats, mice, hamsters, and monkeys, saccharin did not induce cancer in any organ. In two-generation studies involving rats, however, there was evidence that the incidence of bladder tumors was significantly greater in saccharin-treated males of the second generation than in controls; the development of bladder tumors in rats seems to be a species- and organ-specific phenomenon for which there is currently no explanation. In humans, available evidence indicates that the use of artificial sweeteners, including saccharin, is not associated with an increased risk of bladder cancer. Until there is firm evidence of its carcinogenicity in humans, saccharin should continue to be available as a food additive, and reports of adverse health effects associated with its use should be monitored.
- Aspartame. Review of safety issues. Council on Scientific Affairs. JAMA. 1985 Jul 19; 254(3): 400-2
  This report examines the safety issues related to the nutritive sweetener aspartame, including possible toxic effects of aspartame's component amino acids, aspartic acid and phenylalanine, and its major decomposition products, methanol and diketopiperazine, and the potential synergistic effect of aspartame and dietary carbohydrate on brain neurochemicals. Available evidence suggests that consumption of aspartame by normal humans is safe and is not associated with serious adverse health effects. Individuals who need to control their phenylalanine intake should handle aspartame like any other source of phenylalanine.

1984

- Percutaneous transluminal angioplasty. Council on Scientific Affairs. JAMA. 1984 Feb 10; 251(6): 764-8
- The acquired immunodeficiency syndrome. Commentary. Council on Scientific Affairs. JAMA. 1984 Oct 19; 252(15): 2037-43
- Methaqualone: Abuse Limits its Usefulness. JAMA. 1983 Dec 9; 250(22): 3052
- Effects of physical forces on the reproductive cycle. Council on Scientific Affairs. JAMA. 1984 Jan 13; 251(2): 247-50

The Council on Scientific Affairs is aware that physicians, as well as the public in general, have expressed increasing concerns regarding the possible adverse effects of various physical forces on the reproductive organs. Various channels of public communication report anecdotal episodes of suspected cause-and-effect relationships between various physical elements in the environment and harmful effects on reproduction. Many of these episodes have not been substantiated by acceptable scientific research. However, some reports have appeared in the scientific literature that do document adverse reproductive effects on humans and animals at certain levels of some physical forces. At levels above 3,636 m (12,000 ft), adverse reproductive effects have been observed in men and women, in the conceptus, and in certain species of animals. Hyperthermia in excess of 40 degrees C may affect the man and the conceptus, as well as the reproductive capacity of certain animals. However, adverse effects of hypothermia have been observed only in animals. Ionizing radiation can cause injury to the man, woman, and conceptus and to animals, depending on dose and duration of exposure. There have been no well-documented injurious effects to the human reproductive organs resulting from radiofrequency-microwave radiation, but there have been some reports in animals that attributed untoward reproductive limitations to thermal effects. To date, there have been no reports in the scientific literature to implicate electronic and magnetic fields, gravity and acceleration, noise, optical radiation (UV, visible, infrared, and lasers), ultrasound, or vibration as having harmful effects on reproduction in either humans or animals. There is need for more well-designed and controlled studies to be performed in all of these areas of exposure at maximum-tolerated levels to physical force before it can be determined with certainty that no ill effects will accrue to the reproductive cycle, especially in assessing harmful effects from low-level exposure during long periods of time.

- Effects of pregnancy on work performance. Council on Scientific Affairs. JAMA. 1984 Apr 20; 251(15): 1995-7
- Early detection of breast cancer. Council on Scientific Affairs. JAMA. 1984 Dec 7; 252(21): 3008-11
- Exercise programs for the elderly. Council on Scientific Affairs. JAMA. 1984 Jul 27; 252(4): 544-6
- Caffeine labeling. Council on Scientific Affairs. American Medical Association. JAMA. 1984 Aug 10; 252(6): 803-6 (Resolution 74, I-82)
- A physician's guide to asbestos-related diseases. Council on Scientific Affairs. JAMA. 1984 Nov 9; 252(18): 2593-7
- Combined modality approaches to cancer therapy. Council on Scientific Affairs. JAMA. 1984 May 11; 251(18): 2398-407

1983

- Medical evaluations of healthy persons. Council on Scientific Affairs. JAMA. 1983 Mar 25; 249(12): 1626-33
- Fetal effects of maternal alcohol use. JAMA. 1983 May 13; 249(18): 2517-21
- Brain injury in boxing. Council on Scientific Affairs. JAMA. 1983 Jan 14; 249(2): 254-7 (Resolution 145, A-80)
- Sodium in processed foods. JAMA. 1983 Feb 11; 249(6): 784-9 (Resolution 28, I-81)
- Dietary and pharmacologic therapy for the lipid risk factors. JAMA. 1983 Oct 14; 250(14): 1873-9
- Cochlear implants. JAMA. 1983 Jul 15; 250(3): 391-2)
- Automobile-Related Injuries. JAMA. 1983 Jun 17; 249(23): 3216-22.
- Calcium channel blocking agents. Council on scientific affairs. JAMA. 1983 Nov 11; 250(18): 2522-4
- In utero fetal surgery. Resolution 73 (I-81) Council on scientific affairs. JAMA. 1983 Sep 16; 250(11): 1443-4 (Resolution 73 (I-81)
- Estrogen replacement in the menopause. Council on Scientific Affairs. JAMA. 1983 Jan 21; 249(3): 359-61
- Pharmaceutical dissolution of gallstones. JAMA. 1983 Nov 4; 250(17): 2373-4

1982

- Maternal serum alpha-fetoprotein monitoring. Council on Scientific affairs. JAMA. 1982 Mar 12; 247(10): 1478-81
- Genetic counseling and prevention of birth defects. JAMA. 1982 Jul 9; 248 (2): 221-4
- Health effects of Agent Orange and dioxin contaminants. Council on scientific affairs. JAMA. 1982 Oct 15; 248(15): 1895-7
- Drug abuse related to perscribing practices. JAMA. 1982 Feb 12; 247)6): 864-6.
- Health care needs of a homosexual population. Council on Scientific Affairs. JAMA. 1982 Aug 13; 248(6): 736-9
- Dimethyl sulfoxide. Controversy and current status--1981. Council on scientific affairs. JAMA. 1982 Sep 17; 248(11): 1369-71
- Continuous ambulatory peritoneal dialysis. Council on Scientific Affairs. JAMA. 1982 Nov 12; 248(18): 2340-1

1981

- Marijuana. Its health hazards and therapeutic potentials. Council on Scientific Affairs. JAMA. 1981 Oct 16; 246(16): 1823-7
- Hypnotic Drugs and Treatment of Insomnia. JAMA. 1981 Feb 20; 245(7): 749-50.
- Physician-supervised exercise programs in rehabilitation of patients with coronary heart disease. Council on Scientific Affairs. JAMA. 1981 Apr 10; 245(14): 1463-6
- Medical care for indigent and culturally displaced obstetrical patients and their newborns. Committee on Maternal, Adolescent, and Child Health. Council on Scientific Affairs. JAMA. 1981 Mar 20; 245(11): 1159-60
- Carcinogen regulation. Council on Scientific Affairs. JAMA. 1981 Jul 17; 246(3): 253-6
- Organ donor recruitment. Council on Scientific Affairs. JAMA. 1981 Nov 13; 246(19): 2157-8

American

Medical

Association

American Medical Association

- Electronic fetal monitoring. Council on Scientific Affairs. JAMA. 1981 Nov 20; 246(20): 2370-3

1980
- Smoking and Health. JAMA. 1980 Feb 22-29; 243(8): 779-81
- Hypoglycemic treatment. Guidelines for the non-insulin-dependent diabetic. Council on Scientific Affairs. JAMA. 1980 May 23-30; 243(20): 2078-9

1979
- Indications for aortocoronary bypass graft surgery, 1979. Council on Scientific Affairs. JAMA. 1979 Dec 14; 242(24): 2709-11
- American Medical Association concepts of nutrition and health. Council on Scientific Affairs. JAMA. 1979 Nov 23; 242(21): 2335-8

1978
- Adoption of International System of Units for Clinical Chemistry. JAMA. 1978 Dec 8; 240(24): 2664
- Health evaluation of energy-generating sources. AMA Council on Scientific Affairs. JAMA. 1978 Nov 10; 240(20): 2193-5

Council on Scientific Affairs: Unpublished Reports

The following list CSA reports requested by the House of Delegates. They are listed by the meeting they were first presented by a representative of the Council on Scientific Affairs.

1992

1992 Annual Meeting:

Confidential Health Service for Adolescents
    Recommendations for Ensuring the Health of the
    Adolescent Athlete
Police Chase and Chase-Related Inuries
    (Res. 106, A-91)
Food and Drug Administration Regulations
    Regarding the Inclusion of Added L-Glutamic Acid
    Content on Food Labels (Res. 187, A-91)
Benzodiazepine Education (Res. 413, I-91)
U.S. Nuclear Regulatory Regulations Affecting
    Outpatient Treatment with Radiopharmaceuticals
    (Res. 22 & 23, A-91)
Perinatal Addiction: Issues in Care and Prevention
    (Res. 233, A-90)
Family Violence: Adolescents as Victims and
    Perpetrators

1992 Annual Informational Reports:

Improving Patient-Records
Feasibility of Assuring Confidentiality and Security
    of Computer-Based Patient Records
Modern Component Usage in Transfusion
    Therapy, 1992

1992 Interim Meeting:

Autologous Blood Transfusion
Performance Testing
Silicone Gel Breast Implants
Clinical Preventive Services: Implications for
    Adolescent, Adult and Geriatric Medicine

1992 Interim Informational Reports:

Rapid Laboratory Tests for the Identification of
    Mycobacterium Tuberculosis

Interim 1992 Joint Report Of CSA/CMS:

Payment for Patients Enrolled in Clinical Trials
    (Res. 115, I-91)

1991

Annual 1991:

Commercial Weight Loss Systems and Program
The Impact of the Marketing-Distribution System
    for Clozapine on Patient Access
Carrier Screening for Cystic Fibrosis
Adding "Tobacco Contribution" to Death
    Certificates
Physicians and Retirement

Annual 1991 Informational Reports:

Treatment of Depression by Primary Care
    Physicians: Pharmacological Approaches
Treatment of Depression by Primary Care
    Physicians: Psychotherapeutic Treatments
    for Depression
The Recognition and Treatment of Depression in
    Medical Practice
Comorbidity

Interim 1991:

Health Claims by Maufacturers of Breakfast Cereal
Biotechnologies Targeting the Diseases of the
    Aged
The Use of Pulse Oximetry During Conscious
    Sedation
U.S. Nuclear Regulatory Regulations Affecting
    Outpatient Treatment with Radiopharmaceuticals
Financial Incentives for Autopsies
Over the Counter Availability of Veterinary
    Medications
Physicians and Family Caregivers: A Model for
    Partnership
Children and Youth with with Disabilities
Food Safety: Federal Inspection Programs
Silicone Breast Implants

Interim 1991 Informational Reports:
Carpal Tunnel Syndrome
Diagnostic Evaluation of the Differential Diagnosis
    of Thyroid Nodules
Systemic Therapy for Breast Cancer

Interim 1991 Joint Reports Of CSA/CME

Federal Research Grant Indirect Cost Policy

Interim 1991 Joint Reports Of CSA/CMS

Seat Lift Chairs

1990

Annual 1990:

Mandatory Random Drug Testing in Competitive
    Sports
Organ Transplantation
Statement of Concern Regarding Destructive
    Themes Contained in Rock Music

Annual 1990 Informational Reports::

Alternatives to Animal Use in Biomedical Research
Alternative Psychological Methods in Patient Care
Ultrasonographic Evaluation of the Fetus

Annual 1990 Joint Reports Of CSA/CMS:

Radiographic Contrast Media-Interim Report

Interim 1990:

Physician and Medical Students Support for HIV
    Education: Programs for Adolescents
The Need for Increased Research and
    Development in Nuclear Fusion to Reduce
    Environmental Pollution
Drug Testing
The Etiology of Depression in Adults
Genetic Testing and the Potential Basis for Job
    Discrimination
Economic and Public Policy Issues Involving
    Bovine Somatrotropin

Interim 1990 Informational Reports:

Home Total Parenteral Nutrition
Infant Mortality and Access to Care
Extra Low Frequency Electric and Magnetic Field
    and the Question of Cancer

Interim 1990 Joint Reports Of CSA/CME:

Technology Assessment in Medicine
Radiographic Contrast Media

1989

Annual 1989:

Global Climate Change: The Greenhouse Effect
Mammographic Criteria for Surgical Biopsy of
    Nonpalpable Breast Lesions
The Viability of Cancer Clinical Research

Annual 1989 Information Reports:

Recognition of Childhood Sexual Abuse as a
    Factor in Adolescent Health Issues
Health Effects of Video Display Terminals:
    An Update

Interim 1989 Policy Reports

Nationwide Reporting of Elevated Blood Lead
    Levels
Potential Health Effects of the Biological Defense
    Research Program of the Department of
    Defense
DATTA Evaluations
Viability of Clinical Research: Coverage and
    Reimbursement
Stewardship of the Environment

Interim 1989 Joint Reports Of The CSA/CEJA:

Scientific Fraud and Misrepresentation

Interim 1989 Informational Reports:

HIV Infection and Disease-Monographs for
    Physicians and Other Health Care Workers
Establishing Mammographic Criteria for
    Recommending Surgical Biopsy

1988

Annual 1988:

Disseminating Scientific Health Information to the
    Public
Reducing Transmission of Human
    Immunodeficiency Virus (HIV) Among and
    Through Intravenous Drug Abusers

Annual 1988 Informational Reports:

Venomous Snakebites in the United States and
Canada

Interim 1988:

Recommendations for HIV Testing
Fraud and Misrepresentation in Science

Interim 1988 Informational Reports:

Hyperthyroidism in the Elderly
HTLV-I Testing of Blood Donors
The Health Hazards of Lead in Drinking Water
Effects of Pregnancy on Work Performance

1987

Annual 1987

Issues in employee drug testing
Religious Exemptions from Immunizations

Annual 1987 Informational Reports

Classification of the Clinical Spectrum of HIV
    Infection in Adults
Serologic Tests for Human Immunodeficiency
    Virus (HIV)
AIDS and the Obstetrician/Gynecologist:
    Commentary
Epidemiology of Acquired Immunodeficiency
    Syndrome: A Brief Overview
Pediatric Acquired Immunodeficiency Syndrome
The Challenge of AIDS for Physicians Today
Real and Perceived Risks of AIDS in the Family
    and Household
Clinical Trials of Drugs for the Treatment of AIDS
Real and Perceived Risks of AIDS in the Health
    Care and Work Environment
Blood Transfusions and AIDS
Biology of HIV Infection
Treatment of Infertility
Issues in Health Fraud: Colonic Irrigation
Evaluation of Routine Infant Circumcision
Commercial Hair Analysis
Acid Rain Update

Interim 1987

Firearms as a Public Health Problem in the US:
    Injuries and Deaths
AIDS Education
Accuracy of the ELISA and the Western Blot
    Serologic Tests for HIV Infection
Smoking Cessation

Interim 1987 Informational Reports:

Ozone Report

American

Medical

Association

American
Medical
Association

1986

Annual 1986

AIDS and School Discrimination
    (Resolutions 96 and 97, I-85)
Safe Use of Radioactive Materials in Medical
    Practice (Resolution 66, A-85)
Herpes Simplex and School Children
The Heimlich Maneuver - Interim Report
    (Resolution 52, I-85)
Drugs and Athletes - Progress Report
OTC Diet Preparations Containing
    Phenylpropanolamine
    (Resolution 100, I-85)

Annual 1986 Informational Reports

Glucocorticoid-Induced Osteonecrosis
Statement on Liver Transplantation

Interim 1986

The Heimlich Maneuver (Resolution 52, I-85)
Discrimination Against AIDS Patients
    (Resolution 97, I-85)
Warning Labels on Over-the-Counter Iron
    Preparations and Dietary Supplements
Consumption of Lean Beef (Resolution 145, A-86

Interim 1986 Informational Reports

Cocaine: Phenomenology and Treatment of Abuse
Medical Aspects of Pre-Adolescent Participation in
    Sports
Health Fraud Report

1985

Annual 1985

Autopsies: Interim Report
    (Substitute Resolution 11, A-84)

Annual 1985 Informational Reports

Acid Rain
Formaldehyde in Manufactured Housing
Harmful Effects of UVA and UVB Light

Interim 1985

Effects of Pesticide Exposure
Antibiotics in Animal Feeds
Drugs and Athletes-Interim Report
Anti-abortion Film "Silent Scream"
    (Resolution 143, A-85)

Interim 1985 Informational Reports

Opioid Abuse and Dependence: Diagnosis,
    Referral and Treatment
Toxic Shock Syndrome

1984

Annual 1984

FDA Regulation of Drugs and Medical Devices
    (Resolution 71, I-83)
Prescription Abuse Data Synethesis (PADS)
    Project and the AMA
Prescription Drug Abuse Activity

Interim 1984

Chelation Therapy
Nicotine Chewing Gum for Cessation of Smoking
The Health Effects of "Agent Orange" and
    Polychlorinated Dioxin Contaminants

Annual 1983

Choking: The Heimlich Maneuver (Abdominal
    Thrust) vs. Back Blows
Update on Venereal Disease
Current Issues in Pediatric Immunization

Interim 1983

Pharmaceutical Marketing,
    (Substitute Resolution 77, A-82)
Nonsmoking in Hospitals
AMA's Role in Technology Assessment
    (Resolution 131 (A-83)
Drug Substitution -- Definition of Terms
A Guide to the Hospital Management of Injuries
    Arising From Exposure to or Involving Ionizing
    Radiation

1982

Annual 1982

Council on Scientific Affairs Responses to the
    National Center for Health Care Technology
    and Office of Health Research, Statistics and
    Technology
Infant Formula Marketing (Resolution 155, A-81)

Interim 1982

Revision of AMA Guides to Impairment
Addition of Thiamine to Alcoholic Beverages
    (Resolution 140, A-81)
AMA Involvement in Prevention and Treatment of
    Child Abuse and Neglect
    (Substitute Resolution 75, A-81)
Physician Mortality and Suicide: Results and
    Implications of the AMA-APA Pilot Study
Pneumococcal, Influenza and Hepatitis-B Vaccine
    (Resolution 75, A-82)

1981

Annual 1981

Risks of Nuclear Energy and Low-Level Ionizing
    Radiation
The 1980 Report of the Joint National Commission
    on Detection, Evaluation and Treatment of High
    Blood Pressure
Evaluation of Iridology
Acupuncture

Interim 1981

Prescription of Tranquilizers and Antidepressants
    for Women (Board of Trustees Report X, I-80)

1980

Annual 1980

Infant Nutrition (Resolution 111, I-78)
Progress in Adoption of SI Units
Biological Effects of Non-Ionizing Magnetic and
    Electromagnetic Radiation
Encouragement of Physician Investigator Training

Interim 1980

Indications and Contraindications for Exercise
	Testing
The Nutritive Quality of Processed Foods:
	General Policies for Nutrient Additions
Importance of Diagnostic Computerized
	Tomographic Scanning
Health Care Technology Assessment -- 1980
Alcoholism as a Disability

1979

Annual 1979

Statement on the Role of Dietary Management in
	Hypertensive Control
Recommendations for AMA Involvement in
	Alcoholism Activities
Physical Fitness and Physical Education
Reliability of Laboratory Procedures

Interim 1979

Food Safety and the Food, Drug, and Cosmetic
	Act
Saccharin Availability
Evaluation of Community Mental Health Centers
Dietary Sodium and Potassium
Sentinel Deaths
Chymopapain
The Chronic Mental Patient: Commentary on the
	Final Report of the President's Commission on
	Mental Health

1978

Annual 1978

Use of Barbiturates in Medical Practice
Heroin Reclassification
The Medical Implications of Motorcycle Helmet
	Usage
Reliability of Laboratory Procedures

Interim 1978

Status of Multiphasic Health Evaluation -- 1978
Recommendations on Drug Development and
	Drug Regulation
Care for the Chronically Mentally Ill in the
	Community: Progress Report
Community Mental Health Centers
Principles of Quality Mental Health Care
Present Status of the Medical Autopsy
Shortage of Human Growth Hormone
Symptomatic and Supportive Care for Patients
	with Cancer
Staging of Cancer
CHILDSAFE Project
Recommendations for AMA Involvement in
	Alcoholism Activities and Commentary on
	NIAAA's "National Plan to Combat Alcohol
	Abuse and Alcoholism"
AMA Committee on Medical Aspects of Sports

1977

Annual 1977

Guidelines for Recombinant DNA Research
Use of Amphetamines in the Treatment of Obesity

Interim 1977

Statement on Parent and Newborn Interaction
Patient Instructional Leaflets
Airbags, Seatbelts, and Prevention of
	Vehicle-Related Injuries
Physicians and Sex Therapy Clinics

*Contact for free copies of Council on
Scientific Affairs Reports: Brenda Stewart
Council on Scientific Affairs
American Medical Association 515 N. State
St., Chicago, IL 60610
312-464-5046*

Division of Health Care Technology

The AMA is nationally recognized as a leader in
the evaluation of the drugs, devices, procedures,
and techniques used in the practice of
medicine. Through its DATTA program, in the
Department of Technology Assessment, the AMA
provides the most authoritative information
available to enchance the appropriate utilization of
health care technology and communicates and
represents the physician's viewpoint to third-party
payers, self-insurers, HMO's, hospitals, national
associations, and the federal government. In
addition, the Division of Health Care Technology
has major initiatives in the area of outcomes
research, database analysis, cost-effectiveness
analysis, technology transfer, and drug and device
regulatory policy.

The American Medical Association's Diagnostic and Therapeutic Technology Assessment Program

Richard J. Jones. JAMA. 1983 July 15: 250(3):
387-8.

The Diagnostic and Therapeutic Technology
Assessment (DATTA) program was inaugurated in
1982, with invitations extended to all medical
specialty and state medical societies that are
represented in the AMA House of Delegates. They
were asked to submit the names of physicians
whose judgment could be valued in the
assessment of their specialty or in the analysis of
related clinical problems. In addition, members of
the previous expert panels that had served the
AMA through the Council on Scientific Affairs were
nominated to serve. After reviewing the nominees,
the Council on Scientific Affairs appointed 483
physicians to the DATTA roster. A complete
curriculum vitae and bibliography were solicited
from each nominee so that his special interests
and particular expertise could be made available
on file.

The operation of the DATTA program by AMA
staff is supervised by a subcommittee of three
members of the Council on Scientific Affairs. The
Council reviewed several questions that had come
to the AMA from external sources. It also
generated questions of its own for inclusion in the

American

Medical

Association

American

Medical

Association

initial mailing in January of 1983 of six questions of broad interest to the medical profession.

Questions will be considered from any source as long as they are clearly stated in writing and focused so that a clear opinion can be rendered. They should be accompanied by appropriate bibliographic references or suitable documentation that will help to justify the question. The selection of questions will be determined by staff under the direction of the subcommittee of the Council on Scientific Affairs, which will reserve the right to accept or reject questions.

A panel of at least 20 specialists, selected for their knowledge and experience in the clinical area under examination, receives the question, which has been carefully worded in appropriate scientific and technical terms. Each correspondent is asked to respond as to whether the practice is (1) established (with clinical limitation, if any are needed for general use), (2) investigational (used under research protocol), (3) unacceptable, (4) indeterminate, or if there is (5) no opinion (because the respondent has no knowledge of the technology).

Comments are also invited with regard to the experimental basis for the rating, pros and cons of the technology, specific knowledge of controlled trials, and inherent risks as perceived by the respondent. The bibliographic resources of the AMA's library are available to each panel member. The AMA staff is expected concomitantly to research each question and be cognizant of existing assessments (in preparation or extant) from other organizations, including appropriate medical specialty societies.

Responses are based on a consensus of the panelists. When a consensus cannot be reached a special study, conference, or report may be called for by the Council on Scientific Affairs. Approved responses will be returned to the questioner and may be disseminated to the profession and the public through publication in JAMA. Each response will be accompanied by the following statement: "The above response is provided as a service of the American Medical Association. It is based on current scientific and clinical information and does not represent endorsement by the AMA of particular diagnostic and therapeutic procedures or treatment."

It is apparent from this description that these responses to questions are the general opinion held by the clinical specialists in that branch of medicine who should be most knowledgeable about the practice in that area. This opinion should not be considered a final judgment on the ultimate utility or inadequacy of a particular procedure, but rather an indication of how it is viewed at this particular time by knowledgeable practitioners. All of these opinions will, of course, be highly temporal and subject to revision on the basis of new information and experience.

It would be counterproductive if these opinions should lead to a reduction in investigative efforts to establish the sensitivity and specificity of a new method of diagnosis or treatment. All physicians can recall the initial rejection of a novel technique (such as hemodialysis for kidney disease) that later became accepted after the addition of a new element (the artificial arteriovenous shunt).

The Council on Scientific Affairs appreciates that the best way to establish the superiority of one technology over another, for diagnosis or treatment of a particular disease process, is based on research data that are ultimately published in peer-reviewed medical journals. The Journal of the American Medical Association, since its inception, has served along with the other peer-reviewed medical journals as a forum for the publication of data on new and innovative medical technologies.

It is hoped that the DATTA program can facilitate the wide distribution of important information in support of new technologies when that is merited. It should encourage research work at an earlier stage, when proof of utility may not be as apparent to the objective outside observer, as to the investigator who is involved in the developmental research.

In the final analysis, the real proof of the effectiveness of this program will depend on the care that is used in evaluating reports from respondents and in wording the responses to these questions. The first products of this new program are presented in this issue of JAMA. Because these are opinions, it is appropriate to present them in JAMA in close proximity to the usual "Questions And Answers" section. It should be recognized that these responses have only been somewhat more extensively peer-reviewed than the responses of the other experts whose opinions are presented in the section.

Diagnostic and therapeutic technology assessment (DATTA) Opinions.

Diagnostic and therapeutic technology assessment. Surrogate markers of progressive HIV disease.
JAMA. 1992 Jun 3; 267(21): 2948-52

Diagnostic and therapeutic technology assessment. Endoscopic balloon dilation of the prostate.
JAMA. 1992 Feb 26; 267(8): 1123-4, 1127-8

Diagnostic and therapeutic technology assessment. Measurement of bone density with dual-energy X-ray absorptiometry (DEXA).
JAMA. 1992 Jan 8; 267(2): 286-8, 290-4

Diagnostic and therapeutic technology assessment. Vasoactive intracavernous pharmacotherapy for impotence: intracavernous injection of prostaglandin E1. JAMA. 1991 Jun 26; 265(24): 3321-3
The DATTA panelists consider PGE1 to be a useful addition to the family of vasoactive agents used to treat organic impotence. It is associated with fewer side effects than either papaverine or phentolamine. Although most patients can achieve an erection with PGE1, some will not, and the other vasoactive agents may be of benefit in these cases. Synergy has been demonstrated when papaverine and PGE1 are used together, and a combination of the two in reduced dosages may be effective in producing an erection with a reduction in side effects. Intracavernosal therapy should be prescribed and monitored by a urologist who is experienced in the treatment of impotence and who is able to treat any of the potential side effects. Whether long-term use of local injections will produce

additional complications is yet to be determined.

Diagnostic and therapeutic technology assessment. Reassessment of automated percutaneous lumbar diskectomy for herniated disks. JAMA. 1991 Apr 24; 265(16): 2122-3, 2125
Although the safety of the APLD procedure is clearly established both by reports in the published literature and by a consensus of the DATTA panelists, there was no consensus among the DATTA panelists on the effectiveness of the procedure. The average 75% success rate reported in the larger studies contrasts with the 95% success rate reported for laminectomy and diskectomy. For APLD, careful patient selection is essential. Candidates must have failed an adequate trial of conservative therapy (bed rest and limitation of activity) and have disk herniation documented by appropriate imaging studies. These studies are important because they can demonstrate not only the degree of herniation, but also whether it is contained within the annulus and if any free fragments are present. For herniated lumbar disks with nuclear material outside and contiguous with the annulus, a statistically significant consensus of DATTA panelists believed that APLD is an inappropriate procedure. Another study has shown that the procedure can be taught to other surgeons without compromising patient safety, and, as reported, this holds with large numbers of cases. In appropriately selected patients, the clinical trade-off of APLD appears to be between a procedure with a 75% success rate with low risk and rapid recovery vs one with a 95% success rate and a more prolonged recovery. A research question is whether APLD could be extended to patients who have undergone previous surgery whose disks reherniate after a successful laminectomy. Conversely, does an APLD procedure that fails to relieve symptoms complicate subsequent laminectomy? It is recognized that there is a need for prospective, controlled, randomized clinical trials comparing APLD with laminectomy to resolve these and other issues.

Diagnostic and therapeutic technology assessment. Pancreatic transplantations. JAMA. 1991 Jan 23-30; 265(4): 510-4

Diagnostic and therapeutic technology assessment. Allogenic bone marrow transplantation for chronic myelogenous leukemia. JAMA. 1990 Dec 26; 264(24): 3208-11

Diagnostic and therapeutic technology assessment. Dorsal rhizotomy. JAMA. 1990 Nov 21; 264(19): 2569-70, 2572, 2574

Diagnostic and therapeutic technology assessment. Alpha-interferon and chronic myelogenous leukemia. JAMA. 1990 Oct 24-31; 264(16): 2137-40

Diagnostic and therapeutic technology assessment. Prophylactic treatment for opportunistic infections in HIV-positive patients: aerosolized pentamidine. JAMA. 1990 May 9; 263(18): 2510-4
The DATTA panelists considered aerosolized pentamidine to be both safe and effective for primary and secondary prophylaxis of PCP. T4 helper cell counts offer guidance as to the best candidates for primary prophylaxis. Patients with a T4 helper cell count of fewer than 200/mm3 are the most appropriate group to receive primary prophylaxis with aerosolized pentamidine. However, T4 helper cell counts are not an exclusive criterion for aerosolized pentamidine prophylaxis. Some DATTA panelists suggested that certain patients, such as those with Kaposi's sarcoma and lymphomas and those with concomitant human T-cell lymphotropic virus type 1 infection, might be considered candidates for aerosolized pentamidine regardless of T4 helper cell counts. There is no current literature to support this, and this opinion is based solely on clinical experience. Perhaps the use of other markers of immune function (beta 2-microglobulin, neopterin) in conjunction with T4 helper cell counts will give a better indication of when to start primary prophylaxis. Aerosolized pentamidine is not the only potential prophylactic regimen for PCP. Other drugs, including pyrimethamine and sulfadoxine, sulfamethoxazole and trimethoprim, and dapsone, are currently being evaluated. Prior diagnosis and therapy for patients with M tuberculosis must occur before initiation of the use of aerosolized pentamidine. This and other appropriate environmental precautions should reduce transmission of M tuberculosis to health care workers and other patients. Whether any prophylactic treatment of an opportunistic infection will prolong survival in HIV-infected individuals has yet to be proved. The assumption is made, however, that a reduction in opportunistic infections should lower mortality and improve the quality of life.

Diagnostic and therapeutic technology assessment. Transrectal ultrasonography--reassessment. JAMA. 1990 Mar 16; 263(11): 1563-8

Diagnostic and therapeutic technology assessment. Chorionic villus sampling: a reassessment. JAMA. 1990 Jan 12; 263(2): 305-6
The Canadian and National Institute of Child Health and Human Development trials as well as other nonrandomized studies indicate that CVS is both safe and effective. Fetal loss rates have been slightly higher with CVS (6 to 8 more losses per 1000 procedures), but none of these results were statistically significant. Chorionic villus sampling also probably has a slightly higher procedure failure rate than amniocentesis. The DATTA panelists are now confident that the safety of CVS approaches that of amniocentesis and that the higher procedure failure rate is offset by the opportunity of earlier diagnosis with CVS. Transcervical CVS is often preferred by women because it offers an opportunity for early prenatal diagnosis and early intervention if necessary. It is performed as an outpatient procedure and is relatively simple for the patient; however, the practitioner requires special training in CVS. Modifications of the sampling technique are also under investigation. Transabdominal CVS can also be performed early in pregnancy with a fine-bore needle under ultrasonic guidance. It may be used in cases where the placenta is inaccessible to the transcervical approach or there is vaginal infection.

Diagnostic and therapeutic technology assessment. Laminectomy and microlaminectomy for treatment of lumbar disk herniation. JAMA. 1990 Sep 19; 264(11): 1469-72

Diagnostic and therapeutic technology assessment. Vasoactive intracavernous pharmacotherapy for impotence: papaverine and phentolamine. JAMA. 1990 Aug 8; 264(6): 752-4

American
Medical
Association

American
Medical
Association

Diagnostic and therapeutic technology assessment. Rigid and flexible sigmoidoscopies. JAMA. 1990 Jul 4; 264(1): 89-92

Diagnostic and therapeutic technology assessment. Autologous bone marrow transplantation--reassessment [published erratum appears in JAMA 1990 Jul 18;264(3):338] JAMA. 1990 Feb 9; 263(6): 881-7

Diagnostic and therapeutic technology assessment. Continuous subcutaneous insulin infusion. JAMA. 1989 Sep 1; 262(9): 1239-43

Diagnostic and therapeutic technology assessment. Chemonucleolysis for herniated lumbar disk [see comments] JAMA. 1989 Aug 18; 262(7): 953-6
The DATTA panelists did not achieve a definitive consensus on the use of chymopapain chemonucleolysis for a protruding lumbar disk contained by the annulus. Concerns about safety, especially the risk of anaphylaxis and the risk of damage to the spinal cord, were frequent. The effectiveness of this procedure for this indication was also questioned by many of the panelists. The panel did agree that chemonucleolysis is unacceptable as either safe or effective for use in patients with a herniated lumbar disk that is extruding nucleus pulposus through the annulus. Accordingly, diagnostic imaging of any suspect disk must be performed before chemonucleolysis can be deemed appropriate for any individual patient. Current imaging techniques are not infallible and cannot confer an absolute sense of security when seeming to indicate a nonextruded protruding disk.

Diagnostic and therapeutic technology assessment. Continuous peritoneal insulin infusion and implantable insulin infusion pumps for diabetic control. JAMA. 1989 Dec 8; 262(22): 3195-8

Diagnostic and therapeutic technology assessment (DATTA). Noninvasive electrical stimulation for nonunited bone fracture [published erratum appears in JAMA 1989 Jun 9;261(22):3246] JAMA. 1989 Feb 10; 261(6): 917-9

Diagnostic and therapeutic technology assessment. Traveler's diarrhea. JAMA. 1989 Sep 1; 262(9): 1243

Diagnostic and therapeutic technology assessment. Home monitoring of uterine activity. JAMA. 1989 May 26; 261(20): 3027-9

Diagnostic and therapeutic technology assessment. Intrauterine devices [published erratum appears in JAMA 1990 Jan 12;263(2):238] [see comments] JAMA. 1989 Apr 14; 261(14): 2127-30
The DATTA panelists emphasized the critical importance of patient selection when considering IUDs for contraception. The IUD is an acceptable method of contraception, especially for those women who are in the middle to older reproductive years, unable to take oral contraceptives, in a stable monogamous relationship, and not at risk for sexually transmitted diseases. Within these constraints, the panelists gave overwhelming support to the IUD as a safe and effective

method of contraception. The minority opinion (two panelists) that these devices were not established for safety or effectiveness was based on concerns over possible infectious complications.

Diagnostic and therapeutic technology assessment. Gastric restrictive surgery JAMA. 1989 Mar 10; 261(10): 1491-4

Diagnostic and therapeutic technology assessment. Percutaneous lumbar diskectomy for herniated disks [published erratum appears in JAMA 1989 May 26;261(20):2958] [see comments] JAMA. 1989 Jan 6; 261(1): 105-9
Percutaneous diskectomy, particularly using Onik's nucleotome, has promise. It is too early, however, to decide if the percutaneous approach to reducing lumbar disk herniation will achieve a permanent place in the surgical armamentarium. Nevertheless, it is clear that patient selection is important. At the minimum, an adequate trial of conservative therapy must be followed by diagnostic imaging that documents a herniation that can be treated in this fashion and correlates with the patient's neurological signs and symptoms. If free fragments are found, a laminectomy of some sort will be required to remove the offending material. Patients who are at risk for general anesthesia or may be allergic to chymopapain were mentioned by the panel as special subpopulations for whom the procedure may be indicated despite the lack of wide experience with it. The rapidly rising popularity of automated percutaneous lumbar diskectomy via the nucleotome will hopefully be followed in the near future with larger studies with long-term follow-up.

Diagnostic and therapeutic technology assessment. Maternal serum alpha-fetoprotein testing and Down's syndrome. JAMA. 1988 Sep 23-30; 260(12): 1779-82

Diagnostic and therapeutic technology assessment. Radial keratotomy for simple myopia. JAMA. 1988 Jul 8; 260(2): 264-7
There was a lack of consensus among DATTA panelists about the safety and, especially, the effectiveness of radial keratotomy. For patients with a preoperative refractive error greater than -6.00 D, DATTA panelists believed that radial keratotomy has not been established as safe or effective. Concerns about effectiveness focused on the lack of predictability of the results and the continuing change in the refractive error following surgery. Daily fluctuations in visual acuity and the occurrence of anisometropia were other reported adverse events that contributed to the concern expressed by DATTA panelists. Concern over the safety and effectiveness of the procedure became greater as the magnitude of the preoperative refractive error increased. Nevertheless, there is a subpopulation of myopic patients who regard their myopia as a sufficiently severe handicap for them to undergo radial keratotomy. Such carefully chosen patients who have the procedure performed may achieve emmetropia and be free of corrective lenses.

Diagnostic and therapeutic technology assessment. Transrectal ultrasonography in prostatic cancer [published erratum appears in JAMA 1988 Aug 12;260(6):792] JAMA. 1988 May 13; 259(18): 2757-9
The DATTA panelists believe that transrectal ultrasound is established as safe for the screening and staging of prostatic cancer. The majority did not believe, however, that the effectiveness of the procedure has been established yet for

either screening or staging. The panelists and the literature indicate, however, that transrectal ultrasound may well have a significant role to play in the future treatment of prostatic cancers.

Diagnostic and therapeutic technology assessment. Penile implants for erectile impotence. JAMA. 1988 Aug 19; 260(7): 997-1000

Three semirigid penile prostheses (Small-Carrion, Finney Flexirod, and Jonas Silicone-Silver) and a multicomponent inflatable penile prosthesis (Scott) were considered safe and effective treatment for impotence unresponsive to medical management. Each of these prostheses has its own advantages and disadvantages. The entire semirigid prosthesis group is surgically easier to implant than the inflatable models and, except for fracturing of the silver wires in the Jonas model, has a low incidence of mechanical failure. However, the semirigid models are not as aesthetically pleasing or as sexually satisfying to both partners as are inflatable devices. Multicomponent inflatable penile prostheses have had a history of mechanical failure; however, improved design and materials have reduced this problem. Several new concepts in penile prostheses have recently been developed: the self-contained inflatable prosthesis and an articulating prosthesis made of a spring-loaded cable that runs through a series of plastic segments. The self-contained inflatable prosthesis contains a fluid reservoir within the device itself. This eliminates the need for a separate reservoir, pump, and connective tubing (AMS Hydroflex, Flexiflate). There are not yet enough long-term data available to evaluate these new single-component devices.

Diagnostic and therapeutic technology assessment. Immunoaugmentative therapy. JAMA. 1988 Jun 17; 259(23): 3477-8

The scientific evidence to date, as well as the history of IAT, will allow no other conclusion than that IAT is unequivocally dangerous to its patients and of no proved value as a treatment for cancer. Physicians who know of patients receiving IAT must be aware of the high risk those people are incurring for life-threatening infections of several types.

Diagnostic and therapeutic technology assessment. BCG immunotherapy in bladder cancer: a reassessment.
JAMA. 1988 Apr 8; 259(14): 2153-5

The DATTA panelists considered BCG immunotherapy to be efficacious in reducing recurrences of transitional cell carcinoma of the bladder. It has reduced recurrences in some patients in whom chemotherapeutic agents have failed, and in recent trials it has performed better than doxorubicin in preventing recurrences and in treatment of CIS. The DATTA panelists urged close evaluation of patients undergoing BCG therapy to guarantee that the tumor does not progress during treatment. Adverse reactions to BCG were not considered serious enough to jeopardize its use.

Diagnostic and therapeutic technology assessment. Ureteral stone management: the use of ureteroscopy with extracorporeal shockwave lithotripsy or ultrasonic lithotripsy [published erratum appears in JAMA 1988 Jul 15;260(3):343] JAMA. 1988 Mar 4; 259(9): 1382-4

Diagnostic and therapeutic technology assessment. Ureteral stone management: II. Ureteroscopy and ultrasonic lithotripsy. JAMA. 1988 Mar 11; 259(10): 1557-9

Diagnostic and therapeutic technology assessment. Coronary rehabilitation services. JAMA. 1987 Oct 9; 258(14): 1959-62

Diagnostic and therapeutic technology assessment. Chorionic villus sampling. JAMA. 1987 Dec 25; 258(24): 3560-3

Chorionic villus sampling has a promising future as a means of early detection of fetal abnormalities. It has widespread application in Europe, and more than 6000 procedures have been performed in the United States. Universal acceptance of the procedure has been delayed because of uncertainties over the true fetal loss rate. Information available today indicates that the fetal loss rate should be in the same range as that for amniocentesis--approximately 1% or less. Confirmation of these estimates awaits release of the data from the large clinical trials currently under way. Modifications of the sampling technique are also under investigation. Transabdominal CVS can also be performed early in pregnancy (six to 15 weeks) with a fine-bore needle and cannula under ultrasonic guidance. It remains to be seen if this offers any advantages or incurs additional risks over transcervical CVS.

Diagnostic and therapeutic technology assessment. Mammographic screening for breast cancer. JAMA. 1987 Sep 11; 258(10): 1387-9

Diagnostic and therapeutic technology assessment. Ablation of accessory pathways in the Wolff-Parkinson-White syndrome. JAMA. 1987 Jul 24-31; 258(4): 542-4

Diagnostic and therapeutic technology assessment. Ablation of accessory pathways in the Wolff-Parkinson-White syndrome. JAMA. 1987 Jul 17; 258(3): 384-6

Diagnostic and therapeutic technology assessment. Cardiokymography. JAMA. 1987 Jun 5; 257(21): 2973-4

Cardiokymography is one of several noninvasive techniques able to detect coronary artery disease. It can qualitatively determine abnormal left ventricular motion, and, based on animal models, this can be directly related to abnormalities in the left coronary artery. Abnormal motion of the anterolateral, posterolateral, or inferior wall is not detected. The sensitivity and specificity of the technique in detecting coronary artery disease in a high-risk group are similar to those of thallium scintigraphy. No comparison has been made with tomographic thallium imaging or echocardiography. Cardiokymography is generally used along with exercise ECG. Most DATTA panelists considered the device safe but believed its effectiveness had not been established. Many cited greater familiarity with radionuclide methods and satisfaction with the amount of information provided by current techniques. Forty percent (8/20) of the panelists considered this technique unacceptable. A major concern was the possibility of missing coronary artery disease that had not affected the anterior wall of the left ventricle. Panelists who offered an opinion represent the following areas of medical specialty: cardiovascular diseases (20) and cardiovascular surgery/thoracic surgery (two). Their board certification includes the American Board of Internal Medicine (18) and the American Board of Thoracic Surgery (two). Fifteen physicians had no opinion regarding safety and 17 physicians had no opinion regarding effectiveness.

American

Medical

Association

American Medical Association

Diagnostic and therapeutic technology assessment. Bacillus Calmette-Guerin immunotherapy in bladder cancer. JAMA. 1987 Mar 6; 257(9): 1238-40

Diagnostic and therapeutic technology assessment. Autologous bone marrow transplantation. JAMA. 1986 Jul 4; 256(1): 98-101

Diagnostic and therapeutic technology assessment. Garren gastric bubble. JAMA. 1986 Dec 19; 256(23): 3282-4

Diagnostic and therapeutic technology assessment. Angelchik antireflux prosthesis. JAMA. 1986 Sep 12; 256(10): 1358-60
In summary, the DATTA panelists felt that the Angelchik prosthesis is effective in relieving gastroesophageal reflux and that the device, along with other types of surgical procedures, is indicated when medical management has failed and when objective evidence of incompetence of the lower esophageal sphincter is present. Because the procedure is rapid and requires little dissection, it might be most useful in the elderly and high-risk patient. Notwithstanding such support from the DATTA panelists for the device's efficacy, the majority of DATTA panelists felt that concerns about the safety of the device compromise its clinical utility. Such concern arose from past reports of complications and the panelists' own experience with migration or erosion of the device. Thus, these panelists could not recommend the device's routine use. Additionally, some DATTA panelists considered the development of the Angelchik prosthesis to be unnecessary, as standard surgical techniques, eg, fundoplication, give adequate results. The improved safety statistics reported since 1982 may remove some of these reservations in the future.

Diagnostic and therapeutic technology assessment. Stereotactic cingulotomy. JAMA. 1985 Nov 15; 254(19): 2817-8

Diagnostic and therapeutic technology assessment. Diagnostic intraoperative ultrasound. JAMA. 1985 Jul 12; 254(2): 285-7

Diagnostic and therapeutic technology assessment. Endoscopic topical therapy of gastrointestinal tract hemorrhage. JAMA. 1985 May 10; 253(18): 2734-5

Diagnostic and therapeutic technology assessment. Endoscopic electrocoagulation of gastrointestinal tract hemorrhage. JAMA. 1985 May 10; 253(18): 2733-4

Diagnostic and therapeutic technology assessment. Endoscopic thermal coagulation of gastrointestinal tract hemorrhage. JAMA. 1985 May 10; 253(18): 2733

Diagnostic and therapeutic technology assessment. Endoscopic laser photocoagulation of gastrointestinal tract hemorrhage. JAMA. 1985 May 10; 253(18): 2732-3

Diagnostic and therapeutic technology assessment. Enhanced computed tomography in head trauma. JAMA. 1985 Dec 20; 254(23): 3370-1

Diagnostic and therapeutic technology assessment. Macular drusen. JAMA. 1985 Oct 11; 254(14): 1994

Diagnostic and therapeutic technology assessment. Age-adjusted diagnosis of hypertension. JAMA. 1985 Oct 11; 254(14): 1994

Diagnostic and therapeutic technology assessment. Sperm penetration assay. JAMA. 1985 Oct 11; 254(14): 1993-4

Diagnostic and therapeutic technology assessment. Continuous arteriovenous hemofiltration. JAMA. 1985 Mar 1; 253(9): 1325-6

Diagnostic and therapeutic technology assessment. Bone marrow transplantation in childhood leukemia. JAMA. 1984 Apr 27; 251(16): 2155

Diagnostic and therapeutic technology assessment. Implanted electrospinal stimulator for scoliosis. JAMA. 1984 May 25; 251(20): 2723

Diagnostic and therapeutic technology assessment. Endoscopic transurethral nephrolithotomy. JAMA. 1984 Dec 21; 252(23): 3302

Diagnostic and therapeutic technology assessment. Percutaneous nephrolithotomy. JAMA. 1984 Dec 21; 252(23): 3301-2

Diagnostic and therapeutic technology assessment. Noninvasive extracorporeal lithotripsy. JAMA. 1984 Dec 21; 252(23): 3301

Diagnostic and therapeutic technology assessment. Gastric restrictive surgery for morbid obesity. JAMA. 1984 Jun 8; 251(22): 3011

Diagnostic and therapeutic technology assessment. Diaphanography (transillumination of the breast) for cancer screening. JAMA. 1984 Apr 13; 251(14): 1902

Diagnostic and therapeutic technology assessment. Cranial electrostimulation. JAMA. 1984 Feb 24; 251(8): 1094

Diagnostic and therapeutic technology assessment. Cardiokymography for noninvasive cardiological diagnosis. JAMA. 1984 Feb 24; 251(8): 1094

Diagnostic and therapeutic technology assessment. Whole-body hyperthermia treatment of cancer. JAMA. 1984 Jan 13; 251(2): 272

Diagnostic and therapeutic technology assessment. CO2 laser treatment of gynecologic malignant neoplasms. JAMA. 1983 Aug 5; 250(5): 672

Diagnostic and therapeutic technology assessment. Mandatory ECG before elective surgery. JAMA. 1983 Jul 22; 250(4): 540

Diagnostic and therapeutic technology assessment. Diathermy. JAMA. 1983 Jul 22; 250(4): 540

Diagnostic and therapeutic technology assessment. Chelation therapy. JAMA. 1983 Aug 5; 250(5): 672

Diagnostic and therapeutic technology assessment. Radial keratotomy. JAMA. 1983 Jul 15; 250(3): 420

Diagnostic and therapeutic technology assessment. Quantitative EEG (Fast Fourier Transform Analysis) monitoring. JAMA. 1983 Jul 15; 250(3): 420

Diagnostic and therapeutic technology assessment. Biofeedback. JAMA. 1983 Nov 4; 250(17): 2381

Diagnostic and therapeutic technology assessment. Implantable infusion pump. JAMA. 1983 Oct 14; 250(14): 1906

Diagnostic and therapeutic technology assessment. 24-hour ambulatory EEG monitoring. JAMA. 1983 Dec 23-30; 250(24): 3340

Technology News is developed and distributed in conjunction with DATTA evaluations and provides information and analyses of current issues involving medical technology.

Contact for single copies of DATTA evaluations at no charge:
AMA Department of Technology Management
800/AMA-3211 ext. 4531

Medical Education

Council on Medical Education is composed of ten physicians, one resident and one student, and addresses all facets of education, from medical school and residency programs to continuing education and allied health education. Its primary charge is to study and evaluate medical education in order to provide an adequate supply of well-qualified physicians to meet the medical needs of the public. The council also serves as the parent council for committees dealing with more specific areas of medical education. It meets four times a year.

Liason Committee on Medical Education (LCME) is the national authority for the accreditation of medical education programs leading to the M.D. degree in U.S. and Canadian medical schools. The LCME is recognized for this purpose by the U.S. Secretary of Education, by the Council on Postsecondary Accreditation, by the U.S. Congress in various health-related laws, and by state, provincial (Canada), and territorial medical licensure boards.

Accreditation Council for Graduate Medical Education (ACGME)

All of the administration and professional support services provided to the ACGME and its component Residency Review Committee for the accreditation of all residency programs in the U.S. are included in this program. Key activities encompass the training and effective utilization of on-site surveyors; the conduct of all surveys within the expected time frame; the provision of administrative support to the RRC's; the conduct of research and the provision of liaison and representation with relevant agencies, offices, organizations and individuals. The ACGME carries out its accreditation mission by serving as the deliberative body through which standards for residency programs as well as procedures for accreditation are established. As part of the accreditation process, the ACGME maintains oversight of committees of volunteer physicians in each of 24 specialty areas. These committees, called Residency Review Committees, normally make the accreditation decisions within their areas of expertise. In contested accreditation decisions, the ACGME serves as the final decision-making body. Departments specific to the activities of the field staff, the RRC activities and the research and adminstration involved in accreditating the programs round out the elements of this program.

Accreditation Council for
Graduate Medical Education
515 N. State Street, Chicago, IL 60610
312/464-4920

Specialties accredited by the ACGME include:
Allergy and Immunology
Ambulatory Care/See: Internal Medicine
Anesthesiology
Colon and Rectal Surgery
Critical Care
Dermatology
Emergency Medicine
Family Practice
Internal Medicine
Neurological Surgery
Neurology
Nuclear Medicine
Obstetrics/Gynecology
Ophthalmology
Orthopaedic Surgery
Otolaryngology
Pathology
Pediatrics
Pediatric Surgery
Physical Medicine and Rehabilitation
Plastic Surgery
Preventive Medicine
Psychiatry
Radiology
Surgery
Thoracic Surgery
Transitional Year (Rotating Intern) Review Committee
Urology
Vascular Surgery

American Medical Association

American
Medical
Association

Departmental publications include:

FREIDA (Fellowship and Residency Electronic Interactive Database Access) is an expanded computerized version of the *Directory of Graduate Medical Education Programs*, and is published and updated annually. It is available in two formats. Continuing attention will be placed on liaison activities with key leaders, researchers, and organizations in medical education. The FRIEDA Hotline at 312/464-4886 should be contacted with questions regarding data cotained within the service.

Directory of Graduate Medical Education Programs, also known as "The Green Book," contains the official list of ACGME accredited programs, a summary of graduate medical education statistical data, the standards for program accreditation in each specialty, requirements for board certification, and a summary of licensure regulations for each state.

Division of Undergraduate Medical Education

This division's goal is to provide educational materials and guidance to those persons interested in a career in medicine. The Department of Medical Student Services produces several aids to proceed toward that goal including their videotape called "Science and Art in the Name of Healing" that presents the rewards of a medical career, and brochures that introduce the rewards of a career in medicine to students thinking about a committment to medicine. These include "Got That Healing Feeling", "Medicine: A Chance to Make a Difference" and "You the Doctor"

Division of Continuing Medical Education

Accreditation Council for Continuing Medical Education (ACCME): Fostering the AMA's commitment to excellence in the provision of Continuing Medical Education (CME) for physicians, both nationally and internationally, is a central focus of this area. This is done by developing appropriate policies, participating in the establishment of effective accreditation standards and procedures with the Accreditation Council for Continuing Medical Education (ACCME), sponsoring high-quality CME programs, communicating timely and accurate information on CME, and supporting and cooperating with other organizations and institutions that share the AMA's interest in meeting the needs of the profession for continuing medical education of the highest quality. Greater attention will be placed on a comprehensive registry of Continuing Medical Education to enhance clinical competence and local, regional, and national CME activities to promote the visibility of the AMA.

Physician Recognition Award (PRA) initiative is also a part of the CME division's job. Established by the house of Delegates in 1968, the Physician's Recognition Program provides certificates to physicians who qualify by completing required amounts of continuing education of acceptable quality.

Divisional Publications Include:
Directory of Continuing Medical Education (CME) A unique, biennial resources for continuing medical education (CME) planners, the Directory consolidates a variety of information needed for planning, accrediting, and delivering CME opportunities for physicians. The Directory lists accredited state and national CME sponsors and provides a detailed Federation meeting calendar. It includes information on accreditation policies and guidelines, credentialing requirements, research, and special activities. The Directory provides information on AMA's long-standing involvement in continuing medical education and positions the Association as a key national leader on CME issues.

Division of Allied Health Education and Accreditation

The AMA, through the Committee on Allied Health Education Accreditation (CAHEA), leads 26 medical specialty and 25 allied health organizations in a cooperative venture to assess and enhance the quality of the education of allied health professional - persons who work closely with physicians in providing patient care. The quality of patient care is improved when the allied health personnel who assist, facilitate, and complement the work of physicians have been appropriately educated. Departments of Accreditation Services and Allied Health Education are also a part of this area.

Divisional publications include:
The *Allied Health Education Directory* provides information on over 2,800 educational programs accredited by the CAHEA and includes information on 1,500 sponsoring institutions. The Directory includes national statistics on programs, institutions, enrollments, attrition, and graduates. It also provides data reflecting program director perspectives on allied health personnel supply and demand.

Health Policy Development

- Health Policy Programs
- Legislative Activities
- Health Policy Management

The Health Policy Development area seeks to provide an environment that allows physicians the maximum professional autonomy in the delivery of medical services to their patients. Specific areas that are of key concern to physicians include physician payment, medical review, and long-term care financing. Progressive recommendations for AMA policy are developed through this area by the Council on Medical Service. Tangible products such as *Current Procedural Terminology (CPT)* and the "Health Insurance Claim Form" are useful to the profession through practical applications. Increased attention from this area is to be placed on strengthening the AMA's role and presence in implementation of physician payment reform and managed care, as well as in medical coding and nomenclature.

Council on Medical Service is composed of ten physicians, one resident and one student, the Council deals with socioeconomic issues in health care such as national health insurance and health care financing. planning and organization. The Council meets six times a year.

Health Policy Programs

The Association's health policy research program is designed to provide the factual research information and policy alternatives needed for effective representation of physicians. Key research projects include: Medicare physician payment methods, tracking of Medicare expenditures, health system reform, international health systems comparisons, medical practice costs, the economic impact of clinical laboratories, physician manpower, and access to health care. In addition, the research program is responding to the growing technical complexity of national health policy issues by providing increased support to the Association in the form of internal consulting, information for physician leaders, and assistance in policy development. The research program continues to provide an authoritative source of information on medical practice in the United States through a socioeconomic monitoring system data collection program and a publication series. The departments of Health Care Review and Carrier Relations, Health Care Financing and Organization, Coding and Nomenclature, and Medical Service are a part of this division.

Divisional publications include:
New Medicare Physician Payment System: Resources for Organized Medicine
Medicare Carrier Review: What Every Physician Should Know About 'Medically Unnecessary' Denials
Current Procedural Terminaology (CPT)

Division of Health Policy Research

The AMA's health policy research program is designed to provide the factual research information and policy alternatives needed for effective representation of physicians. This area responds to the growing technical complexity of natonal health policy issues by providing increased support to the AMA in the form of internal consulting, information on physician leaders, and assistance in policy development. The research program continues to provide an authoritative source of information on medical practice in the United States through a data collection program and subsequent publication series.

The **Center for Health Policy Research** is the hub of this division. They assist in answering many of the basic questions involved in socioeconomic studies and concerns. Other departments in the area include the Department of Public Policy Studies, the Department of Socioeconomic Research Information, the Department of Policy Development Studies, the Department of Reference Base Studies and the Department of Medical Review

Divisional publications include:
Physicians Marketplace Statistics is an annual reference volume representing Socioeconomic Monitoring System (SMS) data on physician income, professional expenses, fees, and selected practice characteristics. The publication was developed in response to requests from users of *Socioeconomic Characteristics of Medical Practice* who wanted more detailed specialty and geographic breakdowns of information.

Socioeconomic Characteristics of Medical Practice is an annual reference volume containing SMS data on physician income, professional expenses, and selected practice characteristics.

Department of Practice Parameters
The *Directory of Practice Parameters*, an annual publication, is a bibliography of practice parameters produced by physician organizations and others. Developed in cooperation with the Practice Parameters Partnership and Practice Parameters Forum, this 158-page document is the only complete source of information on practice parameters, and is available both in a printed and CD-Rom formats. By controlling the contents of the Directory, the AMA maintains a strategically central role in the development, dissemination, and implementation of practice parameters. The Directory also offers a subscription to "Practice Parameter Update", which is available separately as well.

Office of Quality Assurance and Medical Review: The central focus of this office is to strengthen the AMA's postiion as a leader in the efforts of organized medicine to assure and improve the quality of medical care. This is accomplished by assuring that practice parameters are developed and implemented in consonance with the professional standards of the medical profession. The benefits of these activities include more effective clinical practice and appropriate utilization of health care resources.

Office publications include:
Guides to Uses of Mortality Data in QA Activities
Q.A. Review
Principles of Medical Record Documentation - (Brochure)

American Medical Association

American
Medical
Association

Legislative Activities

These activities help to establish the Association's legislative credibility and presence at both the federal and state levels. Key activities include monitoring and analyzing federal and state legislation and regulations, developing policy positions on legislative proposals through the involvement of the Council on Legislation and others, and advocating such positions to appropriate governmental bodies. The current focus of this area is on the Association's major objectives, including health system reform and access to health care for all Americans, promotion of public health and decreased use of tobacco, continued implementation of physician payment reform, clinical laboratory reform, and reduced administrative hassles under Medicare. This is achieved through testimony, Congressional appearances, regulatory comments, and meetings with government officials and their staffs.

Council on Legislation is composed of ten physicians, one resident and one student. It addresses federal legislation and AMA policies that deal with national legislative issues. The council serves as the principle source of membership input into the development of legislative policy by the Board, and meets six times per year and at House of Delegates sessions.

Health Policy Management

This area works closely with the Council on Long Range Planning and Development to manage AMA's environmental tracking and assessment initiatives; to identify issues and strategies relating to AMA membership, organizational structure, and representation; to develop strategies to enhance the process of policy develpment and implementation; and to participate in the identification, analysis, and development of the long-range policy.

The communication and advocacy support activity focuses on articulating and promoting AMA policy to the various audiences, including government, business, policymakers, physicians, and the public. Emphasis is on the production of advocacy pieces on specific issues for use in addressing the various audiences. Activities and products include Advocacy Briefs, development of AMA "basic messages," and implementation of a patient/physician advocacy communications plan to assist the Federation in promoting AMA health policy. Offices of Policy Planning and Analysis, Policy Communication and Advocacy, and Policy Development and Coordination, plus the Department of Long Range Policy Analysis make up the components of this area.

Council on Long Range Planning and Development consists of an appointed membership of eight physicians, one resident and one student. Purpose of the council is to advise the Board and House of Delegates on the long-term course of the AMA as an organization by dealing with recommendations on membership, organizational structure and major trends. It also evaluates other planning activites in the AMA.

Sample articles include:
The future of general internal medicine. Council on Long Range Planning and Development in Cooperation with the American College of

Physicians, the American Society of Internal Medicine, and the Society of General Internal Medicine. JAMA. 1989 Oct 20; 262(15): 2119-24
The American Medical Association Council on Long Range Planning and Development has been publishing a series of reports that assess trends in the environment of medicine and their impact on physicians and health care provision. The Council believes that each specialty in medicine has unique characteristics and will respond differently to changes in the health care arena. This report, developed in cooperation with the American College of Physicians, the American Society of Internal Medicine, and the Society of General Internal Medicine, provides an overview and environmental analysis of the specialty of general internal medicine. The Council first reviews socioeconomic data pertinent to general internal medicine. This is followed by a review of key issues pertinent to internists that relate to such topics as graduate medical education, reimbursement, scope of practice, manpower, and competition. In the conclusions, the Council suggests activities for the medical profession to pursue in response to the identified environmental trends.

The future of adult cardiology. Council on Long Range Planning and Development in cooperation with the American College of Cardiology. JAMA. 1989 Nov 24; 262(20): 2874-8
During the past several years, the American Medical Association's Council on Long Range Planning and Development has identified trends in the environment of medicine that are likely to affect physicians, their practices, and the provision of medical care in the future. In the course of its environmental analysis studies, the Council has recognized that each medical specialty is uniquely subject to anticipated changes in the environment of medicine. As part of an ongoing series of analyses prepared by the Council, this report focuses on environmental trends that are likely to influence the practice of adult cardiology. The report outlines the current state of cardiology, the forces for change in the environment, and the implications regarding the changes.

The future of general surgery. Council on Long Range Planning and Development. JAMA. 1989 Dec 8; 262(22): 3178-83
During the past several years, the American Medical Association's Council on Long Range Planning and Development has identified trends in the environment of medicine that are likely to affect physicians, their practices, and the provision of medical care in the future. In the course of its environmental analysis studies, the Council has recognized that each medical specialty is uniquely subject to anticipated changes in the environment of medicine. As part of an ongoing series of analyses prepared by the Council, this report focuses on environmental trends that are likely to influence the practice of general surgery. The report outlines the current state of general surgery, the forces for change in the environment, and the implications regarding these changes. The Council concludes that there are certain challenges and many positive indicators for the future of general surgery.

The future of psychiatry. Council on Long Range Planning and Development. JAMA. 1990 Nov 21; 264(19): 2542-8
The American Medical Association Council on Long Range Planning and Development has been publishing a series of reports that assess trends in the environment of medicine and their impact on physicians and health care provision. The Council believes each specialty in medicine will respond

differently to changes in the health care arena. This report, developed in cooperation with the American Psychiatric Association, provides an overview and environmental analysis of the specialty of psychiatry. Socioeconomic data pertinent to psychiatry are reviewed first, followed by a review of scientific and clinical developments in the specialty. Next, the changing provision patterns of psychiatric care, the emerging patient populations served by psychiatrists, and recent developments in graduate medical education in psychiatry are reviewed. The Council also addresses changes in the financing of psychiatric care. In conclusion, the Council suggests implications of these and other environmental trends for psychiatry.

Divisional publications Include:
AMA Policy Compendium is an annually updated catalog of active AMA policy adopted by the House of Delegates arragned by policy topic by year of adoption. Over 2000 sections of AMA policy are arranged here.

American

Medical

Association

Government and Political Affairs

- Government Affairs
- Political Affairs/AMPAC

American Medical Association: Washington Office

AMA's Washington, DC office lobbies with Congress, and works with state and specialties societies, and group practices on legislation affecting physician's practices and patients. It represents the profession before the executive branch of the federal government and various regulatory agencies.

American Medical Association
1101 Vermont Ave., NW, Washington, DC 20005
202/789-7400
FAX 202/789-7485;

Government Affairs

Providing effective advocacy of the Association's policies and positions before Congress and the Executive Branch is the primary purpose of the activities of this area. These are undertaken to ensure the continued availablity of high-quality medical care, to represent and protect the interest of the professionand the public, and to minimize regulatory contraints on the practice of medicine. Divisions of Congressional Affairs, Federal Affairs and an office of Issues Management help this area acheive its goals.

Political Affairs

The primary objectives in this area are to provide innovative political action techniques, including direct contributions, in-kind services and independent expenditure support to congressional candidates, and state-of-the-art political education programs to stimulate legislative and political grassroots involvement.

American Medical Political Action Committee (AMPAC) is a bipartisan political action committee established by the AMA over 30 years ago. AMPAC members participate in political fund-raising, campaign management, and various grassroots activities. Their goal is to persuade legislators to pass, defeat or amend legislation of interest to physicians and, at the same time, for the well-being of their patients.

To Contact AMPAC:
1101 Vermont Ave., NW,
Washington, DC 20005
202/789-7462
FAX 202/789-7469

Office of Political Education offers programs designed to encourage and train physicians and their spouses who are interested in becoming active in political and legislative grassroots activites, such as voter participation projects. They organize and sponsor training initiatives for physician political training, campaign management and campaign strategy.

Office Publications Include:
Stethoscope
Talking Points

American

Medical

Association

Federation Relations and Membership

- Membership
- Specialty Societies and Professional Relations
- State and County Relations

Federation of Medicine Partners of the American Medical Association

County, state and specialty societies are partners with the American Medical Association in the federation of medicine and their members and staff rely upon AMA cooperation.

Several state and county medical societies have made a special commitment to the AMA. They require their members to belong to the AMA as well as to their county and state society. This special commitment contributes significantly to the AMA's membership strength.

The following are unified societies:

Unified States

Delaware(1986)
Illinois(1951)
Mississippi(1985)
Montana(1989 dropped in 1991)
Oklahoma(1950)
Pennsylvania(1989)

Unified Counties

Muskegon(MI)
Genesee(NY)
Chattanooga/Hamilton(TN)
Hill(TX)
Nueces(TX)
Panola(TX)
Runnels(TX)
Genesse/Niagara/Orleans(NY)

Special Society

American Association of Clinical Urologists

National Leadership Conference is a meeting for key Federation staff and elected officials, is designed to serve as an annual focal point for discussions of major national health policy issues. In recent years, the National Communications Conference has been held in conjunction with this meeting.

National Leadership Conference:
1994: February 11-13; San Francisco, CA

Membership

In 1992 the AMA is launched a long-term membership campaign to achieve a 50 percent market share by the year 2000. The campaign is based on a strategy of differentiating AMA members from nonmembers and also highlights members' adherence to the AMA Principles of Medical Ethics. The campaign is multifaceted and involves advertising in national news weeklies and medical journals, patient brochures, enhancement of the membership certificate, new products targeted to specific membership segments, outreach to group practices, new reduced dues categories and payment options, improved communications. and a national member-get-a-member program.

The campaign supplements the ongoing activities of Membership marketing from the AMA and the American Medical Political Action Committee (AMPAC). The Association continues to work with state, county, and specialty societies to improve AMA and AMPAC membership by providing tailored marketing plans and consultation, resources for retention and recruitment activities, and incentive programs. Peer-to-peer recruitment programs aimed at physicians, students, and residents will continue as will efforts to recruit and retain physicians through the direct program.

Divisional Publications include:
Member Matters

Contact the Members Service Center: 800/AMA-3211

Specialty Society and Professional Relations

Department of Resident Physician Services
Establishing direct access to the AMA's policy-making process for resident physicians, mainstreaming them into organized medicine, and providing information to this group are the central focus of these activities. Key projects include the Resident Physicians Section (RPS), which provides an orderly representative framework, organizational-strengthening activities to foster grassroots support, and publications and communications to highlight AMA policies and the benefits of membership involvement. Special attention will be directed toward educating residents about graduate medical education issues and national health policies to train them as young physician leaders.

Burroughs Wellcome Resident Physicians Program
Made possible through a grant from Burroughs Wellcome, fifty residents receive stipends for travel and lodging to attend the Annual and Interim Meetings and participate in the policymaking process. The program requires an application and resident selection is based on a demonstrated commitment, i.e., volunteer work to the civic or medical community.

For information on Burroughs Wellcome contact: 800/621-8335

Department of Medical Student Services
These activities provide a direct voice for medical students in the AMA's policymaking process and serve the identified needs of this group by providing high-quality products and services. Key projects that address these needs include the provision of support for the Medical Student Section (MSS) and state and local section organizational development. Continued activities include a successful government relations internship program designed to expose medical students to legislative and political processes and AMA policy promotion grants for medical student

American Medical Association

American
Medical
Association

groups working on projects and activities that promote AMA policy.

Department of Hospital Medical Staff Services
The AMA's Hospital Medical Staff Section (HMSS) is dedicated to addressing the needs and concerns of organized hospital medical staffs and their physician members. The semi-annual Assembly Meetings are the only national forum convened exclusively for hospital medical staffs. Through the HMSS, each hospital medical staff has an opportunity to participate in AMA's policy-making process. Through the Assembly meetings, educational programs, and publications, the HMSS keeps hospital medical staffs informed of current trends, conditions, and concerns affecting physicians and medical staffs. Major emphasis will be on strengthening AMA communications to hospital medical staffs, increasing participation in the HMSS, and developing membership marketing strategies through the HMSS.

Departmental publications include:
Bylaws: A Guide for Hospital Medical Staffs
*Delineation of Clinical Privileges: A Guide
    for Hospital Medical Staffs"*

Department of Young Physicians Services is designed to meet the identified needs of AMA members who are under age 40 or within the first five years of medical practice. The primary way in which these needs are served include the establishment of the Young Physician Section (YPS) as a national forum for policy deliberation and direct access to the AMA House of Delegates for young physicians.

Women in Medicine Services initiatives consist of general outreach activities with women physicians/medical students, including providing information, support, and assistance to the Federation on Women in Medicine issues and programs; liaison activities with the AMA Board of Trustees, Councils, Section, and other special groups; site visits by Women in Medicine staff and Advisory Panel members; participation in related national and Federation meetings; and implementing the annual Women in Medicine Month campaign. The Women in Medicine project is also headed up by this area.

Office of Specialty Society Relations activities include building and maintaining primary liaison and contact between the AMA and the national medical specialty societies represented in the AMA House of Delegates, building legislative policy consensu, and fostering a sense of unity between the AMA and specialty societies.

State and County Relations
This area emphasizes the building and maintaining of a strong relationship between the Federation and the AMA and to interact with the Federation to build consensus and to minimize potential conflict. These groups provide consultative resources for problem resolution, convey policy and program initiatives, and informs the Federation of necessary action with respect to legislative, federal administrative, and socioeconomic issues.

Federation Network (FEDNET) is a computer bulletin board service which provides county, state, and national specialty organizations with instantaneous news updates and calls for grassroots legislaative action. It is the Associations primary method for transmitting important communications on an immediate basis tot he Federation. The system is routinely utilized by approximately 100 medical societies.

Governance and Corporate Services

- Corporate Services
- EVP Office Administration
- Board of Trustees
- House of Delegates
- Office of International Medicine

AMA Officers 1992-1993

President (1992-93)
John L. Clowe, MD+

President Elect (term will be 1993-94)
Joseph T. Painter, MD+

Immediate Past President (1991-92)
John J. Ring, MD

Secretary-Treasurer
William E. Jacott, MD+
(also Secy. of Board of Trustees)

Speaker, House of Delegates
Daniel H. Johnson Jr., MD

Vice Speaker, House of Delegates
Richard F. Corlin, MD

Chairman, Board of Trustees
Raymond Scalettar, MD+

Vice Chairman, Board of Trustees
Lonnie R. Bristow, MD+

Resident Trustee
Mary Ann Contogiannis, MD

Student Trustee
Melissa J. Garretson

Corporate Services

Department of Meeting Planning and Management aims its planning and management activities at ensuring that the meeting site environment for all AMA-sponsored meetings is conducive to comfortable, cost effective, and productive meetings. Other key activities within the program are designed to provide cost-efficient travel services, high-quality registration services, and a convenient low-cost In-House Meeting program. Attention will continue to be placed on maintaining the current high levels of quality and efficiency for the srvices provided.

The purpose of the annual meeting is to present a forum for the delegates representing various specialty groups to constructively meet to develop policy. This is not a scientific meeting, nor are there vendor booths present.

Annual Meeting
June 13-17, 1993 - Chicago, IL
June 12-16, 1994 - Chicago, IL
June 11-15, 1995 - Chicago, IL

Interim Meeting
December 5-8, 1993 - New Orleans, LA
December 4-7, 1994 - Honolulu, HI
December 3-6, 1995 - Washington, DC

Division of Corporate Facilities
The management of the AMA's corparate facilities located in Chicago, Washington, DC, and New York, are key objectives consistent with general management and administration guidelines. The primary obejctive is to maintain these properties in the most cost-effective manner while protecting the Association's assets and provide an attractive, comfortable, and safe environment for employees. Departments of Building and Facilities Planning and Food Services add to the effort toward obtaining these goals.

Division of Office Services
This area, in addition to providing high-quality, cost-effective communications systems for the AMA and all its operating units, also sees as a primary objective enhancing employee productivity and espirit de corps by providing a cafeteria and an on-site catering operation that serves refreshments at a reasonable cost in a comfortable envirronment. The Departments of Communications, of Word Processing and Records Management, of Distribution Services, and of Reprographic Services are parts of this division.

Office of Officer Services
This program provides resources and staff support to enable the Board of Trustees to fulfill its essential functions. This contact can also provide biographical Information on Officers.

Board of Trustees:
Within the policy guidelines set by the House of Delegates, the board of Trustees maintains primary fiduciary and oversight responsibility for the affairs of the Association. Board members maintain active public speaking schedules and make numerous official appearances to represent the AMA before other organizations, government bodies, the media and the general public. The Board's public appearance program serves to maintain and enhance relationships within the profession, throughout the Federation, and with external groups and organizations. It advances the aims, purposes, and policies of the AMA as well as affording opportunities to gain a better understanding of the needs of the memebership in order to provide appropriate resources and leadership guidance.

The AMA Board of Trustees
Lonnie R. Bristow, MD+;
Mary Ann Contogiannis, MD;
Nancy W. Dickey, MD+;
Palma E. Formica, MD;
Melissa J. Garretson;
William E. Jacott, MD+;
Robert E. Mc Afee, MD;
Thomas R. Reardon, MD;
Raymond Scalettar, MD+;

American Medical Association

American Medical Association

House of Delegates

This area provides high-quality, cost-effective communications systems for the transmission of both voice and hard copy, including printing services, for the House of Delegates, the Board of Trustees, and all operating units of the Association and an effective records storage as primary objectives. Further efforts aimed at increasing the effectiveness of internal and external communications are to be implemented here. New technologies, such as electronic mail, voice messaging, and video conferencing, will be further evaluated and expanded if they provide cost-effective enhancements to communications. In addition, office communication procedures and policies will continue to be reviewed and revised to achieve maximum utilization of AMA staff and financial resources.

Office of International Medicine

Directing its activities toward enhancing the AMA's impact on the level and quality of health care world wide and its ability to influence international health policy, the International Medicine serves an important role. Emphasis of this area is centered on its collaboration with the World Medical Association(WMA) which includes the AMA/WMA Child Survival Action program in collaboration with the US Agency for International Development, the Centers for Disease Control, and Southeast Asian Medical Societies. The AMA cooperates with the World Health Organization, United Nations, Peace Corps, US agencies, National Council for International Health, and medical and public health schools on various health programs. The Association intervenes in cases of human rights violations in cooperation with WMA, American Association for Advancement of Science, Amnesty International, and Physicians for Human Rights. The AMA's corporate art program also falls within this area.

AMA Art Collection

Images, in the form of words or pictures, have a profound place in our world. They are a means of communicating information, sharing ideas, storing memories, delighting us. It has been said that a picture is worth a thousand words, and if that saying is true, the AMA collection is worth volumes. As a "contemporary" collection of American art this group of drawings, paintings, photographs, prints, and sculpture reflect preoccupations and concerns of artists in the late 20th century in these United States. Within this collection are not only a range of techniques, but more importantly, a range of emotions and thoughts that mirror our contemporary world, and make comment on the culture of the current moment. Since ours is a time with a mix of thought on design, there is no one answer, direction, or point of view, and no one artist has a corner on what is correct and accepted as the sole standard of excellence. There is instead throughout the current art world, and so reflected in the AMA collection, a shared ability on the part of artists to respond artistically and intellectually to a complex world.

Like the artworks, which cover a cross section of contemporary directions, the artists, both men and women, represent a geographic cross section from all over the country. Each artist represented in the collection has established a reputation and has shown his or her work at museums and serious galleries. While the majority have solid academic backgrounds, and a knowledge of art history, individuals among the group have chosen to veer from the norms of the past. What is "pictured" is less central for artists who are interested in abstract forms or abstract ideas, such as Christian Eckhart or Marcia Hafif. Also included in the collection are artists who continue to acknowledge traditional standards and who work within established conventions: for these artists who have used recognizable imagery to create cityscapes or figure studies, such as Richard Haas or Leslie Machinest, what is pictures is still very important. Still other artists, such as the team of Helen Mayer and Newton Harrison, have mixed a concern for science into their palette, and have turned our attention to the ecology of our planet, making what is pictured a new way of addressing serious questions of the earth's survival.

The philosophic points raised visually in AMA's artworks can be gently implied - like the dark quiet of Lois Lane's paintings, or shouted with bright energy - like the works by Nancy Graves or John Torreano. There is humor, seriousness, sheer beauty, a sense of history, even a taste for technology and mysticism in our sampling.

Since nothing is off-limits, no area of study or imagination or material, anything is possible for the artist. When at his or her best, the artist becomes the conjurer who can open up our world by offering his or her vision. Such visions can be very tied to the real, like the sculptural reliefs of John Ahearn or the landscapes of Mel Pekarsky or they can be illusions like the drawings of Alan Saret or the recording of the real world into a more perfect world system by Matt Mullican.

To anchor this abundance of differing directions in our late twentieth century, and to suggest that art has always presented many possibilities, the AMA collection includes two nineteenth century examples of excellence in American art: the traditional nature studies of John James Audobon and the revolutionary ornamentation of the architect Louis H. Sullivan. There is much to think about, as well as to look at, in the AMA Art Collection. (AMA Art Collection Handbook)

Communications and Publishing

- Scientific Publications
- Publishing
- Public Relations
- AMNews
- Group on Special Projects
- Consumer Affairs and Corporate Relations

Scientific Publications

With a worldwide audience of more than 1 million recipients in 146 countires, the journals of the American Medical Association - the weekly JAMA and ten monthly specialty journals - seek to fulfill their goals of publishing peer-reviewed clinical and investigative articles in major medical disciplines, providing continuing education for physicians, offering a forum for debate on controversial issues that affect medicine, as well as informing readers about nonclinical aspects of medicine. Various departments function within this area, including the JAMA Programs and International Activities, Editorial Services and Administration, Editorial Affairs and Editorial Processing.

Department of Specialty Journals provides a contact at AMA headquarters for the editorial staffs of the various specialty journals who are located accross the country.

AMA Journals

American Journal of Diseases of Children
Archives of Dermatology
Archives of Family Medicine
Archives of General Psychiatry
Archives of Internal Medicine
Archives of Neurology
Archives of Ophthalmology
*Archives of Otolaryngology - Head and
    Neck Surgery*
Archives of Pathology and Laboratory Medicine
Archives of Surgery
Journal of the American Medical Association

The *Journal of the American Medical Association* (JAMA) has several issues that appear regularly to address pre-defined needs: A brief description of each type of issue follows:

Medical Education defines the state of medical education in a given year. Sections on Undergraduate And Graduate Education, Continuing Medical Education and Allied Health Education and Accreditation make up the body of the issue. Many statistical tables, appendices, and articles of topical interest add to the usefulness of this annual volume.

Contempo takes the opinions of physicians in the field and has them describe the most interesting developments in their field over the previous year. Each issue varies in content, but the basic premise remains the same year to year.

Continuing Education Opportunities for Physicians is compiiled under the direction of the Council on Medical Education of the American Medical Association and by the AMA Division of Continuing Medical Education. The scope of the listing is the accredited CME opportunities for the designated 6-month period of a given issue.

Pulse is prepared by the *Pulse* editors and JAMA staff and is published monthly from September through May as an special section in JAMA. It provides a forum for the ideas, opinions, and news that affect medical students and showcases student writing, research, and artwork.

AMA Official Call is published semi-annually after the AMA Annual and Interim House of Delegates meetings. It includes number of representatives from state associations, members of the House of Delegates, alternative delegates, with their state or organizational affiliation, current AMA officials, and members of the councils and reference committees of the AMA.

Index: Published in the last issue of each volume (twice a year), this source indexes materials from that current volume, and some materials that are not included in other indexing sources, such as the Book Reviews, Poetry, and the JAMA covers.

Reference Directories can be found regularly in JAMA to aid in basic references to addresses of government and specialty organizations and meetings that are helpful to the health care professional. See the table of contents in each JAMA to locate the latest directory in each classification.:

- *Meetings in the United States:* is published in the first issue in every month. It is a list of meetings of medical interest, with notations as to language (if not English), display of exhibits, whether the meeting is scientific or administrative in nature, and the sponsoring organization of the event. It is not intended to be a complete list and tends to cover meetings held within, approximately, a six month period.
- *Meetings Outside the United States*: is published once per volume (twice a year), and contains similar information as the United States meeting listing.
- *State Associations and Examinations and Licensure*: is published once per volume (twice a year). Phone numbers of the Associations are not included, but addresses, information on each state association's annual meeting and the chief executive's names are. Medical Specialty Board examination date information is also included.
- *Organizations of Medical Interest*: An alphabetical listing of many specialty organizations and their addresses, including voting membership number, contact phone number, president, annual meeting date and location.

JAMA is available in several formats.
Computer fulltext database
MEDIS by Mead Data Central
9393 Springboro Pike, P.O. Box 933,
Dayton, OH 45401
800/543-6862

American
Medical
Association

American
Medical
Association

On-line databases with
both JAMA and AMNews full text
Information Access Company's "Health
Periodicals" Database
--Accessible through Dialog file 149 and Data-Star
label HLTH
Information Access Company (IAC)
362 Lakeside Drive, Foster City, CA 94404
800/227-8431

Full text CD-Rom version of JAMA available as
part of the Medical Compact Library from:
Maxwell Electronic Publishing (MEP)
1224 Mount Auburn St. Cambridge, MA 02138
617/661-2995 or 800/342-1338

The JAMA Cover
Until 1964, the JAMA cover simply listed the
contents of each issue. For a brief history on the
development the covers of JAMA:
Breo, DM. Therese Southgate, MD - The women
behind "The Cover". JAMA 1990 Apr.18: 263(15):
2107-12.

Cover essay:
JAMA. 1992 Oct 14: 268(14): 1808
M. Therese Southgate, MD

Her likeness is perhaps the most instantly
recogniziable in all of Western painting, her
portrait the most famous. It has inspired poetry,
reams of prose (not always so inspired), and even
other paintings. The author has been analyzed by
Freud, and the relationship among painter, sitter,
and sitter's husband has been speculated upon.
The mysterious smile has been dissected,
parodied, analyzed, and satirized. Her neck and
bosom have been probed with a laser beam. She
has even been criticized. Yet, after nearly 500
years she has yet to reveal her secret. All that is
known for sure is that her name is Lisa di Antonio
Maria Gherardine. She is 24 years old and she is
the wife of the prosperous Florentine citizen
Francesco del Giocondo, a man who, but for his
wife, would long ago have been forgotten. In her
portrait, she is known familiarly as Mona Lisa,
sometimes La Gioconda. The artist is the aging,
bearded Leonardo, born half a century earlier in
the nearby town of Vinci (1452-1519).

As the mother of mystery, the quintessential
enigma, neither the Mona Lisa nor its creator has
been spared the scrutiny of the centuries. The
early 20th-century French painter Marchel
Duchamp, for example, put a moustache on the
portrait and renamed it L.H.O.O.Q. Some thought
the act (and the bawdy title) sacrilegious, others
that art had at last been put in its place. Andre
Salmon agreed: "[Her smile] was for too long,
perhaps, the Sun of Art. The adoration of her is
like a decadent Christianity - peculiarly
depressing, utterly demoralising." The sculptor
George Moore said he outgrew her: "her
hesitating smile which held my youth in a little
tether has come to seem to me but a grimace."
And Renoir was simply bored.

The 19th-century Renaissance scholar Walter
Pater, on the other hand, recalls how he
succumbed to her spell: "She is older than the
rocks among which she sits; like the vampire, she
has been dead many times, and learned the
secrets of the grave." And going back to the 16th
century, while the painting was still in the state
Leonardo had intended, Georgio Vasari wrote that
"This figure of Leonard's has such a pleasant
smile that it seems rather divine than human, and
was considered marvellous, an exact copy of
nature." A compliment of another sort came from
whoever stole the portrait from the Louvre in
1911. It was not returned until two years later. But
the sincerest judgment is from Leonardo himself.
He lavished three years on the portrait, meanwhile
relieving the tedium of the sittings by engaging, as
Vasari recounts, "people to play and sing, and
jesters to keep her merry, and remove that
melancholy which painting usually gives to
portraits." When it was finished he decided not to
give it up. He kept it for the remaining 16 years of
his life, even taking it with them to France, where
he died in 1519 at age 67.

Millions have stood before the Mona Lisa in the
Louvre, millions more have stood before it when it
visited New York City and Washington, DC. Every
last manifestation of Leonardo's genius has been
remarked upon - from the innovative pose to the
perfect hands, from the hair on the shoulder
whose tendrils blend with the rocky outcropping
on the left to the highlighted shawl over the left
shoulder that leads to the bridge on the right, from
the deepening blue as the landscape recedes into
the distance to the smoky "sfumato" veil Leonardo
has placed between the viewer and figure.
Parallels have been drawn between woman and
earth, to the female figure as generative
nourished by a background that is nutritive. She
has been thought to be pregnant or to be
recovering from a paralysis of the facial nerve.
She is thought once to have been wearing a
necklace, which Leonardo removed.

There are 500 years of speculation, examination,
and analyses of the Mona Lisa. Yet, in spite of the
fact that the paint has been subject to age and to
sometimes inept cleanings, in spite of the fact that
today one can view the painting only through
glass or in not-so-accurate reproductions, the fact
remains that the Mona Lisa is universally
recognized as a masterpiece and her author as a
universal genius. Yet no one has fathomed the
painting's ultimate mystery: What is a
masterpiece? Perhaps that is why she still smiles.

Publishing

The Publishing group provides for the production,
distribution, and financial support of JAMA,
AMNews, and the ten specialty journals.
Departments here include Custom Publications
and Communications Sales and Activites for
JAMA, AMNews and the Specialty Journals.

*Contact for author or multiple copies of
reprints (i.e. copies of articles from AMA
periodicals on high quality stock):
312-464-2123*

Public Relations

Strengthening the AMA's communications outreach to the news, media, the Federation, the public, and the profession is the key element of the public relations program. The Association -wide adoption of a communications plan enables the AMA to focus its attention on major public health issues(violence, AIDS, substance abuse, and biomedical research), public advocacy, and professionalism. As the public's interest in health and medical information continues to expand, media relations activities, speech-writing, and science news, dissemination will also increase out of Public Relations. The addition of a New York office gives the AMA daily visibility among the major print and broadcast media in the New York City area. Continued emphasis in this area is placed on scheduling Officers and Trustees in key regional cities for media visits during each year. The goal of better communication with Federation public relations staffs will enhance a united front with the various audiences the AMA serves. The Division of Public Information, with its conferences for science writers and health reporters, aids in assuring quality of medical news reporting. The Departments of Internal Communication and Issues Management, and News and Information are also a part of the public relations area.

Department of Physician Licencure and Career Resources aids physicians seeking full time employment opportunities by registering them for the Placement Service by completing an application available through the department. This information is then converted into a professional curriculum vitae and is made available to clients registered with the Recruiting Service. The Placement Service also promotes several career related products, including NCVS.

The Recruiting Service provides physicians and recruiting organizations with a resource to identify prospective candidates for long-term and locum tenens recruitment. As of 1993, the recruitment aspect of the Locum Tenens Service is handled by the Recruiting Service. The Recruiting Service will improve product delivery through the development of an electronic bulletin board service, which will cut printing costs for the Physician Placement Register by fifty percent.

To contact the Physician Placement Register, locate Practices for Sale/Transfer or find out more about Recruiting Services: 800/955-3565

Departmental publications include:
Leaving the Bedside

American Medical News

(AMNews) is the Association's weekly socioeconomic newspaper. It aims to be first and best at interpreting for physicians what is happening and what is ahead in their profession. It provides, timely, credible, and balanced reporting on issues in medicine and health care that is unavailable in a similar format. Articles appear in four sections, The "News" section covers issues, events, and trends in medicine, the "Business" section offers practice managaement

advise and business coverage geared specifically toward physicians' concerns. The "Feature" section includes articles highlighting people, programs, and trends that explore the personal side of medicine. The "Commentary" section includes editorials, letters-to-the-editor, and op-ed pieces. AMNews is indexed annually, and is available full text on-line via Dialog.

Consumer Affairs and Corporate Relations

Educating consumers to lead healthier lives has always been an integral part of the AMA's mission. What distinguishes the present Consumer Affairs program from previous initiatives is its objective to establish a more direct and individual relationship between the Association and consumers. This is being accomplished on a variety of levels and through a diversity of activities including the Consumer Book Program, a weekly television program on consumer health, a test for a consumer health magazine, national health campaigns, and the development of a consumer affinity group.

Division of Consumer Books

Since 1977, more than 10 million copies of AMA consumer books have been purchased, including the *AMA Family Medical Guide*, *AMA Encyclopedia of Medicine*, and the *AMA Home Medical Library*. In September, 1991, the AMA began airing its weekly consumer television programming, "Health Styles" and "Living Well America!". In 1992, an AMA consumer health magazine, *Living Well*, had been tested as an insert in the March issue of *Good Housekeeping* that year and as a freestanding issue on newsstands in April of 1992s. The Fat/Cholesterol Education Program and Women's Health Campaign continue to research wide audiences. A Smoking Cessation Program, "Stop for Good," and Children's Health Campaign has also been launched by this area.

American Medical Radio News provides radio stations, not the public or physicians, with a daily, sixty-second news report and a monthly feature report on a medical or health-related topic. Nearly, 1,000 radio stations receive the reports via telephone or satellite hook-up, one-third of which use the reports three or more times per week. Physicians who wish to rent a FM receiver should contact the Physicians' Radio Network at 203/324-1700.

Contact for general information: 800/448-9384

Division of Television, Radio, and Film Services
American Medical Television
In February of 1992, the AMA entered into a unique partnership with NBC's Division of Cable to provide ten hours a week of physician and consumer television programming on CNBC. Under the partnership agreement, American Medical Television (AMT) will enhance the Association's communications effectiveness. AMT's professional programming mix includes items that emphasize news from areas of interest in Washington D.C., news debate and commentatry regarding clinical issues, and special

American

Medical

Association

American Medical Association

programming on topics impacting the practice of medicine. AMT, through its association with the AMA, is also a primary source of health news and information for the public by delivering four hours of entertaining and useful consumer health and lifestyle programming each week.

Various descriptions of initiatives of this division follow.

• *Women's Health Campaign* is a public health education sponsored by the AMA in conjunction with Feeling Fine, Inc. The program is designed to meet specific health needs of women by providing physicians with information on how to help women patients obtain and maintain good health. In addition, self-instructional materials will be developed, courses will be offered locally, and television programs and public advertisements will be produced.

• *AMA Video Journal* is a bimonthly video newsmagazine that is distributed to Hospital Medical Staff Services (HMSS) representatives in 2,000 hospitals nationwide in addition to the Federation. Each Journal highlights what physicians in the hospital setting need to know about a current medical topic, including clinical, regulatory, and practice issues. The concise eight-to-ten minute format can inform physicians while raising the profile of the AMA in the hospital medical staff setting.

• "Living Well America's" written component is **"Living Well!"**, a consumer health magazine published by Hearst in cooperation with the AMA. It is targeted to adults and provides sound, timely healthcare information of use to Americans and their families. If taken on as a regular AMA pulbication it will provide a means for consumers to communicate with the AMA through reader feedback mechanisms. The magazine will feature articles on nutrition, aging exercise, psychology, child care, disease, and medical research. Content of the magazine will be subject to review by the AMA's medical editor.

• To address the needs of Continuing Medical Education that today's physicians face, several initiaves have been developed including "Video Digest, American Medical Television" (Monthly video subscription offers CME credit.

Contact for more information on AMT programs and services : 800-933-4AMT (800-933-4268)

Physician Advisory Panel on Radio, Television and Motion pictures offers medical and technical assistance to the radio, TV and motion picture industries.

Group on Special Projects

Health Access America is the American Medical Association's proposal to reform the American health care system. This program is the on-going development of the proposal and its promotion. Projects include advertising specific to HAA promotion, the development of print material and video material, press conferences, media tours, congressional seminars, policy research, and various additional promotional projects.

The AMA Plan: Health Access America
(The Following Report was issued by the American Medical Association in January, 1993.)

Key Access Mechanism
• Require phase-in of employer-provided health insurance for all full-time employees and dependents, with tax-based incentives and assistance for employers, and
• expand COBRA continuation coverage to require employers to continue to share payment for 4 months
• require employers to offer enrollment period for employees who lost spouse's coverage
• Encourage individuals to establish health IRAs.

Secondary Mechanism
• Medicaid coverage to all below 100% of poverty, with payment at Medicare levels and national basic benefits coverage.
• State sliding-scale health insurance premium subsidies to those between 100 and 150% of poverty.
• No balance billing below 200% of poverty.
• Federal incentives for state risk pools for medically uninsurable and others to whom coverage in unavailable, including small employers, and
• amend ERISA to require self-insured employers to participate in risk pools
• require that businesses have access to basic benefits insurance at group rates

Insurance
• Prohibit exclusion of pre-existing conditions.
• Require community rating for small groups. Allow employment mobility without health insurance waiting periods.
• Preempt state-mandated benefits laws to make small business basic benefit plans affordable.
• Amend ERISA or tax code so state insurance standards also apply to self-insured plans.
• Make permanent and increase to 100% the self-employed deduction for health insurance costs.
• Require every insurer to offer minimum benefits plans in benefit payment schedule version, UCR version, and prepaid/managed care version.

Cost Containment
• Establish practice parameters developed by the profession to assure appropriate medical care, thus limiting costs; recognize appropriateness of payment delay pending peer-to-peer review for med avcs outside parameters.
• Empower consumer decision-making by providing price/cost information before MD and other provider services are given and health insurance is purchased.
• Limit tax deduction for employer-provider health insurance to 133-150% of cost in geographic are of AMA minimum benefits plan so that economy in health care choice is rewarded.
• Cost-sharing including copayments and deductibles to encourage greater consumer decision making.

Financing

- $9 billion a year from general revenues, after reductions from increased consumer-oriented health care decision-making, liability reform, and administrative cost savings.

Medicare Reform

- Enact Medicare reform by changing it to a prefunded program, with vouchers for individuals to purchase health insurance.
- All Medicare funds to be placed in trust funds to be administered by federal reserve-type board independent of Congressional budget review.
- Medicare must negotiate payment schedule conversion factor for physician services with AMA.
- No charges beyond negotiated rate for those below 200% of poverty.

Long-Term Care

- Expand LTC financing through public-private "asset protection" approach, relying on Medicaid when individual insurance depleted; allow penalty-free withdrawals; and allow 100% deduction for LTC insurance costs.

Liability Reform

- Reduce health care cost through professional liability reform, including federal incentives for state adoption of alternative dispute resolution systems and federal adoption of:
- $250,000 limitation on noneconomic damages
- mandatory offset of collateral sources
- sliding-scale limits on attorney contingency fees
- periodic payment of future awards
- limiting statutes of limitations for minors
- requiring certificate of merit before filing medical liability cases
- medical expert witness criteria.

Other

- Reduce administrative costs: require use of HCFA 1500 form and standard electronic claims.
- Expand federal support for medical education, research, and NIH.
- Encourage health promotion and disease prevention.
- Authorize medical societies to operate programs to review patient complaints about fees and services.
- Regulate conduct of utilization/managed care programs to reduce "Hassle quotient." (PMG)

Publications associated with this program include:

Health Policy Agenda for the American People, a three volume set. A summary report of that publication is also available.

American

Medical

Association

References

ABS *Statistical Abstract of the United States*
U.S. Census Bureau. U.S. Government Printing Office.
Washington, DC: 1992.

ACC *Accreditation Manual*
American Medical Association, Committee on Allied Health
Education and Accreditation. American Medical Association.
Chicago: 1988.

ADK *America's Adolescents: How Healthy Are They?*
Janet E. Gans, PhD, et al. American Medical Association.
Chicago: 1990.

AGE *American Medicine Comes of Age 1840-1920*
Lester S. King, MD. American Medical Association. Chicago:
1984.

ALL *Allied Health Directory*
American Medical Association, Committee on Allied Health
Education and Accreditation. American Medical Association.
Chicago: 1992.

ALT *Reader's Guide to Alternative Health Methods*
Arthur W. Hafner, PhD, editor, et al. American Medical
Association. Chicago: 1993.

ANF *Let's Give America the Facts*
American Medical Association. American Medical
Association. Chicago: 1987.

BED *Leaving the Bedside: The Search for a Nonclinical
Medical Career*
American Medical Association Department of Physician
Licensure and Career Resources. American Medical
Association. Chicago: 1992.

BIB *Bibliography of the History of Medicine*
U.S. Public Health Service. US Department of Health and
Human Services. Bethesda, MD: 1992

BUS *The Business Side of Medical Practice*
American Medical Association, Department of Practice
Service. American Medical Association. Chicago: 1989

BUY *Buying and Selling Medical Practices:
A Valuation Guide*
American Medical Association, Department of Practice
Development Resources. American Medical Association.
Chicago: 1990.

CHD *Child Abuse and Neglect: A Medical
Community Response*
Valerie L. Vivian. American Medical Association.
Chicago: 1985.

CHO *Choosing Your Physician*
American Medical Association. (Brochure).

CLO *Closing Your Practice*
American Medical Association, Department of Practice
Development Resources. American Medical Association.
Chicago: 1988.

CJS *A Proposed Alternative to the Civil Justice System for
Resolving Medical Liability Disputes: A Fault-Based,
Administrative System*
American Medical Association, Specialty Society Medical
Liability Project. American Medical Association. Chicago:
1988.

COM *The Competitive Edge*
American Medical Association Department of Practice
Management. American Medical Association. Chicago: 1987.

CPT *CPT Assistant*
American Medical Association. American Medical
Association. Chicago: (Serial)

DEA *Drug Evaluations Annual 1992*
American Medical Association Division of Drugs and
Toxicology. American Medical Association. Chicago: 1992.

DIR *Directory of Practice Parameters*
American Medical Association Office of Quality Assurance.
American Medical Association. Chicago: 1990.

DOT *Dictionary of Occupational Titles*
U.S. Department of Labor, Employment and Training
Administration. U.S. Department of Labor. 1991.

ENC *American Medical Association Encyclopedia
of Medicine*
Charles B. Clayman MD., editor. American Medical
Association.Chicago: 1989.

ENH *Enhancing the Value of Your Medical Practice*
American Medical Association Department of Practice
Development Resources. American Medical Association.
Chicago: 1990.

EST *Establishing Freestanding Ambulatory Surgery Centers*
American Medical Association Division of Professional
Relations. American Medical Association. Chicago: 1982.

EVL *Guides to the Evaluation of Permanent Impairment*
American Medical Association. American Medical
Association. Chicago: 1990.

FAM *The Role of the Family Physician in Occupational
Health Care*
American Medical Association, Environmental and
Occupational Health Program. American Medical
Association. Chicago: 1984.

FIN *Financing a Medical Practice: Start-Up,
Acquisition, or Expansion*
American Medical Association Department of Practice
Development Resources. American Medical Association.
Chicago: 1991.

FOR *Forms of Medical Practice*
American Medical Association Office of the General
Counsel. American Medical Association. Chicago: 1983.

GME *Directory of Graduate Medical Education Programs*
American Medical Association. American Medical
Association. Chicago: 1992.

GRE *Guidebook For Medical Society Grievance
Committees and Disciplinary Committees*
American Medical Association Office of General Counsel.
American Medical Association. Chicago: 1991.

HDS *Physicians' Resource Guide to Health
Delivery Systems*
American Medical Association, Group on Health Services
Policy. American Medical Association. Chicago: 1988.

HIV *HIV Infection and Disease*
Norbert Rapoza, PhD, editor. American Medical
Association, Division of Drugs and Toxicology. American
Medical Association. Chicago: 1989.

HJV *Physician-Hospital Joint Ventures*
American Medical Association, Office of the General
Counsel, Division of Medicolegal Affairs. American Medical
Association. Chicago: 1986.

HMS *Organization: A Guide for Hospital Medical Staffs*
American Medical Association Department of Hospital
Standards and Procedures, Division of Professional
Relations. American Medical Association. Chicago: 1985.

HOM *Physician Guide to Home Health Care*
American Medical Association, Group on Health Service
Policy. American Medical Association. Chicago: 1989.

ICD *The International Classification of Diseases*
U.S. Health Care Financing Administration. U.S. Department
of Health and Human Services. U.S. Government Printing
Office. Washington, DC: 1989.

LIA *Professional Liability in the '80s*
American Medical Association, Special Task Force on
Professional Liability and Insurance. American Medical
Association. Chicago: 1985.

LIC *U.S. Medical Licensure Statistics and Current
Licensure Requirements*
Catherine M. Bidese. American Medical Association
Department of Physician Licensure and Career Resources.
American Medical Association. Chicago: 1992.

LOC *A Guide to Locum Tenens Recruitment*
American Medical Association.

LTH *Let's Talk About Health Insurance*
American Medical Association Division of Health Policy and
Program Evaluation. American Medical Association.
Chicago: 1985.

MDG *Medical Groups in the United States*
American Medical Association. American Medical
Association. Chicago: 1993.

MEM *Member Matters*
American Medical Association. (Newsletter).

MMP *Measuring Medical Practice*
American Medical Association Division of Health Policy and
Program Evaluation. American Medical Association.
Chicago: 1987.

MPP *Medicare Physician Payment Reform:
The Physicians' Guide*
American Medical Association. American Medical
Association. Chicago: 1992.

MSP *Marketing Strategies for Private Practice*
American Medical Association Department of Practice
Management. American Medical Association. Chicago: 1983.

OHS *Occupational Health Services: A Practical Approach*
Tee L. Guidotti, MD, et al. American Medical Association.
Chicago: 1989.

OME *Guiding Principles for Occupational
Medical Examinations*
American Medical Association Environmental and
Occupational Health Program. American Medical
Association. Chicago: 1984.

PCD *Physician Characteristics and Distribution in the U.S.*
American Medical Association, Division of Survey Data
Resources. American Medical Association. Chicago: 1992.

PHM *Physician Marketplace Statistics 1992*
American Medical Association, Center for Health Policy
Research. American Medical Association. Chicago: 1992.

PMF *Planning Guide for Physicians' Medical Facilities*
American Medical Association. American Medical
Association. Chicago: 1986.

PMG *Physicians' Medicare Guide*
American Medical Association. Commerce Clearinghouse.
Chicago: 1992.

PRO *A Physician's Guide to Professional Corporations*
Alton C. Ward, et al. American Medical Association,
Department of Practice Development Resources. American
Medical Association. Chicago: 1989.

PSM *Compendium of Patient Safety and Medical Risk
Management Programs*
American Medical Association, Specialty Society Medical
Liability Project. American Medical Association. Chicago:
1988.

PSU *Physician Supply and Utilization by Specialty:
Trends and Projections*
William D. Marder, et al. American Medical Association.
Chicago: 1988.

QAR *Q.A. Review*
American Medical Association. American Medical
Association. Chicago: (Serial).

SCA *State and County Medical Associations
Directory of Activities*
American Medical Association, Division of Medical Society
Relations. American Medical Association. Chicago: 1984.

SCM *Socioeconomic Characteristics of Medical
Practice 1992*
Center for Health Policy Research. American Medical
Association. Chicago: 1992.

SMP *Sexual Problems in Medical Practice*
Harold I. Lief, MD (editor). American Medical Association.
Chicago: 1981.

SPI *What Every Physician's Spouse Should
Know...Impairment*
American Medical Association Auxiliary. 1986 (Brochure).

SPP *What Every Physician's Spouse Should
Know...Professional Liability*
American Medical Association Auxiliary. 1986 (Brochure).

SPR *A Compendium of State Peer Review Immunity Laws*
American Medical Association. American Medical
Association. Chicago: 1988.

STY *American Medical Association Manual of Style*
Cheryl Iverson, chair, et al. William and Wilkins. Baltimore:
1989.

USG *The United States Government Manual*
Office of the Federal Register, National Archives and
Records Administration. U.S. Government Printing Office.
Washington, DC: 1992.

VIO *Violence: A Compendium*
George D. Lundberg, MD, et al. American Medical
Association. Chicago: 1992.

WOR *The Physician and Workers' Compensation*
American Medical Association, Environmental and
Occupational Health Program. American Medical
Association. Chicago: 1983.

WRT *Good Scientific Writing*
Charles G. Roland, MD. American Medical Association.
Chicago: 1983.

WIM *Women in Medicine in America: In the Mainstream.*
American Medical Association. American Medical
Association. Chicago: 1991.

INDEX

A

Abbreviated injury scale, 1
Abbreviations
 Medicare specialty codes, 1-2
 specialties (self-designation), 1-2
Abdomen
 ultrasonic imaging, 294
Abdominal Surgeons, American Society of, 2
Abdominal surgery, 2
Abnormalities
 birth defects, 29
 cleft palate, 47
 DES (diethylstilbestrol) and, 65-67
 kidney disease, 125
 wrongful life (bibliography), 26
Abortion
 ACOG policy, 3
 AMA policy, 2
 before and after Roe v Wade (Council on Scientific
  Affairs report), 334
 mortality and morbidity, 2-3
Abortion clinic referrals, 3
Absorptiometry
 bone density measurement (DATTA opinions), 350
 dual photon (Health Technology Assessment Reports),
  288
 dual-energy x-ray (DEXA), 350
 radiographic (Health Technology Assessment Reports),
  287
 single photon (Health Technology Assessment Reports),
  288
Abstracts, 241
Academic Health Centers, Association of, 3
Academic Physiatrists, Association of, 202
Academy of Psychosomatic Medicine, 231
Academy of Rehabilitative Audiology, 21
Accent reduction, 3
Accident prevention
 auto seat belts, 255-256
 drunk driving, 73
 national injury information clearinghouse, 116
 product safety, 223
Accident statistics, 281
Accidents, Traffic
 abbreviated injury scale, 1
 auto seat belts, 255-256
 automobile safety, 21, 255-256
ACCME, see Accreditation Council for Continuing Medical
  Education
"Accomplices" (JAMA "A Piece of My Mind"), 255
Accreditation Association for Ambulatory Health Care, 16-17
Accreditation Council for Continuing Medical Education, 3,
  54, 356
Accreditation Council for Graduate Medical Education, 93,
  355-356
 Transitional Year Review Committee, 290
Accreditation Manual for Hospitals, 108
Accreditation, Medical, 3, see also Allied health education
  and accreditation; Ambulatory care; Continuing medical
  education; Graduate medical education; Medical education;
Accrediting Commission on Education for Health Services
  Administration, 99
ACGME, see Accreditation Council for Graduate Medical
  Education
Acne, 3

Acoustic neuroma (bibliography), 24
Acoustic Neuroma Association, 3
Acquired immunodeficiency syndrome, 9-12
 AMA Health Science Division, 333
 AMA HIV/AIDS Office, 333
 case definition, 12
 health professionals' information and referrals
  (Chicago), 10
 history of the epidemic, 103-104
 HIV monographs, 104
 HTLV III (Council on Scientific Affairs report), 344
 national and statewide hotlines, 9-12
 nutrition and (bibliography), 23
 public education and information, 9-12
 stages of HIV infection, 103-104
 statistics, 10
 surrogate HIV markers (DATTA opinions), 350
Activated prothrombin-complex concentrate (Health
  Technology Assessment Reports), 290
Actual charge (Medicare terminology), 164
Acupuncture, National Commission for the Certification
  for, 4
Acupuncture, 3-4
Ad damnum clause (tort reform glossary), 228
Addiction Medicine, American Society on, 4, 13
Addiction Medicine/Addictionolgy, 4
Adjusted average per capita cost (Medicare terminology),
  164
Adjusted historical payment basis (Medicare terminology),
  164
Administration on Aging (US), 7
Admissions
 preadmission criteria, 221
Adolescence, 4-6
 AIDS hotline, 10
 alcoholism (bibliography), 23
 homeless, 108
 pregnancy, 5
 psychiatry, 229
 school-based health centers, 257
 sexuality, 4-5
 suicide (bibliography), 25
Adolescent Health, Commission on the Role of the School
  and the Community in Improving, 5
Adoption Center, National, 6
Adoption, 6
Advance directives (living wills, powers of attorney), 140
Advancement of Science, American Association for the, 257
Adverse selection (Medicare terminology), 164
Advertising, see also Marketing; Radio; Television
 complaints about, 52
 developing a marketing program, 145
 health fraud, 97
 tobacco (magazines banning), 267-271
Advisors for the Health Professions, National Association
  of, Inc, 42
Aerobics and Fitness Association of America, 84
Aerospace Medical Association, 6, 21
Aerospace Medicine
 certification, 6
 pilot physical examinations, 202
Aesculapius, Staff of, 6-7
Aetna Health Plans, 219
African-American physicians
 Black Psychiatrists of America, 230
 National Medical Association, 80
African-Americans

black-white disparities in care, 172

Agency for Healthcare Policy Research (US)
pain management guidelines, 197

Aging
abuse of, 70-71
elder abuse, 70-71
elderly health (Council on Scientific Affairs reports), 336, 337, 341
exercise and (bibliography), 25
medication and (two bibliographies), 25
nursing homes, 182
organizations, information on, 7
sleep disorders (bibliography), 24
state departments of, 7-9

"Aging and Caring" (JAMA "A Piece of My Mind"), 88

Agoraphobia
bibliography, 23
description, 202

Agricultural Library, National, 134

Agriculture Department (US), 182

Agriculture, 134, 335

AHCPR reports, 287-290

AHEPA Cooley's Anemia Foundation, 55

AIDS Foundation of Chicago, 10

AIDS, see Acquired immunodeficiency syndrome

Air pollution
bibliography, 26
concerned agencies, organizations, 13

Air-fluidized bed therapy (Health Technology Assessment Reports), 287

Aircraft, see Aviation

AL-ANON Family Group Headquarters, 13

Alabama (information on various health and social services in this and other states may be found at the heading, State agencies and organizations)

Alaska (information on various health and social services in this and other states may be found at the heading, State agencies and organizations)

Albany (New York) County Medical Society, 314

Alcohol
drivers and (Council on Scientific Affairs report), 343
drunk driving, 13, 73

Alcohol Education For Youth, 13

Alcohol Information, National Clearinghouse for, 13

Alcoholics Anonymous
physicians in, 113
World Services, 13

Alcoholism
adolescent (bibliography), 23
AMA policy, 13
aversion therapy (Health Technology Assessment Reports), 289
Betty Ford Center, 23
chemical aversion therapy (Health Technology Assessment Reports), 287
drunk driving, 13, 73, 343
electroversion therapy (Health Technology Assessment Reports), 289
employee assistance programs, 77-78
family and (bibliography), 25
impaired physicians, 113-115
organizations listed, 13

Alcoholism, National Council on, 13

Allergy
asthma, 19
organizations listed, 13-14
otolaryngic, 195
testing and immunotherapy (Council on Scientific Affairs reports), 342

Allergy and Immunology, American Academy of, 13, 19

Allergy and Immunology, American Board of, 13, 113

Allergy and Immunology, American College of, 13

Alliance for Engineering in Medicine and Biology, 29

Alliance of American Insurers, 116, 226

Allied health education and accreditation, see also names of specific allied-health professions, e.g., Anesthesiologist's assistants
AMA educational and accreditation activities, 356
Allied Health Education Directory, 16
process, CAHEA role, 14-16
recommended books, 32

Allied Health Personnel in Ophthalmology, American Association of Certified, 190

Allied Health Professions, American Society of, 16

Almond, Eudora B, 68-69

Alopecia Areata Foundation, National, 95

Alopecia areata, 95

Alpha-fetoprotein testing (DATTA opinions), 352

Alpha-interferon (DATTA opinions), 351

ALS (Amyotrophic lateral sclerosis), 17

Alternative medicine, 97

Aluminum toxicity, 288

Alzheimer's disease
bibliography, 24
organizations listed, 16

Alzheimer's Disease and Related Disorders Association, 16, 32

AMA, see American Medical Association

AMA-ERF, 333

AMA-FREIDA, 93

AMACO, 226

Ambulance Association, American, 16

Ambulances, 16

Ambulatory care
accreditation, 16
anesthesiology, 18
free clinics, 49
organizations listed, 16-17
surgery, 16

Ambulatory Care, National Association for, 17

Ambulatory Pediatric Association, 199

Ambulatory Plastic Surgery Facilities, American Association for Accreditation of, Inc, 16-17, 213

American Academy for Cerebral Palsy and Developmental Medicine, 43

American Academy of Allergy and Immunology, 13, 19

American Academy of Anesthesiologists' Assistants, 18

American Academy of Child and Adolescent Psychiatry, 4, 229

American Academy of Clinical Psychiatrists, 229

American Academy of Dermatology, 61

American Academy of Disability Evaluating Physicians, 67

American Academy of Environmental Medicine, 79

American Academy of Facial Plastic and Reconstructive Surgery, 213

American Academy of Family Physicians, 5, 85

American Academy of Medical Acupuncturists, 4

American Academy of Medical Directors, 42, 84

American Academy of Neurological Surgery, 176

American Academy of Neurology, 177

American Academy of Nurse Practitioners, 179

American Academy of Ophthalmology, 127, 190

American Academy of Orthopaedic Surgeons, 194

American Academy of Orthotists and Prosthetists, 194, 229

American Academy of Otolaryngic Allergy, 195

American Academy of Otolaryngology--Head and Neck Surgery
address, 195
"Facial Nerve Problems," 23
resident matching program, 146

American Academy of Pain Medicine, 197

American Academy of Pediatrics

address, 199
adolescent health, 4
"Healthy Children" program, 5
HIV-infected children, 12
immunization information, 113
American Academy of Physical Medicine and Rehabilitation, 202, 248
American Academy of Physician's Assistants, 207
American Academy of Psychiatry and the Law, 229
American Academy of Psychoanalysis, 231
American Academy of Thermology, 290
American Alliance for Health, Physical Education, Recreation and Dance, 9
American Ambulance Association, 16
American Amputee Foundation, Inc, 17
American Art Therapy Association, 19
American Association for Accreditation of Ambulatory Plastic Surgery Facilities, Inc, 16-17, 213
American Association for Hand Surgery, 95
American Association for International Aging, 7
American Association for Laboratory Animal Science, 18
American Association for Medical Systems, 52
American Association for Medical Transcription, 156
American Association for Physicists in Medicine, 212
American Association for Respiratory Care, 251
American Association for the Advancement of Science, 257
American Association for the History of Medicine, 103
American Association for the Study of Liver Disease, 140
American Association for the Study of the Headache, 95
American Association for Thoracic Surgery, 290
American Association of Automotive Medicine, 1
American Association of Blood Banks, 30
American Association of Cardiovascular and Pulmonary Rehabilitation, 234
American Association of Certified Allied Health Personnel in Ophthalmology, 190
American Association of Clinical Urologists, Inc, 295
American Association of Colleges of Nursing, 179
American Association of Electromyography and Electrodiagnosis, 76
American Association of Gynecologic Laparoscopists, 94, 183
American Association of Healthcare Consultants, 52
American Association of Homes for the Aging, 182
American Association of Kidney Patients, 125
American Association of Marriage and Family Therapy, 145
American Association of Medical Society Executives, 84
American Association of Naturopathic Physicians, 176
American Association of Nephrology Nurses and Technicians, 65
American Association of Neurological Surgeons
address, 176
spinal cord injury prevention, 5
American Association of Nurse Attorneys, 178
American Association of Pathologists, 198
American Association of Physicians for Human Rights, 214
American Association of Physicians of India, 81
American Association of Plastic Surgeons, 213
American Association of Poison Control Centers, 213
American Association of Preferred Providers, 222
American Association of Public Health Physicians, 232
American Association of Retired Persons, 251
American Association of Tissue Banks, 290
American Association on Mental Retardation, 172
American Back Society, 23
American Bar Association, 127-128
American Board for Certification in Orthotics and Prosthetics, 194, 229
American Board of Allergy and Immunology, 13, 113
American Board of Anesthesiology
anesthesiologist certification, 18

critical care certification, 55
pain management certification, 197
American Board of Colon and Rectal Surgery, 50
American Board of Dermatology, 61
American Board of Emergency Medicine, 77
American Board of Family Practice
family practice certification, 85
geriatrics board certification, 89
sports medicine certification, 277
American Board of Forensic Psychiatry, 86
American Board of Internal Medicine
cardiovascular disease certification, 39, 102
critical care certification, 55
endocrinology and metabolism certification, 78
geriatrics board certification, 89
hematology certification, 102
infectious disease certification, 115
internal medicine and subspecialy certification, 120
nephrology certification, 176
oncology certification, 189
pulmonary disease certification, 234
rheumatology certification, 252
American Board of Medical Specialties
Doctor Certification Line, 55
specialists' compendium, 273
American Board of Neurological Surgery
critical care certification, 55
neurosurgery certification, 177
American Board of Nuclear Medicine, 177
American Board of Obstetrics and Gynecology, 94, 183
critical care certification, 55
oncology certification, 189
reproductive endocrinology certification, 78
American Board of Ophthalmology, 190
American Board of Orthopaedic Surgery
hand surgery certification, 95
orthopedics certification, 194
American Board of Otolaryngology, 195
American Board of Pathology
blood banking, transfusion medicine, 30
forensic pathology, 30
hematology certification, 102
American Board of Pediatrics
critical care certification, 55
infectious disease certification, 115
pediatric and subspecialty certification, 199
American Board of Physical Medicine and Rehabilitation, 202, 248
American Board of Plastic Surgery
hand surgery certification, 95
plastic surgery certification, 213
American Board of Podiatric Orthopedics, 213
American Board of Podiatric Public Health, 213
American Board of Podiatric Surgery, 213
American Board of Preventive Medicine
aerospace medicine certification, 6, 21
occupational medicine certification, 186
undersea medicine certification, 294
American Board of Professional Psychologists, 231
American Board of Psychiatry and Neurology, 177, 229
American Board of Quality Assurance and Utilization Review Physicians, 235
American Board of Radiology
chemotherapy certification, 43
radiation oncology certification, 189
radiologist certification, 238
American Board of Surgery
critical care certification, 55
hand surgery certification, 95
surgery and subspecialty certification, 283

vascular surgery certification, 297
American Board of Thoracic Surgery, 290
American Board of Urology, 295
American Brittle Bone Society, 195
American Burn Association, 35
American Cancer Society
    national headquarters, 37
    statewide societies, 37-39
American Chiropractic Association, 46
American Cleft Palate Association, 47
American Cleft Palate Educational Foundation, 47
American College Health Association, 50
American College of Allergy and Immunology, 13
American College of Angiology, 39, 102
American College of Cardiology, 39, 102
American College of Chest Physicians, 234
American College of Cryosurgery, 55
American College of Emergency Physicians, 77, 290
American College of Gastroenterology, 87
American College of Healthcare Executives, 84
American College of International Physicians, 122, 123
American College of Legal Medicine, 128
American College of Medical Quality, 200
American College of Nuclear Medicine, 177
American College of Nuclear Physicians, 177
American College of Nurse-Midwives, 172, 178
American College of Nutrition, 182
American College of Obstetricians and Gynecologists
    abortion policy implications, 3
    adolescent pregnancy prevention, 5
    adolescent sexuality, 4-5
    contraception pamphlet, 29
    Dalkon Shield information, 59
    home births, 104
    midwifery, 172
    national headquarters, 94, 222
    pregnancy information, 183
    resident matching program, 146
    "The Abused Woman," 70
American College of Occupational Medicine
    address, 186
    drug abuse testing, 72-73
American College of Physicians
    address, 203
    recommended books, 32
American College of Preventive Medicine, 222
American College of Radiology
    address, 238
    mammography recommendations, 145
American College of Rheumatology, 252
American College of Sports Medicine, 277
American College of Surgeons, 283
American College of Utilization Review Physicians, 200
American Congress of Rehabilitation Medicine, 248
American Council for Drug Education, 71
American Council of Blind Parents, 29
American Council of the Blind, 29
American Council on Life Insurance, 139
American Council on Science and Health, 95, 96
American Council on Transplantation, 193
American Deafness and Rehabilitation Association, 99
American Dental Assistants Association, 59
American Dental Association, 59
American Dental Hygienists Association, 59
American Diabetes Association, 62
American Dietetic Association, 65
American Educational Institute, 54
American Epilepsy Society, 80
American Federation for Medical Accreditation, 3
American Federation of Home Health Agencies, 105

American Fertility Society, 85, 277
American Foundation ("Doctors to All People"), 299
American Geriatrics Society, 88
American Group Practice Association, 94
American Hair Loss Council, 95
American Health Assistance Foundation, 7
American Health Care Association, 182
American Health Information Management Association, 156
American Hearing Research Foundation, 99
American Heart Association
    CPR standards and guidelines, 40
    state affiliates, 100-102
American Holistic Medical Association, 104
American Hospital Association
    CME learning assessment form, 54
    ICD-9 Center, 122
    national headquarters, telephone information, 108
    patients' rights, 199
    Statistics Center, 281
American Indian Physicians, Association of, 80
American Indian physicians, 80
American Industrial Health Council, 115
American Industrial Hygiene Association, 115
American Institute of Ultrasound in Medicine, 294
American Insurance Agency, 116, 226
American Insurers, Alliance of, 116, 226
American Kidney Fund, 125
American Laryngological Association, 127
American Laryngological, Rhinological and Otological
    Society, 127, 252
American Leprosy Foundation, 129
American Leprosy Missions, 129
American Library Association
    library user confidentiality, 53-54
    national headquarters, 136
American Liver Foundation, 140
American Lung Association, 143
American Management Association, 145
American Marketing Association, 145
American Massage Therapy Association, 145
American Medical Association, 313-371, see also *Journal
    of the American Medical Association*
    address, general telephone number, 150
    administrative functions and divisions, 329-331
    Adolescent Health Coalition, 5
    Adolescent Health Department, 333
    Adolescent Health Department, 5, 6
    Allied Health Department (see listings for individual
        allied health professions (e.g., Anesthesiologists'
        assistants) for the telephone numbers to call in this
        department), 356
    Allied Health Education and Accreditation Division, 356
    AMA *Archives of...*, 367
    American Medical News, 369
    American Medical Political Action Committee, 361
    American Medical Radio News, 369
    American Medical Television, 369-370
    AMPAC, 361
    Annual and Interim meeting, future dates and locations,
        365
    Archives, 331
    art collection, 366
    Board of Trustees listed, 365-366
    Book Source, 330
    Burroughs Wellcome Resident Physician's Program, 363
    Center for Health Policy Research, 281, 357
    CME learning assessment form, 54
    Committee on Allied Health Education and
        Accreditation, (CAHEA), 14-16
    communications and publishing activities, 367-371
    Constitution, 327-328

consumer affairs and corporate relations, 369
Consumer Books Division, 369
Continuing Medical Education Division, 356
Corporate Facilities Division, 365
Council on Constitution and Bylaws, 327
Council on Legislation, 358
Council on Long Range Planning and Development, 358
Council on Medical Education, 355
Council on Medical Service, 357
Council on Scientific Affairs (published reports
    listed here by year), 334-349
customer services, 330
Data Resource Development Department, 329
Database Licensing Services Department, 329
DATTA (Diagnostic and Therapeutic Technology
    Assessment) program, 349-350
DATTA opinions (summaries for 1983 to first half, 1992),
    350-355
Diagnostic and Therapeutic Technology Assessment
    program (DATTA), 349-350
Drugs and Toxicology Division, 333
Federation Network (FEDNET), 364
federation relations and membership, 363-364
FEDNET, 364
financial services, 330
Foundations and Administration Office, 333
founding, history, 313-317
governance and corporate services, 365-366
government and political affairs activities, programs, 361
Health Care Technology Division, 349
health fraud collection, 331
health policy activities, programs, 357-359
Health Policy Research Division, 357
Health Science Division, 333
HIV/AIDS Department, 9
HIV/AIDS Office, 333
Hospital Medical Staff Services Department, 364
House of Delegates described, 366
House of Delegates future meetings listed, 365
human resources (personnel), 330
Information Planning and Automation Services, 329
International Medicine office, 366
legislative activities and programs, 358-359
Library and Information Management Division, 330-331
Locum Tenens Service, 369
logo (Staff of Aesculapius), 6-7
Marketing Services, Market Research, and Marketing
    Information Divisions, 330
Masterfile Information Department, 330
medical education activities, 355
Medical Education and Science divisions and
    departments, 333-356
Medical Student Services Department, 363-364
Meeting Planning and Management Department, 365
members service center, 363
Mental Health Department, 333
National Leadership Conference, 363
National Physician Credentials Verification Service, 55,
    329
newspaper (*American Medical News*), 369
Office of the General Counsel, 319
Office Services, 365
officers for 1992-1993 listed, 365
Permissions Office (use of AMA published material), 331
Physician Biographic Records, 329
Physician Data Services Department, 207, 329
Physician Placement Register, 369
Physician Professional Activities Department, 330
physician statistics, 281
Physician's Recognition Award, 356
Placement Service (practice location), 141

Policy Library, 331
Political Education Office, 361
Practice Parameters Department, 357
presidents of AMA listed, 317-319
Preventive Medicine and Public Health Department, 334
public relations activities, 369
publication reprints, 368
publishing group, 368
Quality Assurance and Medical Review Office, 357
Recruiting Service, 369
reprints of publications, 368
Resident Physicians Services, 363
scientific publications, 367
Senior (retired) Physicians Services, 251
Specialty Journals Department, 367
specialty society and professional relations, 363
Specialty Society Relations Office, 364
state and county (medical society) relations, 364
subscriber services, 330
Systems and Programming Division, 329
Technology Management Department, 355
Television, Radio and Film Services Division, 369-370
Undergraduate Medical Education, 3, 356
unified (membership) societies, 363
Video Digest (American Medical Television), 297
Washington Office, 361
Women in Medicine initiatives, 364
Young Physicians Services Department, 364
American Medical Association Alliance (Auxiliary)
    adolescent pregnancy prevention, 5
    Doctor's Day, 68-69
American Medical Association Education and Research
    Foundation, 333
American Medical Association publications, see *American
    Medical News; Journal of the American Medical
    Association*; Publications (AMA)
American Medical Assurance Company, 226
American Medical Care and Review Association, 97, 222
American Medical Directors Association, 84
American Medical Directory
    specialty abbreviations, 1-2
American Medical Electroencephalographic Association, 75
American Medical Golf Association, 20
American Medical Informatics Association, 26, 52
American Medical Joggers Association, 20
American Medical News, 369
American Medical Peer Review Association, 200
American Medical Political Action Committee, 361
American Medical Records Association, 156
American Medical Students Association, 162
American Medical Television, 369-370
    Video Digest, 297
American Medical Tennis Association, 20
American Medical Women's Association, 150, 304
American Medical Writers Association, 311
American Narcolepsy Association, 175
American National Standards Institute
    medical literature references and citations, 238-246
American Near East Refuge Aid, Inc, 71
American Nurses Association, 179
American Occupational Medical Association, 186
American Occupational Therapy Association, 189
American Optometric Association, 192
American Orthopaedic Association, 194
American Orthopaedic Society for Sports Medicine,
    194, 277
American Osteopathic Association, 194
American Otological Society, 195
American Overseas Medical Aid Association
    book donations, 31

equipment donations, 71
American Pain Society, 197
American Pancreatic Association, 197
American Paralysis Association, 197
American Parkinson Disease Association, 197
American Pediatric Surgical Association, 199
American Pharmaceutical Association, 202, 281
American Physical Therapy Association, 203
American Physicians Art Association, 19
American Physicians Poetry Association, 213
American Physicians, Association of, 203
American Physiological Society, 84, 212
American Podiatric Medical Association, 213
American Porphyria Foundation, 214
American Professional Practice Association, 141
American Psychiatric Association
    DSM III, 64
    headquarters information, 230
    resident matching program, 146
American Psychological Association, 231
American Public Health Association, 232
American Red Cross, 30, 68
    AIDS facts, 10
American Reye's Syndrome Association, 252
American Rhinologic Society, 252
American Roentgen Ray Society, 238
American Russian Medical and Dental Society, 81
American School Health Association, 257
American Seminar Institute, 55
American Sleep Disorders Association, 266
American Social Health Association, 265
    AIDS hotline, 10
American Society for Clinical Investigation, 48
American Society for Clinical Nutrition, 182
American Society for Clinical Pharmacology and
    Therapeutics, 201
American Society for Dermatologic Surgery, 61
American Society for Gastrointestinal Endoscopy, 87
American Society for Healthcare Marketing and Public
    Relations, 145
American Society for Laser Medicine and Surgery, 127
American Society for Medical Technology, 163
American Society for Parenteral and Enteral Nutrition, 182
American Society for Pharmacology and Experimental
    Therapeutics, 201
American Society for Photobiology, 202
American Society for Psychoprophylaxis in Obstetrics,
    46, 176
American Society for Surgery of the Hand, 95
American Society for Therapeutic Radiology and Oncology,
    189, 238
American Society of Abdominal Surgeons, 2
American Society of Allied Health Professions, 16
American Society of Anesthesiologists, 18
American Society of Bariatric Physicians, 183
American Society of Cataract and Refractive Surgery, 42
American Society of Clinical Hypnosis, 111
American Society of Clinical Oncology, 189
American Society of Clinical Pathologists, 198
    SI unit conversion guide, 49
American Society of Colon and Rectal Surgery, 50
American Society of Cytology, 58
American Society of Echocardiography, 75
American Society of Extra-Corporeal Technology, 201
American Society of Handicapped Physicians, 68
American Society of Hematology, 30, 102
American Society of Internal Medicine, 120
    "Understanding and Choosing Your Health
        Insurance," 118
American Society of Law and Medicine, 128
American Society of Lipo-Suction Surgery, 140

American Society of Maxillofacial Surgeons, 146
American Society of Nephrology, 125, 176
American Society of Outpatient Surgery, 16
American Society of Plastic and Reconstructive
    Surgeons, 140, 213
American Society of Radiologic Technologists, 238
American Society of Transplant Surgeons, 290
American Society of Tropical Medicine and Hygiene, 293
American Society on Addiction Medicine, 4, 13
American Speech-Language-Hearing Association, 3, 100,
    127, 277
American Spinal Injury Association, 277
American Sudden Infant Death Syndrome Institute, 282
American Thoracic Society, 290
American Thyroid Association, 290
American Tinnitus Association, 290
American Tort Reform Association, 226
American Trauma Society, 290
American Trial Lawyers Association, 226
American Urological Association, 295
American Veterinary Medical Association, 297
Americans With Disabilities Act, 95
Amigos de las Americas, 299
AMPAC, 361
Amputation
    concerned organizations listed, 17
    hyperbaric oxygen for severed limbs (Health
        Technology Assessment Reports), 288
Amputee Foundation, Inc, American, 17
Amputee Services Association, 17
Amyotrophic Lateral Sclerosis Association, 17
Amyotrophic lateral sclerosis, 17
Anabolic-androgenic steroids (Council on Scientific Affairs
    report), 337
Analgesia
    laboratory animals (bibliography), 23, 25
Anatomical charts, 20
Anatomical dolls, 17
Anatomical Gift Association, 193
Anatomy
    medical illustration, 151-152
Anemia, Cooley's, 55
Anemia, Sickle cell, 265
Anesthesia
    laboratory animals (bibliography), 23, 25
Anesthesiologists, American Society of, 18
Anesthesiologist's assistants, 17-18
Anesthesiologists' Assistants Education, Association for, 17
Anesthesiologists' Assistants, American Academy of, 18
Anesthesiology
    ambulatory, 18
    ether first used, 68-69
    medical organizations listed, 18
    nurse anesthetist, 179
Anesthesiology, American Board of,
    anesthesiologist certification, 18
    critical care certification, 55
    pain management certification, 197
Angelchick anti-reflux prosthesis 288, 354
Angiology, American College of, 39, 102
Angiology, 39, 102
Angioplasty
    lower extremity treatments (Health Technology
        Assessment Reports), 289
    percutaneous transluminal (three Health Technology
        Assessment Reports), 289
    percutaneous transluminal coronary (Health Technology
        Assessment Reports), 288
    renal artery stenotic lesions (Health Technology
        Assessment Reports), 289

single-coronary-artery stenotic lesions (Health Technology Assessment Reports), 289

Animal research
 AMA Council on Scientific Affairs report, 339
 baboon liver transplants, 290
 concerned organizations listed, 18
 lab animal care and use (1985-1989 bibliography), 25
 lab animal welfare (1988 bibliography), 25
 lab animal welfare (1988-1989 bibliography), 24
 lab animal welfare (1990 bibliography), 23
 lab animal welfare (1991 bibliography), 23
 pain, anesthesia, analgesia (bibliography), 23, 25

Animal Resource Program Branch, 18
Animal rights and research, 18
Animal therapy (pet therapy), 18, 24

Animals
 bovine somatotropin (bibliography), 24
 growth hormone (bovine somatotropin), 24
 human-pet relations (bibliography), 24
 spongiform encephalopathy transmission (bibliography), 23
 toxoplasmosis (bibliography), 25

Animals in medical education (Council on Scientific Affairs report), 335-336
Animals in research (Council on Scientific Affairs report), 339

Anorexia nervosa
 concerned organizations listed, 19

Anorexia Nervosa and Associated Disorders, 19, 34
Anorexia Nervosa and Related Eating Disorders, 19, 34
Anti-inhibitor coagulant complex (Health Technology Assessment Reports), 290
Anxiety, 19
Aortic arch, 289
APACHE II, 281

Apheresis
 chronic relapsing polyneuropathy (Health Technology Assessment Reports), 288
 Goodpasture's syndrome (Health Technology Assessment Reports), 289
 Guillain Barre syndrome (Health Technology Assessment Reports), 288
 kidney transplants (Health Technology Assessment Reports), 288
 membranous proliferative glomerulonephritis (Health Technology Assessment Reports), 289
 multiple sclerosis (Health Technology Assessment Reports), 289
 rheumatoid arthritis (Health Technology Assessment Reports), 289
 rheumatoid vasculitis therapy (Health Technology Assessment Reports), 289

Applied Physiology and Biofeedback, Association of, 29
Appointments, 211
Approved amount (Medicare terminology), 164
Aquatic Exercise Association, 84
Arbitration (tort reform glossary), 228
Architectural and Transportation Barriers Compliance Board, 95
Archives of...., 367
ArcVentures, Inc, Educational Services, 251
Argon photocoagulation, 127
Arizona (information on various health and social services in this and other states may be found at the heading, State agencies and organizations)
Arkansas (information on various health and social services in this and other states may be found at the heading, State agencies and organizations)

Art
 AMA collection, 366

Art therapists, 19
Art Therapy Association, American, 19

Arteriovenous fistula, 289

Arthritis
 description, organizations listed, 19

Arthritis Foundation, 19
Arthroscopy Association of North America, 19
Artificial organs, 19

Asbestos
 AMA policy, 19
 organizations listed, 19

Asbestos Information Association of North America, 19
Asbestos removal (Council on Scientific Affairs report), 336
Asbestos Victims of America, 19
Asian-American Medical Society, 80
ASIM, see American Society of Internal Medicine
Asklepios, 7
Aspartame, 24, 344

Aspirin
 Reye's syndrome, 252

Assault weapons (Council on Scientific Affairs report), 334
Assisted suicide, see Suicide assistance
Association for Anesthesiologists' Assistants Education, 17
Association for Brain Tumor Research, 32
Association for Macular Diseases, 145
Association for the Advancement of Automotive Medicine, 21
Association for the Advancement of Medical Instrumentation, 61
Association for the Care of Children's Health, 46
Association Medicale Mondiale, 151
Association of Academic Health Centers, 3
Association of Academic Physiatrists, 202
Association of American Indian Physicians, 80

Association of American Medical Colleges
 headquarters information, 158
 medical career information, 42
 registration for medical school entrance exam, 162

Association of American Physicians, 203
Association of Applied Physiology and Biofeedback, 29
Association of Birth Defect Children, 29
Association of Community Cancer Centers, 37
Association of Life Insurance Medical Directors of America, 139
Association of Medical Illustrators, 152
Association of Military Surgeons of the United States, 172
Association of Organ Procurement Organizations, 193
Association of Pakistani Physicians, 81
Association of Philippine Physicians in America, 81
Association of Philippine Surgeons in America, 81
Association of State and Territorial Health Officials, 99
Association of Surgical Technologists, 285
Association of the Schools of Public Health, 232
Association of Trial Lawyer of America, 226
Association of University Programs in Health Administration, 95
Association to Aid Fat Americans, National, 183

Asthma
 lung diseases described, 142
 organizations listed, 19

Asthma and Allergy Foundation of America, 19
Asthma Center, National, 19
Ataxia Foundation, National, 19
Ataxia, 19
Athletic trainer, 20
Athletic Trainers Association, National, 20
Athletics, see Sports

Attorneys
 bar associations listed, 127-128
 fees, 228
 nurse, 178

Audio Digest, 20

Audio Visual Center, National, 20
Audiologist, 20-21
Audiovisuals
    organizations having, 20
    video clinics, 297
Australian Medical Association, 150
Authorship
    medical and scientific writing, 309-311
    medical literature references and citations, 239-240
Autism Society of America, 21
Auto Safety Hotline, 256
Autogenous urine immunization (Health Technology
    Assessment Reports), 289
Autoimmune diseases, 125
Autologous transplantation, see Transplantation
Automobile Accidents, see Accidents, Traffic
Automotive Medicine, American Association of, 1
Automotive Medicine, Association for the Advancement
    of, 21
Autopsy
    AMA Council on Scientific Affairs report, 342
    John F Kennedy, 197-198
Aversion therapy
    alcohol (Health Technology Assessment Reports), 289
    AMA Council on Scientific Affairs report, 341
    chemical (Health Technology Assessment Reports), 287
Aviation
    smoking bans, 266
Aviation medicine
    Aerospace Medical Association, 6, 21
    aerospace medicine certification, 6
    pilot physical examinations, 202
Awards (tort reform glossary), 228
Awards, AMA
    Physician's Recognition Award, 356
AZT Hotline, 10

B

B-mode scan (Health Technology Assessment Reports), 289
Baboon liver transplants, 290
Baby sitting, 23
Bacillus Calmette-Guerin immunotherapy (DATTA opinions),
    353, 354
Back Society, American, 23
Back, 23
Bacterial foodborne infections (bibliography), 26
Balance billing (Medicare terminology), 164
Bar Association, American, 127-128
Bar associations, 127-128
Barbara Bush Foundation for Family Literacy, 140
Bariatric Physicians, American Society of, 183
Bariatrics, 183
Baseline adjustment (Medicare terminology), 164
BASH (Bulimia Anorexia Self Help), 19, 34
Batterers Anonymous, 69
BCG (Bacillus Calmette-Guerin) immunotherapy, 353, 354
Bed therapy
    home air-fluidized (Health Technology Assessment
        Reports), 287
Behavioral offset (Medicare terminology), 164
Bell's Palsy
    Health Technology Assessment Reports, 288, 289
    informational booklet, 23
Bentonite flocculation test (Health Technology Assessment
    Reports), 290
Better Business Bureaus
    complaints about clinics, 52
    Council of, 23

    fraudulent ads in newspapers, 97
    health product and business complaints, 23
    research grants, 37
    "Tips on Choosing a Hospital," 109
Bettman Archive, Inc, 202
Betty Ford Center, 23
Bibliographic citations (ANSI standards), 238-246
Bibliographies
    Current Bibliographies in Medicine from the National
        Library of Medicine (1988-1992), 23-26
    history of medicine, 103
Bile acid malabsorption, 288
Billing, Electronic, 26-28
Billings, John Shaw, 135
Bioethics, 28-29
Biofeedback
    DATTA opinions, 355
    description, organizational information, 29
Bioimpedance, Electrical (Health Technology Assessment
    Reports), 287
Biomedical engineering
    organizations listed, 29
Biomedical Engineering Society, 29
Biotechnology and agriculture (Council on Scientific Affairs
    report), 335
Biotin, 298
Birth, see Childbirth
Birth Control, 29
Birth Defect Children, Association of, 29
Birth defects
    cleft palate, 47
    concerned organizations listed, 29
    DES (diethylstilbestrol) and, 65-67
    kidney disease, 125
    wrongful life (bibliography), 26
Birth, see Childbirth
Blacks
    Black Psychiatrists of America, 230
    black-white disparities in care, 172
    National Medical Association, 80
Blind Parents, American Council of, 29
Blind Students, National Alliance of, 29
Blind, American Council of the, 29
Blindness, 29-30
    statewide societies, 29-30
Blindness, National Society to Prevent, 29-30, 193
Blood
    dialysis (bibliography), 26
    glucose monitors (Health Technology Assessment
        Reports), 289
    intravenous immunoglobulin (bibliography), 24
    organizations listed, 30
    red cell transfusion (bibliography), 25
    substitutes (bibliography), 24
    urine having, 125
Blood bank technologist, 31
Blood Banks, American Association of, 30
Blood pressure
    information, testing, 31
Blood pressure, High, see Hypertension
Blood tests, 31
Blood transfusions
    autologous (Council on Scientific Affairs report), 343
    transfusion medicine certification, 30
Bloodborne pathogens standards, 186-187
B-mode scan (Health Technology Assessment
    Reports), 289
Board certification, see Certification
Board of Trustees, AMA, 365-366

Body height
    growth hormones and short stature (bibliography), 25
Body weight
    height-weight tables, 301
    loss (bibliography), 23
Bolen's test (Health Technology Assessment Reports), 289
Bone marrow transplantation
    autologous (Health Technology Assessment Reports), 287, 288
    childhood leukemia (DATTA opinions), 354
    DATTA opinions 351, 352, 354
    Health Technology Assessment Reports, 288
Bone mineral density (Health Technology Assessment Reports), 287, 288, 289
Bones
    osteoporosis, 195
Book donations, 31
Books
    recommended, for small libraries, 32
    references and citations to (style guidelines), 242-243
Boswell, J Thornton, 197-198
Botulinum toxin (bibliography), 24
Bovine somatotropin (bibliography), 24
Boxing, 32
Brain
    banks, donation, 32
    donors, 16
    electroencephalography, 75
    injuries, 32
    intracranial pressure measurement (Health Technology Assessment Reports), 289
    pediatric disorders, 32
    spongiform encephalopathy transmission (bibliography), 23
    tumor, 32
Brain Research Association, National, 32
Brain Tumor Foundation, National, 32
Brain Tumor Research, Association for, 32
Breast cancer
    bibliography, 24
    concerned organizations listed, 32
    diaphanography (transillumination) (DATTA opinions), 354
    mammography, 145, 338, 353
    thermography to detect (Health Technology Assessment Reports), 289
    transillumination light scanning (Health Technology Assessment Reports), 287, 288
Breast Cancer Organizations, National Alliance of, 32
Breast feeding, 32
Breast implants, 23, 32-34
British Medical Association, 150
Brittle Bone Society, American, 195
Broadcasting, 34
Bronchial infections, 142
Budget neutrality (Medicare terminology), 164
Bulimia
    concerned organizations, 34
Bulimia Anorexia Self Help (BASH), 19, 34
Bureau of Health Care Delivery and Assistance (US), 99
Bureau of Health Professions, 34-35
Bureau of the Census (US), 42
Burn Association, American, 35
Burns, 35
Burroughs Wellcome resident physician program, 363
Bush, Barbara, 140
Business loans, 140-141
"Business Response to AIDS," 9
Bypass, see Surgery

C

Caduceus, 6-7
CAHEA (Committee on Allied Health Education and Accreditation), 14-16
CAIN (Computerized AIDS Information Network), 10
California (information on various health and social services in this and other states may be found at the heading, State agencies and organizations)
California Hispanic American Medical Association, 81
Canadian Medical Association, 150
Cancer, see also specific locations for cancer, e.g, Breast cancer
    colon, rectal (bibliography), 24
    DES (diethylstilbestrol) and, 65-67
    diet and, 65
    information and organizations, 37-39
    melanoma (bibliography), 24
    oral complications of therapies (bibliography), 25
    statewide societies, 37-39
    therapy-related second cancers (bibliography), 23
    whole-body hyperthermia (DATTA opinions), 354
Cancer Information Clearinghouse, 37
Cancer research, 37
Cancer Society, American
    national headquarters, 37
    statewide societies, 37-39
Candlelighters Childhood Cancer Foundation, 37
Capitation (Medicare terminology), 165
Capsulotomies, 288
Captioned Films for the Deaf, 39, 100
Captioning Institute, National, 39, 100
Carbon dioxide lasers
    gynecologic cancer treatments (DATTA opinions), 355
    surgery (Health Technology Assessment Reports), 288, 289
Cardiac catheterization (Health Technology Assessment Reports), 287
Cardiac monitors (Health Technology Assessment Reports), 287
Cardiac output (electrical bioimpedance) (Health Technology Assessment Reports), 287
Cardiac pacemakers (Council on Scientific Affairs report), 344
Cardiac rehabilitation (Health Technology Assessment Reports), 287
Cardiointegram (Health Technology Assessment Reports), 287
Cardiokymography
    DATTA opinions, 353, 354
    Health Technology Assessment Reports, 287, 288, 289
Cardiology, American College of, 39, 102
Cardiology, 39, 102
Cardiopulmonary resuscitation
    description, 39-40
    do-not-resuscitate guidelines, 69, 140
    standards and guidelines for, 40
Cardiovascular and Pulmonary Rehabilitation, American Association of, 234
Cardiovascular disease
    certification, 39
Cardiovascular perfusion, 200-201
Cardiovascular rehabilitation, 234
Cardiovascular system
    modeling in research (bibliography), 25
Cardiovascular technologist, 40-41
Cardiovascular Technology/Pulmonary Technology, National Society for, 41, 75
Cardioverter-defibrillators (Health Technology Assessment Reports), 288

Care Medico, 299
Career information (nonclinical alternatives, physician opinion, etc), 41-42
Carotid body resection (Health Technology Assessment Reports), 288
Carotid endarterectomy (Health Technology Assessment Reports), 287
Carrier (Medicare terminology), 165
Carson, Rachel, 201
Case citations (Legal references), 244-246
Cataplexy, 175
Cataract and Refractive Surgery, American Society of, 42
Cataracts, 42
Catholic Health Association, 95
Catholic Medical Mission Board, Inc, 71
CDC, see Centers for Disease Control
CD4 cell count (AIDS definition), 12
Celiac Sprue Society, 14
Cell photography (Health Technology Assessment Reports), 289
Census information, 42
Center for Alternatives to Animal Testing
Center for Dance Medicine, 59
Center for Health Promotion and Education (CDC), 43
Center for Medical Consumers, 54
Center for Research on Women and Gender, 306
Center for Safety in the Arts, 256
Center for Science in the Public Interest, 54
Center for Study of Multiple Birth, 173, 293
Centers for Disease Control (US), 42
    AIDS definition, 12
    AIDS hotline, 10
    AIDS initiative, 9
    Center for Preventive Services, 291
Cerebral edema, 288
Cerebral Palsy and Developmental Medicine, American Academy for, 43
Cerebral palsy, 43
Certification
    ABMS 800 number, 55
    aerospace medicine, 6
    aviation and aerospace medicine, 21
    blood banking/transfusion medicine, 30
    cardiovascular disease, 102
    cardiovascular disease, 39
    chemotherapy, 43
    critical care, 55
    dermatology, 61
    emergency medicine, 77
    endocrinology and metabolism, 78
    family practice, 85
    forensic psychiatry, 86
    geriatrics, 89
    hand surgery, 95
    hematology, 102
    immunology, 113
    infectious diseases, 115
    national specialty boards listed 275-276
    nephrology, 176
    neurological surgery, 177
    nuclear medicine, 177
    obstetrics and gynecology, 183
    obstetrics and gynecology, 94
    occupational medicine, 186
    oncology, 189
    ophthalmology, 190
    orthopaedic surgery, 194
    orthotics, 194
    otolaryngology, 195
    pain management, 197
    pathology, 198
    pediatrics, 199
    physical medicine and rehabilitation, 202
    podiatric orthopedics, 213
    preventive medicine, 222
    prosthetics, 194
    pulmonary disease, 234
    radiation oncology, 189
    radiology, 238
    rehabilitation, 248
    rheumatology, 252
    specialization in medical practice, 273-275
    sports medicine, 277
    surgery, 283
    thoracic surgery, 290
    undersea medicine, 294
    urology, 295
    vascular surgery, 297
CHAMPUS, 43
Charcot-Marie-Tooth International, 87
Charges, see Fees
Charities Information Bureau, National, 43
Charities, 43
Charity care, see Indigent care
Chelation therapy, 104, 290, 355
Chemical aversion therapy (Health Technology Assessment Reports), 287
Chemonucleolysis (DATTA opinions), 352
Chemotherapy
    description, information sources, 43
Chemotherapy Foundation, 43
Chest Physicians, American College of, 234
Chest physicians, 234
Chest x-rays, 43
Chicago Runaway Switchboard, 4
Child abuse
    AMA Council on Scientific Affairs report, 344
    concerned organizations, state agencies, 43-46
    prevention, 69
    sexual abuse, 17
Child Abuse and Family Violence, National Council on, 69
Child Abuse Hotline, National, 44
Child Abuse, National Committee for Prevention of, 44
Child Abuse, National Council, 44
Child and Adolescent Psychiatry, American Academy of, 4, 229
Child Help USA, 43
Child psychiatry, 229
Child Safety Council, National, 256
Child sexual abuse
    anatomical dolls, 17
Child Welfare League of America, 9
Childbirth
    home births, 104, 172
    midwives, 172, 178
    multiple births, 173
    natural, 46, 176
Childfind Hotline, 173
Childhelps, 44
Children, see also Birth Defects
    anatomical dolls, puppets, etc, 17
    associations promoting health of, 46
    baby sitting, 23
    cancer patients, 37
    handicapped, 95
    HIV-infected, 9, 12
    hospitalized, 44
    immunization, 113
    malnutrition (bibliography), 25
    missing, 46, 173, 252

National Center for Education in Maternal and Child Health, 146
  organ donation, 192-193
  safety, accident prevention, 256
  school-based health centers, 257
  state agencies, 44-46
  vaccine-preventable diseases (bibliography), 26
Children in Hospitals, 44, 199
Children of Aging Parents, 7
Children of Alcoholics Foundation, 13
Children's Defense Fund, 46
Children's Health, Association for the Care of, 46
Children's Hospice International, 108
Children's Transplant Association, 290
China
  book donations, 31
Chinese-American Medical Society, 80
Chiropractic
  organizations and information 46-47
Chiropractic assistant, 46
Chiropractic Association, American, 46
Chiropractic schools, 46-47
Choice in Dying, 83
Cholecystectomy, Laparoscopic, 23, 87
Cholesterol
  JAMA theme issue, 65
  triglyceride, high-density lipoprotein and heart disease (bibliography), 24
Chorionic villus sampling (DATTA opinions), 351, 353
Christian Medical and Dental Society, 47, 150
Chronic Fatigue Association, National, 47
Chronic Fatigue Immune Dysfunction Syndrome Association, 47
Chronic Fatigue Immune Dysfunction Syndrome Society, 47
Chronic fatigue syndrome
  bibliography, 25
  description and concerned organizations, 47
Cingulotomy, Stereotactic, 288, 354
Citations, Bibliographic (ANSI standards), 238-246
Citizens for a Better Environment, 75, 79
Citizens for the Treatment of High Blood Pressure, 31, 111
Civil Aviation Medical Association, 21
Civilian Health and Medical Program of the Uniformed Services (CHAMPUS), 43
Clearinghouse for Alcohol Information, National, 13
Clearinghouse for Drug Abuse Information, National, 50, 71
Clearinghouse for Primary Care Information, National, 223
Clearinghouse on Child Abuse and Neglect, 44
Clearinghouse on Licensure, National, Enforcement and Regulation, National, 137
Cleft Palate Association, American, 47
Cleft Palate Educational Foundation, American, 47
Cleft palate, 47
Cleveland Clinic
  Familial Polyposis Registry, 85
  history, 47-48
CLIA (Clinical Laboratory Improvement Act), 48
Climate
  global warming (bibliography), 24
Clinical Appropriateness Initiative, 219
Clinical dietician, 65
Clinical ecology (Council on Scientific Affairs report), 334
Clinical Hypnosis, American Society of, 111
Clinical Investigation, American Society for, 48
Clinical investigation, 48
Clinical laboratories, see Laboratories
Clinical Laboratory Improvement Act (CLIA), 48
Clinical Nutrition, American Society for, 182
Clinical nutrition, 182
Clinical Oncology, American Society of, 189

Clinical Pathologists, American Society of, 198
  SI unit conversion guide, 49
Clinical Pharmacology and Therapeutics, American Society for, 201
Clinical Psychiatrists, American Academy of, 229
Clinical trials (AIDS), 9, 10
Clinical Urologists, American Association of, Inc, 295
Clinics, Free, 49
Closing of medical practices, 49-50
Clove cigarettes (Council on Scientific Affairs report), 341
Cocaine
  information and concerned organizations, 50
  pregnancy and newborn (bibliography), 24
Cocaine Anonymous, 50
Cocaine Baby Helpline, 50
Cocaine Hotline, 50
Cochlear implants, 25, 288
Code fragmentation (Medicare terminology), 168
Codes, Specialty, see Abbreviations
Coding
  CPT, 55-57
  ICD-9-CM, 120-122
  place of service codes (1500 Claim Form), 116-118
Coinsurance (Medicare terminology), 165
COLA (Commission on Office Laboratory Assessment), 49
Collateral source (tort reform glossary), 228
Collection letters (sample), 28
Collections
  billing fundamentals and, 26-28
  closing medical practices, 49-50
College Health Association, American, 50
College health, 50
College of American Pathologists
  drug abuse testing, 72-73
  headquarters information, 198
  self-instruction manual for office laboratories, 49
  Systematized Nomenclature of Medicine (SNOMED), 271
Colleges of Nursing, American Association of, 179
Colleges, Medical, see Medical schools
Colombian Medical Association, 81
Colon and Rectal Surgery, American Board of, 50
Colon and Rectal Surgery, American Society of, 50
Colon and rectal surgery, 50
Colon cancer (bibliography), 24
Colon disease, 50
Colorado (information on various health and social services in this and other states may be found at the heading, State agencies and organizations)
Coma
  life-support withdrawal, 69
"Coming Home" (JAMA "A Piece of My Mind"), 224-226
Commerce Clearing House, 168
Commerce Department (US)
Commission on Office Laboratory Assessment, 49, 189
Commission on Professional and Hospital Activities, 281
Committee on Allied Health Education and Accreditation, 14-16
Common Procedure Coding System (HCPCS), 55-57
Community Cancer Centers, Association of, 37
Community Health Information Library, 54
Community health nurse, 231
Compassionate Friends, 93
Competency Assurance, National Organization for, 50
Competency assurance, 50
Complaints against nursing homes, 182
Complaints against physicians, 50-52, 208-212
Computed tomography
  head trauma (DATTA opinions), 354
Computer-enhanced perimetry (Health Technology Assessment Reports), 289

Computer Retrieval of Information on Scientific Projects (CRISP), 248
Computer services (AMA), 329
Computerized Severity Index (CSI), 281
Computers
    organizations and journals, 52
    video display terminals, 297
"Computers and Medicine," 52
Confidentiality
    informed consent and, 115-116
    patients' rights, 199
    sex counseling, 263
Conflict of interest
    physician-owned facilities (self-referrals), 248
    research (Council on Scientific Affairs report), 337
Congress of Neurological Surgeons
    headquarters information, 177
    spinal cord injury prevention, 5
Congressional Record, 243
Connecticut (information on various health and social services in this and other states may be found at the heading, State agencies and organizations)
Consent, Informed, 115-116
Constitution of the American Medical Association, 327-328
Consultants, 52
Consumer Health Information Network, 54
Consumer Information Center, 54
Consumer Price Index, 54
Consumer Product Safety Commission (US), 54
Consumer Product Safety Commission, 223, 256
Consumers
    choosing insurance, 118
    health information, 53
    insurance complaints, 118
    product safety, 54
    state health-protection agencies, 54
Contact Lens Association of Ophthalmologists, Inc, 54
Contact lenses, 54
Contingent fees (tort reform glossary), 228
Continuing medical education
    Accreditation Council for, 3
    AMA activities, programs, 356
    gifts to physicians from industry, 89-92
    information, forms, organizations conducting, 54-55
    video clinics, 297
Continuity of care, 199
Continuous positive airway pressure (Health Technology Assessment Reports), 288
Contraception, 29
Contraceptives (Dalkon Shield), 59
Conversion factor (Medicare terminology), 165
Cooley's Anemia, 55
Corneal transplantation (Council on Scientific Affairs report), 339
Cornelia De Lange Syndrome Foundation, 87
Coronary rehabilitation services (DATTA opinions), 353
Coroners, 86
Correctional health care
    bibliography, 24
    detained, incarcerated youth, 336
    National Commission, 55
Correctional Health Care, National Commission on, 55
Cosmetic surgery, see Plastic surgery
Cost control
    AMA's Health Access America provisions, 370
Council of Better Business Bureaus
    cancer research, 37
    headquarters information, 23
    "Tips on Choosing a Hospital," 109
Council of Medical Specialty Societies

"Choosing a Medical Specialty," 273
Council of State Goverments, 137
Council on Graduate Medical Education, 93
Council on Teaching Hospitals, 287
Councils, AMA, see specific names under American Medical Association
Counterpulsation (Health Technology Assessment Reports), 288
County medical societies, 55
Court of Appeals (US)
    case citation (style guidelines), 245
CPR, see Cardiopulmonary resuscitation
CPT, see Current Procedural Terminology
Cranial electrostimulation (DATTA opinions), 354
Credentialing
    AMA National Physician Credentials Verification Service, 329
    information, organizations, databases, 55
Credentials Verification Service, National, 55, 207
Cri Du Chat Syndrome Society, 87
Crile, George Washington, 47-48
CRISP (Computer Retrieval of Information on Scientific Projects), 248
Critical care, 55
Crohn's and Colitis Foundation, 50
Cryo Laboratory Facility, 277
Cryosurgery, 55
Cryosurgery, American College of, 55
CSI (Computerized Severity Index), 281
CT scans, see Computed tomography
Cult Hotline and Clinic, 55
Cults, 55
Current Procedural Terminology, 55-57
    insurance claim coding, 118
    Medicare claim filing, 165
    Medicare manual, 168
Curriculum vitae (suggested outline), 57
"Custodian" (JAMA "A Piece of My Mind")
Customary charge (Medicare terminology), 165
Customary, prevailing and reasonable method (Medicare terminology), 165
Cyclotrons (Council on Scientific Affairs report), 340
Cystic fibrosis, 57
Cystic Fibrosis Foundation, 57
Cytology, American Society of, 58
Cytotechnology, 57-58
Cytotoxic leukocyte test (Health Technology Assessment Reports), 289

D

D.E.B.R.A. of America, Inc, 61
"Daddy" (JAMA "A Piece of My Mind"), 252-253
Dalkon Shield, 59
Damage awards (tort reform glossary), 228
Damage limits (tort reform glossary), 228
Dance Association, National, 84
Dance medicine, 59
Darien Book Aid Plan, 31
Data services (AMA), 329
DATTA opinions, 350-355
Davis, Nathan Smith, 314, 324
DEA registration number, 72
Deafness, 100
    captioning services, 39
    Helen Keller Center, 29
Deafness and Rehabilitation Association, American, 99
Deafness Research Foundation, 100
"Debbie," 81-82

DEBRA of America, Inc, 61

Debridement
mycotic toenails (Health Technology Assessment Reports), 288

Decubitus ulcer treatments (Health Technology Assessment Reports), 289

Deductible (Medicare terminology), 165

Defense Department (US)
CHAMPUS office, 43

Defibrillators (Health Technology Assessment Reports), 288

Delaware (information on various health and social services in this and other states may be found at the heading, State agencies and organizations)

Delivery
home births, 104, 172
midwives 172, 178
multiple births, 173
natural, 46, 176

Dementia (Council on Scientific Affairs report), 343

Dental Assistants Association, American, 59

Dental Association, American, 59

Dental associations, State, 59-61

Dental Hygienists Association, American, 59

Dental implants (bibliography), 25

Dental occupations, 59

Dental services director, 83

Dentistry
public health, 231
restorative materials (bibliography), 23

Dentistry for the Handicapped, National Foundation of, 95

Depressant use
impaired physicians, 113-114

Depression, 24, 172

Depressive and Manic Depressive Association, National, 172

Dermatologic Surgery, American Society for, 61

Dermatology
organizations, 61
sun- ultraviolet light (bibliography), 25

Dermatology, American Academy of, 61

Dermatology, American Board of, 61

DES (Diethylstilbestrol), 65-67

Desoxyribonucleic acid (Health Technology Assessment Reports), 290

Detained and incarcerated youth (Council on Scientific Affairs report), 336

Developmental disabilities (bibliography), 25

Devices, Medical
donations of medical supplies, 71
Health Technology Assessment Reports, 287-290
information and organizations, 61-62
manufacturers and distributors, 115

Diabetes
external open-loop pump for insulin (Health Technology Assessment Reports), 288
information and organizations, 62
modeling in research (bibliography), 25

Diabetes Association, American, 62

Diabetes Information Clearinghouse, National, 62

Diagnostic and Statistical Manual of Mental Disorders (DSM III), 64

Diagnostic and Therapeutic Technology Assessment (DATTA) opinions, 350-355

Diagnostic medical sonographer, 64

Dialysis (bibliography), 26

Dialysis technician, 64-65

Diaphanography (DATTA opinions), 354

Diarrhea
traveler's (DATTA opinions), 352

Diathermy
DATTA opinions, 355
Health Technology Assessment Reports, 289

Diet
cancer and (Council on Scientific Affairs report), 334
information and organizations, 65
vitamin sources in food, 297-298

Dietary fiber and health (Council on Scientific Affairs report), 338

Dietetic Association, American, 65

Diethylstilbestrol (DES), 65-67

Dietician, Clinical, 65

Digestive Diseases Education and Information Clearinghouse, National, 67

Direct Relief International, 71

Directory Service, US, 86

Directory of Medical Schools Worldwide, 86

Disabilities
alcoholism, 13
information and organizations, 95
Mobility International (aid in traveling), 291
physicians' 68
wheelchair exercises, 301

Disability Evaluating Physicians, American Academy of, 67

Disability evaluation, 67, 186-187

"Disability Evaluation Under Social Security," 67

Disability Examiners, National Association of, 67

Disaster medical care, 68

Discipline of physicians, 50-52

Disease classification, 120-122

Disease Information Hotline (CDC), 43

Disease Staging, 281

Disease statistics, 281

Diskectomy (DATTA opinions), 351, 352

District of Columbia (information on various health and social services for the District of Columbia may be found at the heading, State agencies and organizations)

Divers Alert Network (DAN), 68, 258

Diving, 68

DNA (Health Technology Assessment Reports), 290

DNR (Do-Not-Resuscitate Orders), 69, 140

DOC, see Doctors Ought to Care

Doctor Certification Line, 55

Doctor's Day (March 30), 68-69

Doctors of the World, 299

Doctors Ought to Care, 203

"Doctors to All People," 299

Doctors Without Borders, 68, 299

Dogs
guide dogs for blind, 29
hearing, 100

Dolls, Anatomical, 17

Domestic violence
information and organizations, 69-71

Domestic Violence, National Coalition Against, 44, 69

Domestic Violence Hotline, National, 70

Donations
book, 71
medical supplies, 71
physician volunteerism, 298-299

Donor cards, 193

Doppler imaging (Council on Scientific Affairs report), 335

Doppler sonography, 294

Down's syndrome
alpha-fetoprotein testing (DATTA opinions), 352

Down's Syndrome Society, National, 87

Driving safety, 255-256

Drug abuse
Betty Ford Center, 23
cocaine, pregnancy and newborn (bibliography), 24
cocaine, 50
employee assistance programs, 77-78

impaired physicians, 113-115
information and concerned organizations, 71-72
pregnancy and, 72
testing for, 72-73
Drug abuse in athletes (Council on Scientific Affairs report), 340
Drug Abuse Information, National Clearinghouse for, 50, 71
Drug and Alcohol Hotline Information and Referral Service, 71
Drug Education, American Council of, 71
Drug Enforcement Administration (US)
physician registration number, 72
Drug industry
gifts to physicians, 89-92
Drug Information Association, 72
Drug sensitivity assay (Health Technology Assessment Reports), 290
Drug statistics, 281
Drug testing (Council on Scientific Affairs report), 342
Drugs
depressant, narcotic, stimulant use by physicians, 113-114
elderly and medication (two bibiliographies), 25
evaluation and information, 72
indigent program, 72
orphan (rare diseases), 193
prescriptive privileges for controlled substances by nurses (by state), 179-180
Drunk driving
information and concerned organizations, 13, 73
Drunk Driving, National Commission Against, 13, 73
DSM III, 64
Dual photon absorptiometry (Health Technology Assessment Reports), 288
Durable powers of attorney, 140
Dyslexia (Council on Scientific Affairs report), 338
Dyslexia Society, Orton, 73
Dysphagia
role of speech-language pathologists (Health Technology Assessment Reports), 287
Dystrophic Epidermolysis Bullosa Research Association, 61

E

Ear, see also Hearing impairment and loss; Otolaryngology
American Otological Society, 195
EAR Foundation, 88
Earnings of physicians, 207
Easter Seal Society, National, 29, 75
Eating disorders, 19
ECFMG, 75, 86, 123
ECG, see Electrocardiography
Echocardiography, American Society of, 75
Ecology, 75
Ectodermal Dysplasia, National Foundation for, 61
EDTA (ethylenediamine tetraacetic acid), 104, 290
Education in Maternal and Child Health, National Center for, 146
Education, Medical, see Medical education
Education, Medical, Continuing, see Continuing medical education
Education, Medical, Graduate, see Graduate medical education
Educational Commission for Foreign Medical Graduates, 75, 86, 123
Educational Institute, American, 54
EEG, see Electroencephalography
Elder abuse, see Aging
Elderly, see Aging

Elders, M Joycelyn, 283
Electrical bioimpedance (Health Technology Assessment Reports), 287
Electrical nerve stimulation, Transcutaneous (Health Technology Assessment Reports), 288
Electrical stimulation
cranial, 354
endocardial (Health Technology Assessment Reports), 288
nerve (transcutaneous; Health Technology Assessment Reports), 288, 289
neuromuscular (Health Technology Assessment Reports), 288
nonunited bone fracture (DATTA opinions), 352
Electrocardiograph technician, 75
Electrocardiography
mandatory before elective surgery (DATTA opinions), 355
Electrocoagulation, 288, 354
Electroencephalography
information and organizations, 75
open heart surgery (Health Technology Assessment Reports), 289
quantitative (fast Fourier transform analysis) (DATTA opinions), 355
twenty-four-hour monitoring (DATTA opinions), 355
video monitoring (Health Technology Assessment Reports), 287
Electromagnetic fields (bibliography), 24
Electromyography, 75-76
Electromyography and Electrodiagnosis, American Association of, 76
Electroneurodiagnostic technologist, 76
Electronic billing, 26-28
Electronic claim (Medicare terminology), 165
Electrospinal stimulator (DATTA opinions), 354
Electrostimulation, Cranial, 354
Electrotherapy (Health Technology Assessment Reports), 288, 289
Electroversion therapy (Health Technology Assessment Reports), 289
Eli Lilly and Co, 65-67
Emergency identification cards, 113
Emergency medical services
cardiac care, 40
Emergency medical technician, 76-77
Emergency Medical Technicians, National Association of, 77
Emergency medicine, 77
Emergency Medicine Alliance, 109
Emergency Medicine, American Board of, 77
Emergency Physicians, American College of, 77, 290
Employee Assistance Professionals Association, 78
Employee assistance programs, 77-78
Employee Assistance Society of North America, 78
Employee drug testing (Council on Scientific Affairs report), 343
Employee physical examinations, 183-186
Employees of physicians, see Office staff
Employers Insurance of Wausau, 102
Encephalopathies, Spongiform (bibliography), 23
"Encourage Information Therapy" (JAMA "A Piece of My Mind"), 53-54
End-stage renal disease
hemoperfusion (Health Technology Assessment Reports), 288
laboratory tests (Health Technology Assessment Reports), 288
Endarterectomy, Carotid (Health Technology Assessment Reports), 287
Endocardial electrical stimulation (pacing), 288

Endocrine Society, 78
Endocrinology, 78
Endodontist, 79
Endometriosis, 79
Endometriosis Association, 79
Endoscopy
    balloon dilation of prostate (DATTA opinions), 350
    electrocoagulation (Health Technology Assessment
        Reports), 288
    electrocoagulation of gastrointestinal tract hemorrhage
        (DATTA opinions), 354
    laser photocoagulation (Health Technology Assessment
        Reports), 287
    laser photocoagulation of gastrointestinal tract
        hemorrhage (DATTA opinions), 354
    thermal coagulation of gastrointestinal tract hemorrhage
        (DATTA opinions), 354
    topical therapy of gastrointestinal tract hemorrhage
        (DATTA opinions), 354
    transurethral nephrolithotomy (DATTA opinions), 354
    ulcer therapy (bibliography), 25
Endothelial cell photography (Health Technology
    Assessment Reports), 289
Engineering, Biomedical, 29
English language
    international (foreign) medical graduate proficiency,
        122-123
Environmental health
    ecology, 75
    global warming (bibliography), 24
    household pollutants (bibliography), 26
    indoor air pollution (two bibliographies), 26
    information and organizations, 79
    infectious medical waste, 163-164
    medical waste disposal (bibliography), 23
    occupational pollutants (bibliography), 26
    radon (bibliography), 26
    volcano effects (bibliography), 24
Environmental Medicine, American Academy of, 79
Environmental Protection Agency (US), 79
    air pollution information, 13
Epidermolysis bullosa, 61
Epilepsy
    information and concerned organizations, 80
    stereotaxic depth electrodes (Health Technology
        Assessment Reports), 289
    surgery for (bibliography), 24
Epilepsy Foundation of America, 80
Epilepsy Society, American, 80
"Equal, Not Really" (JAMA "A Piece of My Mind"), 301
Equipment, Medical, see Devices, Medical
Esophageal pH monitoring (Health Technology Assessment
    Reports), 288
Ether (first use as anesthesia), 68-69
Ethics
    AMA codes of, 316, 321-327
    AMA Principles of, 80
    bioethics institute, center, commission, 28-29
    complaints against physicians, 50-52
    enforcement, 50-52
    gifts to physicians from industry, 89-92
    information and concerned organizations, 80
    institutional committees (bibliography), 26
    Oath of Hippocrates, 102
    research subjects, 249
    self-referrals, 248
    sex counseling, 262-263
    sexual misconduct, 265
Ethnic physicians associations, 80-81
Ethylenediamine tetraacetic acid (EDTA), 104, 290
Euthanasia, 81-83

Evaluation and management services (Medicare
    terminology), 165
Executive physicians, 83
Exercise
    elderly and (bibliography), 25
    information and concerned organizations, 84
    physiology, 84
Exhibitors, 84
Expert witnesses (tort reform glossary), 228
Explanation of Medicare Benefits, 165
External counterpulsation (Health Technology Assessment
    Reports), 288
Extra-Corporeal Technology, American Society of, 201
Extracorporeal shock wave lithotripsy (Health Technology
    Assessment Reports), 288
Extracranial-intracranial bypass (Health Technology
    Assessment Reports), 287
Eye Bank Association of America, 29, 84
Eye Care Project, National, 84
Eye Research Foundation, National, 84
Eyes
    cataracts, 42
    contact lenses, 54
    donor registry, 193
    information and concerned organizations, 84
    retinitis pigmentosa, 251
Eymann Anatomically Correct Dolls, 17

F

Facial nerve palsy, 289
Facial nerve paralysis (Health Technology Assessment
    Reports), 288
"Facial Nerve Problems," 23
Facial Plastic and Reconstructive Surgery, American
    Academy of, 213
Fair Oaks Hospital (Summit, New Jersey)
    cocaine information, 50
Familial Polyposis Registry, 85
Family
    alcoholism and (bibliography), 25
Family Physicians, American Academy of, 5, 85
Family Practice, American Board of,
    family practice certification, 85
    geriatrics board certification, 89
    information and concerned organizations, 85
    sports medicine certification, 277
Family violence, 69-71
Fasting (Health Technology Assessment Reports), 289
Federal Aviation Administration (US), 21
Federal Licensure Exam (FLEX), 85
Federal Register, 243
Federal Trade Commission (US)
    advertising complaints, 6, 52
    description and information on, 85
    fraudulent ads on radio, television, 97
Federation Council on the Aging, 7
Federation for Medical Accreditation, American, 3
Federation Network (FEDNET), 364
Federation of American Health Systems, 99, 109
Federation of Home Health Agencies, American, 105
Federation of Parents for Drug-Free Youth, National, 71
Federation of State Medical Boards of the United States
    address, telephone number, 137
    credentialing information, 55
    credentials data bank, 207
    FLEX exam, 85
    Special Purpose Examination (SPEX), 273
FEDNET, 364

Fees
    attorney, contingent, 228
    billing and collections, 26-28
    complaints, local information, 207
Fellow (term), 250
Fertility, 85
Fertility Research Foundation, 85
Fertility Society, American, 85, 277
Fetal tissue transplantation, 85, 336
1500 Health Insurance Claim Form (HCFA), 116-118
Fifth Pathway, 86
Films, see Motion pictures
Final rule (Medicare terminology), 165
Financing of health care
    AMA's Health Access America provisions, 371
FIND/SVP, 145
Fire safety (Council on Scientific Affairs report), 341
Fish oils, 24, 25
Fitness Foundation, National, 84
FLEX Exam, 85
Florida (information on various health and social services in
    this and other states may be found at the heading,
    State agencies and organizations)
Fluoxetine (Prozac) (bibliography), 23
Flying Physicians Association, 21
Focus, Inc, 71
Folic acid, 298
Food and Drug Administration (US)
    breast implant hotline, 34, 86
    consumer affairs inquiries, 86
    general description, 86
    medical device malfunction reporting, 61, 80
    Office for Orphan Drugs, 193
    Office of Device Evaluation, 34
    Poison Control Branch, 213
Food and Nutrition Information Center, 182
Food groups, Basic, 182
Foods and nutrition
    AIDS and (bibliography), 23
    bacterial, viral and parasitic foodborne infections
        (bibliography), 26
    basic food groups, 182
    fish oils (bibliography), 24, 25
    malnutrition in children (bibliography), 25
    safety, 182
    seafood safety (bibliography), 23
    vitamin sources in diet, 297-298
Foot care, 213
Ford, Betty (Betty Ford Center), 23
Foreign medical graduates, see International medical
    graduates
Forensic medicine, 86
Forensic Psychiatry, American Board of, 86
Formaldehyde (Council on Scientific Affairs report), 338
Foster care, 86
Foster Parents Plan, Inc, 86
Foundation for Biomedical Research, 18
Foundation for Books to China, 31
Fourier analysis
    quantitative electroencephalography (DATTA
        opinions), 355
Fragile X Foundation, 87
Franconi's syndrome, 125
Frauds, 97, 175
    AMA collection, archives, 331
Free clinics, 49
Freud, Sigmund, 230-231
Friedreich's Ataxia Group in America, 88
Friends of the Americas, 299
Frivolous claims (tort reform glossary), 228

G

Gallaudet College, 100
Gallstones (bibliography), 23
Gaming (Medicare terminology), 165
GAPS (Guidelines for Adolescent Preventive Services), 6
Garren gastric bubble (DATTA opinions), 354
Gastric bubble (DATTA opinions), 354
Gastric freezing (Health Technology Assessment
    Reports), 289
Gastric restrictive surgery (DATTA opinions), 352, 354
Gastroenterology, 87
Gastroenterology, American College of, 87
Gastroesophageal reflux, 289
Gastrointestinal Endoscopy, American Society for, 87
Gastrointestinal system
    surgery for obesity (bibliography), 24
Gastrointestinal tract hemorrhage (DATTA opinions), 354
Gastroplasty Support Group, 183
Gaucher disease, 87
Gaucher Foundation, National, 87
Gay and Lesbian Crisisline, National, 10
Gay physicians and medical students, 214
Gender discrimination, 301-303
Gender disparities in research, 305-306
General practitioner, 87
Genetic disorders and syndromes
    information and concerned organizations, 87-88
    kidney disease, 125
Genetic research (Human Genome Research), 87
Genetics Society of America, 87
Geographic practice cost index (Medicare terminology), 165
Geographic variations in utilization, 280
Georgetown University
    bioethics institute, center, 28, 80
Georgia (information on various health and social services
    in this and other states may be found at the heading,
    State agencies and organizations)
Gerber Hart Library and Archive, 9
Geriatrics, 88
Geriatrics Society, American, 88
Gerontological Society of America, 89
Gift Code (AMA), 89-92
Gilles de la Tourette syndrome, 290
Global charge (Medicare terminology), 166
Global surgical package (Medicare terminology), 166
Global warming (bibliography), 24
Glomerulonephritis, 125
Glucose control device (Health Technology Assessment
    Reports), 289
Glucose monitors (Health Technology Assessment
    Reports), 289
Gluten intolerance, 14
Golf, 20
Government Printing Office Bookstores (US), 92-93
Governors Association, National, 99
Graduate medical education
    Accreditation Council for, 3
    Council on, 93
    information and organizations, 93
Grammar hotlines, 93
Grants for research, 248, 249
Great Britain, 151
Grief Education Institute, 93
Grief support, 93
Group Health Association of America, 95, 97
Group practice, 94
Group Practice Association, American, 94

Growth, 94
Growth hormone, see Hormones
Guide Dog Foundation for the Blind, 29
Guides to the Evaluation of Permanent Impairment, 67
Guillain-Barre syndrome (Health Technology Assessment Reports), 288
Gynecologic Laparoscopists, American Association of, 94, 183
Gynecologic sonography (Council on Scientific Affairs report), 336
Gynecologic ultrasonography, 294
Gynecology, 94

H

Hair loss, 95
Hair Loss Council, American, 95
Haitian Medical Association Abroad, 81
Hal's Pals, 17
Hamady Health Science Library, 54
Hand surgery, 95
Hand Surgery, American Association for, 95
Handicapped Children and Youth, National Information Center for, 95
Handicapped Physicians, American Society of, 68
Handicapped Scuba Association, 258
Handicapped Sports and Recreation Association, National, 301
Handicaps, see Disabilities
Hastings Center, 28, 80
Hawaii (information on various health and social services in this and other states may be found at the heading, State agencies and organizations)
Hazardous waste, 23, 163-164
HCFA, see Health Care Financing Administration (US)
HCFA 1500 Health Insurance Claim Form, 116-118
HCPCS, 55-57
    insurance claim coding, 118
    Medicare coding system, 166
HDL, see Lipoproteins, High-density
Head and Spinal Cord Injury Prevention Program, National, 5
Head injuries, 5, 95
Head Injury Foundation, National, 95
Headache, American Association for the Study of the, 95
Headache Foundation, National, 95
Health Access America, 370-371
Health administration
    American Management Association, 145
    descriptions of executive positions, 83
    Association of State and Territorial Health Officials, 99
    university programs, 95
Health and Human Services Department (US)
    Agency for Health Care Policy and Research (AHCPR) reports, 287-290
    consumer health information, 54
    description of, 95
    Medicare complaints (fraud, abuse), 168
    Office of Disease Prevention and Health, 54
    surgical second opinions, 258
Health Assistance Foundation, American, 7
Health associations, see also names of specific associations and diseases, 95
Health Care Anti-Fraud Association, National, 175
Health Care Association, American, 182
Health Care Exhibitors Association, 84
Health Care Financing Administration (US)
    general description, 96
    Office of Research, Demonstrations and Statistics, 122
    regional offices, 96

Health Council, National, 42, 96
Health councils, 96
Health education
    AMA Council on Scientific Affairs report, 337
    consumer information, 53-54
    minority groups (bibliography), 26
Health Education Center, 54
Health Education, National Center for, 54
Health Fraud, National Council Against, 97
Health fraud, 97
    AMA collection, archives, 331
Health Industry Distributors Association, 62, 80, 115
Health Industry Manufacturers Association, 62, 80, 115
Health Information Center, National, 199
Health Information Management Association, American, 156
Health Insurance Association of America, 118
Health Insurance Claim Form (HCFA, 1500), 116-118
Health Insurance, see Insurance
Health Lawyers Association, National, 129
Health Library (Kaiser Medical Center), 54
Health maintenance organizations, 97-98
Health manpower
    Bureau of Health Professions, 34-35
    shortage areas, 98-99
Health, Physical Education, Recreation and Dance, American Alliance for, 9
Health Physics Society, 212
Health policy, 99
    AMA activities, programs, 357-359
Health Policy Agenda for the American People, 371
Health professional shortage area (Medicare terminology), 166
Health promotion
    minority groups (bibliography), 26
Health reform
    AMA program, Health Access America, 370-371
Health Resources and Services Administration (US)
    Bureau of Health Maintenance Organizations and Resources, 97
Health Services Executives, National Association of, 84
Health Statistics, National Center for, 281
Health systems agencies, 99
Health Technology Assessment Reports, 287-290
Healthcare Anti-Fraud Association, National, 118
Healthcare Consultants, American Association of, 52
Healthcare Executives, American College of, 84
Healthcare Financial Management Association, 96
Healthcare Knowledge Resource, 281
Healthcare Marketing and Public Relations, American Society for, 145
Healthy People 2000, 222
Hearing Aid Society, National, 100
Hearing Association, American Speech-Language-, 3
Hearing Helpline, 100
Hearing impairment and loss
    AIDS hotline, 10
    audiology, 20-21
    cochlear implants (bibliography), 25
    information and concerned organizations, 99
    noise and (bibliography), 25
Hearing Research Foundation, American, 99
Heart Association, American
    CPR standards and guidelines, 40
    state affiliates, 100-102
Heart associations, 100-102
Heart diseases
    echocardiography, 75
    modeling in research (bibliography), 25
    rehabilitation services (DATTA opinions), 353

triglyceride, high-density lipoprotein and (bibliography), 24
"Heart Donor" (JAMA "Poetry and Medicine"), 193
Height
  growth hormones and short stature (bibliography), 25
Height-weight tables, 102
Heimlich maneuver poster, 102
Helen Keller National Center for Deaf/Blind Youths and Adults, 29
Help for Incontinent People, Inc (HIP), 294
Helpern (Milton) Institute of Forensic Medicine, 86
Helsinki Declaration, 249
Hematology, 102
Hematology, American Society of, 30, 102
Hematuria, 125
Hemlock Society, 83
Hemochromatosis Research Foundation Inc, 102
Hemodialysis
  reuse of "single use only" devices (Health Technology Assessment Reports), 288
Hemofiltration
  continuous arteriovenous (DATTA opinions), 354
  Health Technology Assessment Reports, 288
Hemoperfusion (Health Technology Assessment Reports), 288
Hemophilia, 102
Hemophilia Foundation, National, 102
Heparin infusion pump (Health Technology Assessment Reports), 289
Heparin therapy (Health Technology Assessment Reports), 288
Hermes, Staff of, 6-7
HHS Department, see Health and Human Services Department (US)
High Blood Pressure Education Program, National, 111
High Blood Pressure Information Center, 31
Highway safety, 256
Highway Traffic Safety Administration, National, 21
HIP (Help for Incontinent People, Inc), 294
Hippocrates, 102
Hispanic-American physicians, 81
Hispanic-Americans, 172
Hispanic health (Council on Scientific Affairs report), 336
Histologic technicians and technologists 153
Histologic technology, 103
Historical Museum of Medicine and Dentistry, 174
History of medicine, 103
  AMA code of ethics, 321-327
  American Medical Association founding, 313-317
  neurosurgery (bibliography), 25
  women physicians, 303-304
History of Medicine, American Association for the, 103
HIV, see Acquired Immunodeficiency Syndrome
Hobbies and recreation
  physicians' athletic associations, 20
Holistic Medical Association, American, 104
Holistic medicine, 104
Home births, 104, 172
Home health care, 105-106
  AIDS patients, 10
  Council on Scientific Affairs report, 335, 337
Home Care, National Association for, 105
Homecare Education and Research, National Center for, 10
Homeless, 107-108
  behavioral and mental disorders (bibliography), 25
Homeless and runaway youth (Council on Scientific Affairs report), 339
Homeless, National Coalition for, 108
Homeopathic medicine, 108
Homeopathy, 322-323
Homeopathy, National Center for, 108
Homes for the Aging, American Association of, 182

Homosexuals
  American Association of Physicians for Human Rights, 214
  National Gay and Lesbian Crisisline, 10
HOPE, Project, 229
Hormone and Pituitary Program, National, 108
Hormones
  growth, and short stature (bibliography), 25
  growth (bovine somatotropin), 24
Hospice Education Institute, 108
Hospice Organization, National, 108
Hospices, 108
Hospital accreditation, 108
Hospital Association, American
  CME learning assessment form, 54
  ICD-9 Center, 122
  national headquarters, telephone information, 108
  patients' rights, 199
  Statistics Center, 281
Hospital associations, 108-110
Hospital management companies, 109
Hospital medical staff
  AMA activities and programs, 364
  services, 109
Hospital mortality data, 279-280
Hospital procedure statistics, 281
Hospital statistics, 279-281
Hospitals, 108-110
  burn centers, 35
  ethics committees (bibliography), 26
  mortality data, 279-280
  preadmission criteria, 221
  Reference Criteria for Short Stay Hospital Review, 238
  statistics, 279-281
  teaching, 287
  technology assessment (bibliography), 24
House calls, 105
"House Calls" (JAMA "A Piece of My Mind") 105
House of Delegates, AMA, 366
Household Product Safety Hotline, 223
Household products (bibliography), 26
Howard University Center for Sickle Cell Disease, 265
Human experimentation, 249
Human Genome Research, 87
Human Growth Foundation, 94
Human rights
  ethical aspects of research, 249
  organizations, 214
Human tumor stem cell drug sensitivity assay (Health Technology Assessment Reports), 290
Humane Education, National Association for the Advancement of, 18
Humane Society of the United States, 18
Humes, James Joseph, 197-198
Huntington's Disease Society of America, 110
Hurley Medical Center (Flint, Michigan), 54
Huxley Institute for Biosocial Research, 193
Hydronephrosis, 125
Hydrotherapy (Health Technology Assessment Reports), 289
Hyperbaric medicine, 294
Hyperbaric oxygen
  actinomycosis treatment (Health Technology Assessment Reports), 289
  acute traumatic peripheral ischemia (Health Technology Assessment Reports), 289
  arthritis disease treatments (Health Technology Assessment Reports), 289
  chronic peripheral vascular insufficiency (Health Technology Assessment Reports), 288

chronic refractory osteomyelitis (Health Technology Assessment Reports), 289

crush injury (Health Technology Assessment Reports), 289

multiple sclerosis (Health Technology Assessment Reports), 289

organic brain syndrome (senility) (Health Technology Assessment Reports), 289

severed limbs (Health Technology Assessment Reports), 288

soft tissue radionecrosis and osteoradionecrosis (Health Technology Assessment Reports), 289

therapy (Health Technology Assessment Reports), 288

Hyperparathyroidism (bibliography), 24

Hypertension

age-adjusted diagnosis (DATTA opinions), 354

automated blood pressure monitoring (Health Technology Assessment Reports), 288

blood pressure monitoring (Health Technology Assessment Reports), 289

blood pressure monitors (patient-activated) (Health Technology Assessment Reports), 289

description, 110-111

information and concerned organizations, 31, 110-111

kidney disease and, 125

Hyperthermia, 288, 354

Hypnosis, 111, 344

Hypnotherapists, 111

Hypoglycemia Association, National, 111

I

ICD-9-CM, 120-122

Idaho (information on various health and social services in this and other states may be found at the heading, State agencies and organizations)

Identification cards (emergencies), 113

Identification Number, Unique Physician (UPIN), 118

Ileitis and Colitis, National Foundation for, 50

Illinois (information on various health and social services in this and other states may be found at the heading, State agencies and organizations)

Illustration, Medical, 151-152

Immigrant aid societies, 291-292

Immunization

childhood disease prevention (bibliography), 26

guides, 113

international travel, 113, 291

Immunoaugmentative therapy (DATTA opinions), 353

Immunoglobulin, Intravenous (bibliography), 24

Immunology, see also Allergy

organizations, 113

Immunosuppression (Council on Scientific Affairs report), 341

Impaired physicians, 113-115

Impairment evaluation, see Disability evaluation

Implants

anti-gastroesophageal reflux (Health Technology Assessment Reports), 289

breast, 23, 32-34

cardioverter-defibrillators (Health Technology Assessment Reports), 288

chemotherapy pump for liver cancer (Health Technology Assessment Reports), 289

cochlear, 25, 288

dental (bibliography), 25

electrospinal stimulator (DATTA opinions), 354

infusion pumps (DATTA opinions), 355

penile (DATTA opinions), 353

pump for heparin therapy (Health Technology Assessment Reports), 288

silicone (bibliography), 23

stereotaxic depth electrodes (focal epilepsy) (Health Technology Assessment Reports), 289

Impotence

bibliography, 23

Health Technology Assessment Reports, 287

papaverine (DATTA opinions), 351

penile implants (DATTA opinions), 353

phentolamine (DATTA opinions), 351

prostaglandin E1 therapy (DATTA opinions), 350-351

"In His Third Year of Dying" (JAMA "Poetry and Medicine"), 213

Incontinence, Urinary, 25, 294

Incorporation of medical practices, 214-215

Indexing (AMA), 331

Indian-American physicians, 81

Indian physicians, American, 80

Indiana (information on various health and social services in this and other states may be found at the heading, State agencies and organizations)

Indigent care

free clinics, 49

free drugs program, 72

local needs and information, 115

National Eye Care Project, 84

physician volunteerism, 298-299

Industrial Health Council, American, 115

Industrial Hygiene Association, American, 115

Infants

baby sitting, 23

cocaine, pregnancy and (bibliography), 24

Infection control, 186-187

Infections

foodborne (bibliography), 26

Infectious diseases, 115

Infectious Diseases, National Foundation for, 115

Infectious wastes (Council on Scientific Affairs report), 339

Informed consent

AMA policy, 115-116

sex counseling, 263

Informed Homebirth/Informed Birth and Parenting, 104, 172

Infusion pumps (DATTA opinions), 355

Injuries, see Accident prevention

Injury Information Clearinghouse, National, 116

Injury scale, Abbreviated, 1

Inoculations, see Immunization

Inspector General's Office

Medicare complaints (fraud, abuse), 168

Institute of Medicine and public health (Council on Scientific Affairs report), 337

Institute of Ultrasound in Medicine, American, 294

Instrumentation, Medical, 61

Insulin

external open-loop pump (Health Technology Assessment Reports), 288

Insulin infusion (two DATTA opinions), 352

Insurance

AMA's Health Access America provisions, 370

cancer coverage, 37

complaints, 118

fraud, 118

Health Insurance Claim Form (HCFA, 1500), 116-118

organizations listed, 116

state departments of, 118-120

Insurance Agency, American, 116, 226

Insurance claim coding, see Coding

Insurance Consumer Hotline, National, 118

Insurance Information Institute, 118, 226

Insurance, Life, see Life insurance

Interamerican College of Physicians and Surgeons, 271
Interchurch Medical Assistance, Inc, 71
Intern (term), 250
Internal medicine, 120
    recommended books, 32
Internal Medicine, American Board of,
    cardiovascular disease certification, 39, 102
    critical care certification, 55
    endocrinology and metabolism certification, 78
    geriatrics board certification, 89
    hematology certification, 102
    infectious disease certification, 115
    internal medicine and subspecialy certification, 120
    nephrology certification, 176
    oncology certification, 189
    pulmonary disease certification, 234
    rheumatology certification, 252
Internal Medicine, American Society of, 120
   "Understanding and Choosing Your Health
      Insurance," 118
International Aging, American Association for, 7
International Association for Medical Assistance to
    Travelers, 291
International Book Project, 31
International Childbirth Education Association, 46, 176
International Classification of Diseases (ICD-9-CM), 120-122
International College of Surgeons
    address, 284
    medical museum, 174
International cooperation
    AMA Office of International Medicine, 366
    book donations, 31
    donations of medical supplies, 71
    organizations listed, 122
    physician service opportunities abroad, 299
    World Health Organization, 308
    World Medical Association, 308
International Doctors in Alcoholics Anonymous, 113
International health
    global warming (bibliography), 24
    organizations, 122
International Health, National Council for, 122, 299
International Hearing Dog Inc, 100
International medical graduates, 122-123
    Educational Commission for Foreign Medical
      Graduates, 75, 86, 123
    Fifth Pathway, 86
    Virchow-Pirquet Medical Society (graduates of Austrian,
      Czech, German, Hungarian, Slovak and Swiss medical
      schools), 81
International Physicians, American College of, 122, 123
International Reference Organization in Forensic Medicine
    and Sciences, 86
International travel, 113, 291
Internists, see Internal medicine
Interns, see Resident physicians
"Internship: Preparation or Hazing?" (JAMA "A Piece of My
    Mind"), 249-250
Interviews by media, 271-272
Intracranial pressure measurement (Health Technology
    Assessment Reports), 289
Intrauterine devices (DATTA opinions), 352
Intravenous immunoglobulin (bibliography), 24
Invertebrates (bibliography), 25
Iowa (information on various health and social services in
    this and other states may be found at the heading,
    State agencies and organizations)
Iron overload, 123, 288
Iron Overload Diseases Association, 123
Islamic Medical Association, 81
"It's Over, Debbie," (JAMA "A Piece of My Mind"), 81-82

Italian American Medical Association, 81

J

JAMA, see Journal of the American Medical Association
Jewish Hospital, National, 19
Jewish Hospital Asthma Center, National, 143
Jogging, 20
Johns Hopkins AIDS Service, 10
Johns Hopkins School of Hygiene and Public Health
    animal testing alternatives, 18
Johns Hopkins University School of Medicine, 159
Joint Commission on Accreditation of Healthcare
    Organizations, 3
    ambulatory surgery, 16
    Home Care Project, 105
    hospices, 108
    hospital accreditation, 108
    nursing home accreditation, 182
Joseph and Rose Kennedy Institute of Ethics, 28, 80
Journal of the American Medical Association
    cover artwork and essays, 368
    formats (databases, etc), 367, 368
    special, periodic issues described, 367
Journal of the American Medical Association (special
    features)
    "A Piece of My Mind"
      "Accomplices," 255
      "Aging and Caring," 88
      "Coming Home," 224-226
      "Custodian," 192-193
      "Daddy," 252-253
      "Encourage Information Therapy," 53-54
      "Equal, Not Really," 301
      "House Calls," 105
      "Internship: Preparation or Hazing?" 249-250
      "It's Over, Debbie," 81-82
      "Keeping Up With the Literature," 135-136
      "Knee," 207
      "One Snake or Two?" 6-7
      "Quality of Mercy," 107-108
      "Sensitive Subject," 282-283
      "Surprise Party," 171-172
      "Waste," 73
    "Poetry and Medicine"
      "Heart Donor," 193
      "In His Third Year of Dying," 213
      "Learning to Hear," 39
      "Med Tech Explains the Differential," 163
      "Overdose," 282
    theme issues
      African American health, 172
      AIDS articles, 9
      alcohol use and abuse, 13
      allergic and immunologic diseases, 14
      animal rights and research, 18
      boxing, 32
      cholesterol, 65
      emergency cardiac care, 40
      human reproduction, 85
      impaired physicians, 113
      Johns Hopkins, 159
      nuclear weapons, 178
      quality of medical care, 235
      Relative value studies, 168
      sexually transmitted diseases, 265
      smoking, 266
Journals, Medical
    "Keeping Up With the Literature," 135-136

NEJM, 177
  reading habits, 135-136
  references and citations to articles in, 238-246
Justice Department (US)
  Drug Enforcement Administration, 72
  people with disabilities, 95
Juvenile Diabetes Foundation, 62

K

Kaiser Health Library, 54
Kansas (information on various health and social services in
  this and other states may be found at the heading,
  State agencies and organizations)
Kaplan, Stanley H, 251
"Keeping Up With the Literature" (JAMA "A Piece of My
  Mind"), 135-136
Keller, Helen (Center for Deaf/Blind), 29
Kennedy, John F, 197-198
Kennedy (Joseph and Rose) Institute of Ethics, 28, 80
Kentucky (information on various health and social services
  in this and other states may be found at the heading,
  State agencies and organizations)
Keratotomy, Radial (DATTA opinions), 352, 355
Kevorkian, Jack, 82-83
Kidney
  dialysis (bibliography), 26
  disease, 125
  end-stage renal disease (Health Technology Assessment
    Reports), 288
  transplantation and apheresis (Health Technology
    Assessment Reports), 288
Kidney Foundation, National, 193
Kidney Fund, American, 125
Kidney Patients, American Association of, 125
Kidney stones
  bibliography, 25
  extracorporeal shock wave lithotripsy (Health Technology
    Assessment Reports), 288
  Health Technology Assessment Reports, 287, 288
  percutaneous nephrolithotomy (DATTA opinions), 354
  percutaneous ultrasound (Health Technology
    Assessment Reports), 288
  transurethral nephrolithotomy (DATTA opinions), 354
"Knee" (JAMA "A Piece of My Mind"), 207
Kunkel test (Health Technology Assessment Reports), 290

L

La Leche League International, 32
Laboratories
  AMA policy, 48
  animal research, 18
  physician-office, 189
Laboratory Animal Science, American Association for, 18
Laboratory animals
  bibliography (1991 bibliography), 23
  care and use (1985-1989 bibliography), 25
  pain, anesthesia, analgesia (bibliography), 23, 25
  research, 18
  welfare (1988 bibliography), 23, 24, 25
Lactose breath hydrogen test (Health Technology
  Assessment Reports), 289
Lactulose breath hydrogen test (Health Technology
  Assessment Reports), 289
Lamaze, 46, 176
Laminectomy (DATTA opinions), 351
Language

American Speech-Language-Hearing Association, 3, 127
  public speaking guidelines, 271-272
Language disorders, 100
Language pathology
  dysphagia management (Health Technology
    Assessment Reports), 287
Language proficiency
  international (foreign) medical graduates, 122-123
Laparoscopic cholecystectomy 23, 87
Laryngological Association, American, 127
Laryngological, Rhinological and Otological Society,
  American, 127, 252
Laryngology, 127
Laser Medicine and Surgery, American Society for, 127
Laser photocoagulation
  gastrointestinal tract hemorrhage (DATTA opinions), 354
  Health Technology Assessment Reports, 287
Laser trabeculoplasty (Health Technology Assessment
  Reports), 288
Lasers
  carbon dioxide (DATTA opinions), 355
  carbon dioxide (Health Technology Assessment
    Reports), 288, 289
  Council on Scientific Affairs report, 343-344
  neodymium-YAG (Health Technology Assessment
    Reports), 288
  organizations listed, 127
  posterior capsulotomies (Health Technology
    Assessment Reports), 288
Latham Foundation, 18
Law and Medicine, American Society of, 128
Lawsuits, 223-228
Lawyers, 127-129
LCME, (Liaison Committee on Medical Education), 355
Leader Dog for the Blind, 29
League of Nursing, National, 179
Learning Assessment Form (Continuing medical
  education), 54
"Learning to Hear" (from JAMA "Poetry and Medicine"), 39
Legal affairs
  AMA Office of the General Counsel, 319
  court-ordered treatments during pregnancy, 222
  organizations listed, 127-129
  references and citations of cases, 244-246
  what happens when suit is filed, 223-224
Legal Medicine, American College of, 128
Lenses
  ultraviolet absorbing and reflecting (Health Technology
    Assessment Reports), 290
Leonard Wood Memorial Foundation, 129
Leonardo da Vinci, 151-152, 368
Leprosy Foundation, American, 129
Leprosy Missions, American, 129
Lesbian physicians and medical students, 214
Leukemia
  bone marrow transplantation in childhood (DATTA
    opinions), 354
Leukemia Association, National, 129
Leukemia Society of America, 129
Leukemia, Chronic myelogenous (DATTA opinions), 351
Leukocyte test, Cytotoxic (Health Technology Assessment
  Reports), 289
Liability insurance
  Medicare relative value factor, 167
Liability insurer associations, 226
Liability reform
  AMA's Health Access America provisions, 371
Liability risk management, 224
Liaison Committee on Medical Education, 355
Libraries, 129-136
  associations listed, 135-136

consumer health information, 53-54
recommended-book lists, 32
Library Association, American
library user confidentiality, 53-54
national headquarters, 136
Library of Congress (US)
address, telephone number, 134
National Library Service for Blind and Physically
Handicapped, 29
National Translation Center, 290
Licensed practical nurse, 179
Licensure
AMA department, 369
FLEX exam, 85
impaired physicians, 113-115
state boards, 137-139
what physicians need to know, 136-137
Licensure, Enforcement and Regulation, National
Clearinghouse on, 137
Life insurance, 139
Life Insurance, American Council, 139
Life Insurance Medical Directors of America, Association
of, 139
Life-support withdrawal, 69
Light scanning, Transillumination (Health Technology
Assessment Reports), 287, 288
Lilly, Eli, see Eli Lilly and Co
Limitations, Statute of (tort reform glossary), 229
Limiting charge (Medicare terminology), 166
Lion's Club International, 29
eye donor registry, 193
Lipid Diseases Foundation, National, 139
Lipoproteins, High-density (bibliography), 24
Lipo-Suction Surgery, American Society of, 140
Liposuction, 140
Literacy, 140
Literacy Volunteers of America, 140
Literature, Medical, see Journals, Medical
Lithotripsy
extracorporeal shockwave, 288, 353
noninvasive, extracorporeal (DATTA opinions), 354
transurethral urethroscopic (Health Technology
Assessment Reports), 287, 288
ultrasonic (DATTA opinions), 353
Liver cancer
implantable chemotherapy pump (Health Technology
Assessment Reports), 289
Liver Disease, American Association for the Study of, 140
Liver Foundation, American, 140
Liver transplantation, 140, 287, 289, 290
Living at Home, 7
Living Bank, 193
Living Well, 369
Living wills, 140
Lixiscope (Health Technology Assessment Reports), 288
Loans, Business, 140-141
Locality (Medicare terminology), 166
Location of medical practice, 141-142
Locum tenens, 142
Long-term care
AMA's Health Access America provisions, 371
Long, Crawford W, 68-69
Lou Gehrig's disease, see Amyotrophic lateral sclerosis
Louisiana (information on various health and social services
in this and other states may be found at the heading, State
agencies and organizations)
Low-level radioactive wastes (Council on Scientific Affairs
report), 338-339
Lung Association, American, 143
Lung associations
chest x-rays, 43

statewide, 143-144
Lung diseases, 142-144
LUNGLINE, 143
Lupus erythematosus, Systemic, 288
Lupus Foundation of America, Inc, 144
Lyme Borreliosis Foundation, 144
Lyme disease, 26, 144

M

"M.D. Computing," 52
MAAC (Medicare terminology), 166
Macular Diseases, Association for, 145
Macular drusen (DATTA opinions), 354
MADD (Mothers Against Drunk Driving), 13
Magazines without tobacco ads, 267-271
Magnetic resonance imaging
abdomen and pelvis (Council on Scientific Affairs
report), 338
cardiovascular system (Council on Scientific Affairs
report), 339
central nervous system (Council on Scientific Affairs
report), 339-340
head and neck (Council on Scientific Affairs report), 338
Health Technology Assessment Reports, 287, 288
musculoskeletal applications (Council on Scientific
Affairs report), 339
prologue, fundamentals (Council on Scientific Affairs
report), 343
surface/specialty coil devices and gating techniques
(Health Technology Assessment Reports), 287
Magnetic Resonance Imaging, Society for, 145
Maine (information on various health and social services in
this and other states may be found at the heading,
State agencies and organizations)
Malnutrition in children (bibliography), 25
Malpractice, see Professional liability
Mammography, 145, 338, 353
Management Association, American, 145
Manic depressives, 172
Manpower, see Health manpower
Manufacturers of health products, 115
March of Dimes Birth Defects Foundation, 29
March 30 (Doctor's Day), 68-69
Marijuana, 145
Marketing, 145
Marketing Association, American, 145
Marketing research, 145
Marriage and Family Therapy, American Association of, 145
Marriage counseling, 145
Maryland (information on various health and social services
in this and other states may be found at the heading,
State agencies and organizations)
Massachusetts (information on various health and social
services in this and other states may be found at the
heading, State agencies and organizations)
Massage Therapy Association, American, 145
Masterfile (AMA), 330
Matching Program, National Resident, 146
Maternal and Child Health, National Center for Education
in, 146
Maxillofacial Surgeons, American Society of, 146
Maxillofacial surgery, 146
Maximum actual allowable charge (Medicare
terminology), 166
Mayo, Charles Horace, 146-148
Mayo, William James, 146-148
Mayo Clinic, 146-148
MCAT review courses, 251

McLean Hospital Brain Bank (Belmont, Massachusetts), 16, 32
"M.D. Computing," 52
Meat safety, 182
"Med Tech Explains the Differential" (JAMA "Poetry and Medicine"), 163
Medecins Sans Frontieres, 68, 299
Media interviews, 271-272
Medic Alert Foundation, 113
    organ donor program, 193
Medicaid
    HCFA administration, 96
    program description, 149
Medical Acupuncturists, American Academy of, 4
Medical and Dental Association, National, 81
Medical assistant, 149-150
Medical associations, 150-151, 203
Medical boards (licensure), 137-139
Medical Books for China, 31
Medical Care and Review Association, American, 97, 222
Medical career information, 41-42
Medical colleges, see Medical schools
Medical Colleges, Association of American
    headquarters information, 158
    medical career information, 42
    registration for medical school entrance exam, 162
Medical Device Register, 62
Medical devices, see Devices, Medical
Medical directive forms, 140
Medical Directors, American Academy of, 42, 84
Medical Directors Association, American, 84
Medical education, see also Continuing medical education; Graduate medical education
    accreditation, 3
    adolescent health, 4-5
    AMA activities, council, divisions, etc, 356
    AMA Department of Undergraduate Medical Education, 3
    animal use, 18
    early, in the United States, 313-314
    international medical graduates, 122-123
    national accrediting bodies, 355-356
    nutrition programs, 182
    review courses, 251
    risks of impairment for physicians, 114-115
Medical Electroencephalographic Association, American, 75
Medical Equipment Suppliers, National Association of, 62, 80
Medical examiners (state boards), 137-139
Medical Examiners, National Association of, 86, 198
Medical Examiners, National Board of, 137, 162
Medical Golf Association, American, 20
Medical Group Management Association, 84, 94
    audiovisuals, 20
Medical illustration, 151-152
Medical illustrators, 152
Medical Illustrators, Association of, 152
Medical informatics (Council on Scientific Affairs report), 335
Medical Informatics Association, American, 26, 52
Medical Information Bureau, 156
Medical Instrumentation, Association for the Advancement of, 61
Medical Joggers Association, American, 20
Medical journals, see Journals, Medical
Medical laboratory technician, 152-153
Medical libraries, 129-136
Medical Library Association, 136
    Code of Ethics, 53-54
Medical literature, see Journals, Medical
Medical meetings, see Meetings
Medical payment schedule (Medicare terminology), 166
Medical Peer Review Association, American, 200

Medical Political Action Committee, American, 361
Medical practice acts (statutes cited by state), 154-155
Medical practice management, see Practice management; other headings beginning with Practice...
Medical Quality, American College of, 200
Medical record administrator, 157
Medical record coding, see Coding
Medical record technician, 157-158
Medical records
    access by patients, 115-116
    closing medical practices, 49-50
    confidentiality, 115-116
    copies of, 155-156
    CPT coding, 55-57
    documentation, 156-157
    retention by physicians, 155-156
    transfer of, 155-156
Medical Records Association, American, 156
Medical review
    AMA office of, 357
    preadmission criteria, 221
    Reference Criteria for Short Stay Hospital Review, 238
    sample criteria, 257
Medical school entrance examination, 162
Medical schools
    accreditation, 3
    foreign, 86
    listings by state, 158-162
Medical Science Knowledge Program, 162
Medical societies, 150-151, 203
    AMA federation relations, 363
    American Association of Medical Society Executives, 84
    American Medical Association founding, 313-317
    county, 55
    ethnic, 80
    member misconduct, discipline, 50-52
    state listings 277-279
    unified membership with AMA, 363
Medical Society Executives, American Association of, 84
Medical Society of the State of New York
    AMA code of ethics, 321-327
Medical sonographer, 64
Medical Specialties, see Specialties, Medical
Medical Specialties, American Board of,
    Doctor Certification Line, 55
    specialists' compendium, 273
Medical specialty societies
    AMA activities and programs, 363, 364
Medical Specialty Societies, Council of
    "Choosing a Medical Specialty," 273
Medical staff
    AMA activities and programs, 364
Medical Staff Services, National Association of, 109
Medical students
    career information, 42
    gifts from industry, 89-92
    reading habits, 135-136
    risks of impairment, 114
    suicide, 282-283
Medical Students Association, American, 162
Medical supplies, see Devices, Medical
Medical Systems, American Association for, 52
Medical technologists and medical technology, 163
Medical Technology, American Society for, 163
Medical Tennis Association, American, 20
Medical Transcription, American Association for, 156
Medical waste, 163-164
Medical Women's Association, American, 150, 304
Medical Writers Association, American, 311
Medical writing, 309-311

Medicare
  carrier listings by state, 168-171
  complaints, 168
  fraud, 168
  general description of program, 168
  glossary of terms, 164-168
  HCFA administration, 96
  HMOs, 97-98
  hospital mortality data, 279-280
  non-par (non-participating physician), 166
  par (participating physician), 167
  payment schedule, 166
  reform (AMA's Health Access America provisions), 371
  specialty codes, 1-2
Medicare carriers (listed by state), 168-171
Medicare Economic Index, 166
Medications, see Drugs
Medicines du Monde, 299
MediQual Systems, 280
Medisgroups, 280
MEDWATCH, 46, 173
Meetings, 171
Melanoma (bibliography), 24
Melodic intonation therapy (Health Technology Assessment
  Reports), 289
Memorial Sloan-Kettering Institute for Cancer Research, 37
Meniere's disease, 88
Mental health, 171-172
  depression (bibliography), 24
  destructive behaviors and developmental disabilities
    (bibliography), 25
  diagnostic manual (DSM III), 64
  disorders of the homeless (bibliography), 25
  employee assistance programs, 77-78
  human-pet relations (bibliography), 24
  impaired physicians, 113-115
  panic attacks, 19
  panic disorder, agoraphobia (bibliography), 23
  postpartum depresssion (bibliography), 24
  seasonal affective disorder (bibliography), 24
Mental Health Association, National, 172
Mental Retardation, American Association on, 172
Mentally Ill, National Alliance for the, 172
Mercury, Staff of, 6-7
Mercy, 107-108
Metabolic disorders
  kidney stones, 125
  specialty certification, 78
Metropolitan Life Insurance Company
  height-weight tables, 301
Mexican Medical Association, 150
Mexico-US border environmental health commission
  (Council on Scientific Affairs report), 337
Michigan (information on various health and social services
  in this and other states may be found at the heading,
  State agencies and organizations)
Michigan Coalition Against Domestic Violence, 70
Microfilm (medical records), 156
Midwives, 172, 178
Migraine headaches, 95
Military medicine, 172
Military Surgeons of the United States, Association of, 172
Milton Helpern Institute of Forensic Medicine, 86
Minnesota (information on various health and social services
  in this and other states may be found at the heading, State
  agencies and organizations)
Minority groups
  health care and access, 172
  health education and promotion (bibliography), 26
Misconduct by physicians, 50-52

Missing and Exploited Children, National Center for, 4, 46,
  173, 252
Missing Child Hotline, 4, 46, 173, 252
Mississippi (information on various health and social
  services in this and other states may be found at the
  heading, State agencies and organizations)
Missouri (information on various health and social services
  in this and other states may be found at the heading,
  State agencies and organizations)
Mobility International, 95
Modern Talking Picture Service, 39
Mona Lisa (JAMA cover), 368
Montana (information on various health and social services
  in this and other states may be found at the heading,
  State agencies and organizations)
Morbidity and Mortality Weekly Report, 43
Mortality data (hospitals'), 279-280
Mothers Against Drunk Driving, 13, 73
Mothers of Twins Club, National Organization of, 293
Motion pictures
  captioning services for deaf, 39, 100
Mouth cancer, 25
MRI, see Magnetic resonance imaging
Multiple births, 173
Multiple Sclerosis Society, National, 173
Muscle disorders, 173
Muscular Dystrophy Association, 173
Musculoskeletal and Skin Diseases, National Institute of
  Arthritis and, 19
Museum of Health and Medicine, National, 174
Museum of History and Technology, National, 202
Museum of Ophthalmology, 174
Museums, Medical, 174
Myasthenia Gravis Foundation, 173
Mycoplasma completion fixation test (Health Technology
  Assessment Reports), 290
Mycotic toenails, 288

N

Narcolepsy and Cataplexy Foundation of America, 175
Narcolepsy Association, American, 175
Narcotic Educational Foundation of America, 175
Narcotics
  impaired physicians, 114
Narcotics Anonymous, 175
National Adoption Center, 6
National Agricultural Library (US), 134, 182
  Rural Information Center Health Services, 253
National AIDS Hotline, 10
National AIDS Information Clearinghouse, 10
National AIDS Testing, 10
National Alliance for the Mentally Ill, 172
National Alliance of Blind Students, 29
National Alliance of Breast Cancer Organizations, 32
National Alopecia Areata Foundation, 95
National Association for the Advancement of Humane
  Education, 18
National Association for Ambulatory Care, 17
National Association for Home Care, 105
National Association for Prenatal Addiction and Education
  cocaine baby helpline, 50
National Association for Sickle Cell Disease, 265
National Association of Advisors for the Health Professions,
  Inc, 42
National Association of Disability Examiners, 67
National Association of Emergency Medical Technicians, 77
National Association of Health Services Executives, 84

National Association of Medical Equipment Suppliers, 62, 80
National Association of Medical Examiners, 86, 198
National Association of Medical Staff Services, 109
National Association of People With AIDS, 10
National Association of Physician Broadcasters, 34, 207
National Association of Private Geriatric Care Managers, 105
National Association of Residents and Interns, 140, 250
National Association of State Boards of Education, 5
National Association to Aid Fat Americans, 183
National Asthma Center, 19
National Ataxia Foundation, 19
National Athletic Trainers Association
National Audio Visual Center, 20
National Board of Medical Examiners, 137
    medical school entrance exam test centers, 162
National Brain Research Association, 32
National Brain Tumor Foundation, 32
National Cancer Institute (US), 37
National Captioning Institute, Inc, 39, 100
National Center for Education in Maternal ahd Child
    Health, 146
National Center for Health Education, 54
National Center for Health Statistics (US), 122, 281
National Center for Homecare Education and Research, 10
National Center for Homeopathy, 108
National Center for Human Genome Research (US), 87
National Center for Missing and Exploited Children,
    4, 46, 173, 252
National Center for Stuttering, 282
National Charities Information Bureau, 43
National Child Abuse Hotline, 44
National Child Safety Council, 256
National Chronic Fatigue Association, 47
National Clearinghouse for Alcohol Information, 13
National Clearinghouse for Drug Abuse Information, 50, 71
National Clearinghouse for Primary Care Information, 223
National Clearinghouse on Licensure, Enforcement and
    Regulation, 137
National Coalition Against Domestic Violence, 44, 69
National Coalition Against the Misuse of Pesticides, 201
National Coalition for the Homeless, 108
National Commission Against Drunk Driving, 13, 73
National Commission for the Certification for Acupuncture, 4
National Commission on Certification of Physician's
    Assistants, 207
National Commission on Correctional Health Care, 55
National Commission on the Role of the School and the
    Community in Improving Adolescent Health, 5
National Committee for Prevention of Child Abuse, 44
National Committee on Youth Suicide Prevention, 4
National Council Against Health Fraud, 97
National Council for International Health, 122, 299
National Council on Alcoholism, 13
National Council on Child Abuse, 44
National Council on Child Abuse and Family Violence, 69
National Council on Patient Information and Education, 199
National Dance Association, 84
National Depressive and Manic Depressive Association
National Diabetes Information Clearinghouse, 62
National Digestive Diseases Education and Information
    Clearinghouse, 67
"National Directory of Alcoholism, Drug Abuse Treatment
    Programs," 72
National Domestic Violence Hotline, 70
National Down's Syndrome Society, 87
National Easter Seal Society, 29, 75
National Eye Care Project, 84
National Eye Institute (US), 84
National Eye Research Foundation, 84
National Federal of Parents for Drug-Free Youth, 71
National Fitness Foundation, 84

National Foundation for Ectodermal Dysplasia, 61
National Foundation for Ileitis and Colitis, 50
National Foundation for Infectious Diseases, 115
National Foundation of Dentistry for the Handicapped, 95
National Gaucher Foundation, 87
National Gay and Lesbian Crisisline, 10
National Governors Association, 99
National Handicapped Sports and Recreation
    Association, 301
National Head and Spinal Cord Injury Prevention
    Program, 5
National Head Injury Foundation, 95
National Headache Foundation, 95
National Health Care Anti-Fraud Association, 175
National Health Council, 42, 96
National Health Information Center, 199
National Health Lawyers Association, 129
National Health Service Corps (US), 98-99, 253
National Healthcare Anti-Fraud Association, 118
National Hearing Aid Society, 100
National Heart, Lung and Blood Institute (US), 102
National Hemophilia Foundation, 102
National High Blood Pressure Education Program, 111
National Highway Traffic Safety Administration, 21, 256
National Hormone and Pituitary Program, 108
National Hospice Organization, 108
National Hypoglycemia Association, 111
National Information Center for Handicapped Children and
    Youth, 95
National Information Center for Orphan Drugs and Rare
    Diseases, 193
National Injury Information Clearinghouse, 116
National Institute of Alcohol Abuse and Alcoholism (US), 13
National Institute of Allergy and Infectious
    Diseases (US), 13
National Institute of Arthritis and Musculoskeletal and Skin
    Diseases (US), 19, 195
National Institute of Child Health (US), 46
National Institute of Dental Research (US), 59
National Institute of Diabetes, Digestive and Kidney
    Disease, (US), 125
National Institute of Environmental Health Sciences
    (US), 75, 79
National Institute of Mental Health (US), 172
    Anti-Social and Violent Behavior Branch, 71, 238
National Institute of Neurological Disorders and Stroke,
    (US), 32, 281
National Institute on Aging (US), 7
National Institute on Drug Abuse (US), 71-72
    cocaine hotline, 50
National Institutes of Health (US), (see also individual
    institutes, above)
    AMA support, 249
    general description, major components, 175-176
    liver transplants, 140, 290
    National High Blood Pressure Education Program, 111
    Office of Research on Women's Health, 305-306
National Insurance Consumer Hotline, 118
National Jewish Hospital, 19
National Jewish Hospital Asthma Center, 143
National Kidney Foundation, 193
National League of Nursing, 179
National Leukemia Asosciation, 129
National Library of Medicine (US), 134
    Audio-Visual Section, 20
    prints and photographic collection, 202
National Library Service for Blind and Physically
    Handicapped, 29
National Lipid Diseases Foundation, 139
National Medical and Dental Association, 81
National Medical Association, 80, 150

National Medical Association (former name of AMA), 313
National Medical School Review, 251
National Mental Health Association, 172
National Multiple Sclerosis Society, 173
National Museum of Health and Medicine, 174
National Museum of History and Technology, 202
National Neurofibromatosis Foundation, 176
National Odd Shoe Exchange, 17
National Organization for Competency Assurance, 50
National Organization for Rare Disorders, 193, 238
National Organization of Mothers of Twins Club, 293
National Osteoporosis Foundation, 195
National Parkinson Foundation, 197
National Phlebotomy Association, 30
National Physician Credentials Verification Service, 55, 207
National Practitioner Data Bank, 55, 207
    Bureau of Health Professions (telephone number), 35
National PTA, 10
National Reference Center for Bioethics Literature, 28, 80
National Registry of Emergency Medical Technicians, 77
National Rehabilitation Information Center, 248
National Research Council, 248
National Resident Matching Program, 146, 250
National Retinitis Pigmentosa Foundation, 251
National Reye's Syndrome Foundation, 252
National Rural Health Association, 253
National Safe Workplace Institute, 265
National Safety Council, 13, 256
    accident statistics, 281
    drunk driving brochure, 73
    medical information on microfilm, 113
National Science Foundation, 257
National Scoliosis Foundation, 258
National Second Opinion Program, 284
National Self-Help Clearinghouse, 259
National Society for Cardiovascular Technology/Pulmonary
    Technology, 41, 75
National Society to Prevent Blindness, 29
    organ donation, 193
    state societies listed, 29-30
National Spinal Cord Injury Association, 277
National Standards Institute, American
    medical literature references and citations, 238-246
National Stroke Association, 281
National Sudden Infant Death Syndrome Foundation, 282
National Tay Sach's and Allied Diseases Foundation, 88
National Tuberous Sclerosis Association, 293
National VD Hotline, 265
National Vitiligo Foundation, 298
National Wheelchair Athletic Association, 301
National Woman Abuse Prevention Center, 70
National Woman Abuse Prevention Project, 70
Natural childbirth, 46, 176
Naturopathic Physicians, American Association of, 176
Naturopathy, 176
NBFM review course, 251
Near East Refuge Aid, American, Inc, American, 71
Nebraska (information on various health and social
    services in this and other states may be found at the
    heading, State agencies and organizations)
Neodymium-YAG laser (Health Technology Assessment
    Reports), 288
Nephrolithotomy (DATTA opinions), 354
Nephrology
    nurses and technicians, 65
    organizations, 176
Nephrology, American Society of, 125, 176
Nephrology Nurses and Technicians, American Association
    of, 65
Nephrotic syndrome, 125

Network for Continuing Medical Education, 297
Neurofibromatosis Foundation, National, 176
Neurological diagnosis, 76
Neurological Surgeons, American Association of
    address, 176
    spinal cord injury prevention, 5
Neurological Surgeons, Congress of, 5, 177
Neurological surgery, 176-177
    history (bibliography), 25
Neurological Surgery, American Academy of, 176
Neurological Surgery, American Board of,
    critical care certification, 55
    neurosurgery certification, 177
Neurology
    information and organizations, 177
    resident matching program, 146
Neurology, American Academy of, 177
Neuroma, Acoustic 3, 24
Neuromuscular electrical stimulation (Health Technology
    Assessment Reports), 288
Neurosurgery, see Neurological surgery
Nevada (information on various health and social services
    in this and other states may be found at the heading,
    State agencies and organizations)
New England Journal of Medicine, 177
New Hampshire (information on various health and social
    services in this and other states may be found at the
    heading, State agencies and organizations)
New Jersey (information on various health and social
    services in this and other states may be found at the
    heading, State agencies and organizations)
New Mexico (information on various health and social
    services in this and other states may be found at the
    heading, State agencies and organizations)
New York (information on various health and social
    services in this and other states may be found at the
    heading, State agencies and organizations)
New York State Medical Association, 322-326
New York State Medical Society, 314-315
Newman Cosmetic Surgery Center, 140
Niacin, 298
Noise and hearing loss (bibliography), 25
Non-participating physicians (Medicare terminology), 166
North Carolina (information on various health and social
    services in this and other states may be found at the
    heading, State agencies and organizations)
North Dakota (information on various health and social
    services in this and other states may be found at the
    heading, State agencies and organizations)
Northwestern University Memorial Hospital (Chicago,
    Illinois)
    cocaine baby helpline, 50
    spinal cord injury care, 277
Notice of proposed rulemaking (Medicare terminology),
    166-167
Nuclear energy, 177
Nuclear Medicine, American Board of, 177
Nuclear Medicine, American College of, 177
Nuclear medicine technologist, 177-178
Nuclear Physicians, American College of, 177
Nuclear power (Council on Scientific Affairs report), 339
Nuclear war, 178
Nurse anesthetist, 179
Nurse Attorneys, American Association of, 178
Nurse-Midwives, American College of, 172, 178
Nurse Practitioners, American Academy of, 179
Nurses Association, American, 179
Nurses' associations, 179, 180-182
Nursing, 178-182
    occupational health, 186

prescriptive privileges for controlled substances (by state), 179
public health (staff, community health), 231
self-care role (bibliography), 24
Nursing homes, 182
Nutrition, see Foods and Nutrition
Nutrition, American College of, 182

O

Oath of Hippocrates, 102
Obesity
gastric restrictive surgery (DATTA opinions), 354
gastrointestinal surgery for (bibliography), 24
information and concerned organizations, 183
treatment (Council on Scientific Affairs report), 340-341
"Obitiatry," 82-83
OBRA, 167
Obsessive Compulsive Disorder Foundation, 183
Obstetricians and Gynecologists, American College of
abortion policy implications, 3
"The Abused Woman," 70
adolescent pregnancy prevention, 5
adolescent sexuality, 4-5
contraception pamphlet, 29
Dalkon Shield information, 59
home births, 104
midwifery, 172
national headquarters, 94, 222
pregnancy information, 183
resident matching program, 146
Obstetrics and gynecology
information and organizations, 183
resident matching program, 146
Obstetrics and Gynecology, American Board of, 94, 183
critical care certification, 55
oncology certification, 189
reproductive endocrinology certification, 78
Occupational health
guidelines for physicians, 183-186
indoor air pollution (bibliography), 26
industrial health, 115
sick building syndrome, 265
video display terminals, 297
Occupational Hearing Service, 100
Occupational Medical Association, American, 186
Occupational medicine, 186
Occupational Medicine, American College of
address, 186
drug abuse testing, 72-73
Occupational Safety and Health Administration (US)
bloodborne pathogens standards, 186-187
regional offices, 187
Occupational therapy, 188-189
Occupational therapy assistant, 188-189
Occupational Therapy Association, American, 189
Odd Shoe Exchange, National, 17
Office laboratories, 189
Office of Drug Control Policy (US), 71
Office of Health Technology Assessment (US), 287
Office of Inspector General (US HHS Department)
Medicare complaints (fraud, abuse), 168
Office on Smoking and Health, 266
Office staff
closing medical practices, 49-50
medical assistants, 149-150
personnel policies in medical practices, 216-217
physician's assistants, 203-207

Ohio (information on various health and social services in this and other states may be found at the heading, State agencies and organizations)
Oklahoma (information on various health and social services in this and other states may be found at the heading, State agencies and organizations)
Omnibus Budget Reconciliation Act of 1989, 167
Oncology, 189
"One Snake or Two?" (JAMA "A Piece of My Mind"), 6-7
Ophthalmic medical technician, 189-190
Ophthalmology
information and organizations, 190
medical museum, 174
Ophthalmology, American Academy of, 127, 190
Ophthalmology, American Board of, 190
Optometric assistant, 192
Optometric Association, American, 192
Optometric associations, 190-192
Optometry, 190-192
Oral oncology, 189
Oral surgery, 146
Oregon (information on various health and social services in this and other states may be found at the heading, State agencies and organizations)
Organ donation, 192-193
Organ Procurement Organizations, Association of, 193
Organ Transplant Fund, 193
Organs, Artificial, 19
Orphan drugs, 193
Orphan Drugs and Rare Diseases, National Information Center for, 193
Orthomolecular Medical Society, 193
Orthopaedic Association, American, 194
Orthopaedic Society for Sports Medicine, American, 194, 277
Orthopaedic Surgeons, American Academy of, 194
Orthopaedic Surgery, American Board of,
hand surgery certification, 95
orthopedics certification, 194
Orthopaedics, 194
Orthopedics, see also headings beginning with Orthopaedic above
podiatric, 213
Orthotic assistant, 194
Orthotics and Prosthetics, American Board for Certification in, 194, 229
Orthotists and Prosthetists, American Academy of, 194, 229
Orton Dyslexia Society, 73
OSHA, see Occupational Safety and Health Administration (US)
Osteopathic Association, American, 194
Osteopathic schools (listed by state), 194-195
Osteopathy, 194-195
Osteoporosis, 195
Osteoporosis Foundation, National, 195
Ostomy, 195
Otolaryngic Allergy, American Academy of, 195
Otolaryngology, 127, 195
Otolaryngology, American Board of, 195
Otolaryngology--Head and Neck Surgery, American Academy of
address, 195
"Facial Nerve Problems," 23
resident matching program, 146
Otological Society, American, 195
Otology, 195
Outlier (Medicare terminology), 167
Outpatient Surgery, American Society of, 16
"Overdose" (JAMA "Poetry and Medicine"), 282
Overseas Medical Aid Association, American
book donations, 31

equipment donations, 71
Oxygen therapy
    decubitus ulcers (Health Technology Assessment
        Reports), 289
    persistent skin lesions (Health Technology Assessment
        Reports), 289

P

Pacing (Health Technology Assessment Reports), 288
Paget's Disease Foundation, 197
Pain
    information and concerned organizations, 197
    laboratory animals (bibliography), 23, 25
    transcutaneous electrical nerve stimulation (Health
        Technology Assessment Reports), 289
Pain Society, American, 197
Pakistani Physicians, Association of, 81
Pan American Development Foundation, 71
Pan American Medical Association, 151
Pancreatic Association, American, 197
Pancreatic transplantation, 288, 351
Panic Attack Sufferers' Support Group, 197
Panic attacks, 19
Panic disorder (bibliography), 23
Pantothenic acid, 298
Papaverine (DATTA opinions), 351
Paralysis Association, American, 197
Paramedic, 76-77
Parasitic foodborne infections (bibliography), 26
Parent-Teachers Association, National, 10
Parenteral and Enteral Nutrition, American Society for, 182
Parenteral antineoplastics (Council on Scientific Affairs
    report), 344
Parents Anonymous Hotline, 44
Parkinson Disease Association, American, 197
Parkinson Foundation, National, 197
Participating physicians (Medicare terminology), 167
Partnership in medical practices, 215-216
Pass Group (Panic Attack Sufferers' Support Group), 19
Paternity testing, 197, 344
Pathologists, American Association of, 198
Pathologists, College of American
    drug abuse testing, 72-73
    headquarters information, 198
    self-instruction manual for office laboratories, 49
    Systematized Nomenclature of Medicine (SNOMED), 271
Pathology, 197-198
Pathology, American Board of,
    blood banking, transfusion medicine, 30
    forensic pathology, 30
    hematology certification, 102
Patient compensation fund (tort reform glossary), 228
Patient complaints, 208-212
Patient education, 199
    self-care (bibliography), 24
Patient identification cards, 113
Patient Information and Education, National Council on, 199
Patient Management Categories, 281
"Patient Medication Instruction Sheets," 72
Patient Puppets, 17
Patient satisfaction, 208-212
Patient support groups, 258-259
Patients' rights
    AMA's Patient Bill of Rights, 199
    informed consent, 115-116
    medical records, 155-156
Peace Corps (US), 299
Pediatric dentistry, 189

Pediatric Surgical Association, American, 199
Pediatrics, see also Children
    adolescent health, 4
    HIV-infected children, 12
Pediatrics, American Academy of
    "Healthy Children" program, 5
    address, 199
    adolescent health, 4
    HIV-infected children, 12
    immunization information, 113
Pediatrics, American Board of,
    critical care certification, 55
    infectious disease certification, 115
    pediatric and subspecialty certification, 199
Peer review, 199-200
    statistical analysis in, 280
Peer review organizations, 199-200
Penile implants (DATTA opinions), 353
Pennsylvania (information on various health and social
    services in this and other states may be found at the
    heading, State agencies and organizations)
Pension plans, see Retirement
People-to-People Health Foundation, 122
People With AIDS, National Association of, 10
People's Medical Society, 214
Percutaneous transluminal angioplasty, 288, 289
Percutaneous ultrasound (Health Technology Assessment
    Reports), 288
Perfusionists, 200-201
Perimetry, Computer-enhanced (Health Technology
    Assessment Reports), 289
Periodic payment of damages (tort reform glossary), 228
Periodicals
    magazines without tobacco ads, 267-271
Peroneal muscular atrophy, 87
Persistent vegetative state, 140, 336
Personnel policies, see Office staff
Pesticide cancer risk, agricultural workers (Council on
    Scientific Affairs report), 340
Pesticides, 75, 79, 201
Pesticides, National Coalition Against the Misuse of, 201
Pets, 18, 24
pH monitoring (esophageal) (Health Technology
    Assessment Reports), 288
Pharmaceutical Association, American, 202, 281
Pharmaceutical Manufacturers Association, 202
    Commission on Drugs for Rate Disorders, 193
    drug program for indigent, 72
Pharmacist assistant, 201
Pharmacology and Experimental Therapeutics, American
    Society for, 201
Pharmacy, 201-202
Pharmacy services director, 83-84
Pharmacy technician, 201
Phentolamine (DATTA opinions), 351
Philanthropic Association of Virginia, 37
Philippine Physicians in America, Association of, 81
Philippine Surgeons in America, Association of, 81
Phlebotomy Association, National, 30
Phobia Society of America, 202
Phobias, 202
Photobiology, American Society for, 202
Photocoagulation, 127, 287, 354
Photographs, Medical, 202
Photography
    endothelial cells (Health Technology Assessment
        Reports), 289
Photokymography (Health Technology Assessment
    Reports), 289
Photoplethysmography (Health Technology Assessment
    Reports), 289

Physiatrists, 202
Physical examinations
    airmen, 202
    healthy persons, 202
    occupational, 183-186
    return-to-work, 186
Physical fitness, 25, 84
Physical medicine, 202
Physical Medicine and Rehabilitation, American Academy
    of, 202, 248
Physical Medicine and Rehabilitation, American Board
    of, 202, 248
Physical therapist assistant, 202-203
Physical therapy, 202-203
Physical Therapy Association, American, 203
Physician-assisted suicide, see Suicide assistance
Physician biographical records, 329
Physician Broadcasters, National Association of, 34, 207
Physician Committee for Responsible Medicine, 214
Physician credentials, see Credentialing
Physician Credentials Verification Service, National 55, 207
Physician earnings, 207
Physician Executive Management Center, 42
Physician Identification Number, Unique (UPIN), 118
Physician Insurers Association of America, 226
Physician Link (AIDS hotline), 10
Physician mortality project (Council on Scientific Affairs
    report), 341
Physician-patient communication, 208-212
Physician-patient relationship, 207-212
    patients' rights, 199
    sex counseling and treatments, 263-264
Physician Payment Review Commission, 167, 168
"Physician Profile," 329
Physician statistics, 281
Physician work (Medicare terminology), 167
Physicians
    athletic associations, 20
    earnings, 207
    ethnic medical associations, 80
    impaired, 113
    legal-degree holders, 128
    reading habits, 135-136
    substitutes (locum tenens), 142
    volunteerism, 298-299
    women in medicine, 301-304
    young (AMA activities and programs), 364
Physicians, American College of
    address, 203
    recommended books, 32
"Physicians and Computers," 52
Physicians Art Association, American, 19
Physician's assistants, 203-207
Physician's Assistants, American Academy of, 207
Physician's Assistants, National Commission on Certification
    of, 207
Physicians' associations, see Medical associations; Medical
    societies
Physician's Desk Reference, 72
Physicians' families
    impaired physicians, 114-115
Physicians for Human Rights, American Association of, 214
Physicians for a National Health Program, 175
Physicians for Social Responsibility, 214
Physicians of India, American Association of, 81
Physicians Poetry Association, American, 213
Physician's Recognition Award, 356
"Physicians' Travel and Meeting Guide," 55
Physicists in Medicine, American Association for, 212
Physics, 212

Physiological Society, American, 84, 212
Physiology, 212
Pilots' physical examinations, 202
Pituitary glands, 108
Placement and recruiting services
    AMA activities and programs, 369
    locum tenens, 142
Planned Parenthood Federation of America, 3, 172
Plasma exchange (Health Technology Assessment
    Reports), 289
Plasma perfusion of charcoal filters (Health Technology
    Assessment Reports), 289
Plasmapheresis, 289, 344
Plastic and Reconstructive Surgeons, American Society
    of, 140, 213
Plastic Surgeons, American Association of, 213
Plastic surgery, 213
    ambulatory surgery accreditation, 16
    liposuction, 140
    resident matching program, 146
Plastic Surgery, American Board of,
    hand surgery certification, 95
    plastic surgery certification, 213
Plenty, 71
PMA Access Hotline, 222
PMS, see Premenstrual syndrome
Pneumonia, 142
Podiatric assistant, 213
Podiatric Medical Association, American, 213
Podiatric Orthopedics, American Board of, 213
Podiatric Public Health, American Board of, 213
Podiatric Surgery, American Board of, 213
Podiatry, 213
Poetry, 213
Poetry and Medicine (JAMA feature), see Journal of the
    American Medical Association (special features)
Poison Control Centers, American Association of, 213
Polio Survivors Association, 213
Poliomyelitis, 213
    post-polio syndrome (bibliography), 25
Polish-American physicians, 81
Political organizations, 214
Polycystic disease of kidneys, 125
Polygraphy (Council on Scientific Affairs report), 343
Polyneuropathy (Health Technology Assessment
    Reports), 288
Polyposis, Familial, 85
Porphyria Foundation, American, 214
Positron emission tomography
    brain chemistry (Council on Scientific Affairs report), 340
    cyclotrons and radiopharmaceuticals (Council on
        Scientific Affairs report), 340
    heart applications (Council on Scientific Affairs
        report), 340
    instrumentation (Council on Scientific Affairs report), 340
    oncology (Council on Scientific Affairs report), 340
Post-Polio League for Information, 213
Post-polio syndrome (bibliography), 25
Posterior capsulotomies (Health Technology Assessment
    Reports), 288
Postgraduate Medical Review Education, Inc, 251
Potsmokers Anonymous, 145
Poultry safety, 182
Powers of attorney, 140
Practice advertising and marketing, 145
Practice closure, 49-50
Practice expense (Medicare terminology), 167
Practice finances
    loans, 140-141
Practice incorporation, 214-215
Practice location, 141-142

Practice management, 214-218
    AMA placement and recruiting services, 369
    partnership, 215-216
    sole proprietorship, 215
Practice parameters, 218-221
    AMA department, 357
Practice purchase and sale, 259-260
Practice start-ups, 216
Practice valuation, 297
Practitioner Data Bank, see National Practitioner Data Bank
Pre-trial screening panels (tort reform glossary), 228
Preadmission criteria, 221
Preferred provider organizations, 221-222
Preferred Providers, American Association of, 222
Pregnancy, 222
    adolescent, 5
    cocaine and (bibliography), 24
    court-ordered medical treatments, 222
    drug abuse and, 72
    older women and (bibliography), 25
    postpartum depresssion (bibliography), 24
    reproductive effects of toxic chemicals (Council on
        Scientific Affairs report), 344
Premenstrual syndrome, 222
Prenatal Addiction and Education, National Association
    for, 50
President's Commission for the Study of Ethical Problems in
    Medicine..., 29
President's Council on Physical Fitness and Sports, 84
Prevailing charge (Medicare terminology), 167
Preventive medicine, 222
Preventive Medicine, American Board of, 222
    aerospace medicine certification, 6, 21
    occupational medicine certification, 186
    undersea medicine certification, 294
Preventive Medicine, American College of, 222
Primary Care Information, National Clearinghouse for, 223
Principles of Medical Ethics, 50-52, 80
Prison health care
    bibliography, 24
    detained, incarcerated youth, 336
    National Commission, 55
Privacy Act Office, 168
Private Geriatric Care Managers, National Association
    of, 105
Private practice, 215
Product safety, 54, 223
Professional component (Medicare terminology), 167
Professional impairment
    disabled physicians, 68
    licensure and discipline, 113-115
Professional liability
    glossary of terms, 228-229
    history, trends, 226-228
    physician-patient communication and, 208-212
    reducing risk of suits (risk management), 224
    "ways to get sued for malpractice," 210
    what happens when suit is filed, 223-224
    wrongful life (bibliography), 26
Professional liability insurance component (Medicare
    terminology), 167
Professional misconduct, 50-52
Professional Practice Association, American, 141
Professional Psychologists, American Board of, 231
Project HOPE, 122, 229
Project Prevention, 4
Prostaglandin E1 (DATTA opinions), 350-351
Prostate cancer, 229
Prosthetics assistant, 229
Prosthetist, 229

Prozac (fluoxetine) (bibliography), 23
Psychiatric Association, American
    DSM III, 64
    headquarters information, 230
    resident matching program, 146
Psychiatry, 229-230
    diagnostic manual (DSM III), 64
    forensic, 86
    resident matching program, 146
Psychiatry and Neurology, American Board of, 177, 229
Psychiatry and the Law, American Academy of, 229
Psychoanalysis, 230-231
Psychoanalysis, American Academy of, 231
Psychological Association, American, 231
Psychology, 231
    human-pet relations (bibliography), 24
    sport (bibliography), 26
Psychoprophylaxis in Obstetrics, American Society
    for, 46, 176
Psychosomatic Medicine, Academy of, 231
Psychosurgery, 288
PTA, 10
Public aid
    Medicaid, 149
Public Citizen Health Research Group, 214, 235
Public health, 231-234
    Healthy People 2000, 222
    officials, 99
    state departments of, 232-234
Public Health Association, American, 232
Public health physician, 231
Public Health Physicians, American Association of, 232
Public Health Service (US), 232
    AIDS facts, 10
    AIDS hotline, 10
    Surgeon General's office, 283
Public Library Association, 136
Public relations and public speaking, 271-272
Publications (AMA)
    American Medical News, 369
    Business Side of Medical Practice, 216
    Buying and Selling Medical Practices: A Valuation
        Guide, 297
    Consumer Books Division, 369
    Continuing Medical Education Directory, 55
    "Continuing Need for Legislative Reform of the
        Medical Liability System..." 226
    Current Procedural Terminology, 55-57
    Directory of Officials and Staff, 55
    Directory of Physicians in the United States, 55
    Directory of Practice Parameters: Guidelines and
        Technology Assessments, 221
    Drug Evaluations, 72
    Financing a Medical Practice Start-Up, 216
    "Got that Healing Feeling," 42
    Guide to the American Medical Association Historical
        Health Fraud and Alternative Medicine Collection, 97
    Guides to the Evaluation of Permanent Impairment, 67
    HIV Infection and Disease: Monographs for Physicians
        and Other Health Care Workers, 104
    Leaving the Bedside: The Search for a Nonclinical
        Medical Career, 42
    Medicare Carrier Review, 171
    Medicare Physician Payment Reform: The Physician's
        Guide, 168
    "Medicine: a Chance to Make a Difference," 42
    Permissions Office (use of AMA published material), 331
    Physician Guide to Home Health Care, 106
    Physician Supply and Utilization by Specialty: Trends
        and Projections, 99
    Physician's Guide to Professional Corporations, 217

Planning Guide for Physicians' Medical Facilities, 217
Reader's Guide to Alternative Health Methods, 97
Socioeconomic Characteristics of Medical Practice, 271
US Medical Licensure Statistics and Current Licensure Requirements, 137
Puerto Rico (information on various health and social services in Puerto Rico may be found at the heading, State agencies and organizations)
Pulmonary diseases, 142, 234
    modeling in research (bibliography), 25
Pulmonary rehabilitation, 234
Pumps, Infusion (DATTA opinions), 355
Purchase of medical practices, 259-260
Pyelonephritis, 125
Pyridoxine, 298

Q

Quality assurance
    AMA office of, 357
    statistical analysis in, 280
Quality Assurance and Utilization Review Physicians, American Board of, 235
Quality assurance coordinator, 235
"Quality of Mercy" (JAMA "A Piece of My Mind"), 107-108
Questionable doctors, 235

R

Rachel Carson Council, Inc, 201
Radial keratotomy (DATTA opinions), 352, 355
Radiation
    tanning salons, 283
    ultraviolet (bibliography), 25
Radiation oncology, 189
Radiation therapy technologist, 237
Radio
    advertising complaints, 6
    physician broadcasters, 34
Radioactive wastes (Council on Scientific Affairs report), 338-339
Radioepidemiological tables (Council on Scientific Affairs report), 341
Radiographer, 237-238
Radiographic absorptiometry (Health Technology Assessment Reports), 287
Radiography
    hand-held x-ray instrument (Health Technology Assessment Reports), 288
Radiologic Technologists, American Society of, 238
Radiologic technology, 237-238
Radiological Society of North America, 238
Radiology, 238
Radiology, American Board of,
    chemotherapy certification, 43
    radiation oncology certification, 189
    radiologist certification, 238
Radiology, American College of
    address, 238
    mammography recommendations, 145
Radiopharmaceuticals (Council on Scientific Affairs report), 340
Radon, 26, 334-335, 342
RAND-AMA practice parameters study, 219
Rape, 238
Rare disease drug treatment (orphan drugs), 193
Rare Disorders, National Organization for, 193, 238

RBRVS, 167, 168
Reading habits and lists, see Journals, Medical
Recreation, see Hobbies and recreation
Recruiting, see Placement and recruiting
Rectal cancer (bibliography), 24
Red cells, see Blood
Red Cross, American, 30, 68
    AIDS facts, 10
Reed, Walter, 293
Reference Center for Bioethics Literature, National, 28, 80
Reference Criteria for Short Stay Hospital Review, 238
References (ANSI standards for citations), 238-246
Referrals
    guidelines for physicians, 246-248
    local physicians, 246
    self-referrals, 248
Referring physicians
    UPIN number, 118
Regional medical programs (bibliography), 24
Registry of Emergency Medical Technicians, National, 77
Rehabilitation, see also Cardiovascular rehabilitation; Pulmonary rehabilitation
    cardiac (Health Technology Assessment Reports), 287
Rehabilitation Information Center, National, 248
Rehabilitation Medicine, American Congress of, 248
Rehabilitative Audiology, Academy of, 21
Rehfuss test (Health Technology Assessment Reports), 289
Relative value scale (Medicare terminology), 167, 168
Relative value unit (Medicare terminology), 167
Renal failure, 125
Renal Physicians Association, 125
Renal tubular acidosis, 125
Reproduction, see Fertility
Reproductive effects of toxic chemicals (Council on Scientific Affairs report), 344
Reproductive endocrinology, 78
Res ipsa loquitur (tort reform glossary), 228-229
Rescue Now, 71
Research, 248
    AMA principles and support for, 249
    animals, 18
    gender disparities, 305-306
    grants, 249
    invertebrate use (bibliography), 25
    modeling, in cardiovascular/pulmonary function and diabetes (bibliography), 25
Research Council, National, 248
Research grants, 248
Residencies, see also Graduate medical education
    AMA electronic database (AMA-FREIDA), 93
    fellowship database, 93
Resident Matching Program, National, 146, 250
Resident physicians, 249-250
    AMA activities and programs, 363
    gifts from industry, 89-92
    National Association of Residents and Interns, 140
    reading habits, 135-136
    risks of impairment, 114
    women, 303-304
Residents and Interns, National Association of, 140, 250
Resolve, Inc, 85
Resource-based relative value scale (Medicare terminology), 167, 168
Respirators
    negative pressure (Health Technology Assessment Reports), 289
Respiratory Care, American Association for, 251
Respiratory therapist, 250-251
Respiratory therapy, 250-251
Respiratory therapy technician, 251

Retinitis pigmentosa, 251
Retinitis Pigmentosa Foundation, National, 251
Retired Persons, American Association of, 251
Retired physicians, 251
Retirement, 217-218, 251
Review courses, 251
Reye's syndrome, 252
Reye's Syndrome Association, American, 252
Reye's Syndrome Foundation, National, 252
Rheumatism, 252
Rheumatology, American College of, 252
Rhinologic Society, American, 252
Rhinology, 252
Rhizotomy (DATTA opinions), 351
Rhode Island (information on various health and social
    services in this and other states may be found at the
    heading, State agencies and organizations)
Riboflavin, 297
Right to die, 81-83
Risk management, 224
    physician-patient communication and, 208-212
Roentgen Ray Society, American, 238
Royal College of Physicians, 151
Royal College of Surgeons, 151
Runaway Hotline, 4, 252
Runaways, 108
Rural health, 252-253
Rural Health Association, National, 253
Rush Lyme Disease Center, 144
Russian Medical and Dental Society, American, 81
RVS, 167, 168
RVU, 167

S

Saccharin (Council on Scientific Affairs report), 344
SAD (seasonal affective disorder), 24
Safe Workplace Institute, National, 265
Safety, 255-256
Safety belts, 255-256
Safety Council, National, 13, 73, 113, 281, 256
Sale of medical practices, 259-260
Saliva as diagnostic fluid (bibliography), 23
"Sample Criteria for Procedure Review," 257
Sarcoidosis Family Aid and Research Foundation, 257
Saturated fatty acids (Council on Scientific Affairs
    report), 336
School-based health programs (Council on Scientific Affairs
    report), 338
School health, 257
School Health Association, American, 257
Schools
    adolescent health improvement, 5
Schools, Medical, see Medical schools
Schools of Public Health, Association of the, 232
Science and Health, American Council on, 95, 96
Science, American Association for the Advancement of, 257
Science Foundation, National, 257
Scientific writing, 309-311
Scleroderma, 257
Scoliosis
    implanted electrospinal stimulator (DATTA opinions), 354
Scoliosis Association, 258
Scoliosis Foundation, National, 258
Screening panels (tort reform glossary), 228
Scuba, 258
Seafood safety (bibliography), 23
Seasonal affective disorder (bibliography), 24
Seat belts, 255-256

Second Opinion Hotline, 258
Second Opinion Program, National, 284
Second opinions, 258, 284
Secondhand smoke, 266
Self-care
    nurses' role (bibliography), 24
Self-help, 258-259
Self-Help Clearinghouse, National, 259
Self Help for Hard of Hearing People, Inc (SHHH), 100
Self-referrals, 248
Selling of medical practices, 259-260
Seminar Institute, American, 55
Senior physicians, 251
"Sensitive Subject" (JAMA "A Piece of My Mind"), 282-283
Seromucoid assay (Health Technology Assessment
    Reports), 289
Serum seromucoid assay (Health Technology Assessment
    Reports), 289
Severity of illness, 279-281
Sex counseling, 260-265
Sex education, 260
Sex Information and Education Council of the US
    (SIECUS), 260
Sexism in medicine, 301-303
Sexual assault, 238, see also Child sexual abuse
Sexual dysfunction
    impotence (bibliography), 23
Sexual harassment in medicine, 301-303
Sexual misconduct, 265
Sexual problems and disorders, 260-265
Sexually transmitted diseases, 265
SHHH (Self Help for Hard of Hearing People, Inc), 100
Shock wave lithotripsy (Health Technology Assessment
    Reports), 288
Shoe exchange (amputees), 17
Shortness (bibliography), 25
Shriners Burns Institute (Cincinnati, Ohio), 35
SI units, 49, 344
Sick building syndrome, 265
Sickle cell anemia, 265
Sickle Cell Disease, National Association for, 265
SIDS (sudden infant death syndrome), 282
SIECUS (Sex Information and Education Council of the
    US), 260
Sigmoidoscopy (DATTA opinions), 352
Silicone gel breast implants, 23, 32-34
Simon Foundation, 294
Single photon absorptiometry (Health Technology
    Assessment Reports), 288
Sjogren's syndrome (bibliography), 26
Sjogren's Syndrome Foundation, Inc, 265
Skin
    sun- ultraviolet light (bibliography), 25
    tanning salons, 283
Skin Diseases, National Institute of Arthritis and
    Musculoskeletal and, 19
Skin ulcers, 289
Skincare Help Line, 3
Sleep, 266
    deprivation (risks of impairment for physicians), 114
    disorders, older people (bibliography), 24
Sleep Disorders Association, American, 266
Sloan-Kettering Institute for Cancer Research, 37
Smithsonian Institution, 202
Smoke detectors (Council on Scientific Affairs report), 341
"Smoke-free" magazines, 267-271
Smokeless tobacco (Council on Scientific Affairs report),
343
Smoking bans on aircraft, 266
Smoking worldwide (Council on Scientific Affairs
    report), 336

Snake (medical symbol), 6-7
Snake bite, 271
SNOMED, 271
Social Health Association, American, 265
    AIDS hotline, 10
Social Security
    disability evaluation, 67
Societies, Medical, see Medical societies
Society for Adolescent Medicine, 5
Society for Investigative Dermatology, Inc, 61
Society for Magnetic Resonance Imaging, 145
Society for Oral Oncology, 189
Society for Vascular Surgery, 297
Society of Ambulatory Anesthesiology, 18
Society of American Gastrointestinal Endoscopic
    Surgeons, 87
Society of Critical Care Medicine, 55
Society of Medical Consultants to the Armed Forces, 172
Society of Medical-Dental Management, 52
Society of Medicine of New York, 322-326
Society of Nuclear Medicine, 177
Society of Professional Business Consultants, 52
Society of Thoracic Surgeons, 290
Sole proprietorship in medical practices, 215
Somatotropin
    bovine (bibliography), 24
    growth hormones and short stature (bibliography), 25
Sonography, 64
South Carolina (information on various health and social
    services in this and other states may be found at the
    heading, State agencies and organizations)
South Dakota (information on various health and social
    services in this and other states may be found at the
    heading, State agencies and organizations)
Southern Medical Association, 151
Spanish language speakers
    AIDS hotline, 10
Spanish speaking physicians, 271
Speaking, Public, 271-272
Special Libraries Association, 136
Special Purpose Examination (SPEX), 273
Specialties, Medical
    abbreviations in American Medical Directory, 1-2
    accreditation by ACGME, 355-356
    choosing (booklet), 273
    compendiums and directories of specialists, 273
    credentials, 207
    history of specialization, 273-275
    resident matching programs, 146
    women physicians, 303-304
Specialty boards, see Certification
Specialty differential (Medicare terminology), 167
Speech disorders, 100
Speech-Language-Hearing Association, American, 3
Speech pathology, 276-277
    audiology, 20-21
    dysphagia management (Health Technology Assessment
        Reports), 287
    referral (800 number), 3
Sperm banks, 277
Sperm penetration assay (DATTA opinions), 354
SPEX (Special Purpose Examination), 273
Spina Bifida Association of America, 88
Spinal cord injuries, 5, 277
Spinal Cord Injury Association, National, 277
Spinal Cord Injury Hotline, 277
Spinal Cord Society, 277
Spinal Injury Association, American, 277
Spinal stimulator (DATTA opinions), 354
Spongiform encephalopathies (bibliography), 23
Sport psychology (bibliography), 26

Sports, see also names of individual sports, e.g., Boxing
    athletic trainers, 20
    medical athletic associations, 20
Sports injuries (women), 277
Sports medicine, 277
Sports Medicine, American College of, 277
Sprinklers (Council on Scientific Affairs report), 341
Staff nurse, 231
Staff of Aesculapius, 6-7
Standard of care (tort reform glossary), 229
Stanley H Kaplan, 251
State agencies and organizations (in most cases, agencies
    for all states are included in the lists below)
    AIDS hotlines, 10-12
    bar associations, 127-128
    blindness prevention, 29-30
    blood pressure testing, 31
    blood tests, 31
    cancer research, 37-39
    chest x-rays, 43
    child abuse and neglect, 43
    child and youth services, 44-46
    consumer health protection, 54
    Council of State Governments, 137
    CPR courses, 40
    dental associations, 59-61
    departments of aging listed, 7-9
    diabetes association affiliates, 62-64
    drug programs for indigent, 72
    free-clinic listings, credentials, 49
    heart associations, 100-102
    hospital associations, 109-110
    insurance regulators, 118-120
    licensure boards, 137-139
    lung associations, 143-144
    medical boards, examiners, ect, 137-139
    medical libraries (regional and resource), 129-136
    medical school listings, 158-162
    medical societies, 277-279
    Medicare carriers, 168-171
    nursing associations, 180-182
    optometric associations, 190-192
    public health departments, 232-234
    self-help centers, 259
    travelers' and immigrant aid societies, 291-292
    workers' compensation offices, 306-308
State and Territorial Health Officials, Association of, 99
State Boards of Education, National Association of, 5
State Governments, Council of, 137
State medical practice acts (referenced by state), 154-155
Statistics, 279
Statute of limitations (tort reform glossary), 229
Statutes
    citation of (style manual), 245-246
Stem cell drug sensitivity assay (Health Technology
    Assessment Reports), 290
Stereotactic cingulotomy, 288, 354
Stimulant use
    impaired physicians, 114
Streptokinase infusion (Health Technology Assessment
    Reports), 288
Stress
    risks of impairment for physicians, 114-115
Stroke, 281
    extracranial-intracranial bypass (Health Technology
        Assessment Reports), 287
Stroke Association, National, 281
Stroke Foundation, 281
Students, see also Medical students
    volunteers interested in medicine, 299

Stuttering, National Center for, 282
Stuttering Resource Foundation, 282
Style manuals
    medical literature references and citations, 238-246
Substitute physicians, see Locum tenens
Sudden infant death syndrome (SIDS), 282
Sudden Infant Death Syndrome Clearinghouse, 282
Sudden Infant Death Syndrome Foundation, National, 282
Sudden Infant Death Syndrome Institute, American, 282
Suicide, 282-283
    adolescent (bibliography), 25
    youth, 4
Suicide assistance, 81-83
Suicide Hotline, 4
Sunlight (bibliography), 25
Suntanning salons, 283
Supplies, Medical, see Devices, Medical
Supreme Court (US)
    case citation (style guidelines), 245
Surfer's Medical Association, 20
Surgeon assistant, 205-206
Surgeon General (US), 283
    AIDS pamphlet, 10
Surgeons, American College of, 283
Surgery, 283-284
    carbon dioxide laser (Health Technology Assessment Reports), 289
    elective, and mandatory electrocardiography (DATTA opinions), 355
    epilepsy treatment (bibliography), 24
    extracranial-intracranial bypass (Health Technology Assessment Reports), 287
    gastric restrictive (DATTA opinions), 354
    global package, 166
    intraoperative ventricular mapping (Health Technology Assessment Reports), 288
    obesity treatment (bibliography), 24
    postoperative pain and nerve stimulation (Health Technology Assessment Reports), 289
    second opinions, 258
    transsexual (Health Technology Assessment Reports), 289
Surgery, Abdominal, 2
Surgery, American Board of,
    critical care certification, 55
    hand surgery certification, 95
    surgery and subspecialty certification, 283
    vascular surgery certification, 297
Surgery of the Hand, American Society for, 95
Surgery, Outpatient, 16
Surgical second opinions, 258, 284
Surgical technologists, 284-285
Surgical Technologists, Association of, 285
"Surprise Party" (JAMA "A Piece of My Mind"), 171-172
Surrogate decision makers, 115-116
Surrogate Parent Foundation, 285
Sweeteners
    aspartame (bibliography), 24
Systematized Nomenclature of Medicine (SNOMED), 271
Systeme International (SI) Units, 49
SysteMetrics, 281
Systemic lupus erythematosus, 288

T

Talbott Recovery Center, 113
Tanning salons, 283
Task Force on Cults, 55
Tay Sach's and Allied Diseases Foundation, National, 88

Tay-Sachs disease, 88
TDD, 100
Teaching Hospitals, Council on, 287
Technetium-99m pertechnetate (Health Technology Assessment Reports), 290
Technical component (Medicare terminology), 168
Technology assessment, 287-290
    Health Technology Assessment Reports, 287-290
    hospital (bibliography), 24
    medical devices, 61, 80
Teenagers, see Adolescence
Telecommunication Device for the Deaf (TDD), 100
Television
    advertising complaints, 6
    AMA (American Medical Television Video Digest), 297
    physician broadcasters, 34
Tennessee (information on various health and social services in this and other states may be found at the heading, State agencies and organizations)
Tennis, 20
Terminal care
    life-support withdrawal, 69
Tetrahydroaminocridine (Alzheimer's disease) Study, 16
Texas (information on various health and social services in this and other states may be found at the heading, State agencies and organizations)
THA (Tetrahydroaminocridine), 16
Therapeutic Radiology and Oncology, American Society for, 189, 238
Thermal coagulation
    gastrointestinal tract hemorrhage (DATTA opinions), 354
Thermography, 290
    breast cancer detection (Health Technology Assessment Reports), 289
    indications other than breast lesions (Health Technology Assessment Reports), 287
Thermology, American Academy of, 290
Thiamine, 297
Thoracic Society, American, 290
Thoracic Surgery, American Association for, 290
Thoracic Surgery, American Board of, 290
Thyroid Association, American, 290
Thyroid gland
    hyperparathyroidism (bibliography), 24
Tinnitus Association, American, 290
Tinnitus maskers (Health Technology Assessment Reports), 289
Tissue Banks, American Association of, 290
Tobacco, see also Smoking
    smokeless (Council on Scientific Affairs report), 343
    smoking bans on aircraft, 266
    smoking worldwide (Council on Scientific Affairs report), 336
Tobacco advertising
    magazines prohibiting, 267-271
Toenails, Mycotic, 288
Tort reform, 226
    AMA's Health Access America provisions, 371
Tort Reform Association, American, 226
Tourette Syndrome Association, 290
Toxoplasmosis (bibliography), 25
Trabeculoplasty (Health Technology Assessment Reports), 288
Tracheitis, 142
Traffic Accidents, see Accidents, Traffic
Transcutaneous electrical nerve stimulation (Health Technology Assessment Reports), 288, 289
Transfusion medicine
    certification, 30
Transfusions, see Blood transfusions

Transillumination light scanning (Health Technology Assessment Reports), 287, 288
Transition asymmetry (Medicare terminology), 168
Transition offset (Medicare terminology), 168
Transitional year, 290
Translations, 290
Transplant Surgeons, American Society of, 290
Transplantation, 290
    autologous bone marrow (Health Technology Assessment Reports), 287, 288
    organ donation, 192-193
Transplantation, American Council on, 193
Transportation Department (US), 256
Transsexual surgery (Health Technology Assessment Reports), 289
Transurethral urethroscopic lithotripsy (Health Technology Assessment Reports), 287, 288
Trauma, 290
Trauma Society, American, 290
Travel
    expenses (industry-paid), 89-92
    foreign travel and immunization, 113, 291
Travelers' and immigrant aid societies, 108, 291-292
Traveler's diarrhea (DATTA opinions), 352
Trial Lawyers of America, Association of, 226
Triglycerides (bibliography), 24
Triological Society, 127
TRIPOD, 100
Tropical medicine, 293
Tropical Medicine and Hygiene, American Society of, 293
Tuberous Sclerosis Association, National, 293
Tumor stem cell drug sensitivity assay (Health Technology Assessment Reports), 290
Turkish American Physicians Association, 81
Twinline, 173, 293
Twins, 293
"200 Ways to Put Your Talent to Work in the Health Field," 42
Typhoid fever, 293

U

Ulcers
    endoscopic therapy (bibliography), 25
Ultrasonography, 294
    AMA Council on Scientific Affairs report, 335
    diagnostic intraoperative (DATTA opinions), 354
    future of (Council on Scientific Affairs report), 335
    heart (Council on Scientific Affairs report), 335
    percutaneous (Health Technology Assessment Reports), 288
    transrectal (DATTA opinions), 351
    transrectal (for prostate cancer) (DATTA opinions), 352-353
Ultrasound, 294
Ultraviolet light
    absorbing and reflecting lenses (Health Technology Assessment Reports), 290
    decubitus ulcer treatment (Health Technology Assessment Reports), 289
Ultraviolet radiation, 25, 283, 339
Unbundle (Medicare terminology), 168
Undergraduate medical education, see Medical education
Undersea and Hyperbaric Medical Society, Inc, 68, 294
Undersea medicine, 294
Uniform donor cards, 193
Unique Physician Identification Number (UPIN), 118
UNISYS Corporation
    National Practitioner Data Bank, 55

United Cerebral Palsy Associations, 43
United Network for Organ Sharing, 193
United Ostomy Association, 195
United Scleroderma Foundation, Inc, 257
United States...(for government agencies, see other part of name; e.g., US Health Care Financing Administration, see Health Care Financing Administration (US))
United States and Canadian Academy of Pathology, 198
United States Pharmacopeial Convention, 72
University of Louisville
    plastic surgery resident matching program, 146
University Programs in Health Administration, Association of, 95
Unproven methods
    AMA archival collection, 331
Upcode (Medicare terminology), 168
UPIN number, 118
Ureteral stones (DATTA opinions), 353
Urinary incontinence, 25, 294
Urine autoinjection (Health Technology Assessment Reports), 289
Urine immunization (Health Technology Assessment Reports), 289
Urological Association, American, 295
Urology, 294-295
Urology, American Board of, 295
US...(for government agencies, see other part of name; e.g., US Health Care Financing Administration, see Health Care Financing Administration (US))
US Directory Service, 86
Us Too (prostate cancer information), 229
USPC, 72
USPHS (US Public Health Service), 232, 283
Utah (information on various health and social services in this and other states may be found at the heading, State agencies and organizations)
Uterine monitoring (DATTA opinions), 352
Utilization of health services
    geographic variation, 280
Utilization review, 200
    preadmission criteria, 221
    Reference Criteria for Short Stay Hospital Review, 238
    statistical analysis in, 280
Utilization Review Physicians, American College of, 200

V

Vaccinations, see Immunization
Vaccine Injury Compensation Program
    Bureau of Health Professions (telephone number), 35
Valuation of medical practices, 297
Value Health Science, 219
Vascular insufficiency (Health Technology Assessment Reports), 288
Vascular surgery, 297
Vascular system
    Doppler sonography, 294
VD Hotline, National, 265
Vegetative state, 140
Venereal diseases, 265
Ventricular mapping (Health Technology Assessment Reports), 288
Vermont (information on various health and social services in this and other states may be found at the heading, State agencies and organizations)
Veterans Affairs Department, (US)
    disabled physicians, 68
Veterans Benefits Administration (US), 297
Veterans, 297

Veterinary Medical Association, American, 297
Veterinary medicine, 297
Video clinics, 297
Video display terminals, 297, 342
Violence against women (Council on Scientific Affairs report), 334
Violence, Domestic, see Familly violence
Viral foodborne infections (bibliography), 26
Virchow-Pirquet Medical Society, 81
Virginia (information on various health and social services in this and other states may be found at the heading, State agencies and organizations)
Vitamin preparations as dietary supplements (Council on Scientific Affairs report), 341
Vitamins, 297-298
Vitiligo Foundation, National, 298
Vocational guidance, see headings beginning with Career...; names of individual medical specialties and allied health professions, e.g., Cardiovascular technology; Obstetrics and gynecology;
Voice Information System and Disease Information Hotline (CDC), 43
Volcanoes, 24
Volume performance standard (Medicare terminology), 166
Volunteerism among physicians, 298-299

W

Washington (information on various health and social services in this and other states may be found at the heading, State agencies and organizations)
Waste disposal 23, 163-164
"Waste" (JAMA "A Piece of My Mind"), 73
Weight-height tables, 102
Weight loss (bibliography), 23
Weights and measures
    SI units, 49
West River Sexual Abuse Treatment Center, 17
West Virginia (information on various health and social services in this and other states may be found at the heading, State agencies and organizations)
Wheat intolerance, 14
Wheelchair Athletic Association, National, 301
Wheelchair exercises, 301
Whirlpool baths (Health Technology Assessment Reports), 289
Whole-body hyperthermia (DATTA opinions), 354
Wilderness Medical Society, 77
Wilms' tumor, 125
Wisconsin (nformation on various health and social services in this and other states may be found at the heading, State agencies and organizations)
Withdrawal of life support, 69, 140
Wolff-Parkinson-White syndrome (DATTA opinions), 353
Woman Abuse Prevention Center, National, 70
Woman Abuse Prevention Project, National, 70
Women
    pregnancy in older women (bibliography), 25
    violence against, 69-71
Women in medicine (women physicians), 301-304
    AMA activities and programs, 364
Women's health, 305-306
Women's Sports Foundation, 277
Wood, Leonard, 129
Worker's compensation, 306-308
World Directory of Medical Schools, 86
World Health Organization, 308
    medical photographs, 202
    "Vaccination Requirements and Health Advice for International Travel," 113

World Medical Association, 151, 308
    biomedical research involving humans, 249
World Medical Journal, 309
World Medical Relief, Inc, 71
World Opportunities International, 71
Writing, Scientific and Medical, 309-311
Wrongful life (bibliography), 26
Wyeth Laboratories
    MEDWATCH (missing/exploited children), 46, 173
Wyoming (nformation on various health and social services in this and other states may be found at the heading, State agencies and organizations)

X

X-rays
    hand-held instrument (Health Technology Assessment Reports), 288
    medical records, 156
Xenografts (Council on Scientific Affairs report), 344
Xeroderma Pigmentosum Registry, 61

Y

Y-Me Breast Cancer Support Program, 32
Yellow fever, 293
Young physicians
    AMA activities and programs, 364
    new practices, 140-141
Youth, see Adolescence; Children
Youth Suicide Prevention, National Committee on, 4
Youth suicide, 4